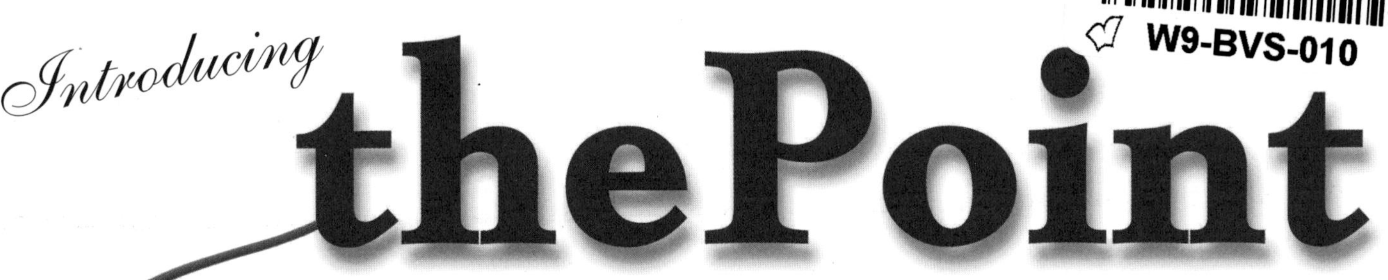

This easy-to-use FREE resource lets you access everything you need.

http://thePoint.LWW.com/goBickley

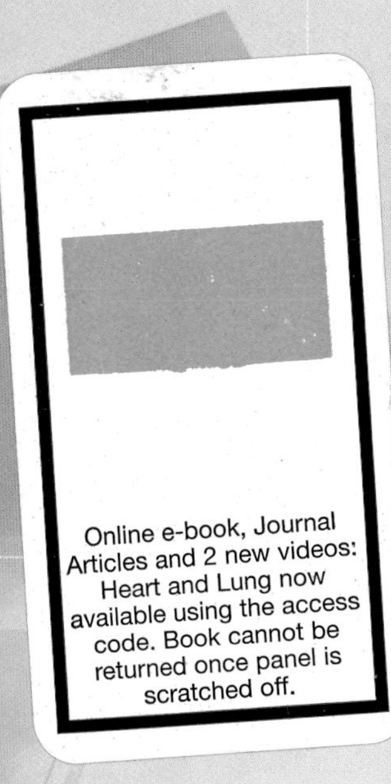

FOR STUDENTS:

- **Head-to-Toe Assessment** video
- **Approach-to-Patient** video
- **Growth Charts**
- more coming soon!

FOR INSTRUCTORS:

- **Test Generator** with hundreds of questions
- **Comprehensive Instructor's Manual**
- **Image Bank** featuring the photos from the text
- **Blackboard and WebCT** ready materials

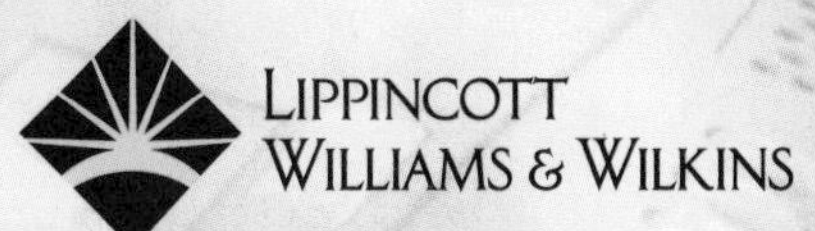

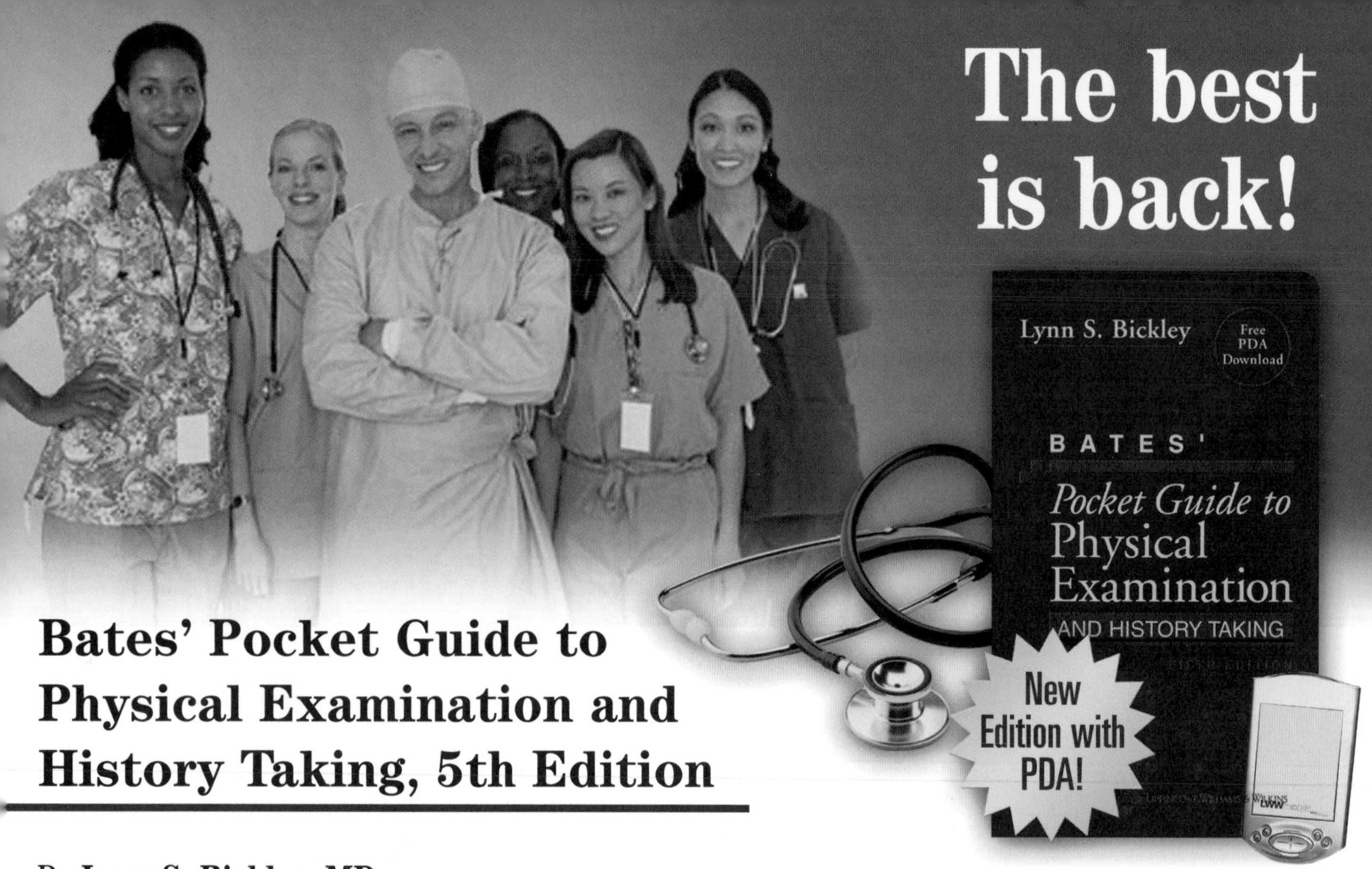

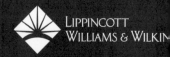

BATES'

Guide to Physical Examination

AND HISTORY TAKING

Chapter 2: Interviewing and the Health History
Elizabeth H. Naumburg, MD
Associate Dean, Advising
Professor, Department of Family Medicine
University of Rochester School of Medicine and Dentistry
Rochester, New York

Chapter 19: The Pregnant Woman
Previous edition contributions by
Joyce E. Thompson, RN, CNM, DrPH, FAAN, FACNM
Lacey Professor of Community Health Nursing
Bronson School of Nursing
Western Michigan University
Kalamazoo, Michigan

BATES'

Guide to Physical Examination

AND HISTORY TAKING

NINTH EDITION

Lynn S. Bickley, MD
Professor of Internal Medicine and Neuropsychiatry
Texas Tech Health Sciences Center
Lubbock, Texas

Peter G. Szilagyi, MD, MPH
Professor of Pediatrics
Chief, Division of General Pediatrics
University of Rochester School of Medicine and Dentistry
Rochester, New York

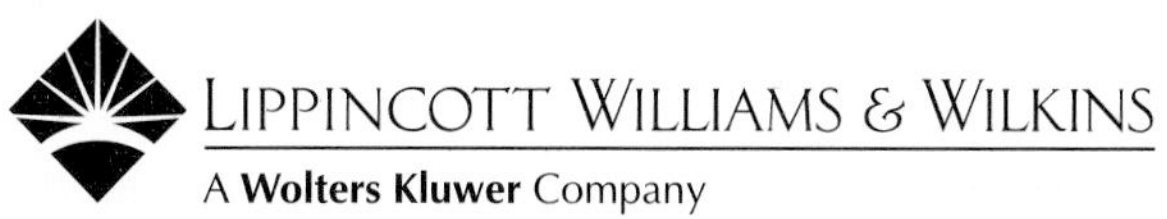
LIPPINCOTT WILLIAMS & WILKINS
A **Wolters Kluwer** Company
Philadelphia • Baltimore • New York • London
Buenos Aires • Hong Kong • Sydney • Tokyo

Senior Acquisitions Editor: Elizabeth Nieginski
Senior Developmental Editor: Renee Gagliardi
Senior Production Editor: Sandra Cherrey Scheinin
Senior Production Manager: Helen Ewan
Managing Editor/Production: Erika Kors
Art Director: Joan Wendt
Art Director, Illustrations: Brett MacNaughton
Interior Illustrator: Ann Rains
Manufacturing Manager: William Alberti
Indexer: Alexandra Nickerson
Compositor: Circle Graphics
Printer: R. R. Donnelley—Willard

9th Edition

9 8 7 6 5 4 3 2

Library of Congress Cataloging-in-Publication Data

Bickley, Lynn S.
Bates' guide to physical examination and history taking.—9th ed. / Lynn S. Bickley, Peter G. Szilagyi.
p. ; cm.
Includes bibliographical references and index.
ISBN 0-7817-6718-0 (alk. paper)
1. Physical diagnosis. 2. Medical history taking. I. Szilagyi, Peter G. II. Bates, Barbara, 1928–2001. III. Title. IV. Title: Guide to physical examination and history taking.
[DNLM: 1. Physical Examination—methods. 2. Medical History Taking—methods. WB 205 B583b 2007]
RC76.B38 2007
616.07'54—dc22

2005023366

Care has been taken to confirm the accuracy of the information presented and to describe generally accepted practices. However, the authors, editors, and publisher are not responsible for errors or omissions or for any consequences from application of the information in this book and make no warranty, express or implied, with respect to the content of the publication.

The authors, editors, and publisher have exerted every effort to ensure that drug selection and dosage set forth in this text are in accordance with the current recommendations and practice at the time of publication. However, in view of ongoing research, changes in government regulations, and the constant flow of information relating to drug therapy and drug reactions, the reader is urged to check the package insert for each drug for any change in indications and dosage and for added warnings and precautions This is particularly important when the recommended agent is a new or infrequently employed drug.

Some drugs and medical devices presented in this publication have Food and Drug Administration (FDA) clearance for limited use in restricted research settings. It is the responsibility of the health care provider to ascertain the FDA status of each drug or device planned for use in his or her clinical practice.

LWW.com

To Gerald W. Murphy, Renaissance teacher and master clinician, whose empathy and acumen have inspired so many.

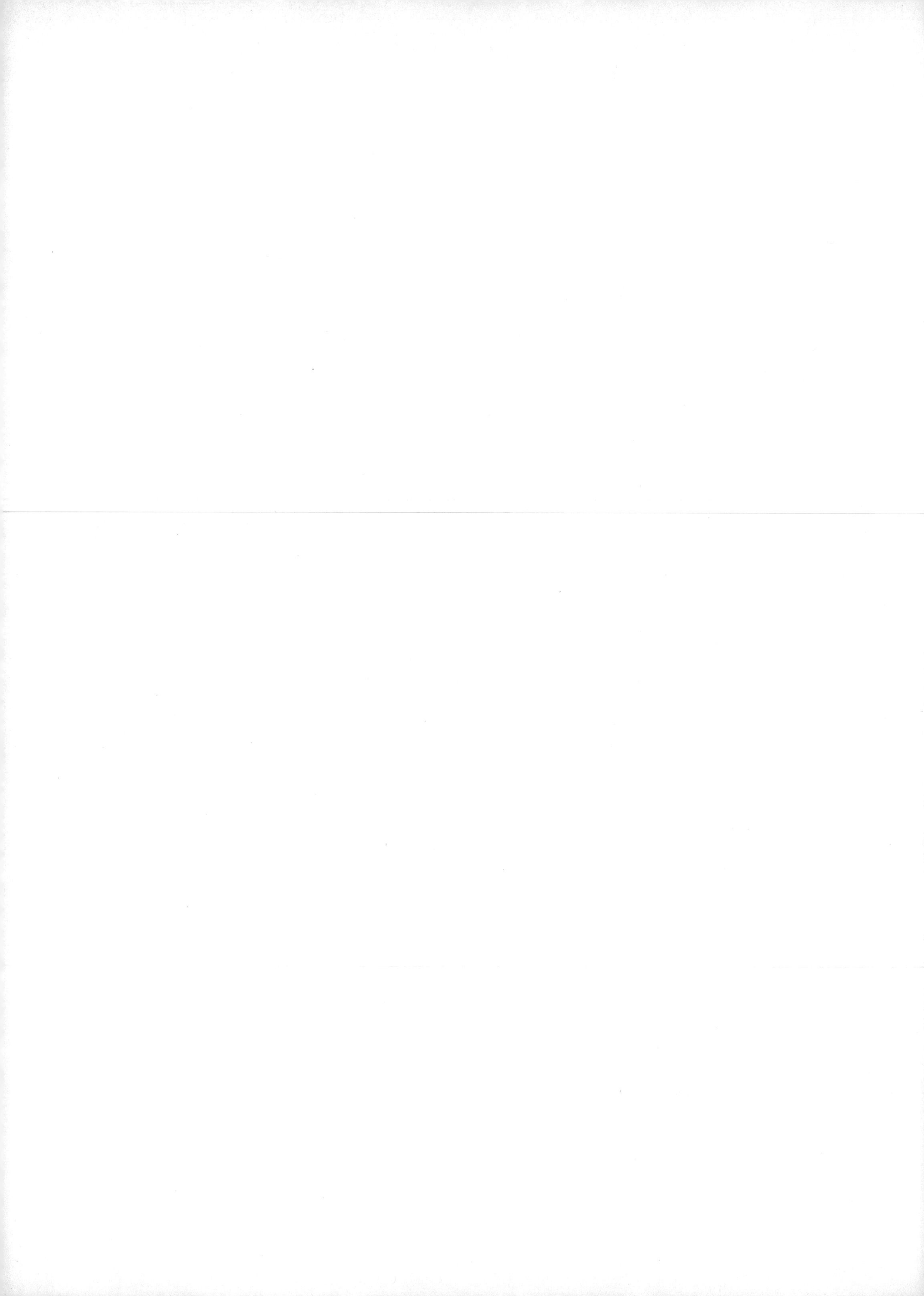

Acknowledgments

For his thoughtful reorganization of *Chapter 18, Assessing Children: Infancy Through Adolescence*, we acknowledge the important contribution of Peter Szilagyi, MD, our pediatrics editor, to this ninth edition of *Bates' Guide to Physical Examination and History Taking*. For her expertise and careful review of *Chapter 20, The Older Adult*, we extend special thanks to Marie Bernard, MD, Professor and Chair, Reynolds Department of Geriatrics at the University of Oklahoma School of Medicine. We also extend our appreciation to Elizabeth Naumburg at the University of Rochester School of Medicine and Dentistry for *Chapter 2, Interviewing and the Health History* and to her colleagues Laurie Donohue, Valerie Gilchrest, Carl Hoffman, Brenda Lee, Anne Nofziger, Steven Lurie, and Nancy Shafer-Clark. We are grateful for the helpful suggestions of Suzanne Cox, MD from the University of Texas Southwestern; of Steven Berk, MD, Jennifer Peterson, MD, Michael Phy, DO, Fiona Prabhu, MD, Randolph Schiffer, MD, and Gary Sutkin, MD, from Texas Tech University Health Sciences Center School of Medicine; and of Susan Stangl, MD, from UCLA. Chloe Alexson, MD, Jeffrey Kaczorowski, MD, and Cheryl Kodjo, MD, MPH, from the University of Rochester School of Medicine and Dentistry have again made valued contributions to illuminating the assessment of children and adolescents.

It has been a pleasure to work with the talented and hard-working acquisitions, editorial, and production teams at Lippincott Williams & Wilkins. Elizabeth Nieginski, Senior Acquisitions Editor, has handled technical matters with unfailing patience and courtesy. Renee Gagliardi, Senior Developmental Editor, has masterminded content and schedules not only for the ninth edition, but also for its growing list of accompanying products, particularly *Bates' Pocket Guide to Physical Examination and History Taking*, 5th edition and the 18-module series *Bates' Visual Guide to Physical Diagnosis and History Taking*, 4th edition. Renee worked with Ancillary Editors Claudia Vaughn and Doris Wray to coordinate the Case Book and the Web site containing the instructor's manual, the test bank of questions, and the new on-line course in physical diagnosis. Sandra Cherrey Scheinin, Senior Production Editor, is again distinguished by her meticulous care in incorporating additions and changes in both substance and format. Brett MacNaughton, Illustration Art Director, has deftly handled coordination of both photographs and illustrations with layout and text. We remain grateful to these editors, as well as to the many other members of Lippincott Williams & Wilkins who have contributed so much to this edition.

For the many small and large tasks that accompany manuscript preparation and submission, we commend Alissia Rollison and Britton Lui, and for invaluable computer expertise, Victor Gonzales.

Contents

CHAPTER 6

The Head and Neck 153

CHAPTER 7

The Thorax and Lungs 241

List of Tables

Introduction

Bates' Guide to Physical Examination and History Taking is designed for students of health care who are learning to talk with patients, to perform their physical examinations, and to apply clinical reasoning to understanding and assessing their problems. The ninth edition has several new features. The book is now divided into three units to facilitate learning: *Foundations of Physical Examination and History Taking, Regional Examinations,* and *Life Span Examinations.* The unit on *Life Span Examinations* includes the new chapter, *The Older Adult.* Citations in each chapter closely align content with evidence from the health care literature.

- In Unit 1, *Foundations of Physical Examination and History Taking,* readers will find in Chapter 1 an overview of the patient interview and physical examination and an example of how these essential components of patient assessment might appear in the written record. *Chapter 2, Interviewing and the Health History,* guides students through the techniques of skilled interviewing, with a special focus on empathic interviewing, cultural competence, and ethics. *Chapter 3, Clinical Reasoning, Assessment, and Plan* completes the cycle of patient assessment. This chapter discusses the steps of clinical reasoning, illustrated by the assessment and plan of an actual case from Chapter 1. It also provides guidelines for evaluating clinical data and preparing a succinct and well-organized patient record.
- Unit 2, *Regional Examinations,* Chapters 4 through 17, begins with the important general survey of the patient and techniques for accurate measurement of the vital signs. Subsequent chapters are devoted to the techniques of examination for each body system. These chapters are arranged in a "head-to-toe" sequence, just as you would examine the patient. Each of these regional examination chapters begins with a review of relevant anatomy and physiology, followed by pertinent health history and information useful for health promotion and counseling. The discussions then continue with the techniques of examination and examples of the written record for the physical examination of that system. Each chapter closes with tables to help students recognize selected abnormalities.
- In Unit 3, *Life Span Examinations,* Chapters 18 through 20, students will find chapters relating to special stages in the life cycle: infancy through adolescence, pregnancy, and aging. The chapter on pediatric assessment elucidates the variations in history taking and examination pertinent to infants through adolescents. The final chapter, *The Older Adult,* details techniques for promoting the special goals of geriatrics: maintaining health and social well-being and optimal levels of function.

We assume that our student readers have had basic courses in human anatomy and physiology. Our sections on these subjects in the *Regional Examinations* chapters are intended to help students apply this knowledge to interpreting symptoms, examining the patient, and understanding physical findings.

Throughout the book, we have emphasized common or important problems rather than the rare and esoteric. Occasionally, a physical sign of a rare disorder has been included when it occupies a solid niche in classic physical diagnosis, or when recognizing the disorder is especially important for the health or even the life of the patient.

Most students learn their examination skills first by practicing on each other. Much of the anatomy and physiology and many of the techniques of examination and abnormal findings are common to both adults and children. Dr. Szilagyi's Chapter 18 helps students adapt their assessment to the remarkable developmental changes spanning infancy through adolescence. The new Chapter 20 casts a similar focus on the unique goals for assessing our growing older population.

THE NINTH EDITION

The ninth edition takes several new departures in *Bates' Guide to Physical Examination and History Taking*. As with previous editions, the changes spring from two sources: the queries of teachers and students, and the goal of making the book easier to read and more efficient to use. The three new units of the book, *Foundations of Physical Examination and History Taking, Regional Examinations,* and *Life Span Examinations,* are designed to bring a more coherent and helpful organization to students learning clinical assessment.

Readers will find both new and substantially revised chapters in the ninth edition:

- *Chapter 20, The Older Adult,* is an entirely new chapter that addresses the demographic imperative to increase not just the life span, but also the "health span" of our older population. It provides students with assessment techniques that will help older patients sustain successful aging to the end of life, enjoying rich and active lives in their homes and communities.
- *Chapter 18, Assessing Children: Infancy Through Adolescence,* has been revised substantially by Peter Szilagyi, MD, our editor for pediatrics. The content now clusters techniques of examination according to the child's developmental stage, whether it be newborn, infancy, early childhood, middle-to-late childhood, or adolescence. The chapter includes a summary of normal child development (e.g., what an infant can do); tips on how to examine children; and many new figures, tables, and boxes of clinical pearls to help you in your examination of children and adolescents.
- As requested by readers, many new tables and photographs have been added to *Chapter 5, The Skin, Hair, and Nails,* to assist beginning examiners with identification of rashes and moles.
- To help students locate the mental status examination, the Nervous System is now divided into *Chapter 16, The Nervous System: Mental Status and Behavior,* and *Chapter 17, The Nervous System: Cranial Nerves, Motor System, Sensory System, and Reflexes.*

All the chapters contain updated information relating to health promotion and counseling. Beginning with this edition, each chapter explicitly reflects an *evidence-based perspective,* listing key citations and references at the close of each chapter. For the first time, all tables are vertical so readers can page through the chapters more easily without turning the book to its side.

As in the eighth edition, each of the regional examination chapters contains sections on Anatomy and Physiology, The Health History, Health Promotion and Counseling, and Techniques of Examination. In this edition, however, Recording Your Findings, which contains samples of the write-up, is more logically placed *after* Techniques of Examination, just before the Tables of Abnormalities. Health history information about symptoms is again incorporated into the regional examination chapter most relevant to those particular symptoms. For example, symptoms and tables pertaining to headache, earache, sinusitis, and difficulty swallowing are found in the Health History and Tables of Abnormalities sections of *Chapter 6, The Head and Neck;* symptoms and a Table of Abnormalities about diarrhea appear in *Chapter 10, The Abdomen.* Throughout the book the sections on Health Promotion and Counseling have been revised and expanded according to new information and guidelines, such as for obesity, cholesterol screening, classification of hypertension, and childhood immunizations.

Chapter 4, Beginning the Physical Examination: General Survey and Vital Signs, is especially useful for students conducting the initial assessment of the patient, particularly nutritional status, measurements of height and weight using body mass index to determine excess weight and obesity, and accurate evaluation of the vital signs. This chapter also contains tables to help clinicians with nutritional assessment, dietary recommendations, and recognition of low-weight conditions such as anorexia nervosa and bulimia.

Color again demarcates chapter sections and tables more clearly, and leads students more easily to insets of key material and special tips for challenging aspects of examination such as taking the blood pressure, assessing the jugular venous pressure, and keeping the patient comfortable during the examination of the pelvis. More than 200 new and revised photographs and drawings have been added to better illustrate key points in the accompanying text.

Even with these changes, readers will recognize the basic core organization of the text. Students may study or review the Anatomy and Physiology sections according to their individual needs. They can study Techniques of Examination to learn how to do the relevant examination, then practice it under faculty guidance, and review it again afterward. Students and faculty also will benefit from identifying common abnormal findings, which appear in two places. The right-hand column of the Techniques of Examination sections presents possible abnormal findings. These are highlighted in red and linked to the adjacent text. Distinguishing these findings from the normal improves learners' observations and clinical acumen. For further information on abnormalities, readers also can turn to the Tables of Abnormalities at the end of each of the regional examination chapters. These tables display or describe various abnormal conditions in a convenient format that allows students to compare and contrast related abnormalities in a single table.

SUGGESTIONS FOR USING THE BOOK

Although the health history and the physical examination are both essential for patient assessment and care, students often learn them separately, sometimes even from different faculty members. Students learning interviewing are advised to return to *Chapter 2, Interviewing and the Health History,* as they gain experience talking with patients of different temperaments and ages. As they begin developing a smooth sequence of examination, students may wish to review the sequence of examination outlined in *Chapter 4, Beginning the Physical Examination: General Survey and Vital Signs.*

Nevertheless, students must learn to integrate the patient's story and the patient's physical findings. We suggest that students study the relevant portions of the Health History as they learn successive parts of the examination. In a few areas, symptoms may lead to examination of more than one body system. For example, chest pain prompts evaluation of both the thorax and lungs and the cardiovascular system. The symptoms of the urinary tract are relevant to the chapters on the abdomen, the prostate, and male and female genitalia.

As students progress through the body systems and regions, they should study the write-ups of the sample patient, Mrs. N, found in Chapter 1 and Chapter 3, and make frequent reference to the sections on Recording Your Findings that display samples of the patient record. This cross-checking will help students learn how to describe and organize information from the interview and physical examination into an understandable written format. Further, studying *Chapter 3, Clinical Reasoning, Assessment, and Plan,* will help students to select and analyze the data they are learning to collect.

Skimming the Tables of Abnormalities makes students more familiar with what they should be looking for and why they are asking certain questions. They should not, however, try to memorize all the detail that is presented. The best time to learn about abnormalities and diseases is when a patient, real or described, appears with a problem. Students should then use this book to try to analyze the concern or finding, and make use of other clinical texts or journals to pursue the patient's problems in as much depth as necessary. Students can refer to the Citations and Additional References at the end of each chapter for additional relevant sources.

RELATED LEARNING MATERIAL

With the ninth edition, we continue the accompanying Case Book, also revised and updated, to help students test their knowledge of symptoms and physical findings by applying principles of clinical reasoning and assessment to a series of common clinical vignettes. Faculty and teachers can again turn to resources available on Lippincott's Connection Web site, including an instructor's manual and a testbank of questions, and a new on-line course covering the basic principles of Physical Examination and History Taking.

In addition, *Bates' Pocket Guide to Physical Examination and History Taking,* 5th edition, 2005 by Lynn Bickley and Peter Szilagyi is an updated, abbreviated version of this text, designed for portability, review, and convenience. The pocket guide does not stand alone; reference to the text and illustrations of *Bates' Guide to Physical Examination and History Taking* is needed for a more comprehensive study and understanding of these subjects.

Bates' Video Guide to Physical Examination, 4th edition, is a completely revised, comprehensive, highly informative series of 18 videotapes keyed to this text. Individual and sets of modules in VHS, DVD, and streaming formats are available from Lippincott Williams and Wilkins. The accompanying front-of-book CD-ROM includes footage from these series, focusing on "Head-to-Toe Examination" and "Approach to the Patient."

EQUIPMENT

Equipment necessary for a physical examination includes the following:

- An ophthalmoscope and an otoscope. If the otoscope is to be used to examine children, it should allow for pneumatic otoscopy.
- A flashlight or penlight
- Tongue depressors
- A ruler and flexible tape measure, preferably marked in centimeters
- A thermometer
- A watch with a second hand
- A sphygmomanometer
- A stethoscope with the following characteristics:
  - Ear tips that fit snugly and painlessly. To get this fit, choose ear tips of the proper size, align the ear pieces with the angle of your ear canals, and adjust the spring of the connecting metal band to a comfortable tightness.
  - Thick-walled tubing as short as feasible to maximize the transmission of sound: about 30 cm (12 inches), if possible, and no longer than 38 cm (15 inches)
  - A bell and a diaphragm with a good changeover mechanism
- Gloves and lubricant for vaginal, rectal, and possibly oral examinations
- Vaginal specula and equipment for cytological and perhaps bacteriological study
- A reflex hammer
- Tuning forks, ideally one of 128 Hz and one of 512 Hz
- Safety pins or other disposable objects for testing two-point discrimination
- Cotton for testing the sense of light touch
- Two test tubes (optional) for testing temperature sensation
- Paper and pen or pencil

UNIT

I

Foundations of Physical Examination and History Taking

CHAPTER

1

Overview of Physical Examination and History Taking

The techniques of physical examination and history taking that you are about to learn embody time-honored skills of healing and patient care. Your ability to gather a sensitive and nuanced history and to perform a thorough and accurate examination deepens your relationships with patients, focuses your assessment, and sets the direction of your clinical thinking. The quality of your history and physical examination governs your next steps with the patient and guides your choices from among the initially bewildering array of secondary testing and technology. Over the course of becoming an accomplished clinician, you will polish these important relational and clinical skills for a lifetime.

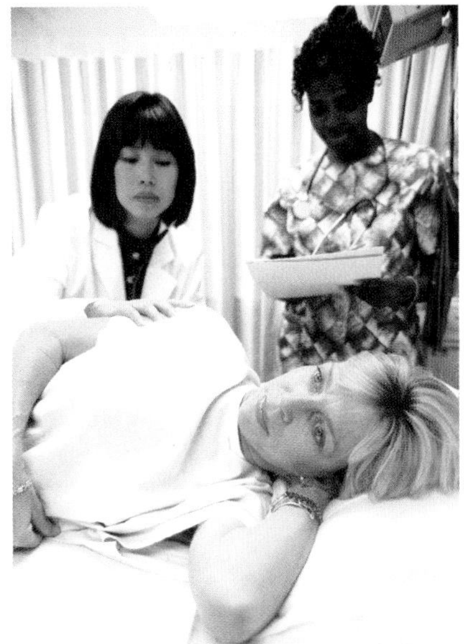

As you enter the realm of patient assessment, you begin integrating the essential elements of clinical care: empathic listening; the ability to interview patients of all ages, moods, and backgrounds; the techniques for examining the different body systems; and, finally, the process of clinical reasoning. Your experience with history taking and physical examination will grow and expand, and will trigger the steps of clinical reasoning from the first moments of the patient encounter: identifying problem symptoms and abnormal findings; linking findings to an underlying process of pathophysiology or psychopathology; and establishing and testing a set of explanatory hypotheses. Working through these steps will reveal the multifaceted profile of the patient before you. Paradoxically, the very skills that allow you to assess all patients also shape the image of the unique human being entrusted to your care.

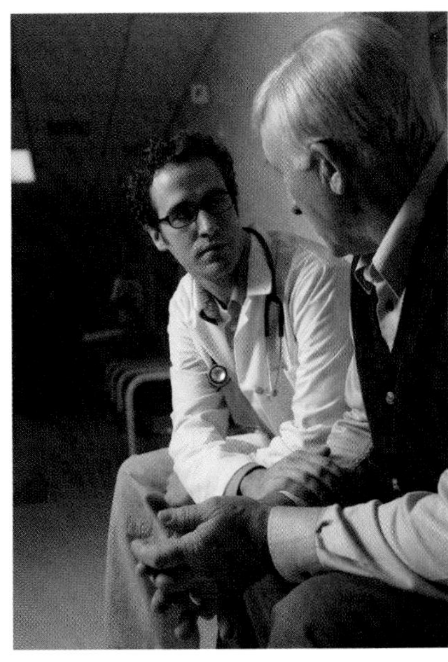

This chapter provides a road map to clinical proficiency in three critical areas: the health history, the physical examination, and the written record, or "write-up." It describes the components of the health history and how to organize the patient's story; it gives an approach and overview to the physical examination and suggests a sequence for ensuring patient comfort; and, finally, it provides an example of the written record, showing documentation of findings from a sample patient history and physical examination. By studying the subsequent chapters and perfecting the skills of examination and history taking described, you will cross into the world of patient assessment—gradually at first, but then with growing satisfaction and expertise.

After you study this chapter and chart the tasks ahead, subsequent chapters will guide your journey to clinical competence.

- *Chapter 2, Interviewing and The Health History*, expands on the techniques and skills of good interviewing.
- *Chapter 3, Clinical Reasoning, Assessment, and Plan*, explores the clinical reasoning process and how to document your evaluation, diagnoses, and plan for patient care.
- *Chapters 4 to 17* detail the anatomy and physiology, health history, guidelines for health promotion and counseling, techniques of examination, and examples of the written record relevant to specific body systems and regions.
- *Chapters 18 to 20* extend and adapt the elements of the adult history and physical examination to special populations: newborns, infants, children, and adolescents; pregnant women; and older adults.

From mastery of these skills and the mutual trust and respect of caring relationships with your patients emerge the timeless rewards of the clinical professions.

THE HEALTH HISTORY

As you read about successful interviewing, you will first learn the elements of the ***Comprehensive Adult Health History.*** The comprehensive history includes *Identifying Data* and *Source of the History, Chief Complaint(s), Present Illness, Past History, Family History, Personal and Social History,* and *Review of Systems.* As you talk with the patient, you must learn to elicit and organize all these elements of the patient's health. Bear in mind that during the interview this information will not spring forth in this order! However, you will quickly learn to identify where to fit in the different aspects of the patient's story.

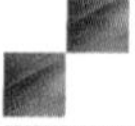

STRUCTURE AND PURPOSES

The Comprehensive vs. Focused Health History. As you gain experience assessing patients in different settings, you will find that new patients in the office or in the hospital merit a *comprehensive health history;* however, in many situations, a more flexible *focused,* or *problem-oriented, interview* may be appropriate. Like a tailor fitting a special garment, you will adapt the scope of the health history to several factors: the patient's concerns and problems; your goals for assessment; the clinical setting (inpatient or outpatient; specialty or primary care); and the time available. Knowing the content and relevance of all components of the comprehensive health history allows you to choose those elements that will be most helpful for addressing patient concerns in different contexts.

These components of the comprehensive adult health history are more fully described in the next few pages. The *comprehensive pediatric health history* appears in Chapter 18. These sample adult and pediatric health histories follow standard formats for written documentation, which you will need to learn. As you review these histories, you will encounter several technical terms for symptoms. Definitions of terms, together with ways to ask about symptoms, can be found in each of the regional examination chapters.

■ Components of the Adult Health History

Identifying Data	▪ *Identifying data*—such as age, gender, occupation, marital status ▪ *Source of the history*—usually the patient, but can be family member, friend, letter of referral, or the medical record ▪ If appropriate, establish *source of referral* because a written report may be needed.
Reliability	Varies according to the patient's memory, trust, and mood
Chief Complaint(s)	The one or more symptoms or concerns causing the patient to seek care
Present Illness	▪ Amplifies the *Chief Complaint;* describes how each symptom developed ▪ Includes patient's thoughts and feelings about the illness ▪ Pulls in relevant portions of the *Review of Systems* (see below) ▪ May include *medications, allergies,* habits of *smoking* and *alcohol,* which are frequently pertinent to the present illness
Past History	▪ Lists childhood illnesses ▪ Lists adult illnesses with dates for at least four categories: medical; surgical; obstetric/gynecologic; and psychiatric ▪ Includes health maintenance practices such as immunizations, screening tests, lifestyle issues, and home safety
Family History	▪ Outlines or diagrams age and health, or age and cause of death, of siblings, parents, and grandparents ▪ Documents presence or absence of specific illnesses in family, such as hypertension, coronary artery disease, etc.
Personal and Social History	Describes educational level, family of origin, current household, personal interests, and lifestyle
Review of Systems	Documents presence or absence of common symptoms related to each major body system

The components of the comprehensive health history structure the patient's story and the format of your written record, but the order shown should not dictate the sequence of the interview. Usually the interview will be more fluid and will follow the patient's leads and cues, as described in Chapter 2.

Subjective vs. Objective Data. As you acquire the techniques of the history taking and physical examination, remember the important differences between ***subjective information*** and ***objective information,*** as summarized in the accompanying table. Knowing these differences helps you apply clinical reasoning and cluster patient information. These distinctions are equally important for organizing written and oral presentations about the patient.

Differences Between Subjective and Objective Data

Subjective Data	Objective Data
What the patient tells you	What you detect during the examination
The history, from Chief Complaint through Review of Systems	All physical examination findings
Example: Mrs. G is a 54-year-old hairdresser who reports pressure over her left chest "like an elephant sitting there," which goes into her left neck and arm.	*Example:* Mrs. G is an older, overweight white female, who is pleasant and cooperative. BP 160/80, HR 96 and regular, respiratory rate 24, afebrile.

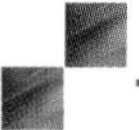

THE COMPREHENSIVE ADULT HEALTH HISTORY

Initial Information

Date and Time of History. The date is always important. You are strongly advised to routinely document the time you evaluate the patient, especially in urgent, emergent, or hospital settings.

Identifying Data. These include age, gender, marital status, and occupation. The ***source of history*** or ***referral*** can be the patient, a family member or friend, an officer, a consultant, or the medical record. Patients requesting evaluations for schools, agencies, or insurance companies may have special priorities compared with patients seeking care on their own initiative. Designating the *source of referral* helps you to assess the type of information provided and any possible biases.

Reliability. This information should be documented if relevant. For example, "The patient is vague when describing symptoms and cannot specify details." This judgment reflects the quality of the information provided by the patient and is usually made at the end of the interview.

Chief Complaint(s). *Make every attempt to quote the patient's own words.* For example, "My stomach hurts and I feel awful." Sometimes patients have no overt complaints, in which case you should report their goals instead. For example, "I have come for my regular check-up"; or "I've been admitted for a thorough evaluation of my heart."

Present Illness. This section of the history is a complete, clear, and chronologic account of the problems prompting the patient to seek care. The narrative should include the onset of the problem, the setting in which it has developed, its manifestations, and any treatments. The principal symptoms should be well-characterized, with descriptions of (1) location; (2) quality; (3) quantity or severity; (4) timing, including onset, duration, and frequency; (5) the setting in which they occur; (6) factors that have aggravated or relieved the symptoms; and (7) associated manifestations. These ***seven attributes*** are invaluable for understanding all patient symptoms (see p. 32). It is also important to include "pertinent positives" and "pertinent negatives" from sections of the *Review of Systems* related to the *Chief Complaint(s)*. These designate the presence or absence of symptoms relevant to the *differential diagnosis,* which refers to the most likely diagnoses explaining the patient's condition. Other information is frequently relevant, such as risk factors for coronary artery disease in patients with chest pain, or current medications in patients with syncope. The *Present Illness* should reveal the patient's responses to his or her symptoms and what effect the illness has had on the patient's life. Always remember, *the data flow spontaneously from the patient, but the task of organization is yours.*

Patients often have more than one complaint or concern. Each merits its own paragraph and a full description.

Medications should be noted, including name, dose, route, and frequency of use. Also list home remedies, nonprescription drugs, vitamins, mineral or herbal supplements, oral contraceptives, and medicines borrowed from family members or friends. It is a good idea to ask patients to bring in all of their medications so you can see exactly what they take. ***Allergies,*** including *specific reactions* to each medication, such as rash or nausea, must be recorded, as well as allergies to foods, insects, or environmental factors. Note ***tobacco*** use, including the type used. Cigarettes are often reported in pack-years (a person who has smoked 1½ packs a day for 12 years has an 18-pack-year history). If someone has quit, note for how long. ***Alcohol and drug use*** should always be investigated (see pp. 50–51 for suggested questions). (Note that *tobacco, alcohol,* and *drugs* may also be included in the *Personal and Social History*; however, many clinicians find these habits pertinent to the *Present Illness.*)

Past History. ***Childhood illnesses,*** such as measles, rubella, mumps, whooping cough, chickenpox, rheumatic fever, scarlet fever, and polio, are included in the *Past History.* Also included are any chronic childhood illnesses.

You should provide information relative to ***Adult Illnesses*** in each of four areas:

- *Medical:* Illnesses such as diabetes, hypertension, hepatitis, asthma, and HIV; hospitalizations; number and gender of sexual partners; and risky sexual practices
- *Surgical:* Dates, indications, and types of operations
- *Obstetric/Gynecologic:* Obstetric history, menstrual history, methods of contraception, and sexual function
- *Psychiatric:* Illness and time frame, diagnoses, hospitalizations, and treatments

Also cover selected aspects of *Health Maintenance,* especially immunizations and screening tests. For *immunizations,* find out whether the patient has received vaccines for tetanus, pertussis, diphtheria, polio, measles, rubella, mumps, influenza, varicella, hepatitis B, *Haemophilus influenza* type B, and pneumococci. For *screening tests,* review tuberculin tests, Pap smears, mammograms, stool tests for occult blood, and cholesterol tests, together with results and when they were last performed. If the patient does not know this information, written permission may be needed to obtain old medical records.

Family History. Under *Family History,* outline or diagram the age and health, or age and cause of death, of each immediate relative, including parents, grandparents, siblings, children, and grandchildren. Review each of the following conditions and record whether they are present or absent in the family: hypertension, coronary artery disease, elevated cholesterol levels, stroke, diabetes, thyroid or renal disease, cancer (specify type), arthritis, tuberculosis, asthma or lung disease, headache, seizure disorder, mental illness, suicide, alcohol or drug addiction, and allergies, as well as symptoms reported by the patient.

Personal and Social History. The *Personal and Social History* captures the patient's personality and interests, sources of support, coping style, strengths, and fears. It should include occupation and the last year of schooling; home situation and significant others; sources of stress, both recent and long-term; important life experiences, such as military service, job history, financial situation, and retirement; leisure activities; religious affiliation and spiritual beliefs; and activities of daily living (ADLs). Baseline level of function is particularly important in older or disabled patients (see p. 852 for the ADLs frequently assessed in older patients). The *Personal and Social History* also conveys lifestyle habits that promote health or create risk such as *exercise and diet,* including frequency of exercise; usual daily food intake; dietary supplements or restrictions; use of coffee, tea, and other caffeine-containing beverages; and *safety measures,* including use of seat belts, bicycle helmets, sunblock, smoke detectors, and other devices related to specific hazards. You may want to include any *alternative health care* practices.

You will come to thread personal and social questions throughout the interview to make the patient feel more at ease.

Review of Systems. Understanding and using *Review of Systems* questions is often challenging for beginning students. Think about asking series of questions going from "head to toe." It is helpful to prepare the patient for the questions to come by saying, "The next part of the history may feel like a million questions, but they are important and I want to be thorough." Most *Review of Systems* questions pertain to *symptoms,* but on occasion some clinicians also include diseases like pneumonia or tuberculosis.

If the patient remembers important illnesses as you ask questions within the *Review of Systems, record or present such illnesses as part of the Present Illness* or *Past History.*

Start with a fairly general question as you address each of the different systems. This focuses the patient's attention and allows you to shift to more specific questions about systems that may be of concern. Examples of starting questions are: "How are your ears and hearing?" "How about your lungs and breathing?" "Any trouble with your heart?" "How is your digestion?" "How about your bowels?" Note that you will vary the need for additional questions depending on the patient's age, complaints, and general state of health and your clinical judgment.

The *Review of Systems* questions may uncover problems that the patient has overlooked, particularly in areas unrelated to the *present illness.* Significant health events, such as a major prior illness or a parent's death, require full exploration. Remember that *major health events should be moved to the Present Illness or Past History in your write-up.* Keep your technique flexible. Interviewing the patient yields a variety of information that you organize into formal written format only after the interview and examination are completed.

Some clinicians do the *Review of Systems* during the physical examination, asking about the ears, for example, as they examine them. If the patient has only a few symptoms, this combination can be efficient. However, if there are multiple symptoms, the flow of both the history and the examination can be disrupted, and necessary note-taking becomes awkward. Listed below is a standard series of review-of-system questions. As you gain experience, the "yes or no" questions, placed at the end of the interview, will take no more than several minutes.

General: Usual weight, recent weight change, any clothes that fit more tightly or loosely than before. Weakness, fatigue, or fever.

Skin: Rashes, lumps, sores, itching, dryness, changes in color; changes in hair or nails; changes in size or color of moles.

Head, Eyes, Ears, Nose, Throat (HEENT): *Head:* Headache, head injury, dizziness, lightheadedness. *Eyes:* Vision, glasses or contact lenses, last examination, pain, redness, excessive tearing, double or blurred vision, spots, specks, flashing lights, glaucoma, cataracts. *Ears:* Hearing, tinnitus, vertigo, earaches, infection, discharge. If hearing is decreased, use or nonuse of hearing aids. *Nose and sinuses:* Frequent colds; nasal stuffiness, discharge, or itching; hay fever; nosebleeds; sinus trouble. *Throat (or mouth and pharynx):* Condition of teeth and gums; bleeding gums; dentures, if any, and how they fit; last dental examination; sore tongue; dry mouth; frequent sore throats; hoarseness.

Neck: "Swollen glands"; goiter; lumps, pain, or stiffness in the neck.

Breasts: Lumps, pain, or discomfort; nipple discharge; self-examination practices.

Respiratory: Cough, sputum (color, quantity), hemoptysis, dyspnea, wheezing, pleurisy, last chest x-ray. You may wish to include asthma, bronchitis, emphysema, pneumonia, and tuberculosis.

Cardiovascular: Heart trouble, high blood pressure, rheumatic fever, heart murmurs; chest pain or discomfort; palpitations, dyspnea, orthopnea, paroxysmal nocturnal dyspnea, edema; results of past electrocardiograms or other cardiovascular tests.

Gastrointestinal: Trouble swallowing, heartburn, appetite, nausea. Bowel movements, stool color and size, change in bowel habits, pain with defecation, rectal bleeding or black or tarry stools, hemorrhoids, constipation, diarrhea. Abdominal pain, food intolerance, excessive belching or passing of gas. Jaundice, liver, or gallbladder trouble; hepatitis.

Urinary: Frequency of urination, polyuria, nocturia, urgency, burning or pain during urination, hematuria, urinary infections, kidney or flank pain, kidney stones, ureteral colic, suprapubic pain, incontinence; in males, reduced caliber or force of the urinary stream, hesitancy, dribbling.

Genital: *Male:* Hernias, discharge from or sores on the penis, testicular pain or masses, scrotal pain or swelling, history of sexually transmitted diseases and their treatments. Sexual habits, interest, function, satisfaction, birth control methods, condom use, and problems. Exposure to HIV infection. *Female:* Age at menarche; regularity, frequency, and duration of periods; amount of bleeding; bleeding between periods or after intercourse; last menstrual period; dysmenorrhea; premenstrual tension. Age at menopause, menopausal symptoms, postmenopausal bleeding. If the patient was born before 1971, exposure to diethylstilbestrol (DES) from maternal use during pregnancy (linked to cervical carcinoma). Vaginal discharge, itching, sores, lumps, sexually transmitted diseases and treatments. Number of pregnancies, number and type of deliveries, number of abortions (spontaneous and induced), complications of pregnancy, birth control methods. Sexual preference, interest, function, satisfaction, any problems, including dyspareunia. Exposure to HIV infection.

Peripheral vascular: Intermittent claudication; leg cramps; varicose veins; past clots in the veins; swelling in calves, legs, or feet; color change in fingertips or toes during cold weather; swelling with redness or tenderness.

Musculoskeletal: Muscle or joint pain, stiffness, arthritis, gout, and backache. If present, describe location of affected joints or muscles, any swelling, redness, pain, tenderness, stiffness, weakness, or limitation of motion or activity; include timing of symptoms (e.g., morning or evening), duration, and any history of trauma. Neck or low back pain. Joint pain with systemic features such as fever, chills, rash, anorexia, weight loss, or weakness.

Psychiatric: Nervousness; tension; mood, including depression, memory change, suicide attempts, if relevant.

Neurologic: Changes in mood, attention, or speech; changes in orientation, memory, insight, or judgment; headache, dizziness, vertigo; fainting, blackouts, seizures, weakness, paralysis, numbness or loss of sensation, tingling or "pins and needles," tremors or other involuntary movements; seizures.

Hematologic: Anemia, easy bruising or bleeding, past transfusions, transfusion reactions.

Endocrine: Thyroid trouble, heat or cold intolerance, excessive sweating, excessive thirst or hunger, polyuria, change in glove or shoe size.

THE PHYSICAL EXAMINATION

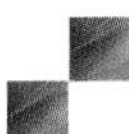

APPROACH AND OVERVIEW

In this section, we outline the ***comprehensive physical examination*** and provide an *overview* of all its components. You will conduct a comprehensive physical examination on most new patients or patients being admitted to the hospital. For more *problem-oriented,* or *focused, assessments,* the presenting complaints will dictate what segments of the examination you elect to perform. You will find a more extended discussion of the approach to the examination, its scope (comprehensive or focused), and a table summarizing the examination sequence in Chapter 4, Beginning the Physical Examination: General Survey and Vital Signs. Information about anatomy and physiology, interview questions, techniques of examination, and important abnormalities are detailed in Chapters 4 through 17 for each of the segments of the physical examination described below.

For an overview of the physical examination, study the following description of the sequence of examination now. *Note that clinicians vary in where they place different segments of the examination, especially the examinations of the musculoskeletal system and the nervous system.* Some of these options are indicated below.

As you develop your own sequence of examination, *an important goal is to minimize how often you ask the patient to change position* from supine to sitting, or from standing to lying supine. Some suggestions for patient positioning during the different segments of the examination are indicated in the right-hand column in *red*.

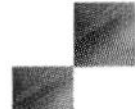

THE COMPREHENSIVE ADULT PHYSICAL EXAMINATION

General Survey. Observe the patient's general state of health, height, build, and sexual development. Obtain the patient's weight. Note posture,

The survey continues throughout the history and examination.

motor activity, and gait; dress, grooming, and personal hygiene; and any odors of the body or breath. Watch the patient's facial expressions and note manner, affect, and reactions to persons and things in the environment. Listen to the patient's manner of speaking and note the state of awareness or level of consciousness.

Vital Signs. Measure the blood pressure. Count the pulse and respiratory rate. If indicated, measure the body temperature.

The **patient is sitting** on the edge of the bed or examining table, unless this position is contraindicated. You should be standing in front of the patient, moving to either side as needed.

Skin. Observe the skin of the face and its characteristics. Identify any lesions, noting their location, distribution, arrangement, type, and color. Inspect and palpate the hair and nails. Study the patient's hands. Continue your assessment of the skin as you examine the other body regions.

Head, Eyes, Ears, Nose, Throat (HEENT). ***Head:*** Examine the hair, scalp, skull, and face. ***Eyes:*** Check visual acuity and screen the visual fields. Note the position and alignment of the eyes. Observe the eyelids and inspect the sclera and conjunctiva of each eye. With oblique lighting, inspect each cornea, iris, and lens. Compare the pupils, and test their reactions to light. Assess the extraocular movements. With an ophthalmoscope, inspect the ocular fundi. ***Ears:*** Inspect the auricles, canals, and drums. Check auditory acuity. If acuity is diminished, check lateralization (Weber test) and compare air and bone conduction (Rinne test). ***Nose and sinuses:*** Examine the external nose; using a light and a nasal speculum, inspect the nasal mucosa, septum, and turbinates. Palpate for tenderness of the frontal and maxillary sinuses. ***Throat (or mouth and pharynx):*** Inspect the lips, oral mucosa, gums, teeth, tongue, palate, tonsils, and pharynx. *(You may wish to assess the cranial nerves during this portion of the examination.)*

The room should be darkened for the ophthalmoscopic examination. This promotes pupillary dilation and visibility of the fundi.

Neck. Inspect and palpate the cervical lymph nodes. Note any masses or unusual pulsations in the neck. Feel for any deviation of the trachea. Observe sound and effort of the patient's breathing. Inspect and palpate the thyroid gland.

Move behind the sitting patient to feel the thyroid gland and to examine the back, posterior thorax, and the lungs.

Back. Inspect and palpate the spine and muscles of the back.

Posterior Thorax and Lungs. Inspect and palpate the spine and muscles of the *upper* back. Inspect, palpate, and percuss the chest. Identify the level of diaphragmatic dullness on each side. Listen to the breath sounds; identify any adventitious (or added) sounds, and, if indicated, listen to the transmitted voice sounds (see p. 260).

Breasts, Axillae, and Epitrochlear Nodes. In a woman, inspect the breasts with her arms relaxed, then elevated, and then with her hands pressed on her hips. In either sex, inspect the axillae and feel for the axillary nodes. Feel for the epitrochlear nodes.

The patient is **still sitting.** Move to the front again.

A Note on the Musculoskeletal System: By this time, you have made some preliminary observations of the musculoskeletal system. You have inspected the hands, surveyed the upper back, and at least in women, made a fair estimate of the shoulders' range of motion. Use these and subsequent observations to decide whether a full musculoskeletal examination is warranted. If indicated, *with the patient still sitting*, examine the hands, arms, shoulders, neck, and temporomandibular joints. Inspect and palpate the joints and check their range of motion. *(You may choose to examine upper extremity muscle bulk, tone, strength, and reflexes at this time, or you may decide to wait until later.)*

Palpate the breasts, while at the same time continuing your inspection.

The patient position is supine. Ask the patient to lie down. You should stand at the *right side* of the patient's bed.

Anterior Thorax and Lungs. Inspect, palpate, and percuss the chest. Listen to the breath sounds, any adventitious sounds, and, if indicated, transmitted voice sounds.

Cardiovascular System. Observe the jugular venous pulsations and measure the jugular venous pressure in relation to the sternal angle. Inspect and palpate the carotid pulsations. Listen for carotid bruits.

Elevate the head of the bed to about 30° for the cardiovascular examination, adjusting as necessary to see the jugular venous pulsations.

Inspect and palpate the precordium. Note the location, diameter, amplitude, and duration of the apical impulse. Listen at the apex and the lower sternal border with the bell of a stethoscope. Listen at each auscultatory area with the diaphragm. Listen for the first and second heart sounds and for physiologic splitting of the second heart sound. Listen for any abnormal heart sounds or murmurs.

Ask the patient to roll partly onto the left side while you listen at the apex. Then have the patient roll back to the supine position while you listen to the rest of the heart. The patient should sit, lean forward, and exhale while you listen for the murmur of aortic regurgitation.

Abdomen. Inspect, auscultate, and percuss the abdomen. Palpate lightly, then deeply. Assess the liver and spleen by percussion and then palpation. Try to feel the kidneys, and palpate the aorta and its pulsations. If you suspect kidney infection, percuss posteriorly over the costovertebral angles.

Lower the head of the bed to the flat position. **The patient should be supine.**

Lower Extremities. Examine the legs, assessing three systems while the patient is still supine. Each of these three systems can be further assessed when the patient stands.

The patient is **supine**.

With the Patient Supine

- *Peripheral Vascular System.* Palpate the femoral pulses and, if indicated, the popliteal pulses. Palpate the inguinal lymph nodes. Inspect for lower extremity edema, discoloration, or ulcers. Palpate for pitting edema.
- *Musculoskeletal System.* Note any deformities or enlarged joints. If indicated, palpate the joints, check their range of motion, and perform any necessary maneuvers.
- *Nervous System.* Assess lower extremity muscle bulk, tone, and strength; also assess sensation and reflexes. Observe any abnormal movements.

With the Patient Standing

The patient is **standing**. You should sit on a chair or stool.

- *Peripheral Vascular System.* Inspect for varicose veins.
- *Musculoskeletal System.* Examine the alignment of the spine and its range of motion, the alignment of the legs, and the feet.
- *Genitalia and Hernias in Men.* Examine the penis and scrotal contents and check for hernias.
- *Nervous System.* Observe the patient's gait and ability to walk heel-to-toe, walk on the toes, walk on the heels, hop in place, and do shallow knee bends. Do a Romberg test and check for pronator drift.

Nervous System. The complete examination of the nervous system can also be done at the end of the examination. It consists of the five segments described below: *mental status, cranial nerves* (including funduscopic examination), *motor system, sensory system,* and *reflexes.*

The patient is **sitting or supine**.

Mental Status. If indicated and not done during the interview, assess the patient's orientation, mood, thought process, thought content, abnormal perceptions, insight and judgment, memory and attention, information and vocabulary, calculating abilities, abstract thinking, and constructional ability.

Cranial Nerves. If not already examined, check sense of smell, strength of the temporal and masseter muscles, corneal reflexes, facial movements, gag reflex, and strength of the trapezia and sternomastoid muscles.

Motor System. Muscle bulk, tone, and strength of major muscle groups. *Cerebellar function:* rapid alternating movements (RAMs), point-to-point movements, such as finger-to-nose (F → N) and heel-to-shin (H → S); gait.

Sensory System. Pain, temperature, light touch, vibration, and discrimination. Compare right with left sides and distal with proximal areas on the limbs.

Reflexes. Including biceps, triceps, brachioradialis, patellar, Achilles deep tendon reflexes; also plantar reflexes or Babinski reflex (see pp. 633–639).

Additional Examinations. The *rectal* and *genital* examinations are often performed at the end of the physical examination. Patient positioning is as indicated.

Rectal Examination in Men. Inspect the sacrococcygeal and perianal areas. Palpate the anal canal, rectum, and prostate. If the patient cannot stand, examine the genitalia before doing the rectal examination.

The patient is **lying on his left side** for the rectal examination.

Genital and Rectal Examination in Women. Examine the external genitalia, vagina, and cervix. Obtain a Pap smear. Palpate the uterus and adnexa. Do a rectovaginal and rectal examination.

The patient is **supine in the lithotomy position**. You should be seated during examination with the speculum, then standing during bimanual examination of the uterus, adnexa, and rectum.

RECORDING YOUR FINDINGS

Now you are ready to review an actual written record documenting a patient's history and physical findings. The history and physical examination form the database for your subsequent *assessment(s)* of the patient and your *plan(s)* with the patient for management and next steps. Your written record organizes the information from the history and physical examination and should clearly communicate the patient's clinical issues to all members of the health care team. You will find that following a standardized format is the most efficient and helpful way to transfer this information. See "Recording the History and Physical Examination: The Case of Mrs. N," for an example.

Your written record should also facilitate clinical reasoning and communicate essential information to the many health professionals involved in your patient's care. Chapter 3, Clinical Reasoning, Assessment, and Plan, will provide more comprehensive information for formulating the *assessment* and *plan* and additional guidelines for documentation.

If you are a beginner, organizing the *Present Illness* may be especially challenging, but do not get discouraged. Considerable knowledge is needed to cluster related symptoms and physical signs. If you are unfamiliar with hyperthyroidism, for example, it may not be apparent that muscular weakness, heat intolerance, excessive sweating, diarrhea, and weight loss all represent a *Present Illness*. Until your knowledge and judgment grow, the patient's story and the seven key attributes of a symptom (see p. 32) are helpful and necessary guides to what to include in this portion of the record.

TIPS FOR A CLEAR AND ACCURATE WRITE-UP

You should write the record as soon as possible, before the data fade from your memory. At first, you will probably prefer to take notes when talking with the patient. As you gain experience, however, work toward recording the *Present Illness*, the *Past History*, the *Family History*, the *Personal and Social History*, and the *Review of Systems* in final form during the interview. Leave spaces for filling in details later. During the *physical examination*, make note immediately of specific measurements, such as blood pressure and heart rate. On the other hand, recording multiple items interrupts the

(continued)

TIPS FOR A CLEAR AND ACCURATE WRITE-UP (Continued)

flow of the examination, and you will soon learn to remember your findings and record them after you have finished.

Several key features distinguish a clear and well-organized written record. Pay special attention to the *order* and the *degree of detail* as you review the record below and later when you construct your own write-ups. Remember that if handwritten, a good record is always legible!

Order of the Write-Up

The order should be consistent and obvious so that future readers, including you, can easily find specific points of information. Keep subjective items of history in the history, for example, and do not let them stray into the physical examination. Offset your headings and make them clear by using indentations and spacing to accent your organization. Create emphasis by using asterisks and underlines for important points. Arrange the *present illness* in chronologic order, starting with the current episode and then filling in the relevant background information. If a patient with long-standing diabetes is hospitalized in a coma, for example, begin with the events leading up to the coma and then summarize the past history of the patient's diabetes.

Degree of Detail

The *degree of detail* is also a challenge. It should be pertinent to the subject or problem but not redundant. Review the record of Mrs. N, then turn to the checklist in Chapter 3 on pp. 81–83. Decide if you think the order and detail included meet the standards of a good medical record.

Recording the History and Physical Examination: The Case of Mrs. N

8/30/05 11:00 AM

Mrs. N is a pleasant, 54-year-old widowed saleswoman residing in Amarillo, Texas.

Referral. None

Source and Reliability. Self-referred; seems reliable.

Chief Complaint: "My head aches."

Present Illness: For about 3 months, Mrs. N has had increasing problems with frontal headaches. These are usually bifrontal, throbbing, and mild to moderately severe. She has missed work on several occasions because of associated nausea and vomiting. Headaches now average once a week, usually related to stress, and last 4 to 6 hours. They are relieved by sleep and putting a damp towel over the forehead. There is little relief from aspirin. No associated visual changes, motor-sensory deficits, or paresthesias.

"Sick headaches" with nausea and vomiting began at age 15, recurred throughout her mid-20s, then decreased to one every 2 or 3 months and almost disappeared.

The patient reports increased pressure at work from a new and demanding boss; she is also worried about her daughter (see *Personal and*

(continued)

Social History). Thinks her headaches may be like those in the past, but wants to be sure because her mother died of a stroke. She is concerned that they interfere with her work and make her irritable with her family. She eats three meals a day and drinks three cups of coffee per day; cola at night.

Medications. Aspirin, 1 to 2 tablets every 4 to 6 hours as needed. "Water pill" in the past for ankle swelling, none recently.

**Allergies.* Ampicillin causes rash.

Tobacco. About 1 pack of cigarettes per day since age 18 (36 pack-years).

Alcohol/drugs. Wine on rare occasions. No illicit drugs.

Past History

Childhood Illnesses. Measles, chickenpox. No scarlet fever or rheumatic fever.

Adult Illnesses. ***Medical:*** Pyelonephritis, 1982, with fever and right flank pain; treated with ampicillin; develop generalized rash with itching several days later. Reports kidney x-rays were normal; no recurrence of infection. ***Surgical:*** Tonsillectomy, age 6; appendectomy, age 13. Sutures for laceration, 1991, after stepping on glass. ***Ob/Gyn:*** G3P3, with normal vaginal deliveries. 3 living children. Menarche age 12. Last menses 6 months ago. Little interest in sex, and not sexually active. No concerns about HIV infection. ***Psychiatric:*** None.

Health Maintenance. ***Immunizations:*** Oral polio vaccine, year uncertain; tetanus shots × 2, 1991, followed with booster 1 year later; flu vaccine, 2000, no reaction. ***Screening tests:*** Last Pap smear, 1998, normal. No mammograms to date.

Family History

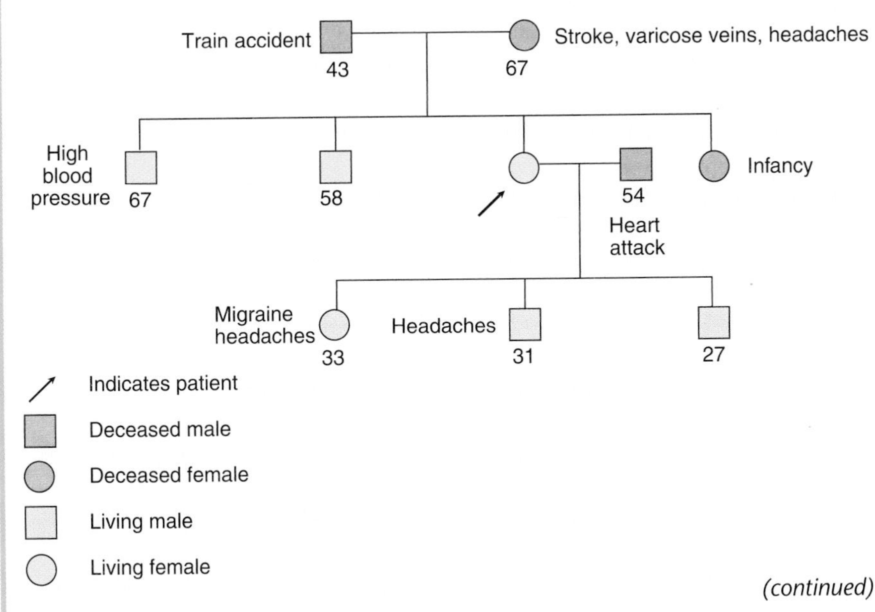

(continued)

The Family History: Can record as a diagram or a narrative. The diagram format is more helpful than the narrative for tracing genetic disorders. The negatives from the family history should follow either format.

*Add an asterisk or underline important points.

or

Father died at age 43 in train accident. Mother died at age 67 of stroke; had varicose veins, headaches

One brother, 61, with hypertension, otherwise well; one brother, 58, well except for mild arthritis; one sister, died in infancy of unknown cause

Husband died at age 54 of heart attack

Daughter, 33, with migraine headaches, otherwise well; son, 31, with headaches; son, 27, well

No family history of diabetes, tuberculosis, heart or kidney disease, cancer, anemia, epilepsy, or mental illness.

Personal and Social History: Born and raised in Lake City, finished high school, married at age 19. Worked as sales clerk for 2 years, then moved with husband to Amarillo, had 3 children. Returned to work 15 years ago because of financial pressures. Children all married. Four years ago Mr. N died suddenly of a heart attack, leaving little savings. Mrs. N has moved to small apartment to be near daughter, Dorothy. Dorothy's husband, Arthur, has an alcohol problem. Mrs. N's apartment now a haven for Dorothy and her 2 children, Kevin, 6 years, and Linda, 3 years. Mrs. N feels responsible for helping them; feels tense and nervous but denies depression. She has friends but rarely discusses family problems: "I'd rather keep them to myself. I don't like gossip." No church or other organizational support. She is typically up at 7:00 A.M., works 9:00 to 5:30, eats dinner alone.

Exercise and diet. Gets little exercise. Diet high in carbohydrates.

Safety measures. Uses seat belt regularly. Uses sunblock. Medications kept in an unlocked medicine cabinet. Cleaning solutions in unlocked cabinet below sink. Mr. N's shotgun and box of shells in unlocked closet upstairs.

Review of Systems

General. Has *gained* about 10 lb in the past 4 years.

Skin. No rashes or other changes.

Head, Eyes, Ears, Nose, Throat (HEENT). See *Present Illness*. No history of head injury. *Eyes:* Reading glasses for 5 years, last checked 1 year ago. No symptoms. *Ears:* Hearing good. No tinnitus, vertigo, infections. *Nose, sinuses:* Occasional mild cold. No hay fever, sinus trouble. **Throat (or *mouth and pharynx):* Some bleeding of gums recently. Last dental visit 2 years ago. Occasional canker sore.

Neck. No lumps, goiter, pain. No swollen glands.

Breasts. No lumps, pain, discharge. Does breast self-exam sporadically.

Respiratory. No cough, wheezing, shortness of breath. Last chest x-ray, 1986, St. Mary's Hospital; unremarkable.

Cardiovascular. No known heart disease or high blood pressure; last blood pressure taken in 1998. No dyspnea, orthopnea, chest pain, palpitations. Has never had an electrocardiogram (ECG).

Gastrointestinal. Appetite good; no nausea, vomiting, indigestion. Bowel movement about once daily, though sometimes has hard stools for 2 to 3 days when especially tense; no diarrhea or bleeding. No pain, jaundice, gallbladder or liver problems.

(continued)

*****Urinary.*** No frequency, dysuria, hematuria, or recent flank pain; nocturia × 1, large volume. Occasionally loses some urine when coughs hard.

Genital. No vaginal or pelvic infections. No dyspareunia.

Peripheral Vascular. Varicose veins appeared in both legs during first pregnancy. For 10 years, has had swollen ankles after prolonged standing; wears light elastic pantyhose; tried "water pill" 5 months ago, but it didn't help much; no history of phlebitis or leg pain.

Musculoskeletal. Mild, aching, low-back pain, often after a long day's work; no radiation down the legs; used to do back exercises but not now. No other joint pain.

Psychiatric. No history of depression or treatment for psychiatric disorders. See also *Present Illness* and *Personal and Social History.*

Neurologic. No fainting, seizures, motor or sensory loss. Memory good.

Hematologic. Except for bleeding gums, no easy bleeding. No anemia.

Endocrine. No known thyroid trouble, temperature intolerance. Sweating average. No symptoms or history of diabetes.

Physical Examination: Mrs. N is a short, overweight, middle-aged woman, who is animated and responds quickly to questions. She is somewhat tense, with moist, cold hands. Her hair is fixed neatly and her clothes are immaculate. Her color is good, and she lies flat without discomfort.

Vital Signs. Ht (without shoes) 157 cm (5′2″). Wt (dressed) 65 kg (143 lb). BMI 26. BP 164/98 right arm, supine; 160/96 left arm, supine; 152/88 right arm, supine with wide cuff. Heart rate (HR) 88 and regular. Respiratory rate (RR) 18. Temperature (oral) 98.6°F.

Skin. Palms cold and moist, but color good. Scattered cherry angiomas over upper trunk. Nails without clubbing, cyanosis.

Head, Eyes, Ears, Nose, Throat (HEENT). *Head:* Hair of average texture. Scalp without lesions, normocephalic/atraumatic (NC/AT). *Eyes:* Vision 20/30 in each eye. Visual fields full by confrontation. Conjunctiva pink; sclera white. Pupils 4 mm constricting to 2 mm, round, regular, equally reactive to light. Extraocular movements intact. Disc margins sharp, without hemorrhages, exudates. No arteriolar narrowing or A-V nicking. *Ears:* Wax partially obscures right tympanic membrane (TM); left canal clear, TM with good cone of light. Acuity good to whispered voice. Weber midline. AC > BC. *Nose:* Mucosa pink, septum midline. No sinus tenderness. *Mouth:* Oral mucosa pink. Several interdental papillae red, slightly swollen. Dentition good. Tongue midline, with 3 × 4 mm shallow white ulcer on red base on undersurface near tip; tender but not indurated. Tonsils absent. Pharynx without exudates.

Neck. Neck supple. Trachea midline. Thyroid isthmus barely palpable, lobes not felt.

Lymph Nodes. Small (<1 cm), soft, nontender, and mobile tonsillar and posterior cervical nodes bilaterally. No axillary or epitrochlear nodes. Several small inguinal nodes bilaterally, soft and nontender.

Thorax and Lungs. Thorax symmetric with good excursion. Lungs resonant. Breath sounds vesicular with no added sounds. Diaphragms descend 4 cm bilaterally.

(continued)

Cardiovascular. Jugular venous pressure 1 cm above the sternal angle, with head of examining table raised to 30°. Carotid upstrokes brisk, without bruits. Apical impulse discrete and tapping, barely palpable in the 5th left interspace, 8 cm lateral to the midsternal line. Good S_1, S_2; no S_3 or S_4. A II/VI medium-pitched midsystolic murmur at the 2nd right interspace; does not radiate to the neck. No diastolic murmurs.

Breasts. Pendulous, symmetric. No masses; nipples without discharge.

Abdomen. Protuberant. Well-healed scar, right lower quadrant. Bowel sounds active. No tenderness or masses. Liver span 7 cm in right midclavicular line; edge smooth, palpable 1 cm below right costal margin (RCM). Spleen and kidneys not felt. No costovertebral angle tenderness (CVAT).

Genitalia. External genitalia without lesions. Mild cystocele at introitus on straining. Vaginal mucosa pink. Cervix pink, parous, and without discharge. Uterus anterior, midline, smooth, not enlarged. Adnexa not palpated due to obesity and poor relaxation. No cervical or adnexal tenderness. Pap smear taken. Rectovaginal wall intact.

Rectal. Rectal vault without masses. Stool brown, negative for occult blood.

Extremities. Warm and without edema. Calves supple, nontender.

Peripheral Vascular. Trace edema at both ankles. Moderate varicosities of saphenous veins both lower extremities. No stasis pigmentation or ulcers. Pulses (2 + = brisk, or normal):

	Radial	Femoral	Popliteal	Dorsalis Pedis	Posterior Tibial
RT	2+	2+	2+	2+	2+
LT	2+	2+	2+	Absent	2+

Musculoskeletal. No joint deformities. Good range of motion in hands, wrists, elbows, shoulders, spine, hips, knees, ankles.

Neurologic. *Mental Status:* Tense but alert and cooperative. Thought coherent. Oriented to person, place, and time. *Cranial Nerves:* II–XII intact. *Motor:* Good muscle bulk and tone. Strength 5/5 throughout (see p. 619 for grading system). *Cerebellar:* Rapid alternating movements (RAMs), point-to-point movements intact. Gait stable, fluid. *Sensory:* Pinprick, light touch, position sense, vibration, and stereognosis intact. Romberg negative. *Reflexes:*

	Biceps	Triceps	Brachio-radialis	Patellar	Achilles	Plantar
RT	2+	2+	2+	2+	1+	↓
LT	2+	2+	2+	2+/2+	1+	↓

OR

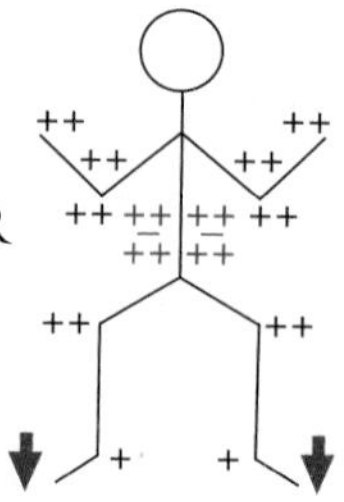

Two methods of recording may be used, depending upon personal preference: a tabular form or a stick picture diagram, as shown below and at right. 2+ = brisk, or normal; see p. 633 for grading system.

Bibliography

Anatomy and Physiology

Agur AMR, Dalley AF, Grant JC, Boileau JC. Grant's Atlas of Anatomy, 11th ed. Philadelphia, Lippincott Williams & Wilkins, 2005.

Berne RM. Physiology, 5th ed. St. Louis, Mosby, 2004.

Buja LM, Krueger GRF, Netter FH. Netter's Illustrated Human Pathology. Teterboro, NJ, Icon Learning Systems, 2005.

Gray H, Standring S, Ellis, H, Berkovitz BKB. Gray's Anatomy: The Anatomical Basis of Clinical Practice, 39th ed. New York, Elsevier–Churchill Livingstone, 2005.

Guyton AC, Hall JE. Textbook of Medical Physiology, 11th ed. Philadelphia, WB Saunders, 2005.

Moore KL, Dalley AF, Agur AMR. Clinically Oriented Anatomy, 5th ed. Baltimore, Lippincott Williams & Wilkins, 2006.

Medicine, Surgery, and Geriatrics

Bailey H, Clain A (eds). Hamilton Bailey's Demonstrations of Physical Signs in Clinical Surgery, 17th ed. Bristol, UK, Wright, 1986.

Barker LR, Burton JR, Zieve PD (eds). Principles of Ambulatory Medicine, 6th ed. Philadelphia, Lippincott Williams & Wilkins, 2003.

Brunicardi FC, Schwartz SI (eds). Schwartz's Principles of Surgery, 8th ed. New York, McGraw-Hill Medical, 2005.

Cassel C, Leipzig RM, Cohen HJ, Larson EB, Meier DE. Geriatric Medicine: An Evidence-based Approach, 4th ed. New York, Springer, 2003.

Cecil RL, Goldman L, Ausiello DA. Cecil Textbook of Medicine, 22nd ed. Philadelphia, WB Saunders, 2004.

Hazzard WR. Principles of Geriatric Medicine and Gerontology, 5th ed. New York, McGraw-Hill Professional, 2003.

Kasper DL, Harrison TR (eds). Harrison's Principles of Internal Medicine, 16th ed. New York, McGraw-Hill, 2005

Mandell GL. Essential Atlas of Infectious Diseases, 3rd ed. Philadelphia, Current Medicine, 2004.

Mandell GL, Gordon R, Bennett JE, Dolin R (eds). Mandell, Douglas, and Bennett's Principles and Practice of Infectious Diseases, 6th ed. Philadelphia, Elsevier–Churchill Livingstone, 2005.

Mandell GL, Mildvan D. Atlas of AIDS, 3rd ed. Philadelphia, Current Medicine, 2001.

Orient JM, Sapira JD (eds). Sapira's Art & Science of Bedside Diagnosis, 3rd ed. Philadelphia, Lippincott Williams & Wilkins, 2005.

Townsend CM, Sabiston DC (eds). Sabiston Textbook of Surgery: The Biological Basis of Modern Surgical Practice, 17th ed. Philadelphia, Elsevier–WB Saunders, 2004.

Youngkin EQ, Davis MS. Women's Health: A Primary Care Clinical Guide, 3rd ed. Upper Saddle River, NJ, Pearson/Prentice Hall, 2004.

Health Promotion and Counseling

Agency for Healthcare Research and Quality. Clinician's Handbook of Preventive Services: Put Prevention Into Practice, 2nd ed. Available at: http://www.ahcpr.gov/clinic/ppiphand.htm. Accessed May 15, 2005.

American Public Health Association. Public Health Links (for public health professionals). Available at: http://www.apha.org/public_health. Accessed May 16, 2005.

Bluestein D. Preventive services: immunization and chemoprevention. Geriatrics 60:35–39, 2005.

National Guideline Clearinghouse. Agency for Healthcare Research and Quality (AHRQ). Available at: http://www.ahrq.gov/clinic/cps3dix.htm. Accessed May 15, 2005.

National Quality Measures Clearinghouse. Agency for Healthcare Research and Quality (AHRQ). Available at: http://www.qualitymeasures.ahrq.gov. Accessed May 15, 2005.

U.S. Preventive Services Task Force. Guide to Clinical Preventive Services, 3rd ed. Available at: http://www.ahrq.gov/clinic/cps3dix.htm. Accessed May 15, 2005.

Zimmerman RK; American Academy of Family Physicians; Advisory Committee on Immunization Practices, American College of Obstetricians and Gynecologists. The 2004 recommended adult immunization schedule. Am Fam Physician 68:2453–2456, 2003.

CHAPTER

2

Interviewing and the Health History

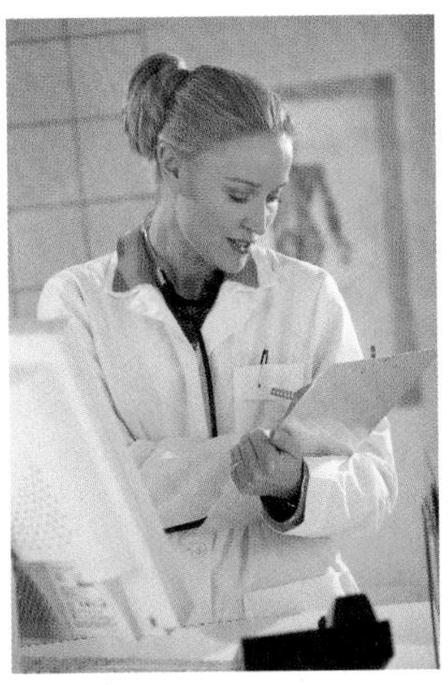

The health history interview is a conversation with a purpose. As you learn to elicit the patient's history, you will draw on many of the interpersonal skills that you use every day, but with unique and important differences. Unlike social conversation, in which you can freely express your own needs and interests and are responsible only for yourself, the primary goal of the clinician–patient interview is to improve the well-being of the patient. At its most basic level, the purpose of conversation with a patient is threefold: to establish a trusting and supportive relationship, to gather information, and to offer information.[1–3]

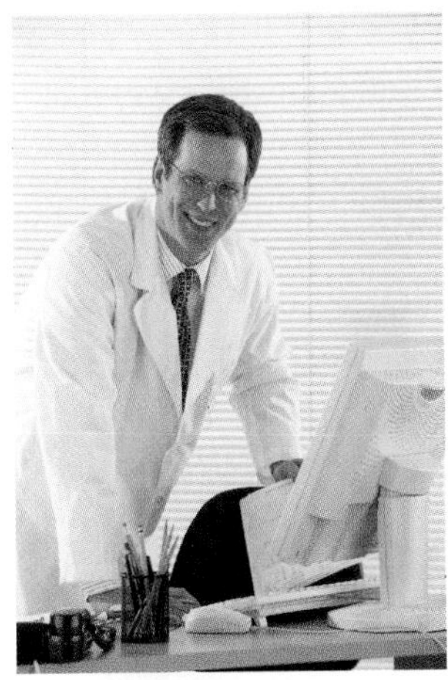

Relating effectively with patients is among the most valued skills of clinical care. As a beginning clinician, you will focus your energies on gathering information. At the same time, by using techniques that promote trust and convey respect, you will allow the patient's story to unfold in its most full and detailed form. Establishing a supportive interaction helps the patient feel more at ease when sharing information and itself becomes the foundation for therapeutic clinician–patient relationships.[4] Because illness can make patients feel discouraged and isolated, "A feeling of connectedness with the doctor, of being deeply heard and understood, reduces this feeling of isolation and despair. This feeling is the very heart of healing."[5]

This chapter introduces you to the essentials of interviewing. It emphasizes the approach to gathering the health history, but covers all the fundamental habits that you will continually use and refine in your conversations with patients. You will learn the guiding principles for skilled interviewing and how to forge trusting patient relationships. You will read about preparing for the interview, the sequence of the interviewing process, important interviewing techniques, and strategies for addressing various challenges that may arise in patient encounters. To help you navigate this journey, look over the Interviewing Milestones, on the next page, that mark the complex tasks of a skilled interview.

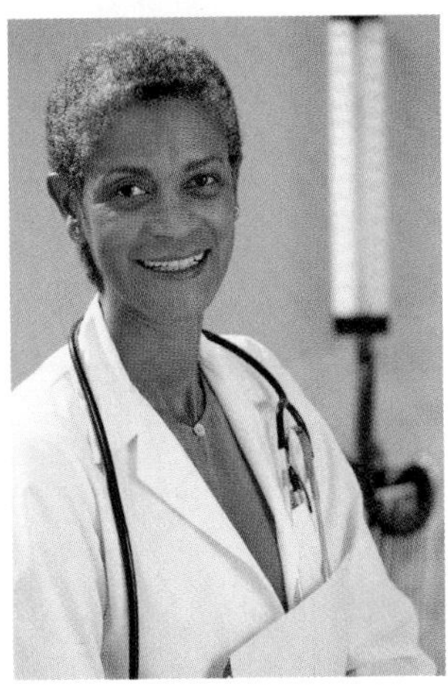

As a clinician facilitating the patient's story, you will come to generate a series of hypotheses about the nature of the patient's concerns. You will then test these various hypotheses by asking for more detailed information. You will also explore the patient's feelings and beliefs about his or her problem. Eventually, as your clinical experience grows, you will respond with your

Interviewing Milestones

Getting Ready: The Approach to the Interview

Taking time for self-reflection. Reviewing the chart. Reviewing your clinical behavior and appearance. Adjusting the environment. Taking notes.

Learning About the Patient: The Sequence of the Interview

Greeting the patient and establishing rapport. Inviting the patient's story. Setting the agenda for the interview. Expanding and clarifying the patient's story. Creating a shared understanding of the patient's concerns. Negotiating a plan. Following up and closing the interview.

Building the Relationship: The Techniques of Skilled Interviewing

Active listening. Guided questioning. Nonverbal communication. Empathic responses. Validation. Reassurance. Partnering. Summarization. Transitions. Empowering the patient.

Adapting Your Interview to Specific Situations

The silent patient. The confusing patient. The patient with impaired capacity. The talkative patient. The angry or disruptive patient. Interviewing across a language barrier. The patient with low literacy. The deaf or hard-of-hearing patient. The blind patient. The patient with limited intelligence. The patient seeking personal advice.

Sensitive Topics that Call for Special Skills

The sexual history. Mental health. Alcohol and drug use. Family violence. Death and dying.

Societal Aspects of Interviewing

Achieving cultural competence. Sexuality in the clinician–patient relationship. Ethical considerations.

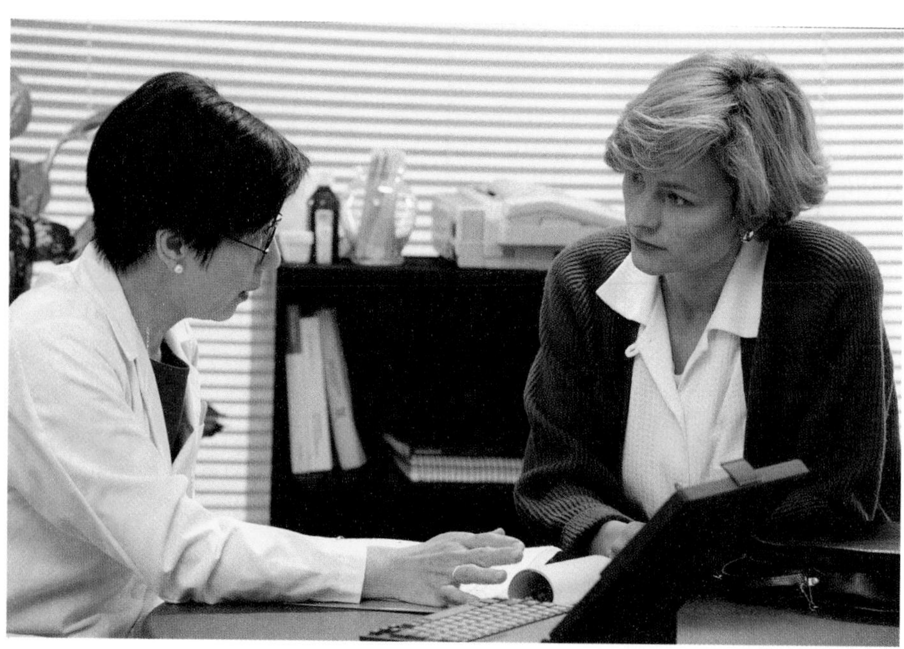

understanding of the patient's concerns. Even if you discover that little can be done, encouraging the patient to discuss the *experience of illness* is itself therapeutic, as shown by the words below from a patient with long-standing and severe arthritis:

> The patient had never talked about what the symptoms meant to her. She had never said: "This means that I can't go to the bathroom by myself, put my clothes on, even get out of bed without calling for help."
>
> When we finished the physical examination I said something like: "Rheumatoid arthritis really has not been nice to you." She burst into tears, and her daughter did also, and I sat there, very close to losing it myself.
>
> She said: "You know, no one has ever talked about it as a personal thing before. No one's ever talked to me as if this were a thing that mattered, a personal event."
>
> That was the significant thing about the encounter. I didn't really have much else to offer. . . . But something really significant had happened between us, something that she valued and would carry away with her.[6]

As you can see from this story, the *process* of interviewing patients requires a highly refined sensitivity to the patient's feelings and behavioral cues and is much more than just asking a series of questions. This process differs significantly from the *format* for the health history presented in Chapter 1 (p. 5). Both are fundamental to your work with patients but serve different purposes:

- The *health history format* is a structured framework for organizing patient information in *written or verbal form* for other health care providers; it focuses the clinician's attention on specific kinds of information that must be obtained from the patient.
- The *interviewing process* that actually generates these pieces of information is much more fluid and demands effective communication and relational skills. It requires not only knowledge of the data that you need to obtain but also the ability to elicit accurate information and the interpersonal skills that allow you to respond to the patient's feelings and concerns.

Underlying the new interviewing skills that you will learn is a mindset that allows you to collaborate with the patient and build a healing relationship.

Different Kinds of Health Histories. As you learned in Chapter 1, the kinds of information you seek varies according to several factors. The scope and degree of detail depend on the patient's needs and concerns, the clinician's goals for the encounter, and the clinical setting (e.g., inpatient or outpatient, amount of time available, primary care or subspecialty).

- For new patients, regardless of setting, you will do a *comprehensive health history* described for adults in Chapter 1.

- For other patients who seek care for specific complaints (e.g., cough, painful urination), a more limited interview tailored to that specific problem may be indicated, sometimes known as a *problem-oriented history.*

In a primary care setting, clinicians frequently choose to address issues of health promotion, such as tobacco cessation or reduction of high-risk sexual behaviors. A subspecialist may do an in-depth history to evaluate one problem that incorporates a wide range of areas of inquiry. Knowing the content and relevance of all the components of a comprehensive health history enables you to select the kinds of information most helpful for meeting both clinician and patient goals. Be assured that you will fully gain the knowledge of what types of information to pursue, and when to pursue them, as you deepen your clinical experience.

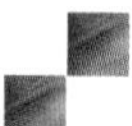

GETTING READY: THE APPROACH TO THE INTERVIEW

Interviewing patients requires planning. You are undoubtedly eager to begin your relationship with the patient, but first consider several steps that are crucial to success: taking time for self-reflection, reviewing the chart, setting goals for the interview, reviewing your behavior and appearance, adjusting the environment, and being ready to take brief notes.

Taking Time for Self-Reflection. As clinicians, we encounter a wide variety of individuals, each one unique. Establishing relationships with people from a broad spectrum of age, social class, race, ethnicity, and states of *health or illness* is an uncommon opportunity and privilege. Being consistently respectful and open to individual differences is one of the clinician's challenges. Because we bring our own values, assumptions, and biases to every encounter, we must look inward to clarify how our own expectations and reactions may affect what we hear and how we behave. *Self-reflection is a continual part of professional development in clinical work. It brings a deepening personal awareness to our work with patients, which is one of the most rewarding aspects of patient care.*

Reviewing the Chart. Before seeing the patient, review the medical record or chart. Doing so helps you gather information and plan what areas you need to explore with the patient. Look closely at identifying data such as age, gender, address, and health insurance, and peruse the problem list, the medication list, and details such as the documentation of allergies. The chart often provides valuable information about past diagnoses and treatments, but do not let the chart prevent you from developing new approaches or ideas. Remember that information in the chart comes from different observers and that standardized forms reflect different institutional norms. Moreover, the chart is not designed to capture the essence of the unique individual you are about to meet. Data may be incomplete, or even disagree with what you learn from the patient—understanding such discrepancies may prove helpful to the patient's care.

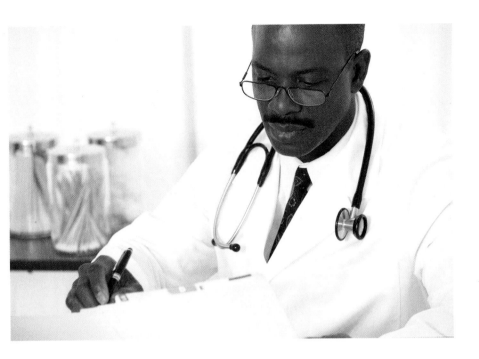

Setting Goals for the Interview. Before you begin talking with the patient, it is important to clarify your goals for the interview. As a student, your goal may be to obtain a complete health history so that you can submit a write-up to your teacher. As a clinician, your goals range from completing forms needed by health care institutions to following up on health care issues to testing hypotheses generated by your review of the chart. *A clinician must balance these provider-centered goals with patient-centered goals.* There can be tension between the needs of the provider, the institution, and the patient and family. Part of the clinician's task is to consider these multiple agendas. By taking a few minutes to think through your goals ahead of time, you will find it easier to strike a healthy balance among the various purposes of the interview to come.

Reviewing Your Clinical Behavior and Appearance. Just as you carefully observe the patient throughout the interview, the patient will be watching you. Consciously or not, you send messages through both your words and your behavior. Be sensitive to those messages and manage them as well as you can. Posture, gestures, eye contact, and tone of voice all convey the extent of your interest, attention, acceptance, and understanding. The skilled interviewer seems calm and unhurried, even when time is limited. Reactions that betray disapproval, embarrassment, impatience, or boredom block communication, as do any behaviors that condescend, stereotype, criticize, or belittle the patient. Although these types of negative feelings are at times unavoidable, as a health care professional, you must take pains not to express them. Guard against these feelings not only when talking to patients but also when discussing patients with your colleagues.

Your personal appearance also affects your clinical relationships. Patients find cleanliness, neatness, conservative dress, and a name tag reassuring. Remember to keep *the patient's perspective* in mind if you want to build the patient's trust.

Adjusting the Environment. Try to make the interview setting as private and comfortable as possible. Although you may have to talk with the patient under difficult circumstances, such as in a two-bed room or the corridor of a busy emergency department, a proper environment improves communication. If there are privacy curtains, ask permission to pull them shut. Suggest moving to an empty room instead of talking in a waiting area. *As the clinician, it is part of your job to make adjustments to the location and seating that make the patient and you more comfortable.* These efforts are always worth the time.

Taking Notes. As a novice, you will need to write down much of what you learn during the interview. Even though experienced clinicians recall much of the interview without taking notes, no one can remember all the details of a comprehensive history. Jot down short phrases, specific dates, or words rather than trying to put them into a final format, but do not let note-taking or written forms distract you from the patient. Maintain good eye contact, and whenever the patient is talking about sensitive or disturbing material, put down your pen. Most patients are accustomed to note-taking, but for those who find it uncomfortable, explore their concerns and explain your need to make an accurate record.

LEARNING ABOUT THE PATIENT: THE SEQUENCE OF THE INTERVIEW

Once you have devoted time and thought to preparing for the interview, you are fully ready to listen to the patient, elicit the patient's concerns, and learn about the patient's health. In general, an interview moves through several stages. *Throughout this sequence you, as the clinician, must always be attuned to the patient's feelings, help the patient express them, respond to their content, and validate their significance.* A typical sequence follows.

The Sequence of the Interview

- Greeting the patient and establishing rapport
- Inviting the patient's story
- Establishing the agenda for the interview
- Expanding and clarifying the patient's story
- Generating and testing diagnostic hypotheses
- Creating a shared understanding of the problem
- Negotiating a plan (includes further evaluation, treatment, and patient education)
- Planning for follow-up and closing the interview

As a student, you will concentrate primarily on gathering the patient's story and creating a shared understanding of the problem. As you become a practicing clinician, reaching agreement on a plan for further evaluation and treatment becomes more important. Whether the interview is comprehensive or focused, you should move through this sequence with close attention to the patient's feelings and affect, always working on strengthening the relationship.

Greeting the Patient and Establishing Rapport. The initial moments of your encounter with the patient lay the foundation for your ongoing relationship. How you greet the patient and other visitors in the room, provide for the patient's comfort, and arrange the physical setting all shape the patient's first impressions.

As you begin, *greet the patient* by name and introduce yourself, giving your own name. If possible, shake hands with the patient. If this is the first contact, explain your role, including your status as a student and how you will be involved in the patient's care. Repeat this part of the introduction on subsequent meetings until you are confident that the patient knows who you are: "Good Morning, Mr. Peters. I am Susannah Martinez, a third-year medical student. You may remember me. I was here yesterday talking with you about your heart problems. I am part of the medical team taking care of you."

Using a formal title to address the patient (e.g., Mr. O'Neil, Ms. Washington) is always best.[7,8] Except with children or adolescents, avoid first names unless you have specific permission from the patient or family. Addressing an unfamiliar adult as "granny" or "dear" can depersonalize and demean. If you are unsure how to pronounce the patient's name, don't be afraid to ask. You can say: "I am afraid of mispronouncing your name. Could you say it for me?" Then repeat it to make sure that you heard it correctly.

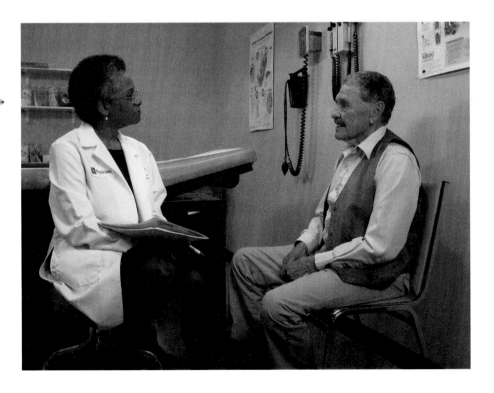

When visitors are in the room, be sure to acknowledge and greet each one in turn, inquiring about each person's name and relationship to the patient. Whenever visitors are present, *you are obligated to maintain the patient's confidentiality*. Let the patient decide if visitors or family members should remain in the room, and ask for the patient's permission before conducting the interview in front of them. For example, "I am comfortable with having your sister stay for the interview, Mrs. Jones, but I want to make sure that this is also what you want" or "Would you prefer if I spoke to you alone or with your sister present?"

Always be attuned to the patient's comfort. In the office or clinic, help the patient find a suitable place for coats and belongings. In the hospital, after greeting the patient, ask how the patient is feeling and if you are coming at a convenient time. Arranging the bed to make the patient more comfortable or allowing a few minutes for the patient to say goodbye to visitors or finish using the bedpan demonstrates your awareness of the patient's needs. In any setting, look for signs of discomfort, such as shifting position or facial expressions showing pain or anxiety. You must attend to pain or anxiety first, both to encourage the patient's trust and to allow enough ease for the interview to proceed.

Consider the best way to *arrange the room* and how far you should be from the patient. Remember that cultural background and individual taste influence preferences about interpersonal space. Choose a distance that facilitates conversation and allows good eye contact. You should probably be within several feet, close enough to be intimate but not intrusive. Pull up a chair and, if possible, sit at eye level with the patient. Move any physical barriers, like desks or bedside tables, out of the way. In an outpatient setting, sitting on a rolling stool, for example, allows you to change distances in response to patient cues. Avoid arrangements that connote disrespect or inequality of power, such as interviewing a woman already positioned for a pelvic examination. Such arrangements are unacceptable. Lighting also makes a difference. If you sit between a patient and a bright light or window, although your view might be good, the patient may have to squint uncomfortably to see you, making the interaction more like an interrogation than a supportive interview.

As you begin the interview, give the patient your undivided attention. Spend enough time on small talk to put the patient at ease, and avoid looking down to take notes or reading the chart.

Inviting the Patient's Story. Now that you have established rapport, you are ready to pursue the patient's reason for seeking health care, designated the *chief complaint*. Begin with ***open-ended questions*** that allow full freedom of response: "What concerns bring you here today?" or "How can I help you?" Helpful open-ended questions are "Was there a specific health concern that prompted you to schedule this appointment?" and "What made you decide to come in to see us today?" Note that these questions encourage the patient to express any possible concerns and do not restrict the patient to a minimally informative "yes" or "no" answer. Sometimes patients do not have a specific complaint or problem—they may want only a blood pressure check or a routine examination. Others may say they just want a physical examination but feel uncomfortable bringing up an underlying concern. In all these situations, *it is still important to start with the patient's story.*[9]

Train yourself to *follow the patient's leads.* Good interviewing technique includes using verbal and nonverbal cues that prompt patients to recount their stories spontaneously. If you intervene too early or ask specific questions prematurely, you risk trampling on the very information you are seeking. You should listen actively and make use of *continuers* (see p. 38), especially at the outset. These include nodding your head and phrases such as "uh huh," "go on," or "I see." Using additional guided questioning (see p. 36) helps you avoid missing any of the patient's concerns.

Listen to the patient's answer *without interrupting.* Studies show that clinicians interrupt patients during office visits after only 18 seconds![10] If patients are allowed to tell their stories, most will finish within 2 minutes. After you have given the patient the opportunity to respond fully, inquire again or even several times, "What else?," "Tell me more," or "Any further concerns?" You may need to lead patients back several times to elicit additional concerns or issues they may want to tell you about.

Establishing an Agenda. The clinician often approaches the interview with specific goals in mind. The patient also has specific questions and concerns. It is important to identify all these issues at the beginning of the encounter. This allows you to use the time available most effectively and ensures that you hear all the patient's issues. As a student, you often have enough time to cover the breadth of both your concerns and those of the patient in one visit. For a clinician, however, time is almost always constrained. As a clinician, you may need to focus the interview by asking the patient which problem is most pressing. For example, "You have told me about several different problems that are important for us to discuss. I also wanted to review your blood pressure medication. We need to decide which problems to address today. Can you tell me which one you are most concerned about?" Once you have agreed on a manageable list, let the patient know that the other problems are also important and will be addressed during a future visit—this reinforces the patient's confidence in your ongoing collaboration. Then proceed with questions such as, "Tell me more about that first problem that you mentioned."

Expanding and Clarifying the Patient's Story. You then guide the patient into elaborating areas of the health history that seem most significant. As a clinician, each symptom has attributes that you must clarify, including context, associations, and chronology. For pain and many other symptoms, understanding these essential characteristics, summarized below as the seven key attributes of a symptom, is critical.

Always pursue the seven attributes. Two mnemonics may help: **OLD CARTS** (**O**nset, **L**ocation, **D**uration, **C**haracter, **A**ggravating/**A**lleviating Factors, **R**adiation, and **T**iming) and **OPQRST** (**O**nset, **P**alliating/**P**rovoking Factors, **Q**uality, **R**adiation, **S**ite, and **T**iming).

THE SEVEN ATTRIBUTES OF A SYMPTOM

1. ***Location.*** Where is it? Does it radiate?
2. ***Quality.*** What is it like?
3. ***Quantity or severity.*** How bad is it? (For pain, ask for a rating on a scale of 1 to 10.)
4. ***Timing.*** When did (does) it start? How long does it last? How often does it come?
5. ***Setting in which it occurs.*** Include environmental factors, personal activities, emotional reactions, or other circumstances that may have contributed to the illness.
6. ***Remitting or exacerbating factors.*** Is there anything that makes it better or worse?
7. ***Associated manifestations.*** Have you noticed anything else that accompanies it?

As you explore these attributes, be sure that you *use language that is understandable and appropriate* to the patient. Although you might ask a trained health professional about dyspnea, the customary term for patients is "shortness of breath." It is easy to slip into using medical language, but beware. Technical language confuses the patient and often blocks communication. Whenever possible, *use the patient's words,* making sure you clarify their meaning.

It is important to establish *the sequence and time course* of each of the patient's symptoms if you are to arrive at accurate assessments. You can encourage a chronologic account by asking such questions as "What then?" or "What happened next?" or "Please start at the beginning, or the last time you felt well, and go step by step." To fill in specific details, guide the patient's story by using different types of questions and the techniques of skilled interviewing described on pp. 35–41. You will need to use some focused questions to elicit specific information that the patient has not already offered (see p. 37). *In general, an interview moves back and forth from open-ended questions to increasingly focused questions and then on to another open-ended question.*

Generating and Testing Diagnostic Hypotheses. Eventually, as you gain experience listening to patient concerns, you will develop the skills of "clinical reasoning." You will *generate and test diagnostic hypotheses* about what disease process might be present. Identifying the various attributes of the patient's symptoms and pursuing specific details are fundamental to recognizing patterns of disease and to generating the differential diagnosis. As you learn more about diagnostic patterns and epidemiology, knowing what data you are listening for and asking about specific details become more automatic. For additional data that contribute to your analysis, use items from relevant sections of the review of systems. (In your oral presentations and written record, add the information gathered from your responses to review of systems questions to the latter paragraphs of the History of Present Illness—this information now constitutes "pertinent positives" and "pertinent negatives"—see Chapter 1, p. 7).

Appropriate questions about symptoms are also suggested in each of the chapters on the regional physical examinations. This is one way that you build evidence for and against various diagnostic possibilities. This kind of clinical thinking is illustrated by the tables on symptoms found in the regional examination chapters and further discussed in Chapter 3, Clinical Reasoning, Assessment, and Plan. The challenge is to not let this kind of inquiry dominate the interview and displace learning about the patient's perspective, conveying concern for the patient's well-being and building the relationship.[5]

Creating a Shared Understanding of the Problem. Recent literature makes it clear that delivering effective health care requires exploring the deeper meanings patients attach to their symptoms. Although the "seven attributes of a symptom" add important details to the patient's history, the **disease/illness distinction model** helps you understand the full range of what every good interview needs to cover.[11] This model acknowledges the very different yet complementary perspectives of the clinician and the patient. ***Disease*** is the explanation that the *clinician* brings to the symptoms. It is the way that the clinician organizes what he or she learns from the patient that leads to a clinical diagnosis. ***Illness*** can be defined as how the *patient* experiences symptoms. Many factors may shape this experience, including prior personal or family health, the effect of symptoms on everyday life, individual outlook and style of coping, and expectations about medical care. The melding of these perspectives forms the basis for planning evaluation and treatment. *The clinical interview needs to take into account both of these views of reality.*

Even a chief complaint as straightforward as sore throat can illustrate these divergent views. The patient may be most concerned about pain and difficulty swallowing, missing time from work, or a cousin who was hospitalized with tonsillitis. The clinician, however, may focus on specific points in the history that differentiate streptococcal pharyngitis from other etiologies, or on a questionable history of allergy to penicillin. To understand the patient's expectations, the clinician needs to go beyond just the attributes of a symptom. Learning about the patient's perception of illness means asking patient-centered questions in the six domains listed below. This information is crucial to patient satisfaction, effective health care, and patient follow-through.[12,13]

EXPLORING THE PATIENT'S PERSPECTIVE

- The patient's thoughts about the nature and the cause of the problem
- The patient's feelings, especially fears, about the problem
- The patient's expectations of the clinician and health care
- The effect of the problem on the patient's life
- Prior personal or family experiences that are similar
- Therapeutic approaches the patient has already tried

The clinician should explore the patient's thoughts about the cause of the problem by saying, for example, "Why do you think you have this stomachache?" To uncover the patient's feelings you might ask, "What concerns you most about the pain?" A patient may worry that the pain is a symptom of serious disease and want reassurance. Alternatively, the patient may be less concerned about the cause of the pain and just want relief. You need to find out what the patient expects from you, the clinician, or from health care in general . . . "I am glad that the pain is almost gone, how specifically can I help you now?" Even if the stomach pain is almost gone, the patient may need a work excuse to take to an employer.

It may be helpful to ask the patient about prior experiences, what has been tried so far, and any related changes in daily activities.

> Clinician: "Has anything like this happened to you or your family before?"
>
> Patient: "I was worried that I might have appendicitis. My Uncle Charlie died of a ruptured appendix."

Explore what the patient has done so far to take care of the problem. Most patients will have tried over-the-counter medications, traditional remedies, or advice from friends or family.

Ask how the illness has affected the patient's lifestyle and level of activity. This question is especially important for patients with chronic illness. "What can't you do now that you could do before? How has your backache (shortness of breath, etc.) affected your ability to work? . . . Your life at home? . . . Your social activities? . . . Your role as a parent? . . . Your function in intimate relationships? . . . The way you feel about yourself as a person?"

Negotiating a Plan. Learning about the disease and conceptualizing the illness give you and the patient the opportunity to create a complete and congruent picture of the problem. This multifaceted picture then forms the basis for planning further evaluation (e.g., physical examination, laboratory tests, consultations) and negotiating a treatment plan. It also plays an important role in building rapport with your patient. More specific techniques for negotiating a plan can be found in Chapter 3. Advanced skills, such as steps for motivating change and the therapeutic use of the clinician–patient relationship, are beyond the scope of this book.

Planning for Follow-Up and Closing. You may find that ending the interview is difficult. Patients often have many questions, and if you have done your job well, they are engaged and affirmed as they talk with you. Let the patient know that the end of the interview is approaching to allow time for the patient to ask any final questions. Make sure the patient understands the mutual plans you have developed. For example, before gathering your papers or standing to leave the room, you can say, "We need to stop now. Do you have any questions about what we've covered?" As you close, reviewing future evaluation, treatments, and follow-up is helpful. "So, you will take the medicine as we discussed, get the blood test before you leave today, and make a follow-up appointment for 4 weeks. Do you have any questions about this?" Address any related concerns or questions that the patient raises.

The patient should have a chance to ask any final questions; however, the last few minutes are not the time to bring up new topics. If that happens (and the concern is not life-threatening), simply assure the patient of your interest and make plans to address the problem at a future time. "That knee pain sounds concerning. Why don't you make an appointment for next week so we can discuss it?" Reconfirming your continued commitment to improving the patient's health is always appreciated.

BUILDING A THERAPEUTIC RELATIONSHIP: THE TECHNIQUES OF SKILLED INTERVIEWING

Building the Relationship. You probably had many reasons to become a health care professional, but one of them was undoubtedly the desire to serve others. To succeed in fulfilling this laudable goal, you must sustain this motivation throughout your rigorous training and transform this goal into a set of behavioral approaches to your patients.

The paradigm that embeds your relationship with the patient into the therapeutic process itself now has many names and models, including the biopsychosocial model and patient-centered care, among others.[5,12,14,15] Comparing these various models reveals common elements that include interest in the patient as a whole person, an empowering approach to the patient role, and involvement of the clinician's self on an emotional and reflective level.[16] There is now robust literature demonstrating that an approach to patient care anchored in these principles is not only more satisfying for the patient and the clinician but also more effective in achieving good health care outcomes.[17]

This section describes the skills that form the basic tools of interviewing. Some of these habits are purely techniques that you can readily put into practice. Some are constructs that will inform your interviewing behaviors. You will employ these interviewing skills to achieve the tasks described earlier in the Sequence of the Interview (see p. 28) more effectively. You need to practice using these tools and find ways to be observed or recorded so that you can receive feedback on your progress. A number of these fundamental skills are listed below and then described in more detail. Pick one or two of them to incorporate into your next patient interview. Then refer back to this chapter to build your repertoire of skills.

The Techniques of Skilled Interviewing

- Active listening
- Guided questioning
- Nonverbal communication
- Empathic responses
- Validation
- Reassurance
- Partnering
- Summarization
- Transitions
- Empowering the patient

Active Listening. Underlying all the various techniques is the habit of *active listening*. Active listening is the process of really attending to what the patient is communicating, being aware of the patient's emotional state, and using verbal and nonverbal skills to encourage the speaker to continue and expand. This takes practice. It is easy to drift into thinking about your next question or the differential diagnosis when you and the patient are best served by your concentration on listening.

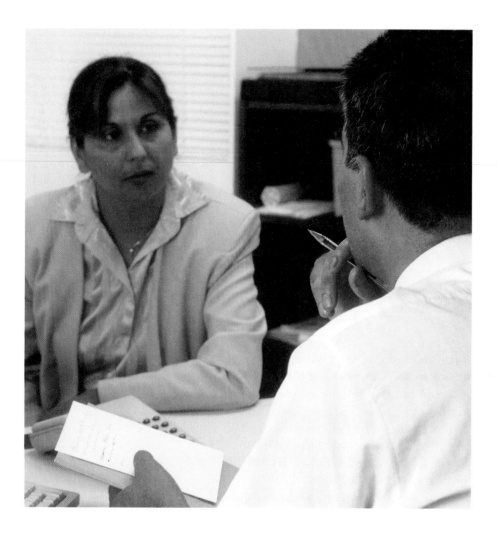

Guided Questioning: Options for Expanding and Clarifying the Patient's Story. There are several ways you can ask for more information from the patient without interfering with the flow of the patient's story. Your goal is to facilitate the patient's fullest communication. Learning the following specific techniques will allow you to guide patients' disclosures, while minimizing the risk for distorting their ideas or missing significant details. This is how you avoid asking a series of specific questions, which takes more time and makes the patient feel more passive.

Guided Questioning: Options for Expanding and Clarifying the Patient's Story

- Moving from open-ended to focused questions
- Using questioning that elicits a graded response
- Asking a series of questions, one at a time
- Offering multiple choices for answers
- Clarifying what the patient means
- Offering continuers
- Using echoing

Moving from Open-Ended to Focused Questions. Your questioning should proceed from general to specific. Start with a truly open-ended question that does not inadvertently include an answer. A possible sequence might be:

"Tell me about your chest pain." (Pause)

"What else?" (Pause)

"Where did you feel it?" (Pause) "Show me."

"Anywhere else?" (Pause) "Did it travel anywhere?" (Pause) "To which arm?"

You should avoid *leading questions* that call for a "yes" or "no" answer. If a patient answers yes to a question such as "Is your pain pressure like . . . ?", you run the risk of turning your words into the patient's words. A better phrasing is "Please describe your pain."

Questioning that Elicits a Graded Response. If necessary, ask questions that require *a graded response* rather than a single answer. "How many steps can you climb before you get short of breath?" is better than "Do you get short of breath climbing stairs?"

Asking a Series of Questions, One at a Time. Be sure to *ask one question at a time.* "Any tuberculosis, pleurisy, asthma, bronchitis, pneumonia?" may lead to a negative answer out of sheer confusion. Try "Do you have any of the following problems?" Be sure to pause and establish eye contact as you list each problem.

Offering Multiple Choices for Answers. Sometimes patients seem quite unable to describe their symptoms without help. To minimize bias, *offer multiple-choice answers:* "Which of the following words best describes your pain: aching, sharp, pressing, burning, shooting, or something else?" Almost any specific question can provide at least two possible answers. "Do you bring up any phlegm with your cough, or is it dry?"

Clarifying What the Patient Means. At times, patients use words that are ambiguous or have unclear associations. To understand their meaning, you need to *request clarification,* as in "Tell me exactly what you meant by 'the flu' " or "You said you were behaving just like your mother. What did you mean?"

Continuers. Without specifying content, you can use posture, gestures, or words to encourage the patient to say more. Pausing with a nod of the head or remaining silent, yet attentive and relaxed, is a *cue for the patient to continue.* Leaning forward, making eye contact, and using phrases like "Mm-hmm," or "Go on," or "I'm listening" all maintain the flow of the patient's story.

Echoing. A simple repetition of the patient's last words, or *echoing,* encourages the patient to express both factual details and feelings, as in the following example:

Patient: "The pain got worse and began to spread." (Pause)

Response: "Spread?" (Pause)

Patient: "Yes, it went to my shoulder and down my left arm to the fingers. It was so bad that I thought I was going to die." (Pause)

Response: "Going to die?"

Patient: "Yes, it was just like the pain my father had when he had his heart attack, and I was afraid the same thing was happening to me."

This reflective technique has helped to reveal not only the location and severity of the pain but also its meaning to the patient. It did not bias the story or interrupt the patient's train of thought.

Nonverbal Communication. Communication that does not involve speech occurs continuously and provides important clues to feelings and emotions. Becoming more sensitive to nonverbal messages allows you to both "read the patient" more effectively and send messages of your own. Pay close attention to eye contact, facial expression, posture, head position and movement such as shaking or nodding, interpersonal distance, and placement of the arms or legs—crossed, neutral, or open. Be aware that nonverbal language is culturally bound.

Just as mirroring your position can signify the patient's increasing sense of connectedness, matching your position to the patient's can signify increased rapport. You can also mirror the patient's *paralanguage,* or qualities of speech, such as pacing, tone, and volume, to increase rapport. Moving closer or physical contact like placing your hand on the patient's arm can convey empathy or help the patient gain control of difficult feelings. Bringing nonverbal communication to the conscious level is the first step to using this crucial form of patient interaction.

Empathic Responses. Conveying empathy greatly strengthens patient rapport. As patients talk with you they may express—with or without words—feelings they may or may not have consciously acknowledged.

These feelings are crucial to understanding their illnesses and to establishing a trusting relationship. *To empathize with your patient, you must first identify the patient's feelings.* This requires a willingness and even interest on your part in hearing about and eliciting emotional content. At first, this may seem unfamiliar or uncomfortable. When you sense important but unexpressed feelings from the patient's face, voice, words, or behavior, inquire about them rather than assuming that you know how the patient feels. You may simply ask, "How did you feel about that?" Unless you let patients know that you are interested in feelings as well as facts, you may miss important insights.

Once you have identified the feelings, respond with understanding and acceptance. Responses may be as simple as "I understand," "That sounds upsetting," or "You seem sad." Empathy may also be nonverbal—for example, offering a tissue to a crying patient or gently placing your hand on the patient's arm to show understanding. When you give an empathic response, be sure that you are responding correctly to what the patient is feeling. If your response acknowledges how upset a patient must have been at the death of a parent, when in fact the death relieved the patient of a longstanding financial and emotional burden, you have misunderstood the situation. Instead of making assumptions, you can ask directly about the patient's emotional response. "I am sorry about the death of your father. What has that been like for you?"

Validation. Another important way to make a patient feel accepted is to legitimize or validate his or her emotional experience. A patient who has been in a car accident but has no physical injury may still be experiencing significant distress. Stating something like, "Being in that accident must have been very scary. Car accidents are always unsettling because they remind us of our vulnerability and mortality. That could explain why you still feel upset," reassures the patient. It helps the patient feel that such emotions are legitimate and understandable.

Reassurance. When you are talking with patients who are anxious or upset, it is tempting to reassure them. You may find yourself saying, "Don't worry. Everything is going to be all right." Although this may be appropriate in nonprofessional relationships, in your role as a clinician, such comments are usually counterproductive. You may fall into reassuring the patient about the wrong thing. Moreover, premature reassurance may block further disclosures, especially if the patient feels that exposing anxiety is a weakness. Such admissions require encouragement, not a cover-up.

The first step to effective reassurance is simply identifying and acknowledging the patient's feelings. This promotes a feeling of connection. The actual reassurance comes much later after you have completed the interview, the physical examination, and perhaps some laboratory studies. At that point, you can interpret for the patient what you think is happening and deal openly with expressed concerns. The reassurance comes from conveying information in a competent manner, making the patient feel confident that problems have been fully understood and will be addressed.

Partnering. When building your relationships with patients, one of the most useful steps is to make explicit your desire to work with them in an ongoing way. When you discuss a diagnosis or express uncertainty about how to explain their symptoms, it is reassuring to state that regardless of what happens with their disease, as their provider, you are committed to a continuing partnership. Even in your role as student, especially in a hospital setting, this support can make a big difference.

Summarization. Giving a capsule summary of the patient's story during the course of the interview can serve several different functions. It indicates to the patient that you have been listening carefully. It can also identify what you know and what you don't know. "Now, let me make sure that I have the full story. You said you've had a cough for 3 days, that it's especially bad at night, and that you have started to bring up yellow phlegm. You have not had a fever or felt short of breath, but you do feel congested with difficulty breathing through your nose." Following with an attentive pause or stating "Anything else?" lets the patient add other information and confirms that you have heard the story correctly.

You can use summarization at different points in the interview to structure the visit, especially at times of transition (see below). This technique also allows you, the clinician, to organize your clinical reasoning and to convey your thinking to the patient, which makes the relationship more collaborative. *It is also a useful technique for learners to use when they draw a blank on what to ask the patient next.*

Transitions. Patients have many reasons to feel vulnerable during a health care visit. To put them more at ease, tell them when you are changing directions during the interview. This gives patients a greater sense of control. As you move from one part of the history to another and on to the physical examination, orient the patient with brief transitional phrases like "Now I'd like to ask some questions about your past health." Make clear what the patient should expect or do next. "Before we move on to reviewing all your medications, was there anything else about past health problems?" "Now I would like to examine you. I will step out for a few minutes. Please get completely undressed and put on this gown." Specifying that the gown should open in the back may earn the patient's gratitude and save you some time.

Empowering the Patient. The clinician–patient relationship is inherently unequal. Your sense of inexperience as a student will predictably and appropriately transition over time to a sense of confidence in your knowledge and skills and power in your role as clinician. But patients have many reasons to feel vulnerable. They may be in pain or worried about a symptom. They may be overwhelmed with the health care system or just unfamiliar with the process that you will come to take for granted. Differences of gender, ethnicity, race, or class may also create power differentials. However, ultimately, patients must be empowered to take care of themselves. They must make lifestyle changes or take the medications you recommend. They must feel confident in their ability to follow through on your advice. Listed next are principles that will help you to share power with your patients. Although many of them have been discussed in other parts of this chapter, the need to empower patients is so fundamental that it is worth summarizing them here. Keep them in mind.

EMPOWERING THE PATIENT: PRINCIPLES OF SHARING POWER

- Inquire about the patient's perspective.
- Express interest in the person, not just the problem.
- Follow the patient's lead.
- Elicit emotional content.
- Share information with the patient (e.g., transitions).
- Make clinical reasoning transparent to the patient.
- Reveal the limits of your knowledge.

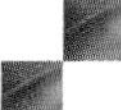

ADAPTING YOUR INTERVIEW TO SPECIFIC SITUATIONS

Interviewing patients may precipitate several behaviors and situations that seem perplexing or even vexing. Your ability to handle these situations will evolve throughout your career. *Always remember the importance of listening to the patient and clarifying the patient's concerns.*

The Silent Patient. Novice interviewers are often uncomfortable with periods of silence and feel obligated to keep the conversation going. Silence has many meanings and many purposes. Patients frequently fall silent for short periods to collect thoughts, remember details, or decide whether you can be trusted with certain information. The period of silence usually feels much longer to the clinician than it does to the patient. The clinician should appear attentive and give brief encouragement to continue when appropriate. During periods of silence, watch the patient closely for nonverbal cues, such as difficulty controlling emotions.

Patients with depression or dementia may lose their usual spontaneity of expression, give short answers to questions, and then fall silent. If you have already tried guiding them through recent events or a typical day, try shifting your inquiry to the symptoms of depression or begin an exploratory mental status examination (see Chapter 16, pp. 573–593).

At times, silence may be the patient's response to how you are asking questions. Are you asking too many short-answer questions in rapid succession? Have you offended the patient in any way by signs of disapproval or criticism? Have you failed to recognize an overwhelming symptom such as pain, nausea, or dyspnea? If so, you may need to ask the patient directly, "You seem very quiet. Have I done something to upset you?"

The Confusing Patient. Some patients present a confusing array of *multiple symptoms.* They seem to have every symptom that you ask about, or "a positive review of systems." With these patients, focus on the meaning or function of the symptom, emphasizing the patient's perspective (see p. 32), and guide the interview into a psychosocial assessment. There is little profit to exploring each symptom in detail. Although the patient may have several illnesses, a somatization disorder may be in play.

At other times, you may feel baffled, frustrated, and confused because you cannot make sense out of the patient's story. The history is vague and difficult to understand, ideas are poorly connected, and language is hard to follow. Even though you word your questions carefully, you cannot seem to get clear answers. The patient's manner of relating to you may also seem peculiar, distant, aloof, or inappropriate. Symptoms may be described in bizarre terms: "My fingernails feel too heavy" or "My stomach knots up like a snake." Perhaps there is a mental status change like psychosis or delirium, a mental illness such as schizophrenia, or a neurologic disorder (see Chapter 17). Consider delirium in acutely ill or intoxicated patients and dementia in the elderly. Such patients give histories that are inconsistent and cannot provide a clear chronology about what has happened. Some may even confabulate to fill in the gaps in their memories.

When you suspect a psychiatric or neurologic disorder, do not spend too much time gathering a detailed history. You will only tire and frustrate both the patient and yourself. Shift to the mental status examination, focusing on level of consciousness, orientation, memory, and capacity to understand. You can work in the initial questions smoothly by asking, "When was your last appointment at the clinic? Let's see . . . that was about how long ago?" "Your address now is. . . ? . . . and your phone number?" You can check these responses against the chart or seek permission to speak with family members or friends and then obtain their perspectives.

The Patient With Altered Capacity. Some patients cannot provide their own histories because of delirium from illness, dementia, or other health or mental health conditions. Others are unable to relate certain parts of the history, such as events related to a febrile illness or a seizure. Under these circumstances, you need to determine whether the patient has "*decision-making capacity*," or the ability to understand information related to health, to make medical choices based on reason and a consistent set of values, and to declare preferences about treatments. The term *capacity* is preferable to the term "*competence*," which is a legal term. You do not need to consult psychiatry to assess capacity unless mental illness impairs decision making. For many patients with psychiatric conditions or even cognitive impairments, their ability to make decisions remains intact.

For patients with capacity, obtain their consent before talking about their health with others. Even if patients can communicate only with facial expressions or gestures, you must maintain confidentiality and elicit their input. Assure patients that any shared history will be kept confidential, and clarify what you can discuss with others. Your knowledge about the patient can be quite comprehensive, yet others may offer surprising and important information. A spouse, for example, may report significant family strains, depressive symptoms, or drinking habits that the patient has denied. Consider dividing the interview into two segments—one with the patient and the other with both the patient and a second informant. Each interview has its own value. Information from other sources often gives you helpful ideas for planning the patient's care, but remains confidential. Also learn the tenets of the *Health Insurance Portability and Accountability Act (HIPAA)* passed by Congress in 1996, which sets strict standards for disclosure for both institutions and providers when sharing patient information. These can be found at http://www.cms.hhs.gov/hipaa/.

For patients with impaired capacity, you will often need to find a *surrogate informant or decision maker* to assist with the history. Check whether the patient has a *durable power of attorney for health care* or a *health care proxy*. If not, in many cases, a spouse or family member who can represent the patient's wishes can fill this role.

Apply the basic principles of interviewing to your conversations with patients' relatives or friends. Find a private place to talk. Introduce yourself, state your purpose, inquire how they are feeling under the circumstances, and recognize and acknowledge their concerns. As you listen to their versions of the history, assess the quality of their relationship with the patient because it may color their credibility. Establish how they know the patient. For example, when a child is brought in for health care, the accompanying adult may not be the primary or even frequent caregiver, just the most available ride. Always seek the best-informed source. Occasionally, a relative or friend insists on being with the patient during your evaluation. Try to find out why, and assess the patient's wishes.

The Talkative Patient. The garrulous rambling patient may be just as difficult as the silent or confused patient. Faced with limited time and the need to "get the whole story," you may grow impatient, even exasperated. Although this problem has no perfect solution, several techniques are helpful. Give the patient free rein for the first 5 or 10 minutes, listening closely to the conversation. Perhaps the patient simply needs a good listener and is expressing pent-up concerns. Maybe the patient's style is to tell stories. Does the patient seem obsessively detailed? Is the patient unduly anxious or apprehensive? Is there a flight of ideas or disorganized thought process that suggests a thought disorder? What about confabulation?

Try to focus on what seems most important to the patient. Show your interest by asking questions in those areas. Interrupt only if necessary, but be courteous. Learn how to be directive and to set limits when needed. Remember that part of your task is structuring the interview to gain important information about the patient's health. A brief summary may help you change the subject yet validate any concerns (see p. 40). "Let me make sure that I understand. You have described many concerns. In particular I heard about two different kinds of pain, one on your left side that goes into your groin and is fairly new, and one in your upper abdomen after you eat that you have had for months. Let's focus just on the side pain first. Can you tell me what it feels like?"

Finally, do not show your impatience. If time runs out, explain the need for a second meeting. Setting a time limit for the next appointment may be helpful. "I know we have much more to talk about. Can you come again next week? We will have a full hour then."

The Crying Patient. Crying signals strong emotions, ranging from sadness to anger or frustration. If the patient is on the verge of tears, pausing, gentle probing, or responding with empathy gives the patient permission to cry. Usually crying is therapeutic, as is your quiet acceptance of the patient's distress or pain. Offer a tissue and wait for the patient to recover. Make a supportive remark like "I am glad that you got that out." Most patients will soon compose themselves and resume their story. Aside from an acute grief or loss, it is unusual for crying to escalate and become uncontrollable.

Crying makes many people uncomfortable. If this is true for you, you will need to learn how to accept displays of emotion so that as a clinician you can support patients at these significant times.

The Angry or Disruptive Patient. Many patients have reasons to be angry: they are ill, they have suffered a loss, they lack their accustomed control over their own lives, and they feel relatively powerless in the health care system. They may direct this anger toward you. It is possible that this hostility toward you is justified . . . were you late for your appointment, inconsiderate, insensitive, or angry yourself? If so, acknowledge the fact and try to make amends. More often, however, patients displace their anger onto the clinician as a reflection of their frustration or pain.

Accept angry feelings from patients. Allow them to express such emotions without getting angry in return. Avoid joining such patients in their hostility toward another provider, the clinic, or the hospital, even when privately you may feel sympathetic. You can validate their feelings without agreeing with their reasons. "I understand that you felt very frustrated by the long wait and answering the same questions over and over. Our complex health care system can seem very unsupportive when you are not feeling well." After the patient has calmed down, help find steps that will avert such situations in the future. Rational solutions to emotional problems are not always possible, however, and people need time to express and work through their angry feelings.

Some angry patients become overtly disruptive. Few people can disturb the clinic or emergency department more quickly than patients who are angry, belligerent, or out of control. Before approaching such patients, alert the security staff—as a clinician, maintaining a safe environment is one of your responsibilities. Stay calm, appear accepting, and avoid being confrontational in return. Keep your posture relaxed and nonthreatening and your hands loosely open. At first do not try to make disruptive patients lower their voices or stop if they are haranguing you or the staff. Listen carefully. Try to understand what they are saying. Once you have established rapport, gently suggest moving to a different location that is more private (and will cause less disruption).

The Interview Across a Language Barrier. Nothing will convince you more of the importance of the history than having to do without one.

If your patient speaks a different language, make every effort to find an interpreter. A few broken words and gestures are no substitute for the full story. The ideal interpreter is a neutral person who is familiar with both languages and cultures. Recruiting family members or friends to serve as interpreters can be hazardous—confidentiality may be violated, meanings may be distorted, and transmitted information may be incomplete. Untrained interpreters may try to speed up the interview by telescoping lengthy replies into a few words, losing much of what may be significant detail.

As you begin working with the interpreter, establish rapport and review what information would be most useful. Explain that you need the interpreter to translate everything, not to condense or summarize. *Make your questions clear, short, and simple.* You can also help the interpreter by outlining your goals for each segment of the history. After going over your plans, arrange the room so that you have easy eye contact and nonverbal communication with the patient. Then speak directly to the patient . . . "How long have you been sick?" rather than "How long has the patient been sick?" Having the interpreter close by the patient keeps you from moving your head back and forth as though you were watching a tennis match.

When available, bilingual written questionnaires are invaluable, especially for the review of systems. First, however, be sure that patients can read in their language; otherwise, ask for help from the interpreter. In some clinical settings, there are speakerphone translators; use them if there are no better options.

GUIDELINES FOR WORKING WITH AN INTERPRETER

- Choose a trained interpreter in preference to a hospital worker, volunteer, or family member.
- Use the interpreter as a resource for cultural information.
- Orient the interpreter to the components you plan to cover in the interview; include reminders to translate everything the patient says.
- Arrange the room so that you and the patient have eye contact and can read each other's nonverbal cues. Seat the interpreter next to the patient.
- Allow the interpreter and the patient to establish rapport.
- Address the patient directly. Reinforce your questions with nonverbal behaviors.
- Keep sentences *short* and *simple.* Focus on the most important concepts to communicate.
- Verify mutual understanding by asking the patient to repeat back what he or she has heard.
- Be patient. The interview will take more time and may provide less information.

The Patient With Low Literacy. Before giving written instructions, assess the patient's ability to read. Literacy levels are highly variable, and marginal reading skills are more prevalent than commonly believed. Explore the many reasons people do not read: language barriers, learning disorders, poor vision, or lack of education. Some people may try to hide their inability to read. Asking about educational level may be helpful, but can be misleading. "I understand that this may be difficult to discuss, but do you have any trouble with reading?" Ask the patient to read whatever instructions you have written. (This will also address any difficulty with your handwriting.) One rapid screen is to hand the patient a written text upside down—most patients who read will turn the page around immediately. Literacy skills may be the reason the patient has not followed through on taking medications or adhered to recommended treatments. Respond sensitively, and remember that illiteracy and lack of intelligence are not synonymous.

The Patient With Impaired Hearing. Communicating with the deaf presents many of the same challenges as communicating with patients who speak a different language. Even people with partial hearing may define themselves as deaf, a distinct cultural group. Find out the patient's preferred method of communicating. Patients may use American Sign Language, a unique language with its own syntax, or various other combinations of signs and speech. Thus, communication is often truly cross-cultural. Ask when hearing loss occurred relative to the development of speech and other language skills. Query about the kinds of schools the patient has attended. These questions help you determine whether the patient identifies with the Deaf culture or the Hearing culture. Written questionnaires are also useful. If the patient prefers sign language, find an interpreter and use the principles identified earlier. Time-consuming handwritten questions and answers may be the only solution, although literacy skills may also be an issue.

Hearing deficits vary. If the patient has a hearing aid, find out if the patient is using it. Make sure it is working. For patients with unilateral hearing loss, sit on the hearing side. A person who is *hard of hearing* may not be aware of the problem, a situation you will have to tactfully address. Eliminate background noise such as television or hallway conversation as much as possible. For patients who have partial hearing or can read lips, face them directly, in good light. Patients should wear their glasses to better pick up visual cues that help them understand you.

Speak at a normal volume and rate and do not let your voice trail off at the ends of sentences. Avoid covering your mouth or looking down at papers while speaking. Remember that even the best lip readers comprehend only a percentage of what is said, so having patients repeat what you have said is important. When closing, write out any oral instructions.

The Patient With Impaired Vision. When meeting with a blind patient, shake hands to establish contact and explain who you are and why you are there. If the room is unfamiliar, orient the patient to the surroundings and report if anyone else is present. It still may be helpful to adjust the light. Encourage visually impaired patients to wear glasses whenever possible. Remember to use words because postures and gestures are unseen.

The Patient With Limited Intelligence. Patients of moderately limited intelligence can usually give adequate histories. In fact, you may even be able to omit their disability from their evaluations. If you suspect problems, however, pay special attention to the patient's schooling and ability to function independently. How far have such patients gone in school? If they didn't finish, why not? What kinds of courses have they taken? How did they do? Have they had any testing done? Are they living alone? Do they need assistance with activities such as transportation or shopping? The sexual history is equally important and often overlooked. Find out if the patient is sexually active and provide information that may be needed about pregnancy or sexually transmitted diseases.

If you are unsure about the patient's level of intelligence, make a smooth transition to the mental status examination and assess simple calculations, vocabulary, memory, and abstract thinking (see Chapter 16, The Nervous System: Mental Status and Behavior).

For patients with severe mental retardation, you will have to turn to the family or caregivers to elicit the history. Identify the person who accompanies the patient, but always show interest in the patient first. Establish rapport, make eye contact, and engage in simple conversation. As with children, avoid "talking down" or using affectations of speech or condescending behavior. The patient, family members, caretakers, or friends will notice and appreciate your respect.

The Patient With Personal Problems. Patients may ask you for advice about personal problems that fall outside the range of your clinical expertise. Should the patient quit a stressful job, for example, or move out of state? Instead of responding, explore the different approaches the patient has considered and related pros and cons, whom else they have discussed the problem with, and what supports are available for different choices. Letting the patient talk through the problem with you is usually much more valuable and therapeutic than any answer you could give.

SENSITIVE TOPICS THAT CALL FOR SPECIFIC APPROACHES

Clinicians talk with patients about various subjects that are emotionally charged or sensitive. These discussions can be particularly difficult for inexperienced clinicians or during evaluations of patients you do not know well. Even seasoned clinicians have some discomfort with certain topics: abuse of alcohol or drugs, sexual practices, death and dying, financial concerns, racial and ethnic experiences, family interactions, domestic violence, psychiatric illnesses, physical deformities, bowel function, and others. These areas are difficult to explore in part because of societal taboos. We all know, for example, that talking about bowel habits is not "polite table talk." Many of these topics evoke strong cultural, societal, and personal values. Mental illness, drug use, and same-sex practices are three obvious examples of issues that can touch on our biases and pose barriers during the interview. This section explores challenges to the clinician in these and other important and sometimes sensitive areas, including domestic violence and the dying patient.

Several basic principles can help guide your response to sensitive topics:

GUIDELINES FOR BROACHING SENSITIVE TOPICS

- *The single most important rule is to be nonjudgmental.* The clinician's role is to learn about the patient and help the patient achieve better health. Disapproval of behaviors or elements in the health history will only interfere with this goal.
- *Explain why you need to know certain information.* This makes patients less apprehensive. For example, say to patients, "Because sexual practices put people at risk for certain diseases, I ask all of my patients the following questions."
- Find opening questions for sensitive topics and learn the specific kinds of data needed for your assessments.
- Finally, consciously acknowledge whatever discomfort you are feeling. Denying your discomfort may lead you to avoid the topic altogether.

Look into other strategies for becoming more comfortable with sensitive areas. Examples include general reading about these topics in medical and lay literature; talking to selected colleagues and teachers openly about your concerns; taking special courses that help you explore your own feelings and reactions; and ultimately, reflecting on your own life experience. Take advantage of all these resources. Whenever possible, listen to experienced clinicians, then practice similar discussions with your own patients. The range of topics that you can explore with comfort will widen progressively.

The Sexual History. Asking questions about sexual behavior can be lifesaving. Sexual behaviors determine risks for pregnancy, sexually transmitted diseases (STDs), and AIDS—good interviewing helps prevent or reduce these risks. Sexual practices may be directly related to the patient's symptoms and integral to both diagnosis and treatment. Many patients have questions or concerns about sexuality that they would discuss more freely if you ask about sexual health. Finally, sexual dysfunction may result from use of medication or from misinformation that, if recognized, can be readily addressed.

You can introduce questions about sexual behavior at multiple points in an interview. If the chief complaint involves genitourinary symptoms, include questions about sexual health as part of "expanding and clarifying" the patient's story. For women, you can ask these questions as part of the Obstetric/Gynecologic section of the Past Medical History. You can bring them into discussions about Health Maintenance, along with diet, exercise, and screening tests, or as part of the lifestyle issues or important relationships covered in the Personal and Social History. Or, in a comprehensive history, you can ask about sexual practices during the Review of Systems. Do not forget this area of inquiry just because the patient is elderly or has a disability or chronic illness.

An orienting sentence or two is often helpful. "To assess your risk for various diseases, I need to ask you some questions about your sexual health and prac-

Two or more affirmative answers to the CAGE Questionnaire suggest alcohol misuse and have a sensitivity that ranges from 43% to 94% and specificity that ranges from 70% to 96%.[21,22] If you detect misuse, you need to ask about blackouts (loss of memory about events during drinking), seizures, accidents or injuries while drinking, job problems, conflict in personal relationships, or legal problems. Also ask specifically about drinking while driving or operating machinery.

Illicit Drugs. As with alcohol, your questions about drugs should generally become more focused if you are to get accurate answers that help you distinguish use from misuse. A good opening question is, "Have you ever used any drugs other than those required for medical reasons?"[23] From there, you can ask specifically about either patterns of use (last use, how often, substances used, amount) or inquire about modes of consumption. "Have you ever injected a drug?" "Have you ever smoked or inhaled a drug?" "Have you ever taken a pill for nonmedical reasons?" As fashions in drugs of abuse change it is important to stay up to date about the most current hazards and risks from overdose.

Another approach is to adapt the CAGE questions to screening for substance abuse by adding "or drugs" to each question. Once you identify substance abuse, continue with further questions like "Are you always able to control your use of drugs?" "Have you had any bad reactions?" "What happened . . . Any drug-related accidents, injuries, or arrests? Job or family problems?" . . . "Have you ever tried to quit? Tell me about it."

Family Violence. Because of the high prevalence of physical, sexual, and emotional abuse, many authorities recommend the routine screening of all female patients for domestic violence. Other patients at increased risk are children and the elderly.[24] As with other sensitive topics, start this part of the interview with general "normalizing" questions: "Because abuse is common in many women's lives, I've begun to ask about it routinely." "Are there times in your relationships that you feel unsafe or afraid?" "Many women tell me that someone at home is hurting them in some way. Is this true for you?" "Within the last year, have you been hit, kicked, punched, or otherwise hurt by someone you know? If so, by whom?" As with other segments of the history, use a pattern that goes from general to specific, less difficult to more difficult.

Physical abuse—often not mentioned by either victim or perpetrator—should be considered in the following settings:

CLUES TO POSSIBLE PHYSICAL ABUSE

- If injuries are unexplained, seem inconsistent with the patient's story, are concealed by the patient, or cause embarrassment
- If the patient has delayed getting treatment for trauma
- If there is a past history of repeated injuries or "accidents"
- If the patient or person close to the patient has a history of alcohol or drug abuse
- If the partner tries to dominate the interview, will not leave the room, or seems unusually anxious or solicitous

When you suspect abuse, it is important to spend part of the encounter alone with the patient. You can use the transition to the physical examination as an excuse to ask the other person to leave the room. If the patient is also resistant, you should not force the situation, potentially placing the victim in jeopardy. Be attuned to diagnoses that have a higher association with abuse, such as pregnancy and somatization disorder.

Child abuse is unfortunately also common. Asking parents about their approach to discipline is a routine part of well-child care (see Chapter 18: Assessing Children: Infancy Through Adolescence). You can also ask parents how they cope with a baby who will not stop crying or a child who misbehaves: "Most parents get very upset when their baby cries (or their child has been naughty). How do you feel when your baby cries?" "What do you do when your baby won't stop crying?" "Do you have any fears that you might hurt your child?" Find out how other caretakers or companions handle these situations as well.

Death and the Dying Patient. There is a growing and important emphasis in health care education on improving clinician training related to death and dying. Many clinicians avoid talking about death because of their own discomforts and anxieties. Work through your own feelings with the help of reading and discussion. Basic concepts of care are appropriate even for beginning students because you will come into contact with patients of all ages near the end of their lives. (For a discussion of end-of-life decision making, grief and bereavement, and advance directives, turn to Chapter 20, The Older Adult, p. 854.)

Kubler-Ross has described five stages in a person's response to loss or the anticipatory grief of impending death: denial and isolation, anger, bargaining, depression or sadness, and acceptance.[25] These stages may occur sequentially or overlap in any order or combination. At each stage, follow the same approach. Be sensitive to the patient's feelings about dying; watch for cues that the patient is open to talking about them. Make openings for patients to ask questions: "I wonder if you have any concerns about the procedure? . . . your illness? . . . what it will be like when you go home?" Explore these concerns and provide whatever information the patient requests. Avoid unwarranted reassurance. If you explore and accept patients' feelings, answer their questions, and demonstrate your commitment to staying with them throughout their illness, reassurance will grow where it really matters—within the patients themselves.

Dying patients rarely want to talk about their illnesses at each encounter, nor do they wish to confide in everyone they meet. Give them opportunities to talk, and listen receptively, but if they stay at a social level, respect their preferences. Remember that illness—even a terminal one—is only one small part of the total person. A smile, a touch, an inquiry about a family member, a comment on the day's events, or even some gentle humor affirms and sustains the unique individual you are caring for. Communicating effectively means getting to know the whole patient; that is part of the helping process.

Understanding the patient's wishes about treatment at the end of life is an important clinician responsibility. Failing to establish communication about end-of-life decisions is widely viewed as a flaw in clinical care. Even if discussions of death and dying are difficult for you, you must learn to ask specific questions. The condition of the patient and the health care setting often determine what needs to be discussed. For patients who are acutely ill and in the hospital, discussions about what the patient wants to have done in the event of a cardiac or respiratory arrest are usually mandatory. Asking about *Do Not Resuscitate (DNR) status* is often difficult when you have no previous relationship with the patient or lack knowledge of the patient's values and life experience. Find out about the patient's frame of reference because the media gives many patients an unrealistic view of the effectiveness of resuscitation. "What experiences have you had with the death of a close friend or relative?" "What do you know about cardiopulmonary resuscitation (CPR)?" Educate patients about the likely success of CPR, especially if they are chronically ill or advanced in age. Assure them that relieving pain and taking care of their other spiritual and physical needs will be a priority.

In general, it is important to encourage any adult, but especially the elderly or chronically ill, to establish a *health proxy,* who can act as the patient's health decision maker (see p. 52). This part of the interview can be a "values history" that identifies what is important to the patient and makes life worth living, and the point when living would no longer be worthwhile. Ask how patients spend their time every day, what brings them joy, and what they look forward to. Make sure to clarify the meaning of statements like, "You said that you don't want to be a burden to your family. What exactly do you mean by that?" Explore the patient's religious or spiritual frame of reference so that you and the patient can make the most appropriate decisions about health care.

SOCIETAL ASPECTS OF INTERVIEWING

Achieving Cultural Competence. Communicating effectively with patients from every background has always been an important professional skill. Nevertheless, disparities in health care resulting from factors such as class, education, ethnicity, and race have fueled renewed efforts to raise the standards of cultural competence among clinicians.[26]

Working well with diverse patients is a career-long process built on genuine interest in learning about others, appreciation of the value of diverse cultures, and the practice of reflecting on how your own perspectives are equally shaped by culture. The following examples illustrate how cultural differences and unconscious bias can unwittingly lead to poor communication and influence the quality of patient care.

CULTURAL COMPETENCE: SCENARIO 1

A 28-year-old taxi driver from Ghana who had recently moved to the United States complained to a friend about U.S. medical care. He had gone to the clinic because of fever and fatigue. He described being weighed, having his temperature taken, and having a cloth wrapped tightly, to the point of pain, around his arm. The clinician, a 36-year-old woman from Washington, D.C., had asked the patient many questions, examined him, and wanted to take blood, which the patient had refused. The patient's final comment was ". . . and she didn't even give me chloroquine!"—his primary reason for seeking care. The man from Ghana was expecting few questions, no examination, and treatment for malaria, which is what fever usually means in Ghana.

In this example, cross-cultural miscommunication is understandable and so less threatening to explore. Unconscious bias leading to miscommunication, however, occurs in many clinical interactions. Consider the scenario below that is closer to daily practice.

CULTURAL COMPETENCE: SCENARIO 2

A 16-year-old high school student came to the local teen health center because of painful menstrual cramps that were interfering with concentrating at school. She was dressed in a tight top and short skirt and had multiple piercings, including in her eyebrow. The 30-year-old male clinician asked the following questions: "Are you passing all of your classes? What kind of job do you want after high school? What kind of birth control do you want?" The teenager felt pressured into accepting birth control pills, even though she had clearly stated that she had never had intercourse and planned to postpone it until she got married. She was an honor student and planning to go to college, but the clinician did not elicit these goals. The clinician glossed over her cramps by saying, "Oh, you can just take some ibuprofen. Cramps usually get better as you get older." The patient will not take the birth control pills that were prescribed, nor will she seek health care soon again. She experienced the encounter as an interrogation, so failed to gain trust in her clinician. In addition, the questions made assumptions about her life and did not treat her health concern with respect. Even though the provider pursued the important psychosocial domains, she received ineffective health care because of conflicting cultural values and unreflected clinician bias.

In both of these cases, the failure stems from mistaken assumptions or biases. In the first case, the clinician did not consider the many variables affecting patient beliefs about health and expectations for care. In the second case, the clinician allowed stereotypes to dictate the agenda instead of listening to the patient and respecting her as an individual. Each of us has our own cultural background and our own biases. These do not simply fade away as we become clinicians.

SOCIETAL ASPECTS OF INTERVIEWING

As you provide care for an ever-expanding and diverse group of patients, you must recognize how culture shapes not just the patient's beliefs, but your own. *Culture* is the system of shared ideas, rules, and meanings that influences how we view the world, experience it emotionally, and behave in relation to other people. It can be understood as the "lens" through which we perceive and make sense out of the world we inhabit. The meaning of culture is much broader than the term "ethnicity." Cultural influences are not limited to minority groups; they are relevant to everyone. They reflect factors like geography, age, religion, gender, sexual orientation, ethnicity, race, and socioeconomic status.

Although learning about specific cultural groups is important, avoid allowing this knowledge to turn into stereotyping rather than understanding. For example, you may have learned that Hispanic patients convey their pain in a more dramatic fashion. However, it is still important for you to evaluate each patient with pain as an individual, not decreasing the amount of analgesic you would typically use, but being aware of your reactions to the patient's style. Work on an appropriate and informed clinical approach to all patients by becoming aware of your own values and biases, developing communication skills that transcend cultural differences, and building therapeutic partnerships based on respect for each patient's life experience. This type of framework, described in the section below, will allow you to approach each patient as unique and distinct.

THE THREE DIMENSIONS OF CULTURAL COMPETENCE

- *Self-awareness.* Learn about your own biases . . . we all have them.
- *Respectful communication.* Work to eliminate assumptions about what is "normal." Learn directly from your patients—they are the experts on their culture and illness.
- *Collaborative partnerships.* Build your patient relationships on respect and mutually acceptable plans.

Self-Awareness. Start by exploring your own cultural identity. How do you describe yourself in terms of ethnicity, class, region or country of origin, religion, and political affiliation? Don't forget the characteristics that we often take for granted—gender, life roles, sexual orientation, physical ability, and race—especially if we are in majority groups. What aspects of your family of origin do you identify with, and how are you different from your family of origin? How do these identities influence your beliefs and behaviors?

A more challenging task in learning about ourselves is to bring our own values and biases to a conscious level. *Values* are the standards we use to measure our own and others' beliefs and behaviors. These may appear to be absolutes. *Biases* are the attitudes or feelings that we attach to perceived differences. Being attuned to difference is normal; in fact, in the distant past, detecting differences may have preserved life. Intuitively knowing members of one's own group is a survival skill that we may have outgrown as a society but that is still actively at work.

Feeling guilty about our biases makes it hard to recognize and acknowledge them. Start with less threatening constructs, like the way an individual relates to time, a culturally determined phenomenon. Are you always on time—a positive value in the dominant Western culture? Or do you tend to run a little late? How do you feel about people whose habits are opposite to yours? Next time you attend a meeting or class, notice who is early, on time, or late. Is it predictable? Think about the role of physical appearance. Do you consider yourself thin, mid-size, or heavy? How do you feel about your weight? What does prevailing U.S. culture teach us to value in physique? How do you feel about people who have different weights?

Respectful Communication. Given the complexity of culture, no one can possibly know the health beliefs and practices of every culture and subculture. Let your patients be the experts on their own unique cultural perspectives. Even if patients have trouble describing their values or beliefs in the abstract, they should be able to respond to specific questions. Find out about the patient's cultural background. Use some of the same questions discussed earlier in the section, Creating a Shared Understanding of the Problem (see p. 33). Maintain an open, respectful, and inquiring attitude. "What did you hope to get from this visit?" If you have established rapport and trust, patients will be willing to teach you. Be aware of questions that contain assumptions. And always be ready to acknowledge your areas of ignorance or bias. "I know very little about Ghana. What would have happened at a clinic there if you had these concerns?" Or, with the second patient and with much more difficulty, "I mistakenly made assumptions about you that are not right. I apologize. Would you be willing to tell me more about yourself and your future goals?"

Learning about specific cultures is valuable because it broadens what you, as a clinician, identify as areas you need to explore. Do some reading about the life experiences of individuals in ethnic or racial groups that live in your area. Go to movies that are filmed in different countries or explicitly present the perspective of different cultures. Learn about the concerns of different consumer groups with visible health agendas. Get to know healers of different disciplines and learn about their practices. Most importantly, be open to learning from your patients. Do not assume that what you have learned about a cultural group applies to the individual before you.

Collaborative Partnerships. Through continual work on self-awareness and seeing through the "lens" of others, the clinician lays the foundation for the collaborative relationship that best supports the patient's health. Communication based on trust, respect, and a willingness to reexamine assumptions allows patients to express aspects of their concerns that may run counter to the dominant culture. These concerns may be associated with strong feelings such as anger or shame. You, the clinician, must be willing to listen to and validate these feelings, and not let your own feelings prevent you from exploring painful areas. You must also be willing to reexamine your beliefs about what is the "right approach" to clinical care in a given situation. Make every effort to be flexible and creative in your plans and respectful of patients' knowledge about their own best interests. By consciously distinguishing what is truly important to the patient's health from what is just the standard advice, you and your patients can construct the unique approach to their health care that is in concert with their beliefs and effective clinical care. Remember that if the patient stops listening, fails to follow your advice, or does not return, your health care has not been successful.

Sexuality in the Clinician–Patient Relationship. Clinicians of both genders occasionally find themselves physically attracted to their patients. Similarly, patients may make sexual overtures or exhibit flirtatious behavior toward clinicians. The emotional and physical intimacy of the clinician–patient relationship may lend itself to these sexual feelings.

If you become aware of such feelings in yourself, accept them as a normal human response, and bring them to conscious level so they will not affect your behavior. Denying these feelings makes it more likely for you to act inappropriately. *Any* sexual contact or romantic relationship with patients is *unethical;* keep your relationship with the patient within professional bounds, and seek help if you need it.

Sometimes clinicians meet patients who are frankly seductive or make sexual advances. You may be tempted to ignore this behavior because you are not sure that it really happened, or you are just hoping it will go away. Calmly but firmly, make it clear that your relationship is professional, not personal. If unwelcome overtures continue, leave the room and find a chaperone to continue the interview. You should also reflect on your image. Has your clothing or demeanor been unconsciously seductive? Have you been overly warm with the patient? Although it is your responsibility to avoid contributing to these problems, usually you are not at fault. Often these problems reflect the patient's discomfort with feeling less powerful.

ETHICS AND PROFESSIONALISM

You may wonder why an introductory chapter on interviewing contains a section on clinical ethics. The potential power of clinician–patient communication calls for guidance beyond our innate sense of morality. *Ethics* are a set of principles crafted through reflection and discussion to define right and wrong. *Medical ethics,* which guide our professional behavior, are neither static nor simple, but several principles have guided clinicians throughout the ages. Although in most situations your gut sense of right and wrong will be all that you need, even as students, you will face decisions that call for the application of ethical principles.

Some of the traditional and still fundamental maxims embedded in the healing professions are listed below.

BUILDING BLOCKS OF PROFESSIONAL ETHICS IN PATIENT CARE

- ***Nonmaleficence or primum non nocere*** is commonly stated as, "First, do no harm." In the context of an interview, giving information that is incorrect or not really related to the patient's problem can do harm. Avoiding relevant topics or creating barriers to open communication can also do harm.

(continued)

BUILDING BLOCKS OF PROFESSIONAL ETHICS IN PATIENT CARE (Continued)

- ***Beneficence*** is the dictum that the clinician needs to "do good" for the patient. As clinicians, your actions need to be motivated by what is in the patient's best interest.
- ***Autonomy*** reminds us that patients have the right to determine what is in their own best interest. This principle has become increasingly important over time and is consistent with collaborative rather than paternalistic clinician–patient relationships.
- ***Confidentiality*** can be one of the most challenging principles. As a clinician, you are obligated not to repeat what you learn from or know about a patient. This privacy is fundamental to our professional relationships with patients. In the daily flurry of activity in a hospital, it is all too easy to let something slip. You must be on your guard.

As students, you are exposed to some of the ethical challenges that you will confront later as practicing clinicians. However, there are dilemmas unique to students that you will face from the time that you begin taking care of patients. The following vignettes capture some of the most common experiences. They raise a variety of ethical and practical issues that are overlapping.

ETHICS AND PROFESSIONALISM: SCENARIO 1

You are a third-year medical student on your first clinical rotation in the hospital. It is late in the evening when you are finally assigned to the patient you are to "work up" and present the next day at preceptor rounds. You go to the patient's room and find the patient exhausted from the day's events and clearly ready to settle down for the night. You know that your intern and attending physician have already done their evaluations. Do you proceed with a history and physical that is likely to take 1 to 2 hours? Is this process only for your education? Do you ask permission before you start? What do you include?

Here you are confronted with the tension between *the need to learn by doing* and *doing no harm to patients.* There is a utilitarian ethical principle that reminds us that if clinicians-in-training do not learn, there will be no future caregivers. Yet the dictums to do no harm and prioritize what is in the patient's best interests are clearly in conflict with that future need. As a student, this dilemma will arise often.

Obtaining *informed consent* is the means to address this ethical dilemma. Making sure the patient realizes that you are in training and new at patient evaluation is always important. It is impressive how often patients willingly let students be involved in their care. It is an opportunity for patients to give back to their caregivers. Even when clinical activities appear to be purely for educational purposes, there may be a benefit to the patient. Multiple caregivers provide multiple perspectives, and the experience of being heard can be therapeutic.

ETHICS AND PROFESSIONALISM: SCENARIO 2

It is after 10 PM, and you and your resident are on the way to complete the required advance directives form with a frail, elderly patient who was admitted earlier that day with bilateral pneumonia. The form, which includes a discussion of Do Not Resuscitate orders, must be completed before the team can sign out and leave for the day. Just then, your resident is paged to an emergency and asks you to go ahead and meet with the patient to complete the form; the resident will cosign it later. You had a lecture on advance directives and end-of-life discussions in your first year of school but have never seen a clinician discuss this with a patient. You have not yet met the patient, nor have you had a chance to really look at the form. What should you do? Do you inform the resident that you have never done this before nor even seen it done? Do you need to inform the patient that this is totally new for you? Who should decide whether you are competent to do this independently?

In this situation, you are being asked to take responsibility for clinical care that exceeds your level of comfort and maybe your competence. This can happen in a number of situations, such as being asked to evaluate a clinical situation without proper back-up or to draw blood or start an IV before you have done one under supervision. For the patient above, you may have many of the following thoughts: "the patient needs to have this completed before going to sleep and so will benefit"; "the risk to the patient from discussing advance directives is minimal"; "you are pretty good with elderly patients and think that you might be able to do this"; "what if the patient actually arrests that night and you are responsible for what happens"; and finally, "if you bother the resident now he or she will be angry and that may affect your evaluation." There is educational value to the learner in being pushed to the limits of his or her knowledge to solve problems and to gain confidence in functioning independently. But what is the right thing to do in this situation?

The principles listed above only partially help you sort this out because only part of your quandary relates to your relationship with the patient. Much of the tension in this scenario has to do with the dynamics of a health care team and your role on that team. You are there to help with the work of the team, but you are primarily there to learn. Current formulations of medical ethics address those issues and others. One such formulation is the Tavistock Principles.[27] These principles construct a framework for analyzing health care situations that extends beyond our direct care of individual patients to complicated choices about the interactions of health care teams and the distribution of resources for the well-being of society. A broadly representative group that initially met in Tavistock Square in London in 1998 has continued to elaborate an evolving document of ethical principles for guiding health care behavior for both individuals and institutions across the health care spectrum. A current iteration of the Tavistock Principles follows.

THE TAVISTOCK PRINCIPLES

Rights: People have a right to health and health care.
Balance: Care of the individual patient is central, but the health of populations is also our concern.
Comprehensiveness: In addition to treating illness, we have an obligation to ease suffering, minimize disability, prevent disease, and promote health.
Cooperation: Health care succeeds only if we cooperate with those we serve, each other, and those in other sectors.
Improvement: Improving health care is a serious and continuing responsibility.
Safety: Do no harm.
Openness: Being open, honest, and trustworthy is vital in health care.

In the second scenario, think about the Tavistock Principles of *openness and cooperation*, in addition to the balance between *do no harm* and *beneficence*. You need to work with your team in a way that is honest and reliable to do the best for the patient. You can also see that there are no clear or easy answers in such situations. What responses are available to you to address these and other quandaries?

You need to reflect on your beliefs and assess your level of comfort with a given situation. Sometimes there may be alternative solutions. For example, in Scenario 1, the patient may really be willing to have the history and physical examination done at that late hour, or perhaps you can renegotiate the time for the next morning. In Scenario 2, you might find another person who is more qualified to complete the form or to supervise when you do it. Alternatively, you may choose to go ahead and complete the form, alerting the patient to your inexperience and obtaining the patient's consent. You will need to choose which situations warrant voicing your concerns, even at the risk of a bad evaluation.

Seek coaching on how to express your reservations in a way that ensures that they will be heard. As a clinical student, you will need settings for discussing these immediately relevant ethical dilemmas with other students and with more senior trainees and faculty. Small groups that are structured to address these kinds of issues are particularly useful in providing validation and support. Take advantage of such opportunities whenever possible.

ETHICS AND PROFESSIONALISM: SCENARIO 3

You are the student on the clinical team that has been taking care of Ms. Robbins, a 64-year-old woman admitted for an evaluation of weight loss and weakness. During the hospitalization, she had a biopsy of a mass in her chest in addition to many other tests. You have gotten to know her well, spending a lot of time with her to answer questions, explain procedures, and learn about her and her family. You have discussed her fears about what

(continued)

ETHICS AND PROFESSIONALISM: SCENARIO 3 (Continued)

"they" will find and know that she likes to know everything possible about her health and medical care. You have even heard her express frustrations with her attending physician at not always being given the "straight story." It is late Friday afternoon, but you promised Ms. Robbins that you would come by one more time before the weekend and let her know if the results of the biopsy were back yet. Just before you go to her room, the resident tells you that the pathology is back from her biopsy and shows metastatic cancer, but the attending physician does not want the team to say anything until he comes in on Monday.

What are you going to do? You feel that it is wrong to avoid the situation by not going to her room. You also believe that the patient's preference and anxiety are best served by finding out then and not waiting for 3 days. You do not want to go against the attending physician's clear instructions, however, both because you respect the fact that it is his patient and because that feels dishonest.

In this situation, telling the patient about her biopsy results is dictated by several ethical principles: the patient's best interests, autonomy, and your integrity. The other part of the ethical dilemma concerns communicating your plan to the attending. Sometimes the most challenging part of such dilemmas tests your will to follow through with the right course of action. Although it may appear to be a lose-lose situation, a respectful and honest discussion with the attending, respectfully articulating what is in the patient's best interest, will usually be heard. Enlist the support of your resident or other helpful attendings if that is possible. Learning how to navigate difficult discussions will be a useful professional skill.

Bibliography

CITATIONS

1. Cohen-Cole SA: The Medical Interview: The Three-Function Approach. St. Louis, Mosby–Year Book, 1991.
2. Bird J, Cohen-Cole SA: The three-function model of the medical interview. Adv Psychosom Med 20:65–88, 1990.
3. Lazare A, Putnam SM, Lipkin M Jr: Three functions of the medical interview. In Lipkin M Jr, Putnam SM, Lazare A, et al (eds): The Medical Interview: Clinical Care, Education, and Research. New York, Springer-Verlag, 1995.
4. Novack DH: Therapeutic aspects of the clinical encounter. In Lipkin M Jr, Putnam SM, Lazare A, et al (eds). The Medical Interview: Clinical Care, Education, and Research, p. 32. New York, Springer-Verlag, 1995.
5. Suchman AL, Matthews DA. What makes the patient-doctor relationship therapeutic? Exploring the connectional dimension of medical care. Ann Intern Med 108(1):125–130, 1988.
6. Hastings C. The lived experiences of the illness: making contact with the patient. In Benne P, Wrubel J (eds): The Primacy of Caring: Stress and Coping in Health and Illness. Menlo Park, CA, Addison-Wesley, 1989.
7. Conant EB. Addressing patients by their first names. N Engl J Med 308(4):226, 1998.
8. Heller ME. Addressing patients by their first names. N Engl J Med 308(18):1107, 1987.
9. Delbanco TL. Enriching the doctor-patient relationship by inviting the patient's perspective. Ann Intern Med 116(5):414–418, 1993.
10. Beckman HB, Frankel RM. The effect of physician behavior on the collection of data. Ann Intern Med 101(5):692–696, 1984.
11. Kleinman A, Eisenberg L, Good B. Culture, illness, and care: clinical lessons from anthropological and cross-cultural research. Ann Intern Med 88(2):251–258, 1978.
12. Smith RC. Patient-Centered Interviewing: An Evidence-Based Method. Philadelphia, Lippincott Williams & Wilkins, 2002.
13. Smith RC, Lyles JS, Mettler J, et al. The effectiveness of an intensive teaching experience for residents in interviewing: a randomized controlled study. Ann Intern Med 128(2):118–126, 1998.

14. Engel GL. The need for a new medical model: a challenge for biomedicine. Science 196(4286):126–129, 1977.
15. Engel GL, Morgan WL Jr. Interviewing the Patient. Philadelphia, WB Saunders, 1973.
16. Bayer–Fetzer Conference on Physician–Patient Communication in Medical Education: Essential elements of communication in medical encounters: the Kalamazoo Consensus Statement. Acad Med 76(4):390–393, 2001.
17. Stewart M. Questions about patient-centered care: answers from quantitative research. In Stewart M, et al (eds): Patient Centered Medicine: Transforming the Clinical Method, pp. 263–268. Abington, UK: Radcliffe Medical Press, 2003.
18. U.S. Preventive Services Task Force. Screening for Depression: Recommendations and Rationale. Rockville, MD, Agency for Healthcare Research and Quality, May 2002.
19. Regier DA, Farmer ME, Rae DS, et al. Comorbidity of mental disorders with alcohol and other drug abuse. Results from the Epidemiologic Catchment Area (ECA) Study. JAMA 264(19): 2511–2518, 1990.
20. Cyr MG, Wartman SA. The effectiveness of routine screening questions in the detection of alcoholism. JAMA 259(1):51–54, 1988.
21. U.S. Preventive Services Task Force: Screening and Behavioral Counseling Interventions in Primary Care to Reduce Alcohol Misuse: Recommendation Statement. Rockville, MD, Agency for Healthcare Research and Quality, April 2004. Available at: http://www.ahrq.gov/clinic/3rduspstf/alcohol/alcomisrs.htm.
22. Ewing JA. Detecting alcoholism: the CAGE questionnaire. JAMA 252(14):1905–1907, 1984.
23. Cocco KM, Carey KB. Psychometric properties of the Drug Abuse Screening Test in psychiatric outpatients. Psychol Assess 10(4):408–414, 1998.
24. U.S. Preventive Services Task Force: Screening for Family and Intimate Partner Violence: Recommendation Statement. Rockville, MD, Agency for Healthcare Research and Quality, March 2004.
25. Kubler-Ross E. On Death and Dying. New York, Macmillan, 1997.
26. Smedley BA, Stith AY, Nelson AR (eds): Committee on Understanding and Eliminating Racial and Ethnic Disparities in Health Care. Unequal Treatment: Confronting Racial and Ethnic Disparities in Health Care. Washington, DC: Institute of Medicine, 2003.
27. Berwick D, Davidoff F, Hiatt H, et al. Refining and implementing the Tavistock principles for everybody in health care. BMJ 323(7313):616–619, 2001.

ADDITIONAL REFERENCES

Building a Therapeutic Relationship: The Techniques of Skilled Interviewing

Billings JA, Stoeckle JD. The Clinical Encounter: A Guide to the Medical Interview and Case Presentation. Chicago, Year Book Medical Publishers, 1989.

Branch WT, Malik TK. Using "windows of opportunities" in brief interviews to understand patients' concerns. JAMA 269(13):1667–1668, 1993.

Fadiman A. The Spirit Catches You and You Fall Down. New York: Farrar, Straus and Giroux, 1997.

Frankel RM, Stein TS. The Four Habits of Highly Effective Clinicians: A Practical Guide. Oakland, CA, Kaiser Permanente Northern California Region Physician Education and Development, 1996.

Inui TS. Establishing the doctor–patient relationship: science, art, or competence? Schweiz Med Wochenschr 128(7):225–230, 1998.

Quill TE, Brody H. Physician recommendations and patient autonomy: finding a balance between physician power and patient choice. Ann Intern Med 125(9):763–769, 1996.

Silverman J, Kurtz S, Draper J. Skills for communicating with patients. Abingdon, UK: Radcliffe Medical Press Ltd, 1998.

Smith RC. The Patient's Story, Integrated Patient-Doctor Interviewing. Boston: Little, Brown, 1996.

Adapting Interviewing Techniques to Specific Situations

Barnett S. Cross-cultural communication with patients who use American Sign Language. Fam Med 34(5):376–382, 2002.

Committee on Disabilities of the Group for the Advancement of Psychiatry: Issues to consider in deaf and hard-of-hearing patients. Am Fam Phys 56(8):2057–2066, 1997.

Goldoft M. A piece of mind: another language. JAMA 268(24): 3482, 1992.

Grantmakers in Health: In the right words: addressing language and culture in providing health care. Issues in Brief 18:1–54, 2003.

Mayeaux EJ Jr, Murphy PW, Arnold C, et al. Improving patient education for patients with low literacy skills. Am Fam Phys 53(1):205–211, 1996.

McDaniel SH, Campbell TL, Hepworth J, et al. Family-Oriented Primary Care, 2nd ed. New York: Springer, 2005.

National Work Group on Literacy and Health. Communicating with patients who have limited literacy skills. Report of the National Work Group on Literacy and Health. J Fam Pract 46(2): 168–176, 1998.

Putsch RW. Cross-cultural communication: the special case of interpreters in health care. JAMA 254(23):3344–3348, 1985.

Rivadeneyra R, Elderkin-Thompson V, Silver RC, et al. Patient centeredness in medical encounters requiring an interpreter. Am J Med 108(6):470–474, 2000.

Sensitive Topics That Call for Specific Approaches

Council on Scientific Affairs, AMA: Health care needs of gay men and lesbians in the U.S. JAMA 275(17):1354–1357, 1996.

End of Life/Palliative Education Resource Center. Available at: http://www.eperc.mcw.edu/index.htm. Accessed February 10, 2005.

Fiellin DA, Reid MC, O'Connor PG. Screening for alcohol problems in primary care: a systematic review. Arch Intern Med 160(13):1977–1989, 2000.

Harrison AE. Primary care of lesbian and gay patients: educating ourselves and our students. Fam Med 28(1):10–23, 1996.

Robinson GE, Stewart DE. A curriculum on physician-patient sexual misconduct and teacher-learner mistreatment. Part 1: Content. Can Med Assoc J 154(1):643–649, 1996.

Societal Aspects of Interviewing

Carrillo JE, Green AR, Betancourt JR. Cross-cultural primary care: a patient-based approach. Ann Intern Med 130:829–834, 1999.

Christakis DA, Feudtner C. Ethics in a short white coat: The ethical dilemmas that medical students confront. Acad Med 68(4):249–254, 1993.

Council on Ethical and Judicial Affairs, American Medical Association: Sexual misconduct in the practice of medicine. JAMA 266(19):2741–2745, 1991.

Doyal L. Closing the gap between professional teaching and practice. BMJ 322(7288):685–686, 2001.

Gabbard GO, Nadelson C. Professional boundaries in the physician-patient relationship. JAMA 273(18):1445–1449, 1995.

Lo B. Resolving Ethical Dilemmas: A Guide for Clinicians. Philadelphia, Lippincott Williams & Wilkins, 2000.

Tervalon M, Murray-Garcia J. Cultural humility versus cultural competence: a critical distinction in defining physician training outcomes in multicultural education. J Health Care Poor Underserved 9(2):117–125, 1998.

Waitzkin H. Doctor-patient communication: clinical implications of social scientific research. JAMA 252(17):2441–2446, 1984.

CHAPTER

3

Clinical Reasoning, Assessment, and Plan

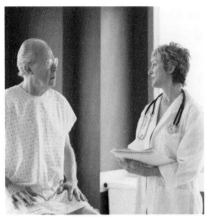

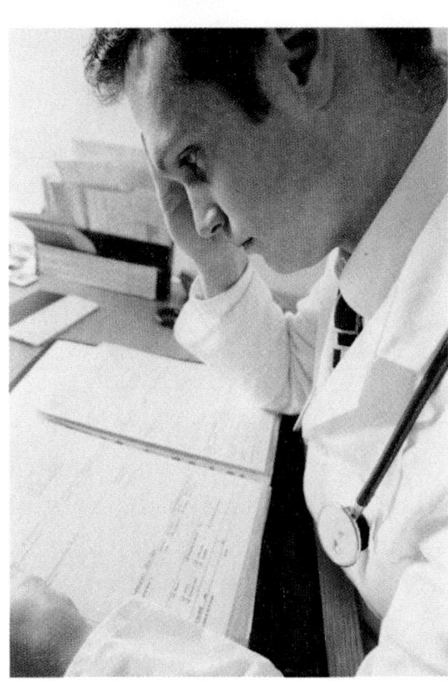

Now that you have gained your patient's trust, gathered a detailed history, and completed the requisite portions of the physical examination, you have reached the critical step of formulating your *Assessment(s)* and *Plan*. You must now analyze your findings and identify the patient's problems. You must also share your impressions with the patient, eliciting any concerns and making sure that he or she understands and agrees to the steps ahead. Finally, you must document your findings in the patient's record in a succinct and legible format. A clear and well-organized record is essential for communicating the patient's story and your clinical reasoning and plan to other members of the health care team.

This chapter follows a step-wise approach designed to help you acquire the important skills of clinical reasoning, assessment, and recording your Assessment and Plan. Review the learning objectives below, which mirror the organization of this chapter, and test your understanding by returning to the history and physical examination of Mrs. N found in Chapter 1, pp. 16–20.

DEVELOPING AN ASSESSMENT AND PLAN: OBJECTIVES FOR LEARNERS

- Understand the process of clinical reasoning and its component steps.
- Analyze this process using the written *Assessment* and *Plan* for Mrs. N (pp. 71–72).
- Address the challenges of clinical data by:
  - Clustering data into single versus multiple problems
  - Sifting through an extensive array of data
  - Assessing the quality of patient information, including how to ensure quality and principles for selecting and analyzing tests
- Integrate clinical reasoning with assessment of clinical data.
- Organize a clear and accurate patient record.

The comprehensive information you have collected, both *subjective* (the history, or what the patient or family has told you) and *objective* (the physical examination and laboratory tests), make up the core elements of your patient observations. This information is primarily factual and descriptive. As you move to *Assessment,* you go beyond description and observation to analysis and interpretation. You select and cluster relevant pieces of information, analyze their possible meanings, and try to explain them logically using principles of biopsychosocial and biomedical science. The *Assessment* and *Plan* include the patient's responses to the problems identified and to your diagnostic and therapeutic plans. A successful *Plan* requires good interpersonal skills and sensitivity to the patient's goals, economic means, competing responsibilities, and family structure and dynamics. Your patient record facilitates clinical thinking, promotes communication and coordination among the many professionals caring for your patient, and documents the patient's problems and management for medicolegal purposes.

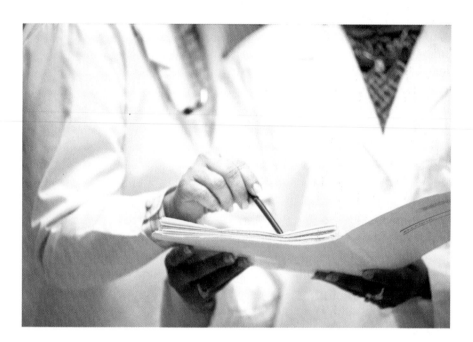

ASSESSMENT AND PLAN: THE PROCESS OF CLINICAL REASONING

Because assessment takes place in the clinician's mind, the process of clinical reasoning often seems inaccessible and even mysterious to the beginning student. Experienced clinicians often think quickly, with little overt or conscious effort. They differ widely in personal style, communication skills, clinical training, experience, and interests. Some clinicians may find it difficult to explain the logic behind their clinical thinking. As an active learner, it is expected that you will ask teachers and clinicians to elaborate on the fine points of their clinical reasoning and decision making.[1,2]

As you gain experience, your thinking process will begin at the outset of the patient encounter, not at the end. Listed below are a set of principles that underlie the process of clinical reasoning and certain explicit steps to help guide your thinking as you analyze the information you have compiled. After reading through this section, review the case of Mrs. N, introduced in Chapter 1, and use this as a sample database to practice the process of clinical reasoning and assessment. As with all patients, focus on finding answers to the questions "What is wrong with this patient?" "What are the problems and diagnoses?" To reach these answers, try following the steps discussed below. Then turn to the *Assessment and Plan* for Mrs. N on pp. 71–72 and compare them with your own insights and clinical thinking.

Identifying Problems and Making Diagnoses: Steps in Clinical Reasoning

- Identify abnormal findings.
- Localize findings anatomically.
- Interpret findings in terms of probable process.
- Make hypotheses about the nature of the patient's problem.
- Test the hypotheses and establish a working diagnosis.
- Develop a plan agreeable to the patient.

- **Identify abnormal findings.** Make a list of the patient's *symptoms,* the *signs* you observed during the physical examination, and any laboratory reports available to you.

- **Localize these findings anatomically.** This step may be easy. The symptom of scratchy throat and the sign of an erythematous inflamed pharynx, for example, clearly localize the problem to the pharynx. For Mrs. N, the complaint of headache leads you quickly to the structures of the skull and brain. Other symptoms, however, may present greater difficulty. Chest pain, for example, can originate in the coronary arteries, the stomach and esophagus, or the muscles and bones of the chest. If the pain is exertional and relieved by rest, either the heart or the musculoskeletal components of the chest wall may be involved. If the patient notes pain only when carrying groceries with the left arm, the musculoskeletal system becomes the likely culprit.[3,4]

  When localizing findings, be as specific as your data allow, but bear in mind that you may have to settle for a body region, such as the chest, or a body system, such as the musculoskeletal system. On the other hand, you may be able to define the exact structure involved, such as the left pectoral muscle. Some symptoms and signs cannot be localized, such as fatigue or fever, but are useful in the next set of steps.

- **Interpret the findings in terms of the probable process.** Patient problems often stem from a *pathologic process* involving diseases of a body structure. There are a number of such processes, variably classified, including congenital, inflammatory or infectious, immunologic, neoplastic, metabolic, nutritional, degenerative, vascular, traumatic, and toxic. Possible pathologic causes of headache, for example, include concussion from trauma, subarachnoid hemorrhage, or even compression from a brain tumor. Fever and stiff neck, or nuchal rigidity, are two of the classic signs of headache from meningitis. Even without other signs, such as rash or papilledema, they strongly suggest an infectious process.

Other problems are *pathophysiologic,* reflecting derangements of biologic functions, such as congestive heart failure or migraine headache. Still other problems are *psychopathologic,* such as disorders of mood like depression or headache as an expression of a somatization disorder.

- **Make hypotheses about the nature of the patient's problem.** Here you will draw on all the knowledge and experience you can muster, and it is here that reading will be most helpful for learning about patterns of abnormalities and diseases, and clustering your patient's findings accordingly.

By consulting the clinical literature, you will embark on the lifelong goal of **evidence-based decision-making.**[5,6]

Until you gain broader knowledge and experience, you may not be able to develop highly specific hypotheses, but proceed as far as you can with the data and knowledge you have. The following steps should help:

STEPS IN CLINICAL DECISION-MAKING

1. *Select the most specific and critical findings to support your hypothesis.* If the patient reports "the worst headache of her life," nausea, and vomiting, for example, and you find a change in mental status, papilledema, and meningismus, build your hypothesis around elevated intracranial pressure rather than gastrointestinal disorders. Although other symptoms are useful diagnostically, they are much less specific.
2. Using your inferences about the structures and processes involved, *match your findings against all the conditions you know that can produce them.* For example, you can match your patient's papilledema with a list of conditions affecting intracranial pressure. Or you can compare the symptoms and signs associated with the patient's headache with the various infectious, vascular, metabolic, or neoplastic conditions that might produce this kind of clinical picture.
3. *Eliminate the diagnostic possibilities that fail to explain the findings.* You might consider cluster headache as a cause of Mrs. N's headaches, but eliminate this hypothesis because it fails to explain the patient's throbbing bifrontal localization with intermittent nausea and vomiting. Also, the pain pattern is atypical for cluster headache—it is not unilateral, boring, or occurring repetitively at the same time over a period of days, nor is it associated with lacrimation or rhinorrhea.
4. *Weigh the competing possibilities and select the most likely diagnosis* from among the conditions that might be responsible for the patient's findings. You are looking for a close match between the patient's clinical presentation and a typical case of a given condition. Other clues help in this selection, too. The *statistical probability* of a given disease in a patient of this age, sex, ethnic group, habits, lifestyle, and locality should greatly influence your selection. You should consider the possi-

(continued)

STEPS IN CLINICAL DECISION-MAKING (Continued)

bilities of osteoarthritis and metastatic prostate cancer in a 70-year-old man with back pain, for example, but not in a 25-year-old woman with the same complaint. The *timing of the patient's illness* also makes a difference. Headache in the setting of fever, rash, and stiff neck that develops suddenly over 24 hours suggests quite a different problem than recurrent headache over a period of years associated with stress, visual scotoma, and nausea and vomiting relieved by rest.

5. Finally, as you develop possible explanations for the patient's problem, *give special attention to potentially life-threatening and treatable conditions* such as meningococcal meningitis, bacterial endocarditis, pulmonary embolus, or subdural hematoma. Here you make every effort to minimize the risk for missing conditions that may occur less frequently or be less probable but that, if present, would be particularly ominous. *One rule of thumb is always to include "the worst case scenario" in your list of differential diagnoses* and make sure you have ruled out that possibility based on your findings and patient assessment.

- **Test your hypotheses.** Now that you have made a hypothesis about the patient's problem, you will usually want to *test your hypothesis.* You are likely to need further history, additional maneuvers on physical examination, or laboratory studies or x-rays to confirm or rule out your tentative diagnosis or to clarify which of two or three possible diagnoses are most likely. When the diagnosis seems clear-cut—a simple upper respiratory infection or a case of hives, for example—these steps may not be necessary.

- **Establish a working diagnosis.** You are now ready to establish a working definition of the problem. Make this at the highest level of explicitness and certainty that the data allow. You may be limited to a symptom, such as "tension headache, cause unknown." At other times, you can define a problem explicitly in terms of its structure, process, and cause. Examples include "bacterial meningitis, pneumococcal," "subarachnoid hemorrhage, left temporoparietal lobe," or "hypertensive cardiovascular disease with left ventricular dilatation and congestive heart failure."

  Although diagnoses are based primarily on identifying abnormal structures, altered processes, and specific causes, you will frequently see patients whose complaints do not fall neatly into these categories. Some symptoms defy analysis, and you may never be able to move beyond simple descriptive categories such as "fatigue" or "anorexia." Other problems relate to the patient's life, rather than to the body. Events such as losing a job or loved one may increase the risk for subsequent illness. Identifying these events and helping the patient develop coping strategies are just as important as managing a headache or a duodenal ulcer.

  Another increasingly prominent item on problem lists is *Health Maintenance.* Routinely listing this category helps you track several important health concerns more effectively: immunizations, screening measures (e.g., mammograms, prostate examinations), instructions regarding nutrition and breast or testicular self-examinations, recommendations about exercise or use of seat belts, and responses to important life events.

- **Develop a plan agreeable to the patient.** You should identify and record a *Plan* for each patient problem. Your *Plan* will flow logically from the problems or diagnoses you have identified and specify which steps are needed next. These steps range from tests to confirm or further evaluate a diagnosis; to consultations for subspecialty evaluation; to additions, deletions, or changes in medication; to arranging a family meeting. You will find that you will follow many of the same diagnoses over time; however, your *Plan* is often more fluid, encompassing changes and modifications that emerge from each patient visit. The *Plan* should make reference to diagnosis, therapy, and patient education.

  Before finalizing your *Plan,* it is important to share your assessment and clinical thinking with the patient and seek out his or her opinions, concerns, and willingness to proceed with any further testing or evaluation. Remember that patients may need to hear the same information multiple times and ways before they comprehend it. You will enhance your relationship with the patient if the patient is an active participant in the plan of care.

THE CASE OF MRS. N: ASSESSMENT AND PLAN

As you study the *Assessment* and *Plan* for Mrs. N, think carefully about the clarity and organization of the clinical record. When creating a record, you do more than simply list the patient's story and your physical findings. You must review and organize your data, evaluate the importance and relevance of each item, and construct a clear, concise, yet comprehensive report. At first, it will be challenging to clearly and logically organize your patient assessment. Let the patient's story and symptoms serve as guides, examine the appropriate areas of the body, and apply the steps of clinical reasoning to deepen your knowledge, judgment, and clinical acumen.

Using Mrs. N's record, make a checklist of the features of a good medical record. Later, compare your list with the checklist on pp. 81–83. The following questions may help:

- Are the data easy to follow, orderly, and presented in a readable format?
- Is there sufficient detail, both positive and negative, to formulate an Assessment and Plan?
- Is there excess repetition of information or redundancy?
- Is the tone professional, avoiding disapproving or moralizing comments?

ASSESSMENT AND PLAN FOR MRS. N

1. **Migraine headaches.** A 54-year-old woman with migraine headaches since childhood, with a throbbing vascular pattern and frequent nausea and vomiting. Headaches are associated with stress and relieved by sleep and cold compresses. There is no papilledema, and there are no motor or sensory deficits on the neurologic examination. The differential diagnosis includes tension headache, also associated with stress, but there is no relief with massage, and the pain is more throbbing than aching. There are no fever, stiff neck, or focal findings to suggest meningitis, and the lifelong recurrent pattern makes subarachnoid hemorrhage unlikely (usually described as "the worst headache of my life").

   Plan:

   - Discuss features of migraine vs. tension headaches.
   - Discuss biofeedback and stress management.
   - Advise patient to avoid caffeine, including coffee, colas, and other carbonated beverages.
   - Start NSAIDs for headache, as needed.
   - If needed next visit, begin prophylactic medication because patient is having more than three migraines per month.

2. **Elevated blood pressure.** Systolic hypertension with wide cuff is present. May be related to obesity, also to anxiety from first visit. No evidence of end-organ damage to retina or heart.

   Plan:

   - Discuss standards for assessing blood pressure.
   - Recheck blood pressure in 1 month, using wide cuff.
   - Review urinalysis.
   - Introduce weight reduction and/or exercise programs (see #4).
   - Reduce salt intake.

3. **Cystocele with occasional stress incontinence.** Cystocele on pelvic examination, probably related to bladder relaxation. Patient is perimenopausal. Incontinence reported with coughing, suggesting alteration in bladder neck anatomy. No dysuria, fever, flank pain. Not taking any contributing medications. Usually involves small amounts of urine, no dribbling, so doubt urge or overflow incontinence.

   Plan:

   - Explain cause of stress incontinence.
   - Review urinalysis.
   - Recommend Kegel's exercises.
   - Consider topical estrogen cream to vagina next visit if no improvement.

4. **Overweight.** Patient 5′2″, weighs 143 lbs. BMI is ~26.

   Plan:

   - Explore diet history, ask patient to keep food intake diary.
   - Explore motivation to lose weight, set target for weight loss by next visit.
   - Schedule visit with dietitian.
   - Discuss exercise program, specifically, walking 30 minutes most days a week.

(continued)

ASSESSMENT AND PLAN FOR MRS. N (Continued)

5. **Family stress.** Son-in-law with alcohol problem; daughter and grandchildren seeking refuge in patient's apartment, leading to tensions in these relationships. Patient also has financial constraints. Stress currently situational. No evidence of major depression at present.

   Plan:

   - Explore patient's views on strategies to cope with sources of stress.
   - Explore sources of support, including Al-Anon for daughter and financial counseling for patient.
   - Continue to monitor for depression.

6. **Occasional musculoskeletal low back pain.** Usually with prolonged standing. No history of trauma or motor vehicle accident. Pain does not radiate; no tenderness or motor-sensory deficits on examination. Doubt disc or nerve root compression, trochanteric bursitis, sacroiliitis.

   Plan:

   - Review benefits of weight loss and exercises to strengthen low back muscles.

7. **Tobacco abuse.** 1 pack per day for 36 years.

   Plan:

   - Check peak flow or FEV_1/FVC on office spirometry.
   - Give strong warning to stop smoking.
   - Offer referral to tobacco cessation program.
   - Offer patch, current treatment to enhance abstinence.

8. **Varicose veins, lower extremities.** No complaints currently.
9. **History of right pyelonephritis, 1982.**
10. **Ampicillin allergy.** Developed rash but no other allergic reaction.
11. **Health maintenance.** Last Pap smear 1998; has never had a mammogram.

    Plan:

    - Teach patient breast self-examination; schedule mammogram.
    - Schedule Pap smear next visit.
    - Provide three stool guaiac cards; next visit discuss screening colonoscopy.
    - Suggest dental care for mild gingivitis.
    - Advise patient to move medications and caustic cleaning agents to locked cabinet, if possible, above shoulder height.

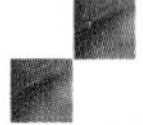

APPROACHING THE CHALLENGES OF CLINICAL DATA

As you can see from the case of Mrs. N, organizing the patient's clinical data poses several challenges. The beginning student must decide whether to cluster the patient's symptoms and signs into one problem or into several problems. The amount of data may appear unmanageable. The quality of the data may be prone to error. Guidelines to help you address these challenges are provided in the following paragraphs.

Clustering Data into Single versus Multiple Problems. One of the greatest difficulties facing students is how to cluster the clinical data. Do selected data fit into one problem or several problems? The patient's *age* may help—young people are more likely to have a single disease, whereas older people tend to have multiple diseases. The *timing* of symptoms is often useful. For example, an episode of pharyngitis 6 weeks ago is probably unrelated to fever, chills, pleuritic chest pain, and cough that prompt an office visit today. To use timing effectively, you need to know the natural history of various diseases and conditions. A yellow penile discharge followed 3 weeks later by a painless penile ulcer suggests two problems: gonorrhea and primary syphilis. In contrast, a penile ulcer followed in 6 weeks by a maculopapular skin rash and generalized lymphadenopathy suggest two stages of the same problem: primary and secondary syphilis.

Involvement of *different body systems* may help you to cluster the clinical data. If symptoms and signs occur in a single system, one disease may explain them. Problems in different, apparently unrelated systems often require more than one explanation. Again, knowledge of disease patterns is necessary. You might decide, for example, to group a patient's high blood pressure and sustained apical impulse together with flame-shaped retinal hemorrhages, place them in the cardiovascular system, and label the constellation "hypertensive cardiovascular disease with hypertensive retinopathy." You would develop another explanation for the patient's mild fever, left lower quadrant tenderness, and diarrhea.

Some diseases involve more than one body system. As you gain knowledge and experience, you will become increasingly adept at recognizing *multisystem conditions* and building plausible explanations that link together their seemingly unrelated manifestations. To explain cough, hemoptysis, and weight loss in a 60-year-old plumber who has smoked cigarettes for 40 years, you probably even now would rank lung cancer high in your differential diagnosis. You might support your diagnosis with your observation of the patient's cyanotic fingernails. With experience and continued reading, you will recognize that his other symptoms and signs can be linked to the same diagnosis. Dysphagia would reflect extension of the cancer to the esophagus, pupillary asymmetry would suggest pressure on the cervical sympathetic chain, and jaundice could result from metastases to the liver.

In another case of multisystem disease, a young man who presents with odynophagia, fever, weight loss, purplish skin lesions, leukoplakia, generalized lymphadenopathy, and chronic diarrhea is likely to have AIDS. Related risk factors should be explored promptly.

Sifting Through an Extensive Array of Data. It is common to confront a relatively long list of symptoms and signs, and an equally long list of potential explanations. One approach is to *tease out separate clusters of observations and analyze one cluster at a time*, as just described. You can also *ask a series of key questions* that may steer your thinking in one direction and allow you to temporarily ignore the others. For example, you may ask what produces and relieves the patient's chest pain. If the answer is exercise and rest, you can focus on the cardiovascular and musculoskeletal systems and set the gastrointestinal system aside. If the pain is substernal, burning, and occurs only after meals, you can logically focus on the gastrointestinal tract. A series of discriminating questions helps you form a decision tree or algorithm that is helpful in collecting and analyzing clinical data and reaching logical conclusions and explanations.

Assessing the Quality of the Data. Almost all clinical information is subject to error. Patients forget to mention symptoms, confuse the events of their illness, avoid recounting facts that are embarrassing, and often slant their stories to what the clinician wants to hear. Clinicians misinterpret patient statements, overlook information, fail to ask "the one key question," jump prematurely to conclusions and diagnoses, or forget an important part of the examination, such as the testicular examination in a young man with asymptomatic testicular carcinoma. You can avoid some of these errors by acquiring the habits of skilled clinicians, summarized below.

TIPS FOR ENSURING THE QUALITY OF PATIENT DATA

- Ask open-ended questions and listen carefully and patiently to the patient's story.
- Craft a thorough and systematic sequence to history taking and physical examination.
- Keep an open mind toward both the patient and the data.
- Always include "the worst-case scenario" in your list of possible explanations of the patient's problem, and make sure it can be safely eliminated.
- Analyze any mistakes in data collection or interpretation.
- Confer with colleagues and review the pertinent medical literature to clarify uncertainties.
- Apply principles of data analysis to patient information and testing.

Symptoms, physical findings, tests, and x-rays should help you reduce uncertainty about whether a patient does or does not have a given condition. Clinical data, including laboratory work, however, are inherently imperfect. You can improve your assessment of clinical data and laboratory tests by applying several key principles for selecting and using clinical data and tests. Learn to apply the principles of *reliability, validity, sensitivity, specificity,* and *predictive value* to your clinical findings and the tests you order. These test characteristics will help you decide how confident you can be of your findings and test results as you assess the presence or absence of a disease or problem.

Displaying Clinical Data. To use these principles, it is important to display the data in the 2 × 2 format diagrammed on the following page. Always using this format will ensure the accuracy of your calculations of sensitivity, specificity, and predictive value. Note that the presence or absence of disease implies use of a *gold standard* to establish whether the disease is truly present or absent. This is usually the best test available, such as a coronary angiogram for assessing coronary artery disease or a tissue biopsy for malignancy.

PRINCIPLES OF TEST SELECTION AND USE

Reliability. Indicates how well repeated measurements of the same relatively stable phenomenon will give the same result, also known as precision. Reliability may be measured for one observer or for more than one observer.

Example: If on several occasions one clinician consistently percusses the same span of a patient's liver dullness, *intraobserver reliability* is good. If, on the other hand, several observers find quite different spans of liver dullness on the same patient, *interobserver reliability* is poor.

Validity. Indicates how closely a given observation agrees with "the true state of affairs," or the best possible measure of reality.

Example: Blood pressure measurements by mercury-based sphygmomanometers are less valid than intra-arterial pressure tracings.

Sensitivity. Identifies the proportion of people who test positive in a group of people known to have the disease or condition, or the proportion of people who are *true positives* compared with the total number of people who actually have the disease. When the observation or test is negative in persons who have the disease, the result is termed *false negative. Good observations or tests have a sensitivity of more than 90%, and help rule out disease because there are few false negatives. Such observations or tests are especially useful for screening.*

Example: The sensitivity of Homan's sign in the diagnosis of deep venous thrombosis (DVT) of the calf is 50%. In other words, compared with a group of patients with deep vein thrombosis confirmed by phlebogram, a much better test, only 50% will have a positive Homan's sign, so this sign, if absent, is not helpful because 50% of patients may have a DVT.

Specificity. Identifies the proportion of people who test negative in a group of people known to be *without* a given disease or condition, or the proportion of people who are "true negatives" compared with the total number of people without the disease. When the observation or test is positive in persons without the disease, the result is termed *false positive.* Good observations or tests have a specificity of more than 90% and help "rule in" disease because the test is rarely positive when disease is absent, and there are few false positives.

Example: The specificity of serum amylase in patients with possible acute pancreatitis is 70%. In other words, of 100 patients without pancreatitis, 70% will have a normal serum amylase; in 30%, the serum amylase will be falsely elevated.

Predictive Value. Indicates how well a given symptom, sign, or test result—either positive or negative—predicts the presence or absence of disease.

(continued)

PRINCIPLES OF TEST SELECTION AND USE (Continued)

Positive predictive value is the probability of disease in a patient with a positive (abnormal) test, or the proportion of "true positives" out of the total population tested.

Example: In a group of women with palpable breast nodules in a cancer screening program, the proportion with confirmed breast cancer would constitute the *positive predictive value* of palpable breast nodules for diagnosing breast cancer.

Negative predictive value is the probability of not having the condition or disease when the test is negative, or normal, or the proportion of "true negatives" out of the total population tested.

Example: In a group of women without palpable breast nodules in a cancer screening program, the proportion without confirmed breast cancer constitutes the *negative predictive value* of absence of breast nodules.

Note that the numbers related to presence or absence of disease, as determined by the gold standard, are always displayed **down the table** in the left and right columns (*present* = *a* + *c*; *absent* = *b* + *d*). Numbers related to the observation or test are always displayed **across the table** in the upper and lower rows (*test positive* = *a* + *b*; *test negative* = *c* + *d*).

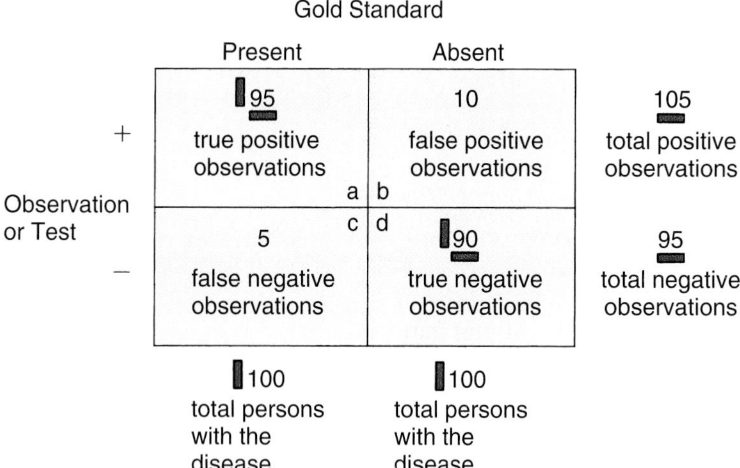

Now you are ready to make your calculations:

$$\textbf{Sensitivity} = \frac{a}{a+c} = \frac{\text{true positive observations (95)}}{\text{total persons with disease }(95+5)} \times 100 = 95\%$$

$$\textbf{Specificity} = \frac{d}{b+d} = \frac{\text{true negative observations (90)}}{\text{total persons with disease }(90+10)} \times 100 = 90\%$$

$$\textbf{Positive predictive value} = \frac{a}{a+b} = \frac{\text{true positive observations (95)}}{\text{total positive observations }(95+10)} \times 100 = 90.5\%$$

$$\textbf{Negative predictive value} = \frac{d}{c+d} = \frac{\text{true negative observations (90)}}{\text{total negative observations }(90+5)} \times 100 = 94.7\%$$

Now return to the table. *The **vertical red bars** designate sensitivity (a/a + c) and specificity (d/b + d), and the **horizontal red bars** designate positive predictive value (a/a + b) and negative predictive value (d/c + d).* The data displayed indicate that the hypothetical test has excellent test characteristics. The sensitivity and specificity of the test are both more than 90%, as are the positive and negative predictive values. Such a test would be clinically useful for assessing a disease or condition in your patient.

Note that the predictive value of a test or observation depends heavily on the *prevalence* of the condition within the population studied. Prevalence is the proportion of people in a defined population at any given point in time who have the condition in question. When the prevalence of a condition is *low*, the positive predictive value of the test will fall. When the prevalence is *high*, the sensitivity, specificity, and positive predictive value are high, and the negative predictive value approaches zero. To work further on these relationships, turn to the tables below on Prevalence and Predictive Value, and practice making the calculations described.

PREVALENCE AND PREDICTIVE VALUE

Two examples further illustrate these principles and show *how predictive values vary with prevalence.* Consider first (*Example 1*) an imaginary population *A* with 1,000 people. The prevalence of disease *X* in this population is high—40%. You can quickly calculate that 400 of these people have *X*. You then set out to detect these cases with an observation or test that is 90% sensitive and 80% specific. Of the 400 people with *X*, the observation reveals .90 × 400, or 360 (the true positives). It misses the other 40 (400 – 360, the false negatives). Out of the 600 people without *X*, the observation or test proves negative in .80 × 600, or 480. These people are truly free of *X*, as the observation suggests (the true negatives). But the observation misleads you in the remaining 120 (600 – 480). These people are falsely labeled as having *X* when they are really free of it (the false positives). These figures are summarized below:

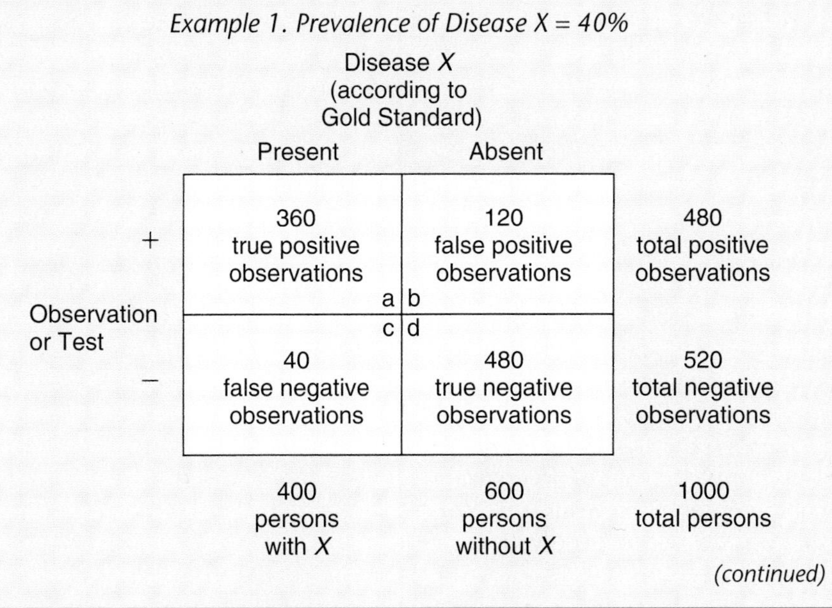

Example 1. Prevalence of Disease X = 40%

		Disease *X* (according to Gold Standard): Present	Disease *X* (according to Gold Standard): Absent	
Observation or Test	+	360 true positive observations (a)	120 false positive observations (b)	480 total positive observations
	–	40 false negative observations (c)	480 true negative observations (d)	520 total negative observations
		400 persons with *X*	600 persons without *X*	1000 total persons

(continued)

PREVALENCE AND PREDICTIVE VALUE (Continued)

As a clinician who does not have perfect knowledge of who really does or does not have disease *X*, you are faced with a total of 480 people with positive observations. You must try to distinguish between the true and the false positives and will undoubtedly use additional kinds of data to help you in this task. Given only the sensitivity and specificity of your observation, however, you can determine the probability that a positive observation is a true positive, and you may wish to explain it to the concerned patient. This probability is calculated as follows:

$$\textit{Positive predictive value} = \frac{a}{a+b} = \frac{\text{true positives (360)}}{\text{total positives (360 + 120)}} \times 100 = 75\%$$

Thus, 3 out of 4 of the people with positive observations really have the disease, and 1 out of 4 does not.

By a similar calculation, you can determine the probability that a negative observation is a true negative. The results here are reasonably reassuring to the involved patient:

$$\textit{Negative predictive value} = \frac{d}{c+d} = \frac{\text{true negatives (480)}}{\text{total negatives (40 + 480)}} \times 100 = 92\%$$

As *prevalence* of the disease in a population diminishes, however, the predictive value of a positive observation diminishes remarkably, while the predictive value of a negative observation rises further. In *Example 2,* in a second population, *B,* of 1,000 people, only 1% have disease *X*. Now there are only 10 cases of *X* and 990 people without *X*. If this population is screened with the same observation, which has a 90% sensitivity and an 80% specificity, here are the results:

Example 2. Prevalence of Disease X = 1%

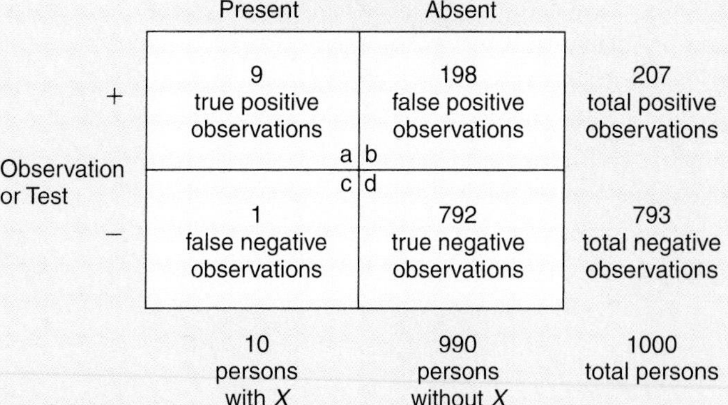

Observation or Test	Disease *X* (according to Gold Standard): Present	Absent	
+	9 true positive observations (a)	198 false positive observations (b)	207 total positive observations
−	1 false negative observations (c)	792 true negative observations (d)	793 total negative observations
	10 persons with *X*	990 persons without *X*	1000 total persons

You are now confronted with possibly upsetting 207 people (all those with positive observations) to detect 9 out of the 10 real cases. The predictive value of a positive observation is only 4%. Improving the specificity of your observation without diminishing its sensitivity would be very helpful, if it were possible. For example, if you could increase the specificity of the observation from 80% to 98% (given the same prevalence of 1% and sensitivity of 90%), the positive predictive value of the observation would improve from 4% to 31%—scarcely ideal but certainly better. Good observations or tests have a sensitivity and specificity of 90%.

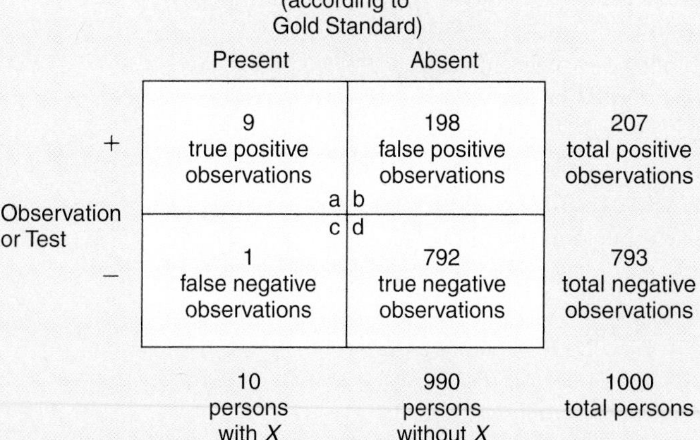

Because prevalence strongly affects the predictive value of an observation, prevalence too influences the assessment process. Because coronary artery disease is much more common in middle-aged men than in young women, you should pursue angina as a cause of chest pain more actively in the former group. The effect of prevalence on predictive value explains why your odds of making a correct assessment are better when you hypothesize a common condition rather than a rare one. The combination of fever, headache, myalgias, and cough probably has the same sensitivity and specificity for influenza throughout the year, but your chance of making this diagnosis correctly by using this cluster of symptoms is much greater during a winter flu epidemic than it is during a quiet August.

Prevalence varies importantly with clinical setting as well as with season. Chronic bronchitis is probably the most common cause of hemoptysis among patients seen in a general medical clinic. In the oncology clinic of a tertiary medical center, however, lung cancer might head the list, while in a group of postoperative patients on a general surgical service, irritation from an endotracheal tube or pulmonary infarction might be most likely. In certain parts of Asia, in contrast, one should think first of a worm called a lung fluke. When you hear hoofbeats in the distance, according to the familiar saying, bet on horses, not on zebras, unless, of course, you're visiting the zoo.

BUILDING YOUR CASE: INTEGRATING CLINICAL REASONING AND ASSESSMENT OF CLINICAL DATA

The concepts of sensitivity and specificity help in both the collection and analysis of data. They even underlie some of the basic strategies of interviewing. Questions with high sensitivity, if answered in the affirmative, may be particularly useful for screening and for gathering evidence to support a hypothesis. For example, "Have you had any discomfort or pain in your chest?" is a highly sensitive question for diagnosing angina pectoris. For patients with this condition, there would be few false-negative responses. Thus, it is a good first screening question. However, because there are many other causes of chest discomfort, it is not all that specific. Pain that is retrosternal, pressing, and less than 10 minutes in duration—each a reasonably sensitive attribute of angina—would add importantly to your growing evidence for the diagnosis. To confirm your hypothesis, a more specific question, if answered in the affirmative, is needed, such as "Is the pain precipitated by exertion?" or "Is the pain relieved by rest?"

Data for testing hypotheses also come from the physical examination. Heart murmurs are good examples of findings with varying sensitivity and specificity. The vast majority of patients with significant valvular *aortic stenosis* have systolic ejection murmurs audible in the aortic area. Presence of a systolic murmur has a high sensitivity for aortic stenosis. This finding is present in most cases. The false-negative rate is low. On the other hand, many other conditions produce systolic murmurs, such as increased blood flow across a normal valve, or the sclerotic changes associated with aging, termed aortic sclerosis, so the finding of a systolic murmur is not very specific. Using such a murmur as your only criterion for diagnosing aortic stenosis would lead to many false positives.

In contrast, a high-pitched, soft blowing decrescendo diastolic murmur best heard along the left sternal border is quite specific for *aortic regurgitation*. Such a murmur is almost never heard in normal people, and it is present in very few other conditions, so there are few false positives.

Combining data from the history and physical examination allows you to test your hypotheses, screen for selected conditions, build your case, and clinch a diagnosis even before obtaining further diagnostic tests. Consider the following list of evidence: cough, fever, a shaking chill, left-sided pleuritic chest pain, dullness throughout the left lower posterior lung field with crackles, bronchial breathing, and egophony. Cough and fever are good screening items for pneumonia, the next items support the hypothesis, and bronchial breathing with egophony in this distribution is very specific for lobar pneumonia. A chest x-ray would confirm the diagnosis.

Absence of selected symptoms and signs is also diagnostically useful, especially when they are usually present in a given condition (i.e., their sensitivity is high). For example, if a patient with cough and left-sided pleuritic chest pain does not have fever, bacterial pneumonia becomes much less likely (except possibly in infancy and old age). Likewise, in a patient with severe dyspnea, the absence of orthopnea makes left ventricular failure less probable as an explanation for shortness of breath.

Skilled clinicians use this kind of logic even if they are unaware of its statistical underpinnings. They start to generate tentative hypotheses as soon as the patient describes the *Chief Complaint,* then build evidence for one or more of these hypotheses and discard others as they continue with the history and examination. In developing a *Present Illness,* they borrow items from other parts of the history, such as the *Past Medical History,* the *Family History,* and the *Review of Systems.* In a 55-year-old man with chest pain, the skilled clinician does not stop with the attributes of pain, but moves on to probe risk factors from coronary artery disease such as family history, hypertension, diabetes, lipid abnormalities, and smoking. In both the history and physical examination, the clinician searches explicitly for other possible manifestations of cardiovascular disease such as congestive heart failure or the claudication or diminished lower extremity pulses of atherosclerotic peripheral vascular disease. By generating hypotheses early and testing them sequentially, experienced clinicians improve their efficiency and enhance the relevance and value of the data they collect. They dig and collect less ore but find more gold.

This sequence of collecting data and testing hypotheses is diagrammed below.

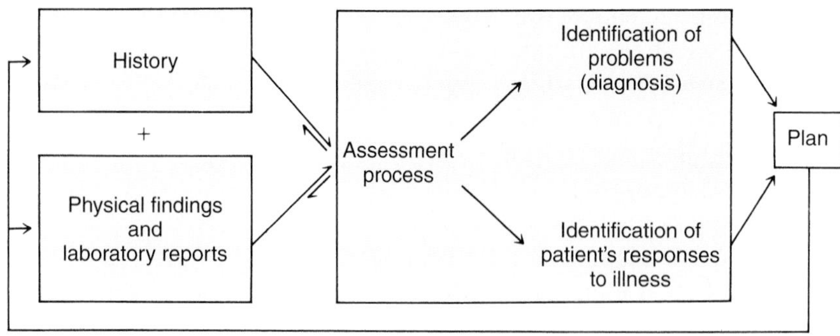

After the plan has been implemented, the process recycles. The clinician gathers more data, assesses the patient's progress, modifies the problem list if indicated, and adjusts the plan accordingly. As you gain experience, the interplay of assessment and data collection will become increasingly familiar. You will come to value the challenges and rewards of clinical reasoning and assessment that make patient care so meaningful.

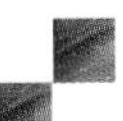

ORGANIZING THE PATIENT RECORD

A clear, well-organized clinical record is one of the most important adjuncts to your patient care. Your skill in recording your patient's history and physical examination should evolve in parallel with your growing skills in clinical reasoning and your ability to formulate the patient's *Assessment* and *Plan*. Your goal should be a clear, concise, but comprehensive report that documents the key findings of your patient assessment and communicates the patient's problems in a succinct and *legible* format to other providers and members of the health care team. Note that a good record provides the supporting data for the problems or diagnoses identified.

Regardless of your experience, certain principles will help you to organize a good record. Think especially about the *order and readability* of the record and the *amount of detail* needed. How much detail to include often poses a vexing problem. As a student, you may wish (or you may be required) to be quite detailed. This helps to build your descriptive skills, vocabulary, and speed—admittedly a painful and tedious process. Pressures of time, however, will ultimately force some compromises.

Run through the following checklist to make sure your record is clear, informative, and easy to follow.

CHECKLIST FOR YOUR PATIENT RECORD

Is the order clear?

Order is imperative. Make sure that future readers, including yourself, can easily find specific points of information. Keep the *subjective* items of the history, for example, in the history; do not let them stray into the physical examination. Did you . . .

- Make the headings clear?
- Accent your organization with indentations and spacing?
- Arrange the *Present Illness* in chronologic order, starting with the current episode, then filling in relevant background information?

Do the data included contribute directly to the assessment?

You should spell out the supporting data—both positive and negative—for every problem or diagnosis that you identify.

(continued)

CHECKLIST FOR YOUR PATIENT RECORD (Continued)

Are pertinent negatives specifically described?

Often portions of the history or examination suggest that an abnormality might exist or develop in that area.

For the patient with notable bruises, record the "pertinent negatives," such as the absence of injury or violence, familial bleeding disorders, or medications or nutritional deficits that might lead to bruising.

For the patient who is depressed but not suicidal, record both facts. In the patient with a transient mood swing, on the other hand, a comment on suicide is unnecessary.

Are there overgeneralizations or omissions of important data?

Remember that data not recorded are data lost. No matter how vividly you can recall selected details today, you will probably not remember them in a few months. The phrase "neurologic exam negative," even in your own handwriting, may leave you wondering in a few months' time, "Did I really do the sensory exam?"

Is there too much detail?

Avoid burying important information in a mass of excessive detail, to be discovered by only the most persistent reader. *Omit most of your negative findings* unless they relate directly to the patient's complaints or to specific exclusions in your diagnostic assessment. *Do not list abnormalities that you did not observe. Instead, concentrate on a few major ones, such as* "no heart murmurs," and try to describe structures in a concise, positive way. You can omit certain body structures even though you examined them, such as normal eyebrows and eyelashes.

"Cervix pink and smooth" indicates you saw no redness, ulcers, nodules, masses, cysts or other suspicious lesions, but this description is shorter and readable.

Are phrases and short words used appropriately? Is there unnecessary repetition of data?

Omit unnecessary words, such as those in parentheses in the examples. This saves valuable time and space.

"Cervix is pink (in color)." "Lungs are resonant (to percussion)." "Liver is tender (to palpation)." "Both (right and left) ears with cerumen." "II/IV systolic ejection murmur (audible)." "Thorax symmetric (bilaterally)."

Omit repetitive introductory phrases such as "The patient reports no . . . " because readers assume the patient is the source of the history unless otherwise specified.
Use short words instead of longer, fancier ones when they mean the same thing, such as "felt" for "palpated" or "heard" for "auscultated."

(continued)

CHECKLIST FOR YOUR PATIENT RECORD (Continued)

Describe what you observed, not what you did. "Optic discs seen" is less informative than "disc margins sharp," even if it marks your first glimpse as an examiner!

Is the written style succinct? Is there excessive use of abbreviations?

Records are scientific and legal documents, so they should be clear and understandable.

Using words and brief phrases instead of whole sentences is common, but abbreviations and symbols should be used only if they are readily understood.

Likewise, an overly elegant style is less appealing than a concise summary.

Be sure your record is legible, otherwise, all that you have recorded is worthless to your readers.

Are diagrams and precise measurements included where appropriate?

Diagrams add greatly to the clarity of the record.

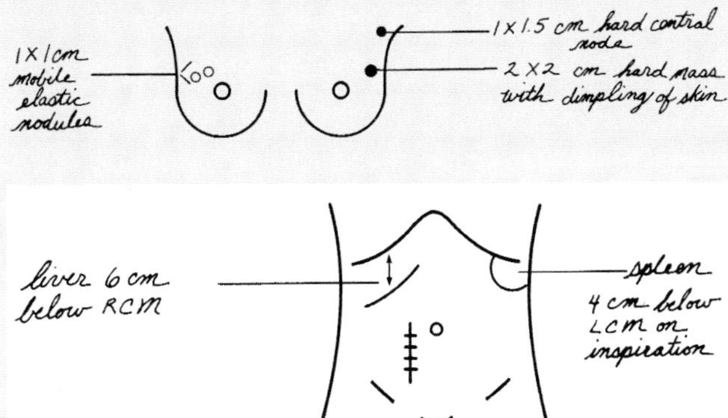

To ensure accurate evaluations and future comparisons, make measurements in centimeters, not in fruits, nuts, or vegetables.

"1 × 1 cm lymph node" versus a "pea-sized lymph node . . ." Or "2 × 2 cm mass on the left lobe of the prostate" versus a "walnut-sized prostate mass."

Is the tone of the write-up neutral and professional?

It is important to be objective. Hostile, moralizing, or disapproving comments have no place in the patient's record. Never use inflammatory or demeaning words, penmanship, or punctuation.

Comments such as "Patient DRUNK and LATE TO CLINIC AGAIN!!" are unprofessional and set a bad example for other providers reading the chart. They also might prove difficult to defend in a legal setting.

Your institution or agency may have printed forms for recording patient information, but you should always be able to create your own record. The record of Mrs. N may be longer than what you might see in patient charts, yet it still does not reflect every question and technique that you have learned to use. The amount of detail varies, depending on the patient's symptoms and signs and the complexity of the clinician's diagnoses and plans for management.

Generating the Problem List. Once you have completed your assessment and written record, you will find it helpful to generate a *Problem List* that summarizes the patient's problems for the front of the office or hospital chart. *List the most active and serious problems first, and record their date of onset.* Some clinicians make separate lists for active or inactive problems; others make one list in order of priority. You will find that on follow-up visits the *Problem List* helps you remember to check the status of problems the patient may not mention. The *Problem List* also allows other members of the health care team to review the patient's health status at a glance.

A sample *Problem List* for Mrs. N is provided below. You may wish to give each problem a number and use the number when referring to specific problems in subsequent notes.

SAMPLE PROBLEM LIST

Date Entered	Problem No.	Problem
1/30/06	1	Migraine headaches
	2	Elevated blood pressure
	3	Cystocele with occasional stress incontinence
	4	Overweight
	5	Family stress
	6	Low back pain
	7	Tobacco abuse
	8	Varicose veins
	9	History of right pyelonephritis
	10	Allergy to ampicillin
	11	Health maintenance

Clinicians organize problem lists differently, even for the same patient. Your problem list for Mrs. N may look somewhat different from the one above. Note that problems can be symptoms, signs, or conditions. Good lists vary in emphasis, length, and detail, depending on the clinician's philosophy, specialty, and role as a provider. The list illustrated here includes problems that need attention now, such as the headaches, as well as problems that need future observation or attention, such as the blood pressure and cystocele. Listing the allergy to ampicillin warns you not to prescribe medications in the penicillin family.

Some of the items noted in the history and physical examination, such as the canker sores and hard stools, do not appear in this problem list because they are relatively common phenomena that do not currently demand attention. Such judgments may prove to be wrong; however, problem lists that are cluttered with relatively insignificant items diminish in value. Some clinicians would find this list too long; others would be more explicit about such problems as "family stress" or "varicose veins."

Writing the Progress Note. A month later, Mrs. N returns for a follow-up visit. The style of the progress note is also quite variable, but it should follow the same standards as the initial assessment. It should be clear, sufficiently detailed, and easy to follow. It should reflect your clinical thinking and delineate your assessment and plan. The following note follows the SOAP note format (**S**ubjective, **O**bjective, **A**ssessment, and **P**lan), but you will see many other styles and interest in making more "patient-centered" medical records.[7] Often clinicians record the history and physical examination, then give each patient problem *Assessment* and *Plan*.

SAMPLE SOAP NOTE

1. Migraine headaches.
   S: Has had only two headaches, both mild and without associated symptoms. These are less troubling. Cannot detect any precipitating factors.
   O: No tenderness over the temporal muscles. No papilledema.
   A: Headaches improved, now without migraine features.
   P: Call if symptoms recur.

CLINICAL ASSESSMENT: THE JOURNEY TO EXCELLENCE

The process of learning about a patient continues far beyond the first few encounters. Your understanding of patient care will grow in depth and complexity throughout your clinical career. Your prowess in history taking, physical examination, clinical reasoning, evidence-based decision-making, and documenting the patient record is launched. Now you must embark on repetitive practice, with supervision, and on the lifelong pursuit of polishing your newly acquired skills.

Bibliography

CITATIONS

1. Peterson MC, Holbrook JH, Von Hales DE, et al. Contributions of the history, physical examination, and laboratory investigation in making medical diagnoses. West J Med 156:163–165, 1992.
2. Hampton JR, Harrison MJ, Mitchell JRA, et al. Relative contributions of history-taking, physical examination, and laboratory investigation to diagnosis and management of medical outpatients. BMJ 2:486–489, 1975.
3. McGee S. Evidence-Based Physical Diagnosis. Philadelphia: WB Saunders, 2001.
4. Schneiderman H. Bedside Diagnosis. An Annotated Bibliography of Literature on Physical Examination and Interviewing, 3rd ed. Philadelphia: American College of Physicians, 1997.
5. Evidence-Based Medicine Working Group. Evidence-based medicine: a new approach to teaching the practice of medicine. JAMA 268(17)2420–2425, 1992. [Launched the Rational Clinical Examination Series.]
6. Guyatt G, Rennie D. Users' Guides to the Medical Literature: A Manual for Evidence-Based Clinical Practice. Chicago: American Medical Association, 2001.
7. Donnelly WJ. Viewpoint: Patient-centered medical care requires a patient-centered medical record. Acad Med 80(1):33–38, 2005.

ADDITIONAL REFERENCES

Alfaro-LeFevre R. Critical Thinking and Clinical Judgment: A Practical Approach, 3rd ed. St. Louis, WB Saunders, 2004.

Carpenito LJ. Nursing Diagnosis: Application to Clinical Practice, 11th ed. Philadelphia, Lippincott Williams & Wilkins, 2005.

Cherry B, Jacob SR. Contemporary Nursing: Issues, Trends, and Management, 3rd ed. St. Louis, Elsevier Mosby, 2005.

Fletcher RH, Fletcher, SW. Clinical Epidemiology: The Essentials, 4th ed. Philadelphia, Lippincott Williams & Wilkins, 2005.

Innui TS. Establishing the doctor–patient relationship: science, art, or competence? Schweiz Med Wochenschr 128:225, 1998.

Laditka JN, Laditka SB, Mastanduno MP. Hospital utilization for ambulatory care sensitive conditions: health outcome disparities associated with race and ethnicity. Soc Sci Med 57(8):1429–1441, 2003.

Nettina SM. The Lippincott Manual of Nursing Practice, 7th ed. Philadelphia, Lippincott Williams & Wilkins, 2001.

Panzer RJ, Bordley DR, Cappuccio J, et al (eds). Diagnostic Strategies in Common Medical Problems, 3rd ed. Philadelphia: American College of Physicians, 2006.

Sackett DL. Evidence-based Medicine: How to Practice and Teach EBM, 2nd ed. New York, Churchill Livingstone, 2000.

UNIT

II

Regional Examinations

CHAPTER

4

Beginning the Physical Examination: General Survey and Vital Signs

Once you understand the patient's concerns and have elicited a careful history, you are ready to begin the physical examination. At first you may feel unsure of how the patient will relate to you. With practice, your skills in physical examination will grow, and you will gain confidence. Through study and repetition, the examination will flow more smoothly, and you will soon shift your attention from technique and how to handle instruments to what you hear, see, and feel. Touching the patient's body will seem more natural, and you will learn to minimize any discomfort to the patient. You will become more responsive to the patient's reactions and provide reassurance when needed. Before long, as you gain proficiency, what once took between 1 and 2 hours will take considerably less time.

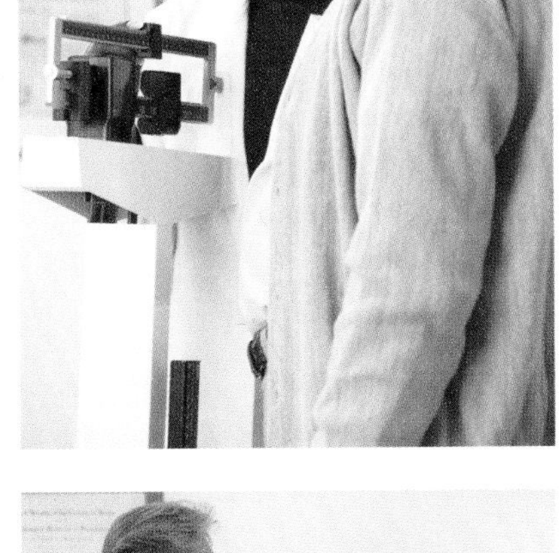

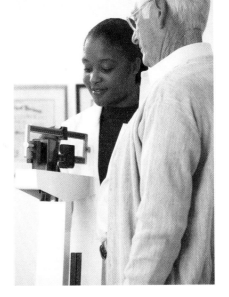

This chapter addresses skills and techniques needed for initial assessment as you begin the physical examination. Under Anatomy and Physiology, you will find information on how to measure height, weight, and Body Mass Index (BMI) and guidelines for nutritional assessment. There is clinical information on the relevant health history and on health promotion and counseling. The section on Techniques of Examination describes the initial steps of the physical examination: preparing for the examination, conducting the general survey, and taking the vital signs. Then follows an example of the written record relevant to the general survey and vital signs.

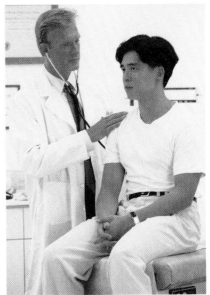

ANATOMY AND PHYSIOLOGY

As you begin the physical examination, you will survey the patient's general appearance and measure the patient's height and weight. These data provide information about the patient's nutritional status and amount of body fat. Body fat consists primarily of adipose in the form of triglyceride and is stored in subcutaneous, intra-abdominal, and intramuscular fat deposits. These stores are inaccessible and difficult to measure, so it will be important to compare your measurements of height and weight with standardized ranges of normal.

In the past, tables of desirable weight-for-height have been based on life insurance data, which often did not adjust for the effects of smoking and selected weight-inducing medical conditions such as diabetes and which tended to overstate desirable weight. Current practice, however, is to use the *Body Mass Index,* which incorporates estimated but more accurate measures of body fat than weight alone. BMI standards are derived from two surveys: the National Health Examination Survey, consisting of three survey cycles between 1960 and 1970, and the National Health and Nutrition Examination Survey, with three cycles from the 1970s to the 1990s.

More than half of U.S. adults are overweight (BMI >25), and nearly one fourth are obese (BMI >30), so assessing and educating patients about their BMI are vital for promoting health. These conditions are proven risk factors for diabetes, heart disease, stroke, hypertension, osteoarthritis, sleep apnea syndrome, and some forms of cancer. Remember that these BMI criteria are not rigid cutpoints but guidelines for increasing risks for health and well-being. Note that people older than age 65 have a disproportionate risk for undernutrition when compared with younger adults.

Height and weight in childhood and adolescence reflect the many behavioral, cognitive, and physiologic changes of growth and development. Developmental milestones, markers for growth spurts, and sexual maturity ratings can be found in Chapter 18, Assessing Children: Infancy Through Adolescence. With aging, some of these changes reverse, as described in Chapter 20, The Older Adult. Height may decrease, posture may become more stooping from kyphosis of the thoracic spine, and extension of the knees and hips may diminish. The abdominal muscles may relax, changing the abdominal contour, and fat may accumulate at the hips and lower abdomen. Be alert to these changes as you assess older patients.

Calculating the BMI. There are several ways to calculate the BMI, as shown in the accompanying table. Choose the method most suited to your practice. The National Institutes of Health and the National Heart, Lung, and Blood Institute caution that people who are very muscular may have a high BMI but still be healthy.[1] Likewise, the BMI for people with low muscle mass and reduced nutrition may appear inappropriately "normal."

If the BMI is 35 or higher, measure the patient's *waist circumference.* With the patient standing, measure the waist just above the hip bones. The patient may have excess body fat if the waist measures:

- ≥35 inches for women
- ≥40 inches for men

■ Methods to Calculate Body Mass Index (BMI)

Unit of Measure	Method of Calculation
Weight *in pounds*, height *in inches*	(1) Body Mass Index Chart (see table below)
	(2) $\dfrac{\left(\dfrac{\text{Weight (lbs)} \times 700^{*}}{\text{Height (inches)}}\right)}{\text{Height (inches)}}$
Weight *in kilograms*, height *in meters squared*	(3) $\dfrac{\text{Weight (kg)}}{\text{Height }(\text{m}^2)}$
Either	(4) "BMI Calculator" at website www.nhlbisupport.com/bmi/bmicalc.htm

*Several organizations use 704.5, but the variation in BMI is negligible. Conversion formulas: 2.2 lbs = 1 kg; 1.0 inch = 2.54 cm; 100 cm = 1 meter.

Source: National Institutes of Health and National Heart, Lung, and Blood Institute: Body Mass Index Calculator. Available at: http://www.nhlbisupport.com/bmi/bmicalc.htm. Accessed December 12, 2004.

■ Body Mass Index Table

	Normal						Overweight					Obese									
BMI	19	20	21	22	23	24	25	26	27	28	29	30	31	32	33	34	35	36	37	38	39
Height (inches)	Body Weight (pounds)																				
58	91	96	100	105	110	115	119	124	129	134	138	143	148	153	158	162	167	172	177	181	186
59	94	99	104	109	114	119	124	128	133	138	143	148	153	158	163	168	173	178	183	188	193
60	97	102	107	112	118	123	128	133	138	143	148	153	158	163	168	174	179	184	189	194	199
61	100	106	111	116	122	127	132	137	143	148	153	158	164	169	174	180	185	190	195	201	206
62	104	109	115	120	126	131	136	142	147	153	158	164	169	175	180	186	191	196	202	207	213
63	107	113	118	124	130	135	141	146	152	158	163	169	175	180	186	191	197	203	208	214	220
64	110	116	122	128	134	140	145	151	157	163	169	174	180	186	192	197	204	209	215	221	227
65	114	120	126	132	138	144	150	156	162	168	174	180	186	192	198	204	210	216	222	228	234
66	118	124	130	136	142	148	155	161	167	173	179	186	192	198	204	210	216	223	229	235	241
67	121	127	134	140	146	153	159	166	172	178	185	191	198	204	211	217	223	230	236	242	249
68	125	131	138	144	151	158	164	171	177	184	190	197	203	210	216	223	230	236	243	249	256
69	128	135	142	149	155	162	169	176	182	189	196	203	209	216	223	230	236	243	250	257	263
70	132	139	146	153	160	167	174	181	188	195	202	209	216	222	229	236	243	250	257	264	271
71	136	143	150	157	165	172	179	186	193	200	208	215	222	229	236	243	250	257	265	272	279
72	140	147	154	162	169	177	184	191	199	206	213	221	228	235	242	250	258	265	272	279	287
73	144	151	159	166	174	182	189	197	204	212	219	227	235	242	250	257	265	272	280	288	295
74	148	155	163	171	179	186	194	202	210	218	225	233	241	249	256	264	272	280	287	295	303
75	152	160	168	176	184	192	200	208	216	224	232	240	248	256	264	272	279	287	295	303	311
76	156	164	172	180	189	197	205	213	221	230	238	246	254	263	271	279	287	295	304	312	320

Source: Adapted from National Institutes of Health and National Heart, Lung, and Blood Institute: Clinical Guidelines on the Identification, Evaluation and Treatment of Overweight and Obesity in Adults: The Evidence Report. June 1998. Available at: www.nhlbi.nih.gov/guidelines/obesity/ob_gdlns.pdf. Accessed December 12, 2004.

Interpreting and Acting on the BMI. Classify the BMI according to the national guidelines in the table below. If the BMI is *above 25*, assess the patient for *additional risk factors* for heart disease and other obesity-related diseases: hypertension, high LDL cholesterol, low HDL cholesterol, high triglycerides, high blood glucose, family history of premature heart disease, physical inactivity, and cigarette smoking. Patients with a BMI over 25 and two or more risk factors should pursue weight loss, especially if the waist circumference is elevated.

Classification of Overweight and Obesity by BMI

	Obesity Class	BMI (kg/m^2)
Underweight		<18.5
Normal		18.5–24.9
Overweight		25.0–29.9
Obesity	I	30.0–34.9
	II	35.0–39.9
Extreme obesity	III	≥40

Source: National Institutes of Health and National Heart, Lung, and Blood Institute: Clinical Guidelines on the Identification, Evaluation, and Treatment of Overweight and Obesity in Adults: The Evidence Report. NIH Publication 98-4083. June 1998.

Assessing Dietary Intake. Advising patients about diet and weight loss is important, especially in light of the many, often contradictory dieting options in the popular press. Review three excellent guidelines for counseling your patients:

See Table 4-1, Healthy Eating: Food Groups and Servings per Day, p. 115. For screening tools, see Table 4-2, Rapid Screen for Dietary Intake, p. 115, and Table 4-4, Nutrition Screening Checklist, p. 117.

- National Institutes of Health and National Heart, Lung, and Blood Institute: Clinical Guidelines on the Identification, Evaluation, and Treatment of Overweight and Obesity in Adults: The Evidence Report. September 1998. Available at: www.nhlbi.nih.gov/guidelines/obesity/ob_gdlns.pdf.[1]
- U.S. Preventive Services Task Force: Screening for Obesity in Adults: Recommendations and Rationale. November 2003. Available at: www.ahrq.gov/clinic/3rduspstf/obesity/obesrr.htm.[2]
- Department of Health and Human Services and the U.S. Department of Agriculture: Nutrition and Your Health. January 2005. Available at: www.health.gov/dietaryguidelines/dga2005/report/.[3]

Diet recommendations hinge on assessment of the patient's motivation and readiness to lose weight and individual risk factors. The *Clinical Guidelines on the Identification, Evaluation, and Treatment of Overweight and Obesity in Adults*[1] recommend the following general guidelines:

- A 10% weight reduction over 6 months, or a decrease of 300 to 500 kcal/day, for people with BMIs between 27 and 35

- A weight loss goal of ½ to 1 pound per week because more rapid weight loss does not lead to better results at 1 year.[1]

These guidelines recommend low-calorie diets of 800 to 1500 kcal per day. Interventions that combine nutrition education, diet, and moderate exercise with behavioral strategies are most likely to succeed (see pp. 95–97). The *Clinical Guidelines* cite evidence supporting the role of moderate physical activity in weight loss and weight loss maintenance programs: it enhances and may assist with maintenance of weight; it increases cardiorespiratory fitness; and it may decrease abdominal fat.

If the BMI falls *below 18.5*, be concerned about possible anorexia nervosa, bulimia, or other medical conditions. These conditions are summarized in Table 4-3, Eating Disorders and Excessively Low BMI, p. 116. (See also pp. 95–97 for health promotion and counseling for overweight or underweight patients.)

THE HEALTH HISTORY

Common or Concerning Symptoms

- Changes in weight
- Fatigue and weakness
- Fever, chills, night sweats

Changes in Weight. Changes in weight result from changes in body tissues or body fluid. Good opening questions include "How often do you check your weight?" "How is it compared to a year ago?" For changes, ask, "Why do you think it has changed?" "What would you like to weigh?" If weight gain or loss appears to be a problem, ask about the amount of change, its timing, the setting in which it occurred, and any associated symptoms.

Rapid changes in weight (over a few days) suggest changes in body fluids, not tissues.

Weight gain occurs when caloric intake exceeds caloric expenditure over time and typically appears as increased body fat. Weight gain may also reflect abnormal accumulation of body fluids. When the retention of fluid is relatively mild, it may not be visible, but several pounds of fluid usually appear as *edema*.

In the overweight patient, for example, when did the weight gain begin? Was the patient heavy as an infant or a child? Using milestones appropriate to the patient's age, inquire about weight at the following times: birth, kindergarten, high school or college graduation, discharge from military service, marriage, after each pregnancy, menopause, and retirement. What were the patient's life circumstances during the periods of weight gain? Has the patient tried to lose weight? How? With what results?

Weight loss is an important symptom with many causes. Mechanisms include one or more of the following: decreased intake of food for reasons such as anorexia, dysphagia, vomiting, and insufficient supplies of food; defective absorption of nutrients through the gastrointestinal tract; increased metabolic requirements; and loss of nutrients through the urine, feces, or injured skin. A person may also lose weight when a fluid-retaining state improves or responds to treatment.

Causes of weight loss include gastrointestinal diseases; endocrine disorders (diabetes mellitus, hyperthyroidism, adrenal insufficiency); chronic infections; malignancy; chronic cardiac, pulmonary, or renal failure; depression; and anorexia nervosa or bulimia (see Table 4-3, Eating Disorders and Excessively Low BMI, p. 116).

Try to determine whether the drop in weight is proportional to any change in food intake, or whether it has remained normal or even increased.

Weight loss with relatively high food intake suggests diabetes mellitus, hyperthyroidism, or malabsorption. Consider also binge eating (bulimia) with clandestine vomiting.

Symptoms associated with weight loss often suggest a cause, as does a good psychosocial history. Who cooks and shops for the patient? Where does the patient eat? With whom? Are there any problems with obtaining, storing, preparing, or chewing food? Does the patient avoid or restrict certain foods for medical, religious, or other reasons?

Poverty, old age, social isolation, physical disability, emotional or mental impairment, lack of teeth, ill-fitting dentures, alcoholism, and drug abuse increase the likelihood of malnutrition.

Throughout the history, be alert for signs of malnutrition. Symptoms may be subtle and nonspecific, such as weakness, easy fatigability, cold intolerance, flaky dermatitis, and ankle swelling. Securing a good history of eating patterns and quantities is mandatory. It is important to ask general questions about intake at different times throughout the day, such as "Tell me what you typically eat for lunch." "What do you eat for a snack?" "When?"

See Table 4-4, Nutrition Screening Checklist, p. 117.

Fatigue and Weakness. Like weight loss, *fatigue* is a nonspecific symptom with many causes. It refers to a sense of weariness or loss of energy that patients describe in various ways. "I don't feel like getting up in the morning" . . . "I don't have any energy" . . . "I just feel blah". . . "I'm all done in" . . . "I can hardly get through the day" . . . "By the time I get to the office I feel as if I've done a day's work." Because fatigue is a normal response to hard work, sustained stress, or grief, try to elicit the life circumstances in which it occurs. Fatigue unrelated to such situations requires further investigation.

Fatigue is a common symptom of depression and anxiety states, but also consider infections (such as hepatitis, infectious mononucleosis, and tuberculosis); endocrine disorders (hypothyroidism, adrenal insufficiency, diabetes mellitus, panhypopituitarism); heart failure; chronic disease of the lungs, kidneys, or liver; electrolyte imbalance; moderate to severe anemia; malignancies; nutritional deficits; and medications.

Use open-ended questions to explore the attributes of the patient's fatigue, and encourage the patient to fully describe what he or she is experiencing. Important clues about etiology often emerge from a good psychosocial history, exploration of sleep patterns, and a thorough review of systems.

Weakness is different from fatigue. It denotes a demonstrable loss of muscle power and will be discussed later with other neurologic symptoms (see pp. 608–609).

Weakness, especially if localized in a neuroanatomic pattern, suggests possible neuropathy or myopathy.

Fever, Chills and Night Sweats. *Fever* refers to an abnormal elevation in body temperature (see p. 112 for definitions of normal). Ask about fever if patients have an acute or chronic illness. Find out whether the patient has used a thermometer to measure the temperature. Bear in mind that errors in technique can lead to unreliable information. Has the patient felt feverish or unusually hot, noted excessive sweating, or felt chilly and cold? Try to distinguish between subjective *chilliness,* and a *shaking chill* with shivering throughout the body and chattering of teeth.

Recurrent shaking chills suggest more extreme swings in temperature and systemic bacteremia.

Feeling cold, goosebumps, and shivering accompany a rising temperature, while feeling hot and sweating accompany a falling temperature. Normally the body temperature rises during the day and falls during the night. When fever exaggerates this swing, *night sweats* occur. Malaise, headache, and pain in the muscles and joints often accompany fever.

Feelings of heat and sweating also accompany menopause. Night sweats occur in tuberculosis and malignancy.

Fever has many causes. Focus your questions on the timing of the illness and its associated symptoms. Become familiar with patterns of infectious diseases that may affect your patient. Inquire about travel, contact with sick people, or other unusual exposures. Be sure to inquire about medications because they may cause fever. In contrast, recent ingestion of aspirin, acetaminophen, corticosteroids, and nonsteroidal anti-inflammatory drugs may mask fever and affect the temperature recorded at the time of the physical examination.

HEALTH PROMOTION AND COUNSELING

Important Topics for Health Promotion and Counseling

- Optimal weight and nutrition
- Exercise
- Blood pressure and diet

Optimal Weight and Nutrition. Less than half of U.S. adults maintain a healthy weight (BMI ≥19 but ≤25). Obesity has increased in every segment of the population, regardless of age, gender, ethnicity, or socioeconomic group. More than half of people with non-insulin-dependent diabetes and roughly 20% of those with hypertension or elevated cholesterol are overweight or obese. Increasing obesity in children has been linked to rising rates of childhood diabetes. Once you detect excess weight or unhealthy nutritional patterns, take advantage of the excellent materials available to promote weight loss and good nutrition. Even reducing weight by

5% to 10% can improve blood pressure, lipid levels, and glucose tolerance and reduce the risk for developing diabetes or hypertension.

Once you have assessed food intake, nutritional status, and motivation to adopt healthy eating behaviors or lose weight, give patients the "nine major messages" of the 2005 Dietary Guidelines Advisory Committee to the Secretaries of HHS and USDA, as summarized and adapted below[3]:

See Table 4-1, Healthy Eating: Food Groups and Servings per Day, p. 115.

- Consume a variety of foods within and among the basic food groups while staying within energy needs.
- Control calorie intake and portion size to manage body weight.
- Maintain moderate physical activity for at least 30 minutes each day, for example, walking 3 to 4 miles per hour.
- Increase daily intake of fruits and vegetables, whole grains, and nonfat or low-fat milk and milk products.
- Choose fats wisely, keeping intake of saturated fat, *trans* fat found in partially hydrogenated vegetable oils, and cholesterol low.
- Choose carbohydrates—sugars, starches, and fibers—wisely for good health.
- Choose and prepare foods with little salt.
- If you drink alcoholic beverages, do so in moderation.
- Keep food safe to eat.

Be prepared to help adolescent females and women of childbearing age increase intake of iron and folic acid. Assist adults older than age 50 to identify foods rich in vitamin B12 and calcium. Advise older adults and those with dark skin or low exposure to sunlight to increase intake of vitamin D.

See Table 4-5, Nutrition Counseling: Sources of Nutrients, p. 117.

Exercise. Fitness is a key component of both weight control and weight loss. Currently, 30 minutes of moderate activity, defined as walking 2 miles in 30 minutes on most days of the week or its equivalent, is recommended. Patients can increase exercise by such simple measures as parking further away from their place of work or using stairs instead of elevators. A safe goal for weight loss is ½ to 2 pounds per week.

Blood Pressure and Diet. With respect to blood pressure, there is reliable evidence that regular and frequent exercise, decreased sodium intake and increased potassium intake, and maintenance of a healthy weight will reduce the risk for developing hypertension as well as lower blood pressure in adults who are already hypertensive. Explain to patients that most of the sodium in our diet comes from salt (sodium chloride). The recommended daily allowance (RDA) of sodium is <2400 mg, or 1 teaspoon, per day. Patients need to read food labels closely, especially the Nutrition Facts panel. Low-sodium foods are those with sodium listed at less than 5% of the RDA of <2400 mg. For nutritional interventions to reduce the risk for cardiac disease, turn to p. 118.

See Table 4-6, Patients With Hypertension: Recommended Changes in Diet, p. 118.

TECHNIQUES OF EXAMINATION

BEGINNING THE EXAMINATION: SETTING THE STAGE

Preparing for the Physical Examination

- Reflect on your approach to the patient.
- Adjust the lighting and the environment.
- Determine the scope of the examination.
- Choose the sequence of the examination.
- Observe the correct examining position and handedness.
- Make the patient comfortable.

Before you begin the physical examination, take time to prepare for the tasks ahead. Think through your approach to the patient, your professional demeanor, and how to make the patient feel comfortable and relaxed. Review the measures that promote the patient's physical comfort and make any adjustments needed in the lighting and the surrounding environment. *Make sure that you wash your hands in the presence of the patient before beginning the examination. This is a subtle yet much appreciated gesture of concern for the patient's welfare.*

Reflect on Your Approach to the Patient. When first examining patients, feelings of insecurity are inevitable, but these will soon diminish with experience. Be straightforward. Identify yourself as a student. Try to appear calm, organized, and competent, even when you feel differently. If you forget to do part of the examination, this is not uncommon, especially at first! Simply examine that area out of sequence, but smoothly. It is not unusual to go back to the bedside and ask to check one or two items that you might have overlooked.

As a beginner, you will need to spend more time than experienced clinicians on selected portions of the examination, such as the ophthalmoscopic examination or cardiac auscultation. To avoid alarming the patient, warn the patient ahead of time by saying, for example, "I would like to spend extra time listening to your heart and the heart sounds, but this doesn't mean I hear anything wrong."

Most patients view the physical examination with at least some anxiety. They feel vulnerable, physically exposed, apprehensive about possible pain, and uneasy about what the clinician may find. At the same time, they appreciate the clinician's concern about their problems and respond to your attentiveness. With these considerations in mind, the skillful clinician is thorough without wasting time, systematic without being rigid, gentle yet not afraid to cause discomfort should this be required. In applying the techniques of inspection, palpation, auscultation, and percussion, the skillful clinician examines each region of the body, and at the same time senses the whole patient, notes the wince or worried glance, and shares information that calms, explains, and reassures.

Over time, you will begin sharing your findings with the patient. As a beginner, avoid interpreting your findings. You are not the patient's primary caretaker, and your views may be conflicting or wrong. As you grow in experience and responsibility, sharing findings will become more appropriate. If the patient has specific concerns, you may even provide reassurance as you finish examining the relevant area. Be selective, however—if you find an unexpected abnormality, you may wish you had kept a judicious silence. At times, you may discover abnormalities such as an ominous mass or a deep oozing ulcer. Always avoid showing distaste, alarm, or other negative reactions.

Adjust the Lighting and the Environment. Surprisingly, several environmental factors affect the calibre and reliability of your physical findings. To achieve superior techniques of examination, it is important to "set the stage" so that both you and the patient are comfortable. As the examiner, you will find that awkward positions impair the quality of your observations. Take the time to adjust the bed to a convenient height (but be sure to lower it when finished!), and ask the patient to move toward you if this makes it easier to examine a region of the body more carefully.

Good lighting and a quiet environment make important contributions to what you see and hear but may be hard to arrange. Do the best you can. If a television interferes with listening to heart sounds, politely ask the nearby patient to lower the volume. Most people cooperate readily. Be courteous and remember to thank the patient as you leave.

Tangential lighting is optimal for inspecting structures such as the jugular venous pulse, the thyroid gland, and the apical impulse of the heart. It casts light across body surfaces that throws contours, elevations, and depressions, whether moving or stationary, into sharper relief.

When light is perpendicular to the surface or diffuse, shadows are reduced and subtle undulations across the surface are lost. Experiment with focused,

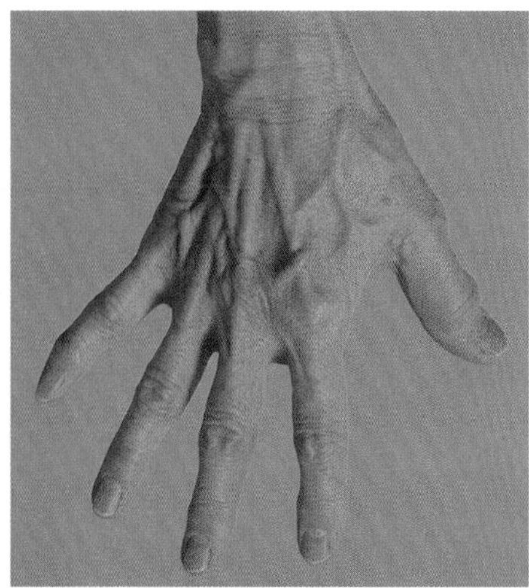

TANGENTIAL LIGHTING

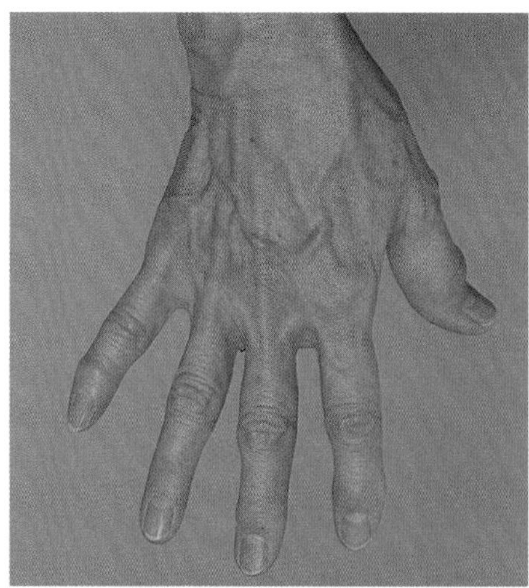

PERPENDICULAR LIGHTING

tangential lighting across the tendons on the back of your hand; try to see the pulsations of the radial artery at your wrist.

Determine the Scope of the Examination: Comprehensive or Focused? With each patient visit, you will ponder "How complete should I make the physical examination?" There is no simple answer to this common question. Chapter 1 provides initial guidelines for selecting a comprehensive examination or a focused examination (see p. 4). Review the table below to clarify your thinking as you enter the realm of patient assessment.

■ ***The Physical Examination: Comprehensive or Focused? General Guidelines***

The Comprehensive Examination	The Focused Examination
▪ Is appropriate for new patients in the office or hospital ▪ Provides fundamental and personalized knowledge about the patient ▪ Strengthens the clinician-patient relationship ▪ Helps identify or rule out physical causes related to patient concerns ▪ Provides baselines for future assessments ▪ Creates platform for health promotion through education and counseling ▪ Develops proficiency in the essential skills of physical examination	▪ Is appropriate for established patients, especially during routine or urgent care visits ▪ Addresses focused concerns or symptoms ▪ Assesses symptoms restricted to a specific body system ▪ Applies examination methods relevant to assessing the concern or problem as precisely and carefully as possible

As you can see, the *comprehensive examination* does more than assess body systems. It is a source of fundamental and personalized knowledge about the patient that strengthens the clinician-patient relationship. Most people seeking your care have specific worries or symptoms. The comprehensive examination provides a more complete basis for assessing patient concerns and answering patient questions.

For the focused examination, you will select the methods relevant to thorough assessment of the targeted problem. The patient's symptoms, age, and health history help determine the scope of your examination, as does your knowledge of disease patterns. Of all the patients with sore throat, for example, you will need to decide who may have infectious mononucleosis and warrants careful palpation of the liver and spleen and who, in contrast, has a common cold and does not need this examination. The clinical thinking that underlies and guides such decisions is discussed in Chapter 3.

What about the *routine clinical check-up*, or *periodic physical examination?* The usefulness of the comprehensive physical examination for the purposes of screening and prevention of illness, in contrast to evaluation of symptoms, has been scrutinized in several studies.[4–6] Findings have validated the importance of physical examination techniques: blood pressure measurement, assessment of central venous pressure from the jugular venous pulse, listening to the heart for evidence of valvular disease, the clinical breast examination, detection of hepatic and splenic enlargement, and the pelvic examination with Papanicolaou smears. Recommendations for examination and screening have been further expanded by various consensus panels and expert advisory groups. Bear in mind, however, that when used for screening (rather than assessment of complaints), not all components of the examination have been validated as ways to reduce future morbidity and mortality.

Choose the Sequence of the Examination. It is important to recognize that *the key to a thorough and accurate physical examination is developing a systematic sequence of examination.* Organize your comprehensive or focused examination around three general goals:

- Maximize the patient's comfort.
- Avoid unnecessary changes in position.
- Enhance clinical efficiency.

In general, move from "head to toe." Avoid examining the patient's feet, for example, before checking the face or mouth. You will quickly see that some segments of the examination are best obtained while the patient is sitting, such as examination of the head and neck and of the thorax and lungs, whereas others are best obtained with the patient supine, such as the cardiovascular and abdominal examinations.

Often you will need to examine a patient *at bed rest,* as often occurs in the hospital, where patients frequently cannot sit up in bed or stand. This often dictates changes in your sequence of examination. You can examine the head, neck, and anterior chest with the patient lying supine. Then roll the patient onto each side to listen to the lungs, examine the back, and inspect the skin. Roll the patient back and finish the rest of the examination with the patient again supine.

With practice, you will develop your own sequence of examination, keeping the need for thoroughness and patient comfort in mind. At first, you may need notes to remind you what to look for as you examine each region of the body, but with a few months of practice, you will acquire a routine sequence of your own. This sequence will become habit and often prompt you to return to a segment of the examination you may have inadvertently skipped, helping you to become thorough.

Turn to Chapter 1, pp. 11–15, to review the examination sequence suggested there, and study the outline of this sequence summarized below. After you study and practice the techniques described in the regional examination chapters, reread these overviews to see how each segment of the examination fits into an integrated whole.

THE PHYSICAL EXAMINATION: SUMMARY OF SUGGESTED SEQUENCE

- General survey
- Vital signs
- Skin: upper torso, anterior and posterior
- Head and neck, including thyroid and lymph nodes
- *Optional:* nervous system (mental status, cranial nerves, upper extremity motor strength, bulk, tone; cerebellar function)
- Thorax and lungs
- Breasts
- Musculoskeletal as indicated: upper extremities
- Cardiovascular, including JVP, carotid upstrokes and bruits, PMI, etc.
- Cardiovascular, for S_3 and murmur of mitral stenosis
- Cardiovascular, for murmur of aortic insufficiency
- *Optional:* thorax and lungs—anterior
- Breasts and axillae
- Abdomen
- Peripheral vascular; *Optional:* skin—lower torso and extremities
- Nervous system: lower extremity motor strength, bulk, tone: sensation; reflexes; Babinskis
- Musculoskeletal, as indicated
- *Optional:* skin, anterior and posterior
- *Optional:* nervous system, including gait
- *Optional:* musculoskeletal, comprehensive
- *Women:* pelvic and rectal examination
- *Men:* prostate and rectal examination

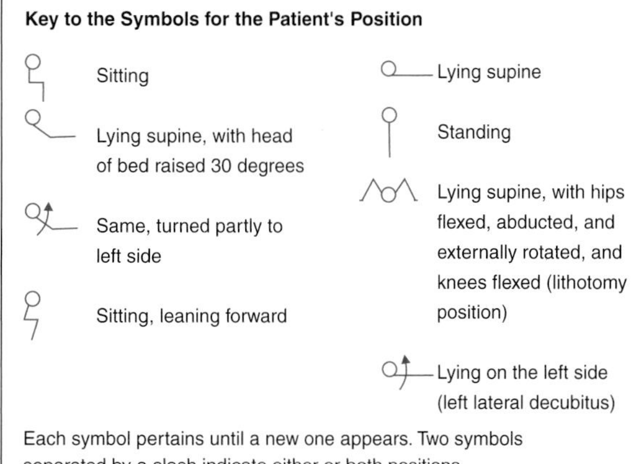

Observe the Correct Examining Position and Handedness. *This book recommends examining the patient from the patient's* ***right side,*** moving to the opposite side or foot of the bed or examining table as necessary. This is the standard position for the physical examination and has several advantages compared with the left side: it is more reliable to estimate jugular venous pressure from the right, the palpating hand rests more comfortably on the apical impulse, the right kidney is more frequently palpable than the left, and examining tables are frequently positioned to accommodate a right-handed approach.

Left-handed students are encouraged to adopt right-sided positioning, even though at first it may seem awkward. It still may be easier to use the left hand for percussing or for holding instruments such as the otoscope or reflex hammer.

Make the Patient Comfortable. Your access to the patient's body is a unique and time-honored privilege of your role as a clinician. Showing concern for privacy and patient modesty must be ingrained in your professional behavior. These attributes help the patient feel respected and at ease. Be sure to close nearby doors and draw the curtains in the hospital or examining room before the examination begins.

You will acquire the art of *draping the patient* with the gown or draw sheet as you learn each segment of the examination in the chapters ahead. *Your goal is to visualize one area of the body at a time.* This preserves the patient's modesty but also helps you to focus on the area being examined. With the patient sitting, for example, untie the gown in back to better listen to the lungs. For the breast examination, uncover the right breast but keep the left chest draped. Redrape the right chest, then uncover the left chest and proceed to examine the left breast and heart. For the abdominal examination, only the abdomen should be exposed. Adjust the gown to cover the chest and place the sheet or drape at the inguinal area.

To help the patient prepare for segments that might be awkward, it is considerate to briefly describe your plans before starting the examination. As you proceed with the examination, keep the patient informed, especially when you anticipate embarrassment or discomfort, as when checking for the femoral pulse. Also try to gauge how much the patient wants to know. Is the patient curious about the lung findings or your method for assessing the liver or spleen?

Make sure your instructions to the patient at each step in the examination are courteous and clear. For example, "I would like to examine your heart now, so please lie down."

As in the interview, be sensitive to the patient's feelings and physical comfort. Watching the patient's facial expressions and even asking "Is it okay?" as you move through the examination often reveals unexpressed worries or sources of pain. To ease discomfort, it may help to adjust the slant of the patient's bed or examining table. Rearranging the pillows or adding blankets for warmth shows your attentiveness to the patient's well-being.

When you have completed the examination, tell the patient your general impressions and what to expect next. For hospitalized patients, make sure the patient is comfortable and rearrange the immediate environment to his or her satisfaction. Be sure to lower the bed to avoid risk for falls and raise the bedrails if needed. As you leave, wash your hands, clean your equipment, and dispose of any waste materials.

THE GENERAL SURVEY

The *General Survey* of the patient's build, height, and weight begins with the opening moments of the patient encounter, but you will find that your observations of the patient's appearance crystallize as you start the physical examination. The best clinicians continually sharpen their powers of observation and description, like naturalists identifying birds from silhouettes backlit against the sky. It is important to heighten the acuity of your clinical perceptions of the patient's mood, build, and behavior. These details enrich and deepen your emerging clinical impression. A skilled observer can depict distinguishing features of the patient's general appearance so well in words that a colleague could spot the patient in a crowd of strangers.

Many factors contribute to the patient's body habitus—socioeconomic status, nutrition, genetic makeup, degree of fitness, mood state, early illnesses, gender, geographic location, and age cohort. Recall that the patient's nutritional status affects many of the characteristics you scrutinize during the *General Survey:* height and weight, blood pressure, posture, mood and alertness, facial coloration, dentition and condition of the tongue and gingiva, color of the nail beds, and muscle bulk, to name a few. Be sure to make the assessment of height, weight, BMI, and risk for obesity a routine part of your clinical practice.

You should now recapture the observations you have been making since the first moments of your interaction and sharpen them throughout your assessment. Does the patient hear you when greeted in the waiting room or examination room? Rise with ease? Walk easily or stiffly? If hospitalized when you first meet, what is the patient doing—sitting up and enjoying television? . . . or lying in bed? . . . What occupies the bedside table—a magazine? . . . a flock of "get well" cards? . . . a Bible or a rosary? . . . an emesis basin? . . . or nothing at all? Each of these observations should raise one or more tentative hypotheses about the patient for you to consider during future assessments.

Apparent State of Health. Try to make a general judgment based on observations throughout the encounter. Support it with the significant details.

Acutely or chronically ill, frail, feeble

Level of Consciousness. Is the patient awake, alert, and responsive to you and others in the environment? If not, promptly assess the level of consciousness (see p. 579).

Signs of Distress. For example, does the patient show evidence of these problems?

- Cardiac or respiratory distress

Clutching the chest, pallor, diaphoresis; labored breathing, wheezing, cough

- Pain

Wincing, sweating, protectiveness of painful area

- Anxiety or depression

Anxious face, fidgety movements, cold and moist palms; inexpressive or flat affect, poor eye contact, psychomotor slowing

Height and Build. If possible, measure the patient's height in stocking feet. Is the patient unusually short or tall? Is the build slender and lanky, muscular, or stocky? Is the body symmetric? Note the general body proportions and look for any deformities.

Very short stature is seen in Turner's syndrome, childhood renal failure, and achondroplastic and hypopituitary dwarfism. Long limbs in proportion to the trunk are seen in hypogonadism and Marfan's syndrome. Height loss occurs with osteoporosis and vertebral compression fractures.

Weight. Is the patient emaciated, slender, plump, obese, or somewhere in between? If the patient is obese, is the fat distributed evenly or concentrated over the trunk, the upper torso, or around the hips?

Generalized fat in simple obesity; truncal fat with relatively thin limbs in Cushing's syndrome and metabolic, or insulin resistance, syndrome

Whenever possible, weigh the patient with shoes off. Weight provides one index of caloric intake, and changes over time yield other valuable diagnostic data. Remember that changes in weight can occur with changes in body fluid status, as well as in fat or muscle mass.

Causes of weight loss include malignancy, diabetes mellitus, hyperthyroidism, chronic infection, depression, diuresis, and successful dieting.

Use weight and height measurements to calculate the BMI (see pp. 90–92).

Skin Color and Obvious Lesions. See Chapter 5, The Skin, Hair, and Nails, for details.

Pallor, cyanosis, jaundice, rashes, bruises

Dress, Grooming, and Personal Hygiene. How is the patient dressed? Is clothing appropriate to the temperature and weather? Is it clean, properly buttoned, and zipped? How does it compare with clothing worn by people of comparable age and social group?

Excess clothing may reflect the cold intolerance of hypothyroidism, hide skin rash or needle marks, or signal personal lifestyle preferences.

Glance at the patient's shoes. Have holes been cut in them? Are the laces tied? Or is the patient wearing slippers?

Cut-out holes or slippers may indicate gout, bunions, or other painful foot conditions. Untied laces or slippers also suggest edema.

Is the patient wearing any unusual jewelry? Where? Is there any body piercing?

Copper bracelets are sometimes worn for arthritis. Piercing may appear on any part of the body.

Note the patient's hair, fingernails, and use of cosmetics. They may be clues to the patient's personality, mood, or lifestyle. Nail polish and hair coloring that have "grown out" may signify decreased interest in personal appearance.

"Grown-out" hair and nail polish can help you estimate the length of an illness if the patient cannot give a history. Fingernails chewed to the quick may reflect stress.

Do personal hygiene and grooming seem appropriate to the patient's age, lifestyle, occupation, and socioeconomic group? These are norms that vary widely, of course.

Unkempt appearance may be seen in depression and dementia, but this appearance must be compared with the patient's probable norm.

Facial Expression. Observe the facial expression at rest, during conversation about specific topics, during the physical examination, and in interaction with others. Watch for eye contact. Is it natural? Sustained and unblinking? Averted quickly? Absent?

The stare of hyperthyroidism; the immobile face of parkinsonism; the flat or sad affect of depression. Decreased eye contact may be cultural, or may suggest anxiety, fear, or sadness.

Odors of the Body and Breath. Odors can be important diagnostic clues, such as the fruity odor of diabetes or the scent of alcohol. (For the scent of alcohol, the CAGE questions, p. 50, will help you determine possible misuse.)

Breath odors of alcohol, acetone (diabetes), pulmonary infections, uremia, or liver failure

Never assume that alcohol on a patient's breath explains changes in mental status or neurologic findings.

People with alcoholism may have other serious and potentially correctable problems such as hypoglycemia, subdural hematoma, or post-ictal state

Posture, Gait, and Motor Activity. What is the patient's preferred posture?

Preference for sitting up in left-sided heart failure, and for leaning forward with arms braced in chronic obstructive pulmonary disease

Is the patient restless or quiet? How often does the patient change position? How fast are the movements?

Fast, frequent movements of hyperthyroidism; slowed activity of hypothyroidism

Is there any apparent involuntary motor activity? Are some body parts immobile? Which ones?

Tremors or other involuntary movements; paralyses. See Table 17-3, Tremors and Involuntary Movements (pp. 653–654).

Does the patient walk smoothly, with comfort, self-confidence, and balance, or is there a limp or discomfort, fear of falling, loss of balance, or any movement disorder?

See Table 17-8, Abnormalities of Gait and Posture (pp. 663–664).

THE VITAL SIGNS

Now you are ready to measure the *Vital Signs*—the blood pressure, heart rate, respiratory rate, and temperature. You may find that the vital signs are already taken and recorded in the chart; if abnormal, you may wish to repeat them yourself. You can also make these important measurements later as you start the cardiovascular and thorax and lung examinations, but often they provide important initial information that influences the direction of your evaluation.

Check either the blood pressure or the pulse first. If the blood pressure is high, measure it again later in the examination. Count the radial pulse with your fingers, or the apical pulse with your stethoscope at the cardiac apex. Continue either of these techniques and count the respiratory rate without alerting the patient; because breathing patterns may change if the patient becomes aware that someone is watching. The temperature is taken with glass thermometers, tympanic thermometers, or digital electronic probes. Further details on techniques for ensuring accuracy of the vital signs are provided in the following pages.

See Table 4-7, Abnormalities of the Arterial Pulse and Pressure Waves (p. 119). See Table 4-8, Abnormalities in Rate and Rhythm of Breathing (p. 120).

BLOOD PRESSURE

Choice of Blood Pressure Cuff (Sphygmomanometer). As many as 50 million Americans have elevated blood pressure.[7] To measure blood pressure accurately, you must carefully choose a cuff of appropriate size. The blood pressure gauge may be either the aneroid or the mercury type. Because an aneroid instrument can become inaccurate with repeated use, it should be recalibrated regularly.

Cuffs that are too short or too narrow may give falsely high readings. Using a regular-size cuff on an obese arm may lead to a false diagnosis of hypertension.

The guidelines below will help you to select the best size blood pressure cuff and also to advise patients wishing to purchase home measurement devices. Urge patients to have such devices checked routinely for accuracy.

SELECTING THE CORRECT BLOOD PRESSURE CUFF

- Width of the inflatable bladder of the cuff should be about 40% of upper arm circumference (about 12–14 cm in the average adult).
- Length of the inflatable bladder should be about 80% of upper arm circumference (almost long enough to encircle the arm).

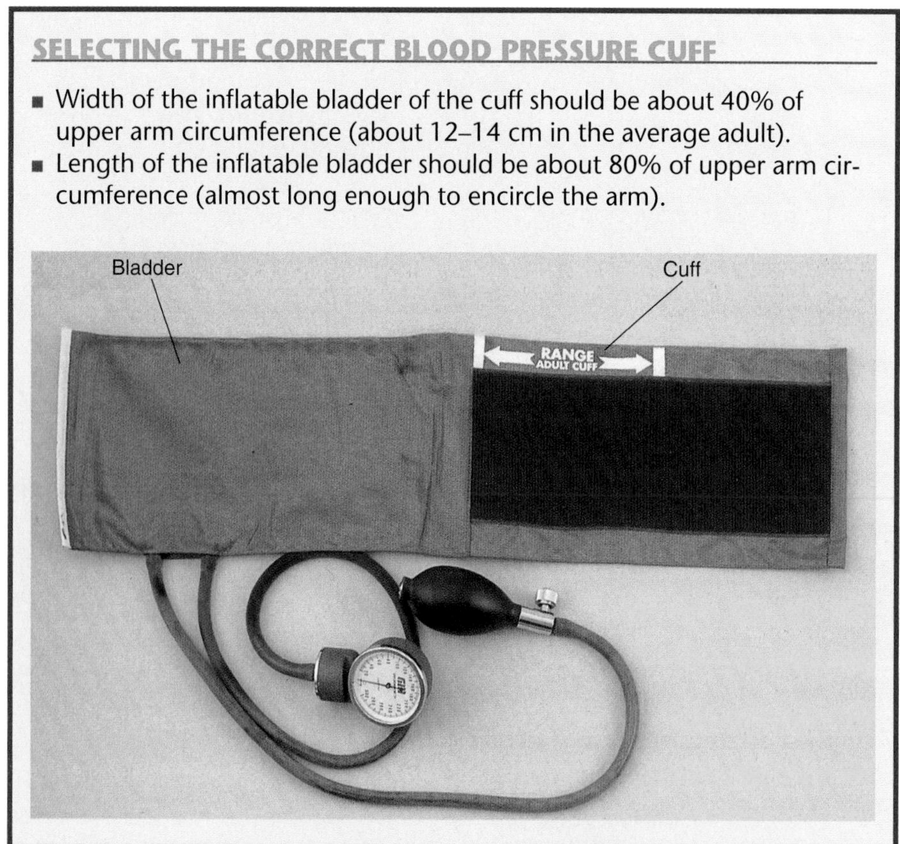

Technique for Measuring Blood Pressure. Before assessing the blood pressure, you should take several steps to make sure your measurement will be accurate. Once these steps are taken, you are ready to measure the blood pressure. Proper technique is important and reduces the inherent variability arising from the patient or examiner, the equipment, and the procedure itself.

GETTING READY TO MEASURE BLOOD PRESSURE

- Ideally, instruct the patient to avoid smoking or drinking caffeinated beverages for 30 minutes before the blood pressure is measured.
- Check to make sure the examining room is quiet and comfortably warm.
- Ask the patient to sit quietly for at least 5 minutes in a chair, rather than on the examining table, with feet on the floor. The arm should be supported at heart level.
- Make sure the arm selected is *free of clothing.* There should be no arteriovenous fistulas for dialysis, scarring from prior brachial artery cutdowns, or signs of lymphedema (seen after axillary node dissection or radiation therapy).
- Palpate the brachial artery to confirm that it has a viable pulse.
- Position the arm so that the brachial artery, at the antecubital crease, is *at heart level*—roughly level with the 4th interspace at its junction with the sternum.
- If the patient is seated, rest the arm on a table a little above the patient's waist; if standing, try to support the patient's arm at the midchest level.

If the brachial artery is much below heart level, blood pressure appears falsely high. The patient's own effort to support the arm may raise the blood pressure.

Now you are ready to measure the blood pressure.

- Center the inflatable bladder over the brachial artery. The lower border of the cuff should be about 2.5 cm above the antecubital crease. Secure the cuff snugly. Position the patient's arm so that it is slightly flexed at the elbow.

A loose cuff or a bladder that balloons outside the cuff leads to falsely high readings.

- To determine how high to raise the cuff pressure, first estimate the systolic pressure by palpation. As you feel the radial artery with the fingers of one hand, rapidly inflate the cuff until the radial pulse disappears. Read this pressure on the manometer and add 30 mm Hg to it. Use of this sum as the target for subsequent inflations prevents discomfort from unnecessarily high cuff pressures. It also avoids the occasional error caused by an *auscultatory gap*—a silent interval that may be present between the systolic and the diastolic pressures.

An unrecognized auscultatory gap may lead to serious underestimation of systolic pressure (e.g., 150/98 in the example on the next page) or overestimation of diastolic pressure.

- Deflate the cuff promptly and completely and wait 15 to 30 seconds.
- Now place the bell of a stethoscope lightly over the brachial artery, taking care to make an air seal with its full rim. Because the sounds to be heard, the *Korotkoff sounds,* are relatively low in pitch, they are heard better with the bell.

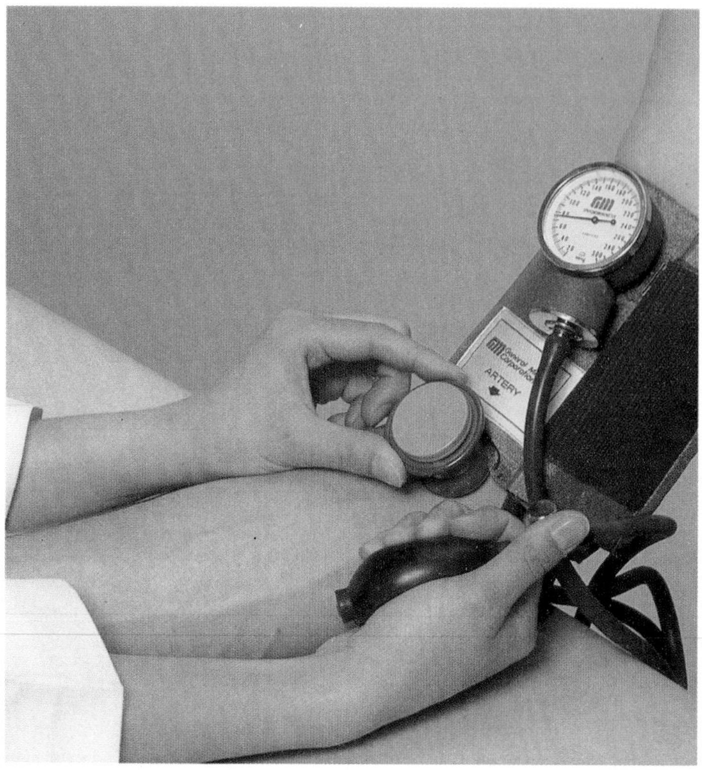

- Inflate the cuff rapidly again to the level just determined, and then deflate it slowly at a rate of about 2 to 3 mm Hg per second. Note the level at which you hear the sounds of at least two consecutive beats. This is the systolic pressure.

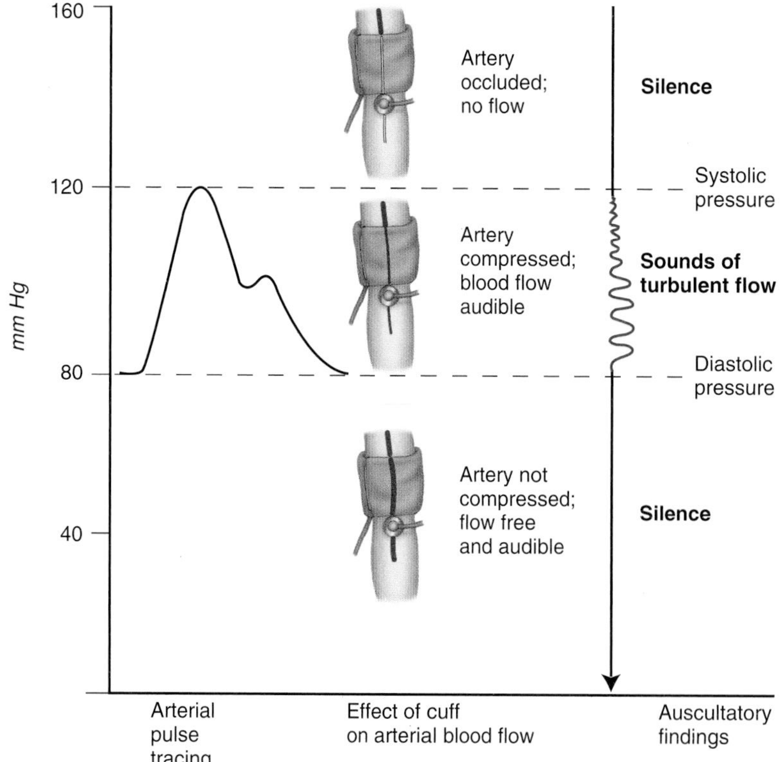

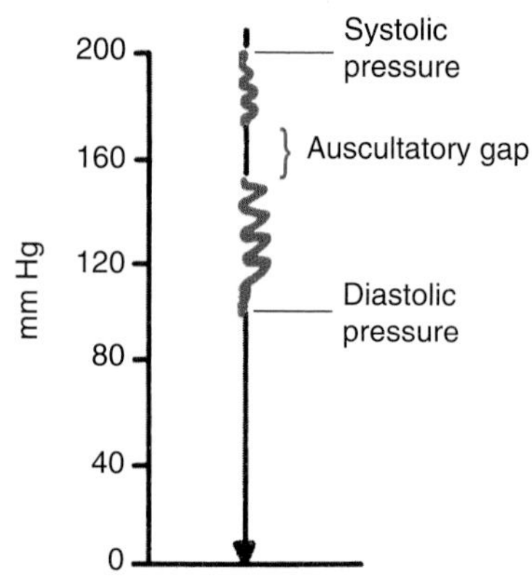

If you find an auscultatory gap, record your findings completely (e.g., 200/98 with an auscultatory gap from 170–150).

An auscultatory gap is associated with arterial stiffness and atherosclerotic disease.[8]

- Continue to lower the pressure slowly until the sounds become muffled and then disappear. To confirm the disappearance of sounds, listen as the pressure falls another 10 to 20 mm Hg. Then deflate the cuff rapidly to zero. The disappearance point, which is usually only a few mm Hg below the muffling point, provides the best estimate of true diastolic pressure in adults.

In some people, the muffling point and the disappearance point are farther apart. Occasionally, as in aortic regurgitation, the sounds never disappear. If there is more than 10 mm Hg difference, record both figures (e.g., 154/80/68).

- Read both the systolic and the diastolic levels to the nearest 2 mm Hg. Wait 2 or more minutes and repeat. Average your readings. If the first two readings differ by more than 5 mm Hg, take additional readings.

- When using a mercury sphygmomanometer, keep the manometer vertical (unless you are using a tilted floor model) and make all readings at eye level with the meniscus. When using an aneroid instrument, hold the dial so that it faces you directly. Avoid slow or repetitive inflations of the cuff, because the resulting venous congestion can cause false readings.

By making the sounds less audible, venous congestion may produce artificially low systolic and high diastolic pressures.

- Blood pressure should be taken in both arms at least once. Normally, there may be a difference in pressure of 5 mm Hg and sometimes up to 10 mm Hg. Subsequent readings should be made on the arm with the higher pressure.

Pressure difference of more than 10–15 mm Hg suggests arterial compression or obstruction on the side with the lower pressure.

Classification of Normal and Abnormal Blood Pressure. In its seventh report in 2003, the Joint National Committee on Prevention, Detection, Evaluation, and Treatment of High Blood Pressure recommended using the mean of two or more properly measured seated blood pressure readings, taken on two or more office visits, for diagnosis of hypertension.[7] Blood pressure measurement should be verified in the contralateral arm.

The Joint National Committee has identified four levels of systolic and diastolic hypertension. Note that either component may be high.

Blood Pressure Classification (Adults Older Than 18 Years)

Category	Systolic (mm Hg)	Diastolic (mm Hg)
Normal	<120	<80
Prehypertension	120–139	80–89
Hypertension		
Stage 1	140–159	90–99
Stage 2	≥160	≥100

Assessment of hypertension also includes its effects on target organs—the eyes, the heart, the brain, and the kidneys. Look for evidence of hypertensive retinopathy, left ventricular hypertrophy, and neurologic deficits suggesting a stroke. Renal assessment requires urinalysis and blood tests.

When the systolic and diastolic levels fall in different categories, use the higher category. For example, 170/92 mm Hg is Stage 2 hypertension; 135/100 mm Hg is Stage 1 hypertension. In *isolated systolic hypertension*, systolic blood pressure is ≥140 mm Hg, and diastolic blood pressure is <90 mm Hg.[9]

Relatively low levels of blood pressure should always be interpreted in the light of past readings and the patient's present clinical state.

A pressure of 110/70 mm Hg would usually be normal, but could also indicate significant hypotension if past pressures have been high.

If indicated, assess *orthostatic*, or *postural, blood pressure* (see Chapter 20, the Older Adult, p. 861). Measure blood pressure and heart rate in two positions—supine after the patient is resting up to 10 minutes, then within 3 minutes after the patient stands up. Normally, as the patient rises from the horizontal to the standing position, systolic pressure drops slightly or remains unchanged, while diastolic pressure rises slightly. Orthostatic hypotension is a drop in systolic blood pressure of ≥20 mm Hg or in diastolic blood pressure of ≥ 10 mm Hg within 3 minutes of standing.[10,11]

A fall in systolic pressure of 20 mm Hg or more, especially when accompanied by symptoms, indicates orthostatic (postural) hypotension. Causes include drugs, loss of blood, prolonged bed rest, and diseases of the autonomic nervous system.

Special Situations

Weak or Inaudible Korotkoff Sounds. Consider technical problems such as erroneous placement of your stethoscope, failure to make full skin contact with the bell, and venous engorgement of the patient's arm from repeated inflations of the cuff. Consider also the possibility of shock.

When you cannot hear Korotkoff sounds at all, you may be able to estimate the systolic pressure by palpation. Alternative methods such as Doppler techniques or direct arterial pressure tracings may be necessary.

To intensify Korotkoff sounds, one of the following methods may be helpful:

- Raise the patient's arm before and while you inflate the cuff. Then lower the arm and determine the blood pressure.
- Inflate the cuff. Ask the patient to make a fist several times, and then determine the blood pressure.

Arrhythmias. Irregular rhythms produce variations in pressure and therefore unreliable measurements. Ignore the effects of an occasional premature contraction. With frequent premature contractions or atrial fibrillation, determine the average of several observations and note that your measurements are approximate.

The Anxious Patient and Isolated Office Hypertension (or "white coat hypertension"). Anxiety is a frequent cause of diastolic blood pressure readings in the office that are higher than those at home or during normal activities, occurring in 12% to 25% of patients.[12,13] This effect may last for several visits. Try to relax the patient and measure the blood pressure again later in the encounter.

Isolated home or ambulatory hypertension, unlike isolated office hypertension, is associated with increased risk for cardiovascular disease.[12–15]

The Obese or Very Thin Patient. For the obese arm, it is important to use a wide cuff of 15 cm. If the arm circumference exceeds 41 cm, use a thigh cuff of 18 cm. For the very thin arm, a pediatric cuff may be indicated.

Use of a cuff that is too small can lead to overestimation of systolic blood pressure in obese patients.

The Hypertensive Patient With Unequal Blood Pressures in the Arms and Legs. To detect coarctation of the aorta, make two further blood pressure measurements at least once in every hypertensive patient:

Coarctation of the aorta arises from narrowing of the thoracic aorta, usually proximal but sometimes distal to the left subclavian artery.

- Compare blood pressures in the arms and legs.
- Compare the volume and timing of the radial and femoral pulses. Normally, volume is equal and the pulses occur simultaneously.

Coarctation of the aorta and *occlusive aortic disease* are distinguished by hypertension in the upper extremities and low blood pressure in the legs and by diminished or delayed femoral pulses.[16]

To determine blood pressure in the leg, use a wide, long thigh cuff that has a bladder size of 18 × 42 cm, and apply it to the midthigh. Center the bladder over the posterior surface, wrap it securely, and listen over the popliteal artery. If possible, the patient should be prone. Alternatively, ask the supine patient to flex one leg slightly, with the heel resting on the bed. When cuffs of the proper size are used for both the leg and the arm, blood pressures should be equal in the two areas. (The usual arm cuff, improperly used on the leg, gives a falsely high reading.)

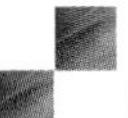

HEART RATE AND RHYTHM

Examine the arterial pulses, the heart rate and rhythm, and the amplitude and contour of the pulse wave.

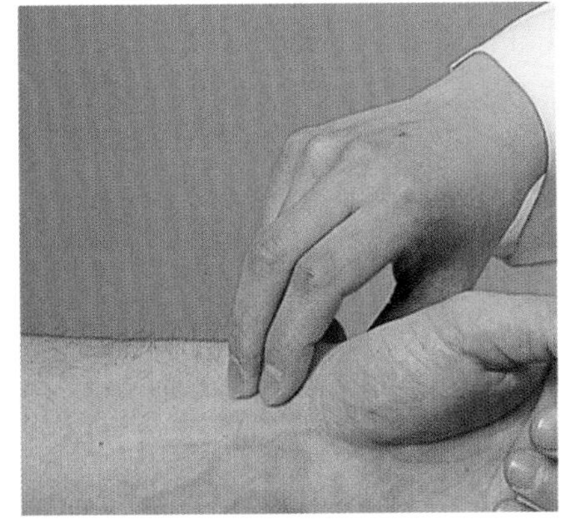

Heart Rate. The radial pulse is commonly used to assess the heart rate. With the pads of your index and middle fingers, compress the radial artery until a maximal pulsation is detected. If the rhythm is regular and the rate seems normal, count the rate for 15 seconds and multiply by 4. If the rate is unusually fast or slow, however, count it for 60 seconds.

When the rhythm is irregular, evaluate the heart rate by cardiac auscultation. Beats that occur earlier than others may not be detected peripherally, and the heart rate can thus be seriously underestimated.

Irregular rhythms include atrial fibrillation and atrial or ventricular premature contractions.

Rhythm. To begin your assessment of rhythm, feel the radial pulse. If there are any irregularities, check the rhythm again by listening with your stethoscope at the cardiac apex. Is the rhythm regular or irregular? If irregular, try to identify a pattern: (1) Do early beats appear in a basically regular rhythm? (2) Does the irregularity vary consistently with respiration? (3) Is the rhythm totally irregular?

See Table 8-1, Selected Heart Rates and Rhythms (p. 324) and Table 8-2, Selected Irregular Rhythms (p. 325).

Palpation of an irregularly irregular rhythm reliably indicates *atrial fibrillation.* For all other irregular patterns, an ECG is needed to identify the arrhythmia.

RESPIRATORY RATE AND RHYTHM

Observe the *rate, rhythm, depth,* and *effort of breathing.* Count the number of respirations in 1 minute either by visual inspection or by subtly listening over the patient's trachea with your stethoscope during your examination of the head and neck or chest. Normally, adults take 14 to 20 breaths per minute in a quiet, regular pattern. An occasional sigh is normal. Check to see if expiration is prolonged.

See Table 4-8, Abnormalities in Rate and Rhythm of Breathing (p. 120).

Prolonged expiration suggests narrowing in the bronchioles.

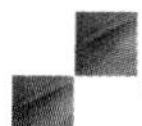

TEMPERATURE

Although you may choose to omit measuring the temperature in ambulatory patients, it should be checked whenever you suspect an abnormality. The average *oral temperature,* usually quoted at 37°C (98.6°F), fluctuates considerably. In the early morning hours, it may fall as low as 35.8°C (96.4°F), and in the late afternoon or evening, it may rise as high as 37.3°C (99.1°F). *Rectal temperatures* are *higher* than oral temperatures by an average of 0.4 to 0.5°C (0.7 to 0.9°F), but this difference is also quite variable. In contrast, *axillary temperatures* are *lower* than oral temperatures by approximately 1°, but take 5 to 10 minutes to register and are generally considered less accurate than other measurements.

Fever or pyrexia refers to an elevated body temperature. *Hyperpyrexia* refers to extreme elevation in temperature, above 41.1°C (106°F), while *hypothermia* refers to an abnormally low temperature, below 35°C (95°F) rectally.

Most patients prefer oral to rectal temperatures. However, taking oral temperatures is not recommended when patients are unconscious, restless, or unable to close their mouths. Temperature readings may be inaccurate and thermometers may be broken by unexpected movements of the patient's jaws.

Rapid respiratory rates tend to increase the discrepancy between oral and rectal temperatures. In this situation, rectal temperatures are more reliable.

For *oral temperatures,* you may choose either a glass or electronic thermometer. When using a glass thermometer, shake the thermometer down to 35°C (96°F) or below, insert it under the tongue, instruct the patient to close both lips, and wait 3 to 5 minutes. Then read the thermometer, reinsert it for a minute, and read it again. If the temperature is still rising, repeat this procedure until the reading remains stable. Note that hot or cold liquids, and even smoking, can alter the temperature reading. In these situations, it is best to delay measuring the temperature for 10 to 15 minutes.

Causes of *fever* include infection, trauma such as surgery or crush injuries, malignancy, blood disorders such as acute hemolytic anemia, drug reactions, and immune disorders such as collagen vascular disease.

If using an electronic thermometer, carefully place the disposable cover over the probe and insert the thermometer under the tongue. Ask the patient to close both lips, and then watch closely for the digital readout. An accurate temperature recording usually takes about 10 seconds.

The chief cause of *hypothermia* is exposure to cold. Other predisposing causes include reduced movement as in paralysis, interference

For a *rectal temperature*, ask the patient to lie on one side with the hip flexed. Select a rectal thermometer with a stubby tip, lubricate it, and insert it about 3 cm to 4 cm (1½ inches) into the anal canal, in a direction pointing to the umbilicus. Remove it after 3 minutes, then read. Alternatively, use an electronic thermometer after lubricating the probe cover. Wait about 10 seconds for the digital temperature recording to appear.

with vasoconstriction as from sepsis or excess alcohol, starvation, hypothyroidism, and hypoglycemia. Elderly people are especially susceptible to hypothermia and also less likely to develop fever.

Taking the *tympanic membrane temperature* is an increasingly common practice and is quick, safe, and reliable if performed properly. Make sure the external auditory canal is free of cerumen. Position the probe in the canal so that the infrared beam is aimed at the tympanic membrane (otherwise the measurement will be invalid). Wait 2 to 3 seconds until the digital temperature reading appears. This method measures core body temperature, which is higher than the normal oral temperature by approximately 0.8°C (1.4°F).

RECORDING YOUR FINDINGS

Your write-up of the physical examination begins with a general description of the patient's appearance, based on the General Survey. Note that initially you may use sentences to describe your findings; later you will use phrases. The style below contains phrases appropriate for most write-ups.

Recording the Physical Examination— The General Survey and Vital Signs

Choose vivid and graphic adjectives, as if you are painting a picture in words. Avoid cliches such as "well-developed" or "well-nourished" or "in no acute distress," because they could apply to any patient and do not convey the special features of the patient before you.

Record the vital signs taken at the time of your examination. They are preferable to those taken earlier in the day by other providers. (Common abbreviations for blood pressure, heart rate, and respiratory rate are self-explanatory.)

"Mrs. Scott is a young, healthy-appearing woman, well-groomed, fit, and in good spirits. Height is 5′4″, weight 135 lbs, BMI 24, BP 120/80, HR 72 and regular, RR 16, temperature 37.5°C."

OR

"Mr. Jones is an elderly male who looks pale and chronically ill. He is alert, with good eye contact but unable to speak more than two or three words at a time due to shortness of breath. He has intercostal muscle retraction when breathing and sits upright in bed. He is thin, with diffuse muscle wasting. Height is 6′2″, weight 175 lbs, BP 160/95, HR 108 and irregular, RR 32 and labored, temperature 101.2°F."

Suggests exacerbation of *chronic obstructive pulmonary disease*

Bibliography

CITATIONS

1. National Institutes of Health and National Heart, Lung, and Blood Institute. Clinical Guidelines on the Identification, Evaluation, and Treatment of Overweight and Obesity in Adults: The Evidence Report. NIH Publication 98-4083. June 1998. Available at: www.nhlbi.nih.gov/guidelines/obesity/ob_gdlns.pdf. Accessed December 12, 2004.
2. U.S. Preventive Services Task Force. Screening for Obesity in Adults: Recommendations and Rationale. Rockville, MD. Agency for Healthcare Research and Quality, November 2003. Available at: www.ahrq.gov/clinic/3rduspstf/obesity/obesrr.htm. Accessed December 12, 2004.
3. 2005 Dietary Guidelines Advisory Committee to the Secretaries of Health and Human Services and the U.S. Department of Agriculture. Nutrition and Your Health. January 2005. Available at: www.health/gov/dietaryguidelines/dga2005/report/. Accessed December 13, 2004.
4. U.S. Preventive Services Task Force. Clinician's Handbook of Preventive Services: Put Prevention Into Practice, 2nd ed. Washington, DC, Office of Public Health and Science, Office of Disease Prevention and Health Promotion, 1998.
5. Hensrud DD. Clinical preventive medicine in primary care: background and practice. Rational and current preventive practices. Mayo Clin Proc 75:165–172, 2000.
6. Culica D, Rohrer J, Ward M, et al. Medical check-ups: who does not get them? Am J Public Health 92(1):8890, 2002.
7. Chobanion AV, Bakris GL, Black HR, et al. The Seventh Report of the Joint National Committee on Prevention, Detection, Evaluation, and Treatment of High Blood Pressure—The JNC 7 Report. JAMA 289(19):2560–2572, 2003. Available at: www.nhlbi.nih.gov/guidelines/hypertension/jncintro.htm.
8. Cavallini MC, Roman MJ, Blank SG, et al. Association of the auscultatory gap with vascular disease in hypertensive patients. Ann Intern Med 124(10):877–883, 1996.
9. Chaudhry SI, Krumholz HM, Foody JM. Systolic hypertension in older persons. JAMA 292(9):1074–1080, 2004.
10. Carlson JE. Assessment of orthostatic blood pressure: measurement technique and clinical applications. South Med J 92(2):167–173, 1999.
11. Consensus Committee of the American Autonomic Society and the American Academy of Neurology. Consensus statement on the definition of orthostatic hypotension, pure autonomic failure, and multiple system atrophy. Neurology 46:1470, 1996.
12. Kaplan NM, Rose BD. Ambulatory blood pressure monitoring and white coat hypertension in adults. Available at: www.utdol.com. Accessed December 11, 2004.
13. Bobrie G, Genes N, Vaur L, et al. Is "isolated home" hypertension as opposed to "isolated office" hypertension a sign of greater cardiovascular risk? Arch Intern Med 161(18):2205–2211, 2001.
14. Clement DL, De Buyzere ML, De Bacquer DA, et al. Prognostic value of ambulatory blood-pressure recordings in patients with treated hypertension. N Engl J Med 348(24):2407–2415, 2003.
15. Rickerby J. The role of home blood pressure measurement in managing hypertension: an evidence-based review. J Hum Hypertens 16(7):469–472, 2002.
16. Brickner ME, Hillis LD, Lange RA. Congenital heart disease in adults. First of two parts. N Engl J Med 342(4):256–263, 2000.

ADDITIONAL REFERENCES

Weight and Nutrition

American Academy of Family Physicians. Nutrition Screening Initiative. Available at: http://www.aafp.org/preBuilt/NSI_DETERMINE.pdf. Accessed December 12, 2004.

Beevers G, Lip GY, O'Brien E. ABC of hypertension. Blood pressure measurement. Part I. Sphygmomanometry: factors common in all techniques. BMJ 322(7292):981–985, 2001.

Beevers G, Lip GY, O'Brien E. ABC of hypertension. Blood pressure measurement. Part II. Conventional sphygmomanometry: technique of auscultatory blood pressure measurement. BMJ 322(7293):1043–1047, 2001.

Ford ES, Wayne G, Dietz WH, Ford ES, Giles WH, Dietz WH. Prevalence of the metabolic syndrome among U.S. adults: findings from the Third National Health and Nutrition Examination Survey. JAMA 287(3):356–359, 2002.

Gail SM, Castracacane VD, Mantazoros. Energy homeostasis, obesity and eating disorders: recent advances in endocrinology. J. Nutr 134:295–298, 2004.

Mehler PS. Bulimia nervosa. N Engl J Med 349(9):875–880, 2003.

Sacks FM, Svetkey LP, Vollmer WM, et al. Effects on blood pressure of reduced dietary sodium and the dietary approaches to stop hypertension (DASH) diet. N Engl J Med 344(1):3–10, 2001.

Samaha FF, Iqbal N, Seshadri P, et al. A low-carbohydrate as compared with a low-fat diet in severe obesity. N Engl J Med 34(21):2074–2081, 2003.

McAlister FA, Straus SE. Evidence-based treatment of hypertension. Measurement of blood pressure: an evidence based review. BMJ 322:908–911, 2001.

Pearson TA, Blair SN, Daniels SR, et al. AHA guidelines for primary prevention of cardiovascular disease and stroke: 2002 update. Circulation 106:388–391, 2002.

Blood Pressure

Perry HM, Davis BR, Price TR, et al, for the Systolic Hypertension in the Elderly Program Cooperative Research Group. Effect of treating isolated systolic hypertension on the risk of developing various types and subtypes of stroke: the Systolic Hypertension in the Elderly Program (SHEP). JAMA 284(4):465–471, 2000.

Tholl U, Forstner K, Anlauf M. Measuring blood pressure: pitfalls and recommendations. Nephrol Dial Transplant 19:766, 2004.

U.S. Preventive Services Task Force. Screening for High Blood Pressure: Recommendations and Rationale. Rockville, MD, Agency for Healthcare Research and Quality, July 2003. Available at: http://www.ahrq.gov/clinic/3rduspstf/hibloodrr.htm. Accessed December 9, 2004.

Writing Group of the PREMIER Collaborative Research Group. Effects of comprehensive lifestyle modification on blood pressure control: main results of the PREMIER clinical trial. JAMA 289(16): 2083–2093, 2003.

TABLE 4-1 Healthy Eating: Food Groups and Servings per Day

Food Group	Women, Some Older Adults, Children Ages 2–6 yrs (about 1,600 cal)*	Active Women, Most Men, Older Children, Teen Girls (about 2,200 cal)*	Active Men, Teen Boys (about 2,800 cal)*
Bread, rice, cereal, pasta (grains) group, especially whole grain	6	9	11
Vegetable group	3	4	5
Fruit group	2	3	4
Milk, yogurt, and cheese (dairy) group—preferably fat free or low fat	2–3**	2–3**	2–3**
Dry beans, eggs, nuts, fish, and meat and poultry group—preferably lean or low fat	2, for a total of 5 oz	2, for a total of 6 oz	3, for a total of 7 oz

Source: Adapted from U.S. Department of Agriculture, Center for Nutrition Policy and Promotion. The Food Guide Pyramid, Home and Garden Bulletin Number 252, 1996.

*These are the calorie levels if low-fat, lean foods are chosen from the 5 major food groups and foods from the fats, oil, and sweets group are used sparingly.

**Older children and teenagers (ages 9–18 yrs) and adults older than the age of 50 need 3 servings daily. During pregnancy and lactation, the recommended number of dairy group servings is the same as for nonpregnant women.

TABLE 4-2 Rapid Screen for Dietary Intake

	Portions Consumed by Patient	Recommended
Grains, cereals, bread group	____	6–11
Fruit group	____	2–4
Vegetable group	____	3–5
Meat/meat substitute group	____	2–3
Dairy group	____	2–3
Sugars, fats, snack foods	____	—
Soft drinks	____	—
Alcoholic beverages	____	<2

Instructions. Ask the patient for a 24-hour dietary recall (perhaps two of these) before completing the form.

Source: Nestle M: Nutrition. In: Woolf SH, Jonas S, Lawrence RS, eds. Health Promotion and Disease Prevention in Clinical Practice. Baltimore, Williams & Wilkins, 1996.

TABLE 4-3 Eating Disorders and Excessively Low BMI

In the United States an estimated 5 to 10 million women and 1 million men suffer from eating disorders. These severe disturbances of eating behavior are often difficult to detect, especially in teens wearing baggy clothes or in individuals who binge then induce vomiting or evacuation. Be familiar with the two principal eating disorders, *anorexia nervosa* and *bulimia nervosa*. Both conditions are characterized by distorted perceptions of body image and weight. Early detection is important, because prognosis improves when treatment occurs in the early stages of these disorders.

Clinical Features

Anorexia Nervosa

- Refusal to maintain minimally normal body weight (or BMI above 17.5 kg/m^2)
- Afraid of appearing fat
- Frequently starving but in denial; lacking insight
- Often brought in by family members
- May present as failure to make expected weight gains in childhood or adolescence, amenorrhea in women, loss of libido or potency in men
- Associated with depressive symptoms such as depressed mood, irritability, social withdrawal, insomnia, decreased libido
- Additional features supporting diagnosis: self-induced vomiting or purging, excessive exercise, use of appetite suppressants and/or diuretics
- Biologic complications
  - *Neuroendocrine changes:* amenorrhea, increased corticotropin-releasing factor, cortisol, growth hormone, serotonin; decreased diurnal cortisol fluctuation, luteinizing hormone, follicle-stimulating hormone, thyroid-stimulating hormone
  - *Cardiovascular disorders:* bradycardia, hypotension, arrhythmias, cardiomyopathy
  - *Metabolic disorders:* hypokalemia, hypochloremic metabolic alkalosis, increased BUN, edema
  - *Other:* dry skin, dental caries, delayed gastric emptying, constipation, anemia, osteoporosis

Bulimia Nervosa

- Repeated binge eating followed by self-induced vomiting, misuse of laxatives, diuretics or other medications, fasting; or excessive exercise
- Often with normal weight
- Overeating at least twice a week during 3-month period; large amounts of food consumed in short period (~2 hrs)
- Preoccupation with eating; craving and compulsion to eat; lack of control over eating; alternating with periods of starvation
- Dread of fatness but may be obese
- Subtypes of
  - *Purging:* bulimic episodes accompanied by self-induced vomiting or use of laxatives, diuretics, or enemas
  - *Nonpurging:* bulimic episodes accompanied by compensatory behavior such as fasting, exercise, but without purging
- Biologic complications

  See changes listed for anorexia nervosa, especially weakness, fatigue, mild cognitive disorder; also erosion of dental enamel, parotitis, pancreatic inflammation with elevated amylase, mild neuropathies, seizures, hypokalemia, hypochloremic metabolic acidosis, hypomagnesemia

Sources: World Health Organization: The ICD-10 Classification of Mental and Behavioral Disorders: Diagnostic Criteria for Research. Geneva, World Health Organization, 1993. American Psychiatric Association: DSM-IV-TR: Diagnostic and Statistical Manual of Mental Disorders, 4th ed. Washington, DC, American Psychiatric Association, 1994. Halmi KA: Eating Disorders: In: Kaplan HI, Sadock BJ, eds. Comprehensive Textbook of Psychiatry, 7th ed. Philadelphia, Lippincott Williams & Wilkins, 1663–1676, 2000. Mehler PS. Bulimia nervosa. N Engl J Med 349(9):875–880, 2003.

TABLE 4-4 Nutrition Screening Checklist

I have an illness or condition that made me change the kind and/or amount of food I eat.	Yes (2 pts)	____
I eat fewer than 2 meals per day.	Yes (3 pts)	____
I eat few fruits or vegetables, or milk products.	Yes (2 pts)	____
I have 3 or more drinks of beer, liquor, or wine almost every day.	Yes (2 pts)	____
I have tooth or mouth problems that make it hard for me to eat.	Yes (2 pts)	____
I don't always have enough money to buy the food I need.	Yes (4 pts)	____
I eat alone most of the time.	Yes (1 pt)	____
I take 3 or more different prescribed or over-the-counter drugs each day.	Yes (1 pt)	____
Without wanting to, I have lost or gained 10 pounds in the last 6 months.	Yes (2 pts)	____
I am not always physically able to shop, cook, and/or feed myself.	Yes (2 pts)	____
	TOTAL	____

Instructions. Check "yes" for each condition that applies, then total the nutritional score. For total scores between 3–5 points (moderate risk) or ≥6 points (high risk), further evaluation is needed (especially for the elderly).

Source: American Academy of Family Physicians: The Nutrition Screening Initiative. Available at: www.aafp.org/PreBuilt/NSI_DETERMINE.pdf. Accessed December 12, 2004.

TABLE 4-5 Nutrition Counseling: Sources of Nutrients

Nutrient	Food Source
Calcium	Dairy foods such as yogurt, milk, and natural cheeses Breakfast cereal, fruit juice with calcium supplements Dark green leafy vegetables such as collards, turnip greens
Iron	Shellfish Lean meat, dark turkey meat Cereals with iron supplements Spinach, peas, lentils Enriched and whole-grain bread
Folate	Cooked dried beans and peas Oranges, orange juice Dark-green leafy vegetables
Vitamin D	Milk (fortified) Eggs, butter, margarine Cereals (fortified)

Source: Adapted from Dietary Guidelines Committee, 2000 Report. Nutrition and Your Health: Dietary Guidelines for Americans. Washington, DC, Agricultural Research Service, U.S. Department of Agriculture, 2000.

TABLE 4-6 Patients With Hypertension: Recommended Changes in Diet

Dietary Change	Food Source
Increase foods high in potassium	Baked white or sweet potatoes, cooked greens such as spinach Bananas, plantains, many dried fruits, orange juice
Decrease foods high in sodium	Canned foods (soups, tuna fish) Pretzels, potato chips, pickles, olives Many processed foods (frozen dinners, ketchup, mustard) Batter-fried foods Table salt, including for cooking

Source: Adapted from Dietary Guidelines Committee, 2000 Report. Nutrition and Your Health: Dietary Guidelines for Americans. Washington, DC, Agricultural Research Service, U.S. Department of Agriculture, 2000.

TABLE 4-7 Abnormalities of the Arterial Pulse and Pressure Waves

Normal

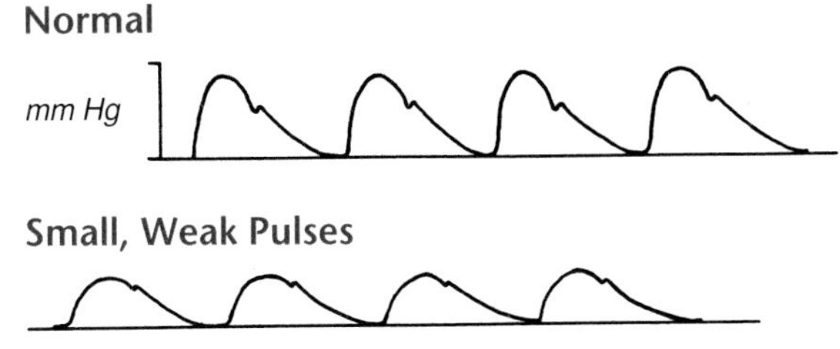

The pulse pressure is about 30–40 mm Hg. The pulse contour is smooth and rounded. (The notch on the descending slope of the pulse wave is not palpable.)

Small, Weak Pulses

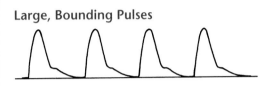

The pulse pressure is diminished, and the pulse feels weak and small. The upstroke may feel slowed, the peak prolonged. Causes include (1) decreased stroke volume, as in heart failure, hypovolemia, and severe aortic stenosis, and (2) increased peripheral resistance, as in exposure to cold and severe congestive heart failure.

Large, Bounding Pulses

The pulse pressure is increased, and the pulse feels strong and bounding. The rise and fall may feel rapid, the peak brief. Causes include (1) an increased stroke volume, a decreased peripheral resistance, or both, as in fever, anemia, hyperthyroidism, aortic regurgitation, arteriovenous fistulas, and patent ductus arteriosus; (2) an increased stroke volume due to slow heart rates, as in bradycardia and complete heart block; and (3) decreased compliance (increased stiffness) of the aortic walls, as in aging or atherosclerosis.

Bisferiens Pulse

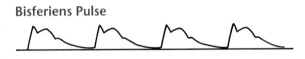

A bisferiens pulse is an increased arterial pulse with a double systolic peak. Causes include pure aortic regurgitation, combined aortic stenosis and regurgitation, and, though less commonly palpable, hypertrophic cardiomyopathy.

Pulsus Alternans

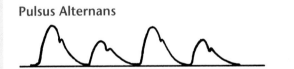

The pulse alternates in amplitude from beat to beat even though the rhythm is basically regular (and must be for you to make this judgment). When the difference between stronger and weaker beats is slight, it can be detected only by sphygmomanometry. Pulsus alternans indicates left ventricular failure and is usually accompanied by a left-sided S_3.

Bigeminal Pulse

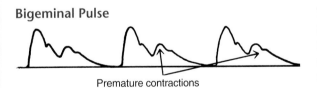

Premature contractions

This is a disorder of rhythm that may masquerade as pulsus alternans. A bigeminal pulse is caused by a normal beat alternating with a premature contraction. The stroke volume of the premature beat is diminished in relation to that of the normal beats, and the pulse varies in amplitude accordingly.

Paradoxical Pulse

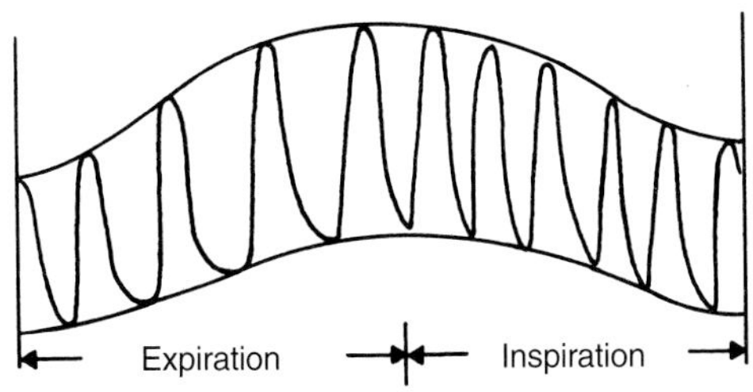

A paradoxical pulse may be detected by a palpable decrease in the pulse's amplitude on quiet inspiration. If the sign is less pronounced, a blood pressure cuff is needed. Systolic pressure decreases by more than 10 mm Hg during inspiration. A paradoxical pulse is found in pericardial tamponade, constrictive pericarditis (though less commonly), and obstructive lung disease.

TABLE 4-8 Abnormalities in Rate and Rhythm of Breathing

When observing respiratory patterns, think in terms of *rate, depth,* and *regularity* of the patient's breathing. Describe what you see in these terms. Traditional terms, such as tachypnea, are given below so that you will understand them, but simple descriptions are recommended for use.

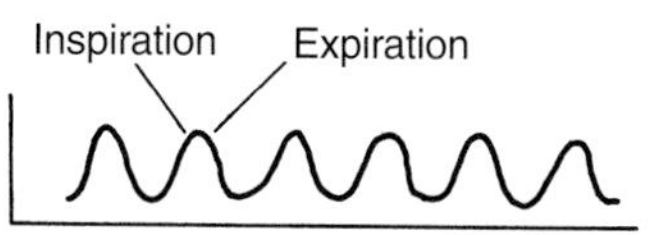

Normal

The respiratory rate is about 14–20 per min in normal adults and up to 44 per min in infants.

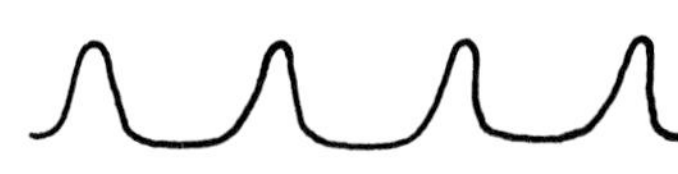

Slow Breathing (*Bradypnea*)

Slow breathing may be secondary to such causes as diabetic coma, drug-induced respiratory depression, and increased intracranial pressure.

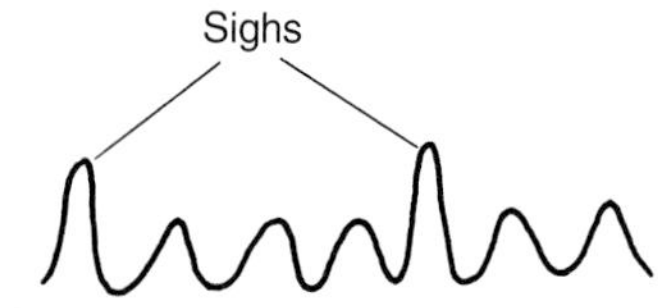

Sighing Respiration

Breathing punctuated by frequent sighs should alert you to the possibility of hyperventilation syndrome—a common cause of dyspnea and dizziness. Occasional sighs are normal.

Rapid Shallow Breathing (*Tachypnea*)

Rapid shallow breathing has a number of causes, including restrictive lung disease, pleuritic chest pain, and an elevated diaphragm.

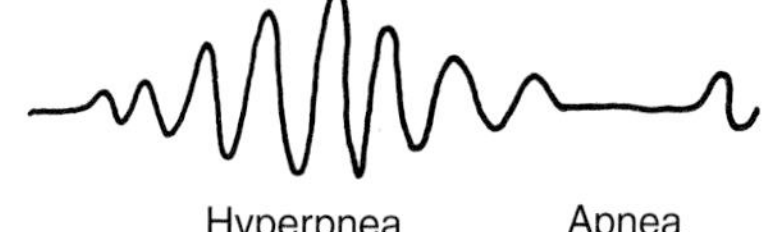

Cheyne-Stokes Breathing

Periods of deep breathing alternate with periods of apnea (no breathing). Children and aging people normally may show this pattern in sleep. Other causes include heart failure, uremia, drug-induced respiratory depression, and brain damage (typically on both sides of the cerebral hemispheres or diencephalon).

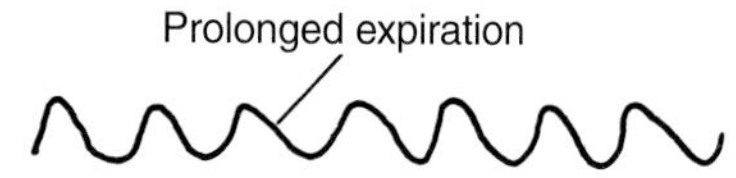

Obstructive Breathing

In obstructive lung disease, expiration is prolonged because narrowed airways increase the resistance to air flow. Causes include asthma, chronic bronchitis, and COPD.

Rapid Deep Breathing (*Hyperpnea, Hyperventilation*)

Rapid deep breathing has several causes, including exercise, anxiety, and metabolic acidosis. In the comatose patient, consider infarction, hypoxia, or hypoglycemia affecting the midbrain or pons. *Kussmaul breathing* is deep breathing due to metabolic acidosis. It may be fast, normal in rate, or slow.

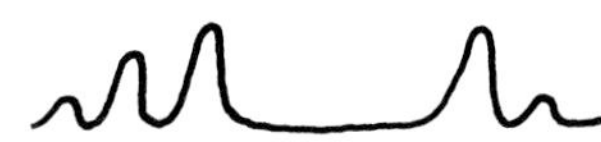

Ataxic Breathing (*Biot's Breathing*)

Ataxic breathing is characterized by unpredictable irregularity. Breaths may be shallow or deep, and stop for short periods. Causes include respiratory depression and brain damage, typically at the medullary level.

CHAPTER

5

The Skin, Hair, and Nails

ANATOMY AND PHYSIOLOGY

The major function of the skin is to keep the body in homeostasis despite the daily assaults of the environment. The skin provides boundaries for body fluids while protecting underlying tissues from microorganisms, harmful substances, and radiation. It modulates body temperature and synthesizes vitamin D. **Hair, nails,** and **sebaceous** and **sweat glands** are considered appendages of the skin. The skin and its appendages undergo many changes during aging. Turn to Chapter 20, The Older Adult (pp. 841–842), to review normal and abnormal changes of the skin with aging.

Skin. The skin is the heaviest single organ of the body, accounting for approximately 16% of body weight and covering an area of roughly 1.2 to 2.3 meters squared. It contains three layers: the epidermis, the dermis, and the subcutaneous tissues.

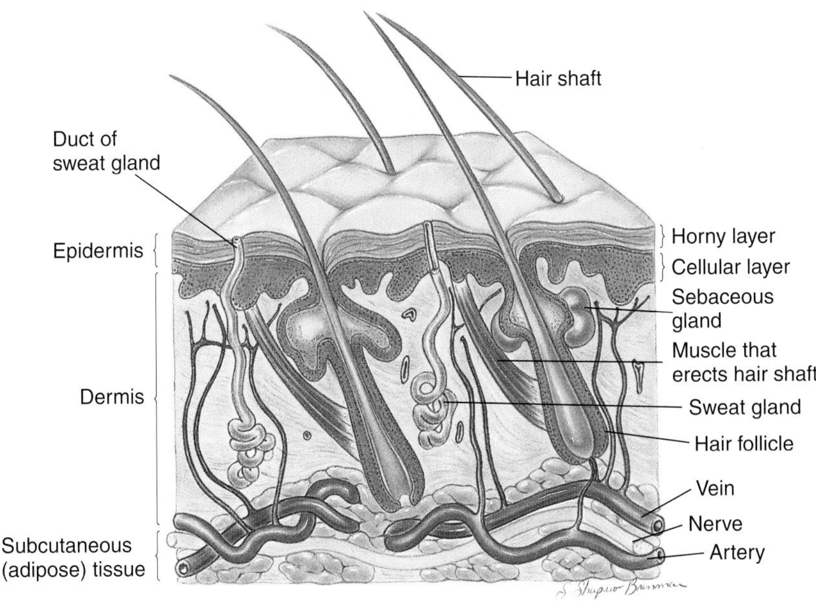

The most superficial layer, the *epidermis,* is thin, devoid of blood vessels, and itself divided into two layers: an outer horny layer of dead keratinized cells and an inner cellular layer where both melanin and keratin are formed. Migration from the inner layer to the top layer of the epidermis takes approximately 1 month.

The epidermis depends on the underlying *dermis* for its nutrition. The dermis is well supplied with blood. It contains connective tissue, sebaceous glands, sweat glands, and hair follicles. It merges below with *subcutaneous tissue,* or *adipose,* also known as fat.

The color of normal skin depends primarily on four pigments: melanin, carotene, oxyhemoglobin, and deoxyhemoglobin. The amount of *melanin,* the brownish pigment of the skin, is genetically determined and is increased by sunlight. *Carotene* is a golden yellow pigment that exists in subcutaneous fat and in heavily keratinized areas such as the palms and soles.

Hemoglobin, which circulates in the red cells and carries most of the oxygen of the blood, exists in two forms. *Oxyhemoglobin,* a bright red pigment, predominates in the arteries and capillaries. An increase in blood flow through the arteries to the capillaries of the skin causes a reddening of the skin, whereas the opposite change usually produces pallor. The skin of light-colored people is normally redder on the palms, soles, face, neck, and upper chest.

As blood passes through the capillary bed, oxyhemoglobin loses its oxygen to the tissues and changes to *deoxyhemoglobin*—a darker and somewhat bluer pigment. An increased concentration of deoxyhemoglobin in cutaneous blood vessels gives the skin a bluish cast known as *cyanosis.*

Cyanosis is of two kinds, depending on the oxygen level in the arterial blood. If this level is low, cyanosis is *central.* If it is normal, cyanosis is *peripheral.* Peripheral cyanosis occurs when cutaneous blood flow decreases and slows, and tissues extract more oxygen than usual from the blood. Peripheral cyanosis may be a normal response to anxiety or a cold environment.

Skin color is affected not only by pigments but also by the scattering of light as it is reflected back through the turbid superficial layers of the skin or vessel walls. This scattering makes the color look more blue and less red. The bluish color of a subcutaneous vein is a result of this effect; it is much bluer than the venous blood obtained on venipuncture.

Hair. Adults have two types of hair: *vellus hair,* which is short, fine, inconspicuous, and relatively unpigmented; and *terminal hair,* which is coarser, thicker, more conspicuous, and usually pigmented. Scalp hair and eyebrows are examples of terminal hair.

Nails. Nails protect the distal ends of the fingers and toes. The firm, rectangular, and usually curving *nail plate* gets its pink color from the vascular *nail bed* to which the plate is firmly attached. Note the whitish moon, or *lunula,* and the free edge of the nail plate. Roughly one fourth of the nail plate (the *nail root*) is covered by the *proximal nail fold.* The *cuticle* extends from this fold and, functioning as a seal, protects the space between the fold and the plate from external moisture. *Lateral nail folds* cover the sides of the nail plate. Note that the angle between the proximal nail fold and the nail plate is normally less than 180°.

Fingernails grow approximately 0.1 mm daily; toenails grow more slowly.

Sebaceous Glands and Sweat Glands. *Sebaceous glands* produce a fatty substance that is secreted onto the skin surface through the hair follicles. These glands are present on all skin surfaces except the palms and soles.

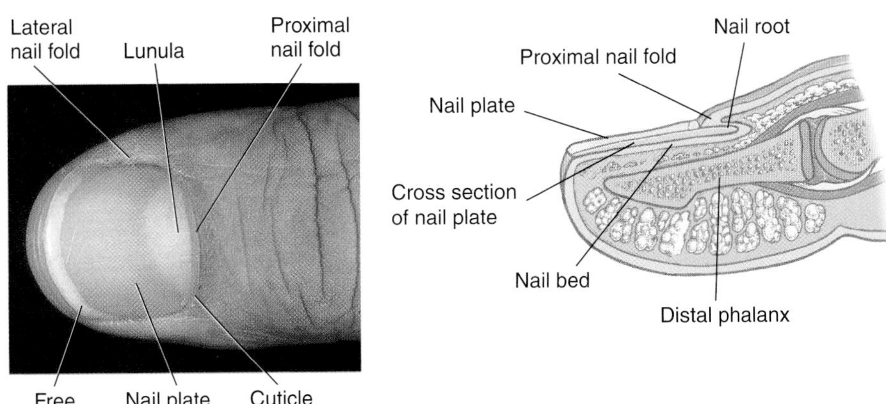

Sweat glands are of two types: eccrine and apocrine. The *eccrine glands* are widely distributed, open directly onto the skin surface, and by their sweat production help to control body temperature. In contrast, the *apocrine glands* are found chiefly in the axillary and genital regions, usually open into hair follicles, and are stimulated by emotional stress. Bacterial decomposition of apocrine sweat is responsible for adult body odor.

THE HEALTH HISTORY

Common or Concerning Symptoms

- Hair loss
- Rash
- Moles

Start your inquiry about the skin with a few open-ended questions: "Have you noticed any changes in your skin?". . . your hair? . . . your nails?. . . "Have you had any rashes? . . . sores? . . . lumps? . . . itching?"

Causes of generalized itching without obvious reason include dry skin, aging, pregnancy, uremia, jaundice, lymphomas and leukemia, drug reaction, and lice.

Ask, "Have you noticed any moles you are concerned about? Do you have any moles that have changed in size, shape, color, or sensation? What about any new moles?" If patients have such moles, pursue any personal or family history of melanoma and results of any prior biopsies of the skin.

Approximately half of *melanomas* are initially detected by the patient.[1]

You may wish to defer further questions about the skin until the physical examination, when you inspect the skin and identify the lesions that the patient is concerned about.

HEALTH PROMOTION AND COUNSELING

Important Topics for Health Promotion and Counseling

- Risk factors for melanoma
- Avoidance of excessive sun exposure

Clinicians play an important role in educating patients about early detection of suspicious moles, protective measures for skin care, and the hazards of excessive sun exposure. Skin cancers are the most common cancers in the United States and usually arise on sun-exposed areas, particularly the head, neck, and hands. Almost all skin cancers are of three types[2, 3]:

- *Basal cell carcinoma,* arising in the lowest, or basal, level of the epidermis, accounts for approximately 80% of skin cancers. These cancers are shiny and translucent, tend to grow slowly, and rarely metastasize.

- *Squamous cell carcinoma,* in the upper layer of the epidermis, accounts for approximately 16% of skin cancers. These cancers are often crusted and scaly with a red inflamed or ulcerated appearance; they can metastasize.

- *Melanoma,* arising from the pigment-producing melanocytes in the epidermis that give the skin its color, accounts for approximately 4% of skin cancers and is the most lethal type. Although rare, melanomas are the most rapidly increasing U.S. malignancy. Lifetime risk for invasive melanoma is now 1 in 65, and is 1 in 37 for noninvasive melanoma. Melanomas can spread rapidly to the lymph system and internal organs. Mortality rates are highest in white men, approximately 3.6% per year, possibly because of lower "skin awareness" and lower rates of self-examination.[4]

Educate your patients about *risk factors for melanoma:* 50 or more common moles; 1–4 or more atypical or unusual moles, especially if dysplastic[5, 6]; red or light hair; actinic lentigenes, or macular brown or tan spots usually on sun-exposed areas, such as freckles; heavy sun exposure; light eye or skin color, especially skin that freckles or burns easily; and family history of melanoma.[4] Early detection of melanoma when less than 3 mm improves prognosis.

The most commonly recommended screening measure for skin cancer is *total-body skin examination* by a clinician, although data on utility of this method for nondermatologists are limited. Although the U.S. Preventive Services Task Force has found insufficient evidence to recommend inspection for routine screening, the American Cancer Society recommends skin examination as part of a routine cancer-related check-up every 3 years for people aged 20–40, and yearly for those older than 40.[7, 8] Only a few studies have shown that *skin self-examination* enhances detection,[9–11] but this low-cost method of patient education can promote health awareness in at-risk patients. (See Techniques for Skin Self-Examination on pp. 128–129.)

There is also value in use of the ***ABCDE method*** for screening moles for melanoma by clinicians and patients. Sensitivity ranges from 50% to 97%, and specificity from 96% to 99%[1,12] (see Table 5-8, Benign and Malignant Nevi, p. 143).

ABCDE: SCREENING MOLES FOR POSSIBLE MELANOMA

- **A** for *asymmetry*
- **B** for irregular *borders,* especially ragged, notched, or blurred
- **C** for variation or change in *color,* especially blue or black
- **D** for *diameter* ≥ *6 mm* or *different from others,* especially if changing, itching, or bleeding
- **E** for *elevation* or *enlargement*

You may also wish to counsel patients about such preventive strategies as reducing sun exposure and using sunscreens (though these are not conclusively validated as effective[9]). Caution patients to minimize direct sun exposure, especially at midday when ultraviolet B rays (UV-B), the most common cause of skin cancer, are most intense. Sunscreens fall into two categories—thick, pastelike ointments that block all solar rays, and light-absorbing sunscreens rated by "sun protective factor" (SPF). The SPF is a ratio of the number of minutes for treated versus untreated skin to redden with exposure to UV-B. An SPF of at least 15 is recommended and protects against 93% of UV-B. (There is no scale for UV-A, which causes photoaging, or UV-C, the most carcinogenic ray but blocked in the atmosphere by ozone.) Water-resistant sunscreens that remain on the skin for prolonged periods are preferable. Be aware, however, that use of sunscreens may give patients a false sense of security and increase sun exposure.

TECHNIQUES OF EXAMINATION

Your examination of the skin, hair, and nails begins with the General Survey and continues throughout the physical examination. Take time, however, to ensure that the patient wears a gown and is draped accordingly to facilitate close inspection of the hair, anterior and posterior surfaces of the body, palms and soles, and webspaces between the fingers and toes.

Inspect the entire skin surface in good light, preferably natural light or artificial light that resembles it. Correlate your findings with observations of the mucous membranes, especially when assessing skin color, because diseases may appear in both areas. Techniques for examining these membranes are described in later chapters.

Artificial light often distorts colors and masks jaundice.

To sharpen your observations, you may wish to turn now to the tables at the end of the chapter to better identify skin colors and patterns and types of lesions that you may encounter during the examination.

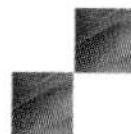

SKIN

Inspect and palpate the skin. Note these characteristics:

Color. Patients may notice a change in their skin color before the clinician does. Ask about it. Look for increased pigmentation (brownness), loss of pigmentation, redness, pallor, cyanosis, and yellowing of the skin.

See Table 5-1, Skin Colors (pp. 132–133).

The red color of oxyhemoglobin and the pallor in its absence are best assessed where the horny layer of the epidermis is thinnest and causes the least scatter: the fingernails, the lips, and the mucous membranes, particularly those of the mouth and the palpebral conjunctiva. In dark-skinned people, inspecting the palms and soles may also be useful.

Pallor from decreased redness in *anemia* and in decreased blood flow, as occurs in fainting or arterial insufficiency

Central cyanosis is best identified in the lips, oral mucosa, and tongue. The lips, however, may turn blue in the cold, and melanin in the lips may simulate cyanosis in darker-skinned people.

Causes of *central cyanosis* include advanced lung disease, congenital heart disease, and abnormal hemoglobins.

Cyanosis of the nails, hands, and feet may be central or peripheral in origin. Anxiety or a cold examining room may cause peripheral cyanosis.

Cyanosis in congestive heart failure is usually peripheral, reflecting decreased blood flow, but in pulmonary edema, it may also be central. Venous obstruction may cause peripheral cyanosis.

Look for the yellow color of jaundice in the sclera. Jaundice may also appear in the palpebral conjunctiva, lips, hard palate, undersurface of the tongue, tympanic membrane, and skin. To see jaundice more easily in the lips, blanch out the red color by pressure with a glass slide.

Jaundice suggests liver disease or excessive hemolysis of red blood cells.

For the yellow color that accompanies high levels of carotene, look at the palms, soles, and face.

Carotenemia

Moisture. Examples are dryness, sweating, and oiliness.

Dryness in hypothyroidism; oiliness in acne

Temperature. Use the backs of your fingers to make this assessment. In addition to identifying generalized warmth or coolness of the skin, note the temperature of any red areas.

Generalized warmth in fever, *hyperthyroidism;* coolness in *hypothyroidism.* Local warmth of inflammation or cellulitis

Texture. Examples are roughness and smoothness.

Roughness in hypothyroidism; velvety texture in hyperthyroidism

Mobility and Turgor. Lift a fold of skin and note the ease with which it lifts up (mobility) and the speed with which it returns into place (turgor).

Decreased mobility in edema, *scleroderma;* decreased turgor in dehydration

Lesions. Observe any lesions of the skin, noting their characteristics:

- Their *anatomic location and distribution* over the body. Are they generalized or localized? Do they, for example, involve the exposed surfaces, the intertriginous or skin fold areas, extensor or flexor areas, or acral (peripheral) areas? Do they involve areas exposed to specific allergens or irritants, such as wrist bands, rings, or industrial chemicals?

Many skin diseases have typical distributions. Acne affects the face, upper chest, and back; psoriasis, the knees and elbows (among other areas); and *Candida* infections, the intertriginous areas. See patterns in Table 5-2, Skin Lesions—Anatomic Location and Distribution (p. 134).

- Their *patterns and shapes.* For example, are they linear, clustered, annular (in a ring), arciform (in an arc), geographic, or serpiginous (serpent or worm-like)? Are they dermatomal, covering a skin band that corresponds to a sensory nerve root (see pp. 605–606)?

Vesicles in a unilateral dermatomal pattern are typical of herpes zoster.[13] See patterns in Table 5-3, Skin Lesions—Patterns and Shapes (p. 135).

- The *types of skin lesions* (e.g., macules, papules, vesicles, nevi). If possible, find representative and recent lesions that have not been traumatized by scratching or otherwise altered. Inspect them carefully and feel them.
- Their *color.*

See Table 5-4, Elevated Skin Lesions (pp. 136–139); Table 5-5, Depressed Skin Lesions (p. 140); Table 5-6, Vascular and Purpuric Lesions of the Skin (p. 141); Table 5-7, Skin Tumors (p. 142); and Table 5-8, Benign and Malignant Nevi (p. 143).

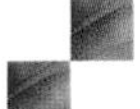

SKIN LESIONS IN CONTEXT

After familiarizing yourself with the basic types of lesions, review their appearances in Tables 5-9 and 5-10 and in a well-illustrated textbook of dermatology. Whenever you see a skin lesion, look it up in such a text. The type of lesions, their location, and their distribution, together with other infor-

See Table 5-9, Skin Lesions in Context (pp. 144–145), and Table 5-10, Diseases and Related Skin Conditions (pp. 146–147).

mation from the history and the examination, should equip you well for this search and, in time, for arriving at specific dermatologic diagnoses.

Evaluating the Bedbound Patient. People who are confined to bed, especially when they are emaciated, elderly, or neurologically impaired, are particularly susceptible to skin damage and ulceration. *Pressure sores* result when sustained compression obliterates arteriolar and capillary blood flow to the skin. Sores may also result from the shearing forces created by bodily movements. When a person slides down in bed from a partially sitting position, for example, or is dragged rather than lifted up from a supine position, the movements may distort the soft tissues of the buttocks and close off the arteries and arterioles within. Friction and moisture further increase the risk.

See Table 5-11, Pressure Ulcers (p. 148).

Assess every susceptible patient by carefully inspecting the skin that overlies the sacrum, buttocks, greater trochanters, knees, and heels. Roll the patient onto one side to see the sacrum and buttocks.

Local redness of the skin warns of impending necrosis, although some deep pressure sores develop without antecedent redness. Ulcers may be seen.

HAIR

Inspect and palpate the hair. Note its quantity, distribution, and texture.

Alopecia refers to hair loss—diffuse, patchy, or total. Sparse hair in hypothyroidism; fine silky hair in hyperthyroidism

See Table 5-12, Hair Loss (p. 149).

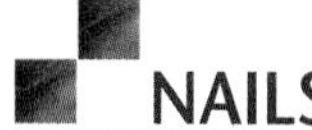

NAILS

Inspect and palpate the fingernails and toenails. Note their color and shape and any lesions. Longitudinal bands of pigment may be seen in the nails of normal people who have darker skin.

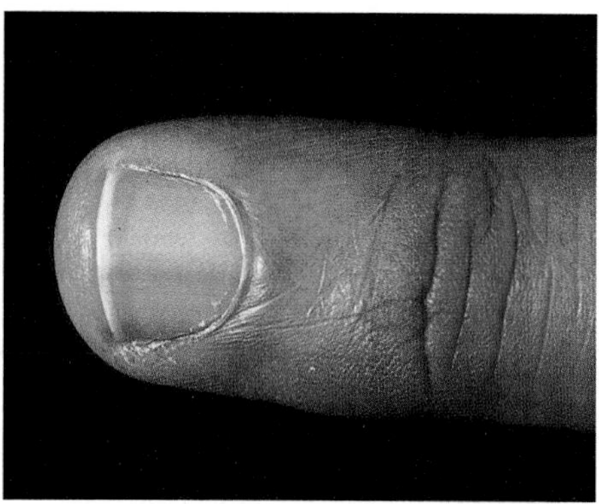

See Table 5-13, Findings In or Near the Nails (pp. 150–151).

SPECIAL TECHNIQUES

Instructions for the Skin Self-Examination. The American Academy of Dermatology recommends regular self-examination of the skin using the techniques below. The patient will need a full-length mirror, a hand-held mirror, and a well-lit room that provides privacy. Teach the patient the **ABCDE** method for assessing moles (see p. 125), and show the patient the photos of benign and malignant nevi in Table 5-8 on p. 143.

PATIENT INSTRUCTIONS FOR THE SKIN SELF-EXAMINATION

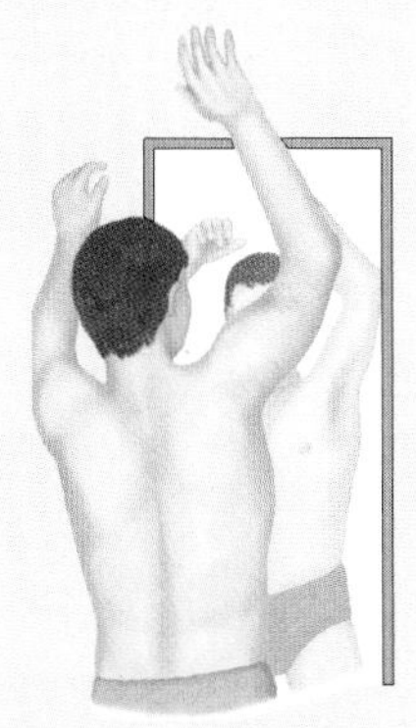

Examine your body front and back in the mirror, then right and left sides with arms raised.

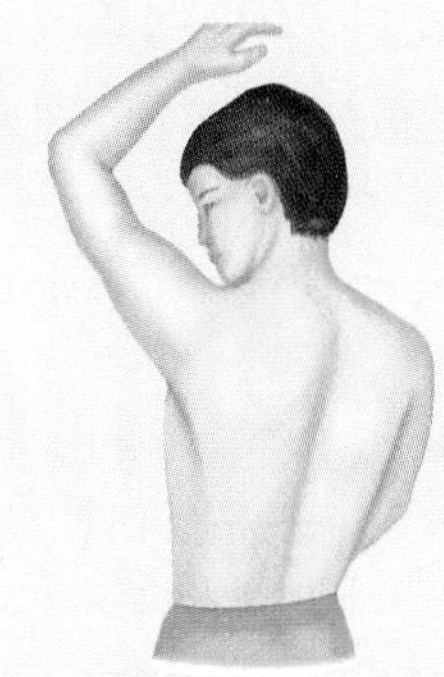

Bend elbows and look carefully at forearms, upper underarms, and palms.

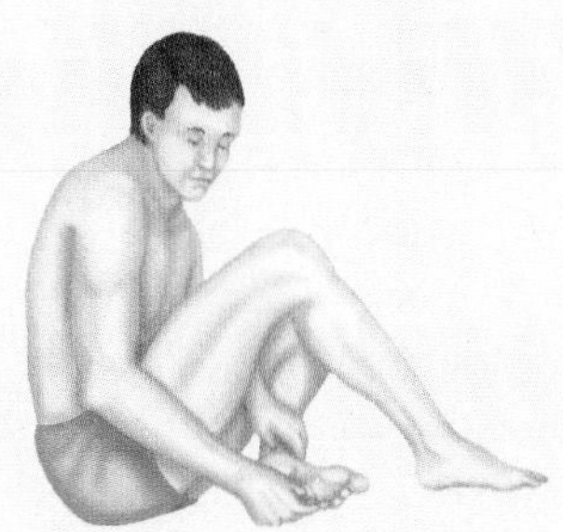

Look at the backs of your legs and feet, the spaces between your toes, and the sole.

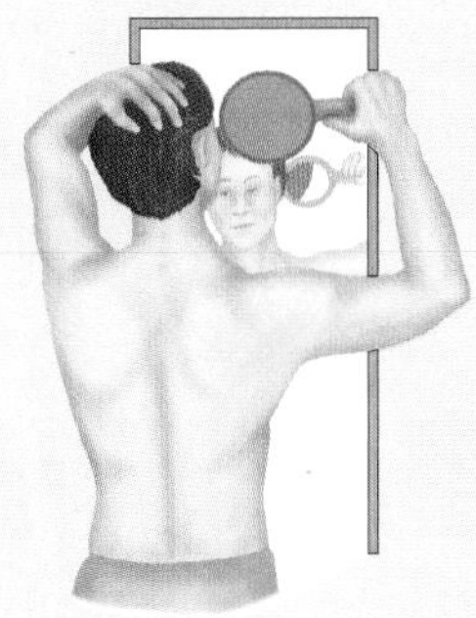

Examine the backs of your neck and scalp with a hand mirror. Part hair for a closer look.

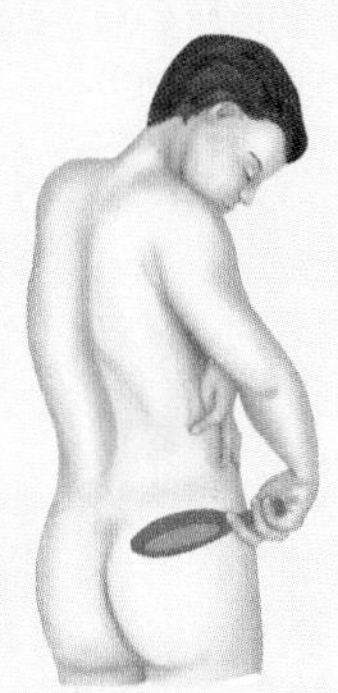

Finally, check your back and buttocks with a hand mirror.

Source: Adapted from American Academy of Dermatology. SkinCancerNet. Available at: http://www.skincarephysicians.com/skincancernet; and from American Academy of Dermatology. How to perform a self-examination. Available at: http://www.aad.org/public/News/DermInfo/SelfExam.htm.

RECORDING YOUR FINDINGS

Note that initially you may use sentences to describe your findings; later you will use phrases. The style below contains phrases appropriate for most write-ups.

Recording the Physical Examination—The Skin	
"Color good. Skin warm and moist. Nails without clubbing or cyanosis. No suspicious nevi. No rash, petechiae, or ecchymoses."	
OR	
"Marked facial pallor, with circumoral cyanosis. Palms cold and moist. Cyanosis in nailbeds of fingers and toes. One raised blue-black nevus, 1 × 2 cm, with irregular border on right forearm. No rash."	Suggests central cyanosis and possible melanoma
OR	
"Facial plethora. Skin icteric. Spider angioma over anterior torso. Palmar erythema. Single pearly papule with depressed center and telangiectasias, 1 × 1 cm, on posterior neck above collarline. No suspicious nevi. Nails with clubbing but no cyanosis."	Suggests possible liver disease and basal cell carcinoma

Bibliography

CITATIONS

1. Whited JD, Grichnik JM. Does this patient have a mole or a melanoma? The rational clinical examination. JAMA 279(9): 696–701, 1998.
2. American Academy of Dermatology. Public Resource Center: 2004 Melanoma fact sheet. Available at: http://www.aad.org/public/News/DermInfo/2004MelanomaFAQ.htm. Accessed January 29, 2005.
3. American Academy of Dermatology. What is skin cancer? Skincare.net. Available at: http://www.skincarephysicians.com/skincancernet/whatis.html. Accessed January 29, 2005.
4. Helfand M, Krages KP. Counseling to Prevent Skin Cancer: A Summary of the Evidence for the U.S. Preventive Services Task Force. Rockville, MD, Agency for Healthcare Research and Quality, 2003. Available at: http://www.ahrq.gov/clinic/3rduspstf/skcacoun/skcounsum.htm. Accessed January 29, 2005.
5. Naeyaert JM, Broches L. Dysplastic nevi. N Engl J Med 349(23):2233–2240, 2003.
6. Tucker MA, Halpern A, Holly EA, et al. Clinically recognized dysplastic nevi: A central risk factor for cutaneous melanoma. JAMA 277(18):1439–1444, 1997.
7. U.S. Preventive Services Task Force. Screening for Skin Cancer: Recommendations and Rationale. [Article originally published in Am J Prev Med 20(3S):44–46, 2001.] Rockville, MD, Agency for Healthcare Research and Quality. Available at: http://www.ahrq.gov/clinic/ajpmsuppl/skcarr.htm. Accessed January 29, 2005.
8. American Cancer Society. Skin cancer, 2005. Available at: http://www.cancer.org/downloads/PRO/SkinCancer.pdf. Accessed January 19, 2005.
9. U.S. Preventive Services Task Force: Counseling to Prevent Skin Cancer: Recommendations and Rationale. Rockville, MD, Agency for Healthcare Research and Quality, 2003. Available at: http://www.ahrq.gov/clinic/3rduspstf/skcacoun/skcarr.htm. Accessed January 28, 2005.
10. Berwick M, Begg CB, Fine JA, et al. Screening for cutaneous melanoma by skin self-examination. J Natl Cancer Inst 88: 17–23, 1996.
11. Robinson JK, Fisher SG, Turrisi RJ. Predictors of skin self-examination performance. Cancer 95(1):135–146, 2002.
12. U.S. Preventive Services Task Force: Screening for Skin Cancer: Summary of the Evidence. [Article originally published in Am J Prev 20(3S):47–58, 2001.] Rockville, MD, Agency for Healthcare Research and Quality, 2001. Available at: http://www.ahrq.gov/clinic/ajpmsuppl/helfand1.htm. Accessed January 29, 2005.
13. Gnann JG, Whitley RJ: Herpes zoster. N Engl J Med 3247(5):340–346, 2002.

ADDITIONAL REFERENCES

Fitzpatrick TB, Freedberg IM. Fitzpatrick's Dermatology in General Medicine, 6th ed. New York, McGraw-Hill, 2003.

Fitzpatrick TB, Wolff K, Johnson RA, Suurmond D. Fitzpatrick's Color Atlas and Synopsis of Clinical Dermatology, 5th ed. New York, McGraw-Hill, 2005.

Grimes P. New insights and new therapies in vitiligo. JAMA 293(6):730–735, 2005.

Habif TP. Clinical Dermatology: A Color Guide to Diagnosis and Therapy, 4th ed. New York, Mosby, 2004.

Habif TP. Skin Disease: Diagnosis and Treatment, 2nd ed. Philadelphia, Elsevier Mosby, 2005.

Hall JC, Sauer GC. Sauer's Manual of Skin Diseases, 8th ed. Philadelphia, Lippincott Williams & Wilkins, 2000.

Hordinsky M, Sawaya M, Roberts JL. Hirsutism and hair loss in the elderly. Clin Geriatr Med 18(1):121–133, 2002.

Lyder CH. Pressure ulcer prevention and management. JAMA 289(2):223–226.

Myers KA, Farquhar DRE. Does this patient have clubbing? JAMA 2001(2863):341–347.

Scanlon E, Stubbs N. Pressure ulcer risk assessment in patients with darkly pigmented skin. Professional Nurse 19(6):339–341, 2004.

Schon MP, Henning-Boehncke W. Psoriasis. N Engl J Med 352(18): 1899–1912, 2005.

Singer AJ, Clark RAF. Cutaneous wound healing. N Engl J Med 341(10):738–746, 1999.

Singh N, Armstrong DG, Lipsky BA. Preventing foot ulcers in patients with diabetes. JAMA 293(2):217–228, 2005.

Swartz MN. Cellulitis. N Engl J Med 350(9):904–912, 2004.

Yancey KB, Egan GA. Pemphigoid: clinical, histologic, immunopathologic, and therapeutic considerations. JAMA 284(3): 350–356, 2000.

TABLE 5-1 Skin Colors

Changes in Pigmentation

A widespread increase in *melanin* may be caused by Addison's disease (hypofunction of the adrenal cortex) or some pituitary tumors. More common are local areas of increased or decreased pigment:

Café-Au-Lait Spot

A slightly but uniformly pigmented macule or patch with a somewhat irregular border, usually 0.5 to 1.5 cm in diameter and of no consequence. Six or more such spots, each with a diameter of >1.5 cm, however, suggest neurofibromatosis (p. 799). (The small, darker macules are unrelated.)

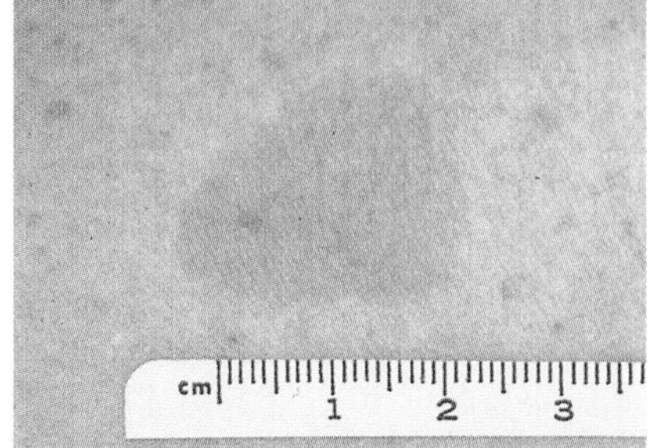

Tinea Versicolor

Common superficial fungus infection of the skin, causing hypopigmented, slightly scaly macules on the trunk, neck, and upper arms (short-sleeved shirt distribution). They are easier to see in darker skin and in some are more obvious after tanning. In lighter skin, macules may look reddish or tan instead of pale.

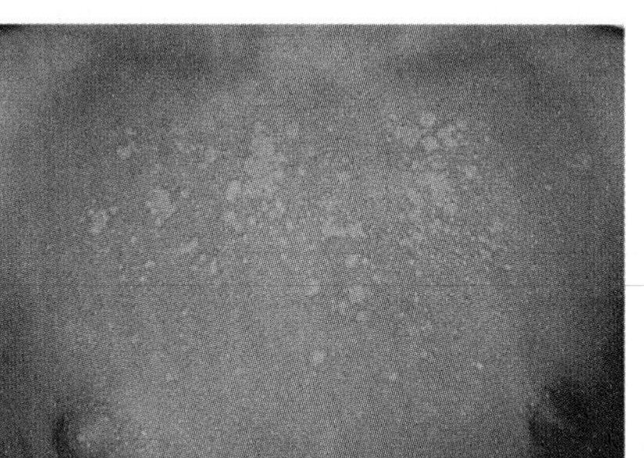

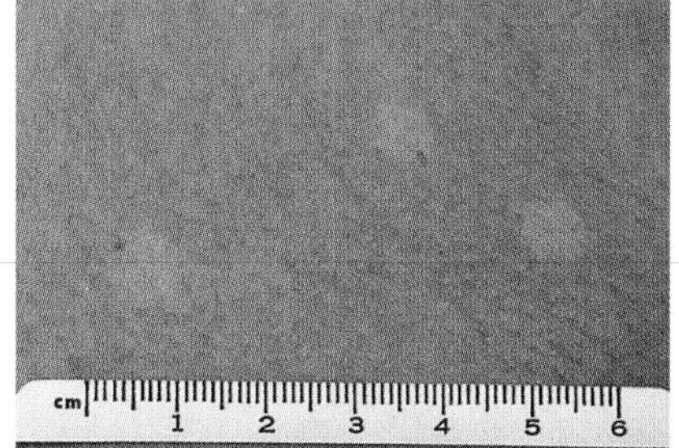

Vitiligo

In vitiligo, depigmented macules appear on the face, hands, feet, extensor surfaces, and other regions and may coalesce into extensive areas that lack melanin. The brown pigment is normal skin color; the pale areas are vitiligo. The condition may be hereditary. These changes may be distressing to the patient.

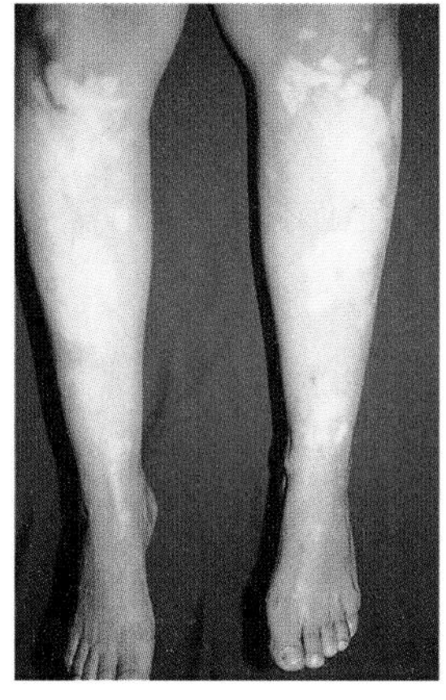

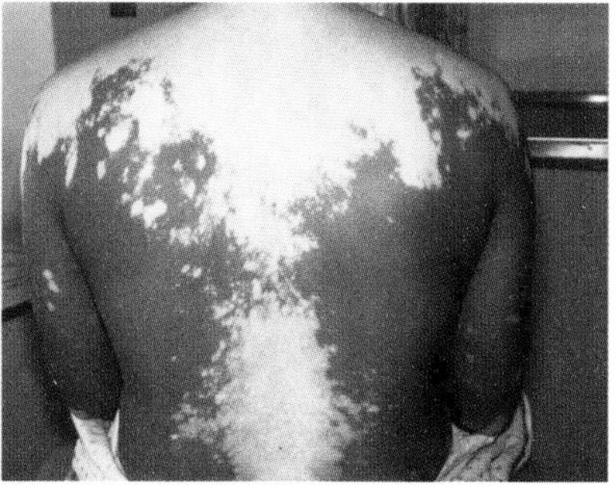

Cyanosis

Cyanosis is the somewhat bluish color that is visible in these toenails and toes. Compare this color with the normally pink fingernails and fingers of the same patient. Impaired venous return in the leg caused this example of peripheral cyanosis. Cyanosis, especially when slight, may be hard to distinguish from normal skin color.

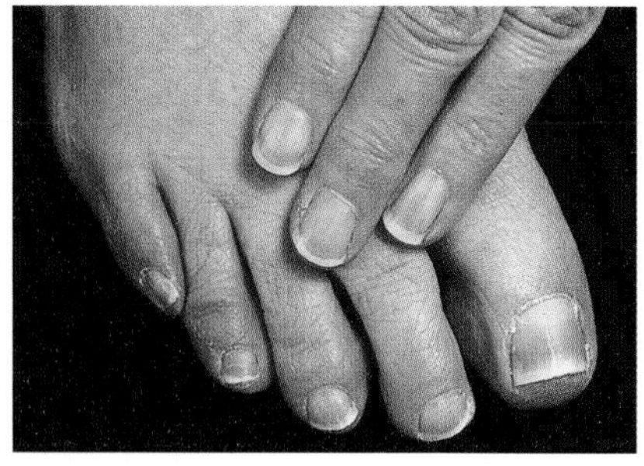

(table continues next page)

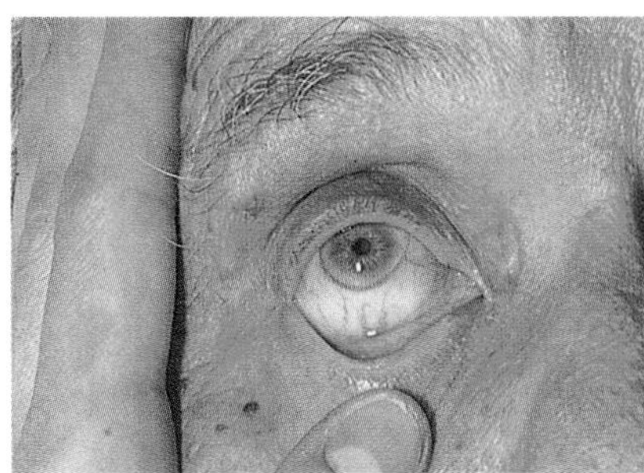

Jaundice

Jaundice makes the skin diffusely yellow. Note this patient's skin color, contrasted with the examiner's hand. The color of jaundice is seen most easily and reliably in the sclera, as shown here. It may also be visible in mucous membranes. Causes include liver disease and hemolysis of red blood cells.

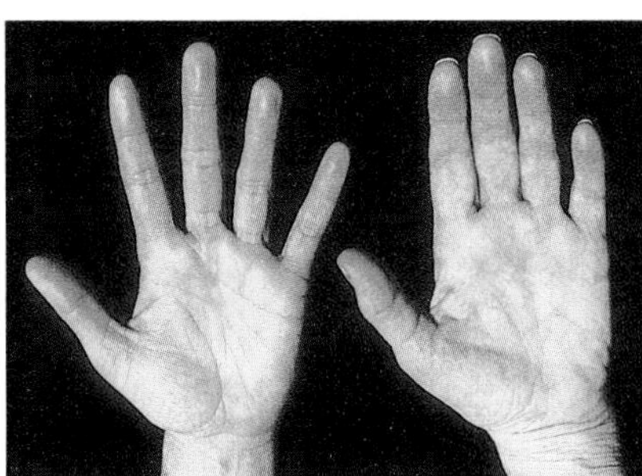

Carotenemia

The yellowish palm of carotenemia is compared with a normally pink palm, sometimes a subtle finding. Unlike jaundice, carotenemia does not affect the sclera, which remains white. The cause is a diet high in carrots and other yellow vegetables or fruits. Carotenemia is not harmful but indicates the need for assessing dietary intake.

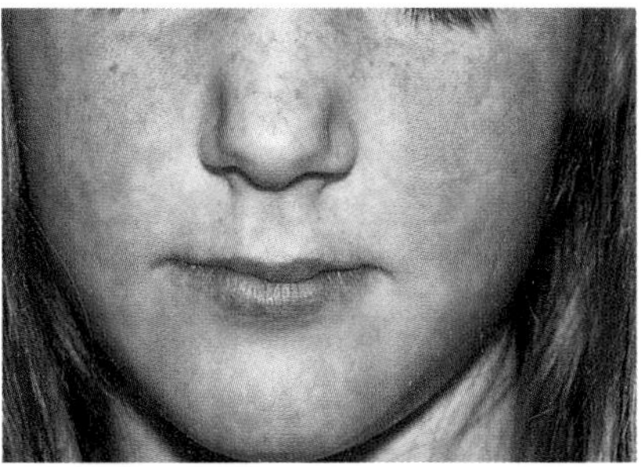

Erythema

Red hue, increased blood flow, seen here as the "slapped cheeks" of erythema infectiosum ("fifth disease").

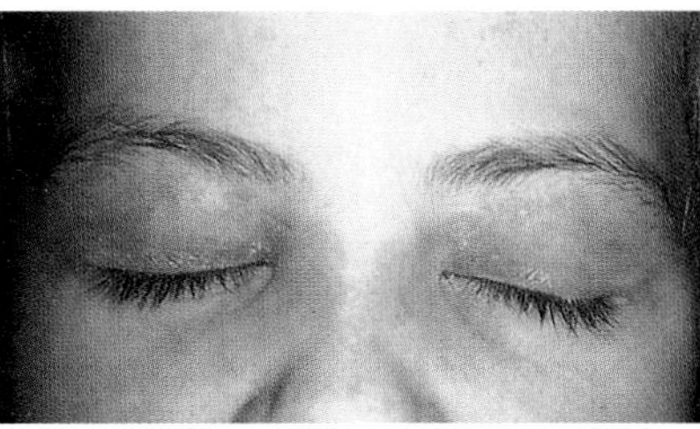

Heliotrope

Violaceous eruption over the eyelids in the collagen vascular disease dermatomyositis.

(Sources of photos: *Tinea Versicolor*—Ostler HB, Mailbach HI, Hoke AW, Schwab IR. Diseases of the Eye and Skin: A Color Atlas. Philadelphia, Lippincott Williams & Wilkins, 2004; *Vitiligo, Erythema*—Goodheart HP. Goodheart's Photoguide of Common Skin Disorders: Diagnosis and Management, 2nd ed. Philadelphia, Lippincott Williams & Wilkins, 2003; *Heliotrope*—Hall JC. Sauer's Manual of Skin Diseases, 8th ed. Philadelphia, Lippincott Williams & Wilkins, 2000)

TABLE 5-2 Skin Lesions—Anatomic Location and Distribution

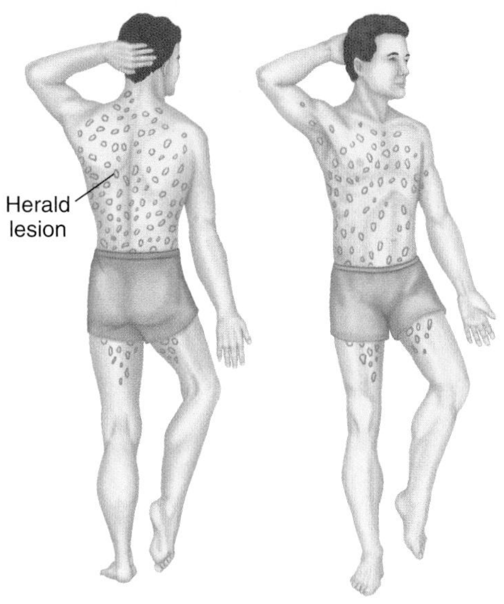

Pityriasis Rosea
Reddish oval ringworm-like lesions

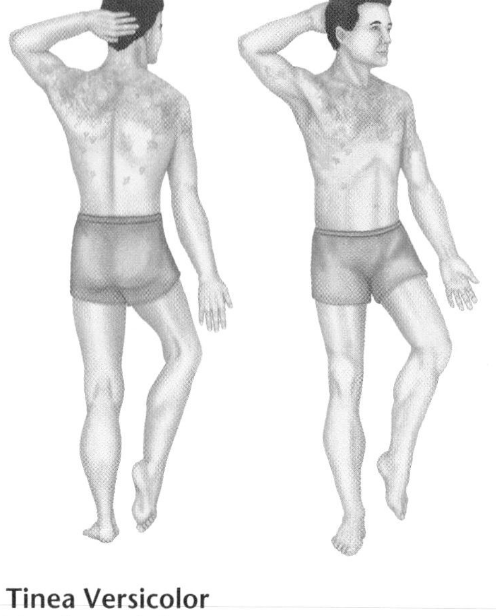

Tinea Versicolor
Tan, flat, scaly lesions

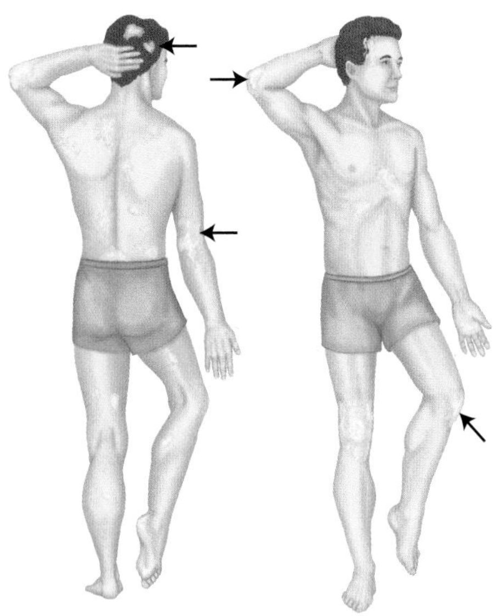

Psoriasis
Silvery scaly lesions, mainly on the extensor surfaces

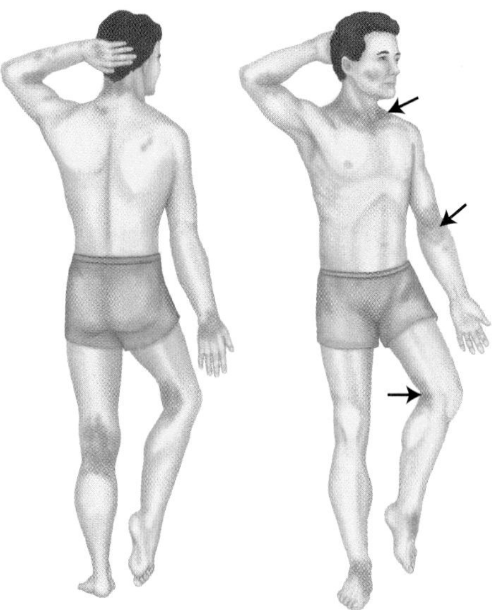

Atopic Eczema (adult form)
Appears mainly on flexor surfaces

(Source: Hall JC. *Sauer's Manual of Skin Diseases*, 8th ed. Philadelphia, Lippincott Williams & Wilkins, 2000)

TABLE 5-3 Skin Lesions—Patterns and Shapes

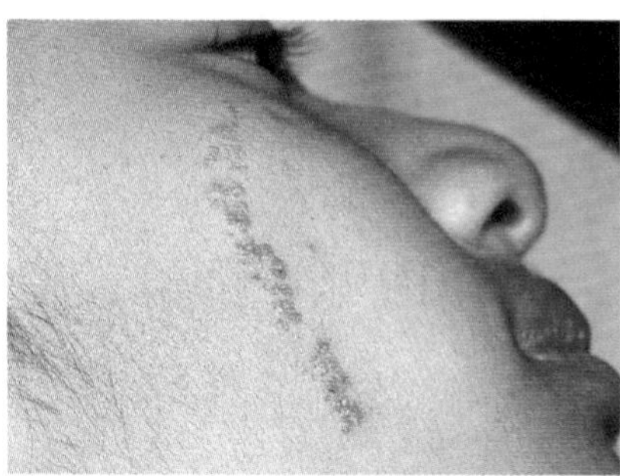

Linear
Example: Linear epidermal nevus

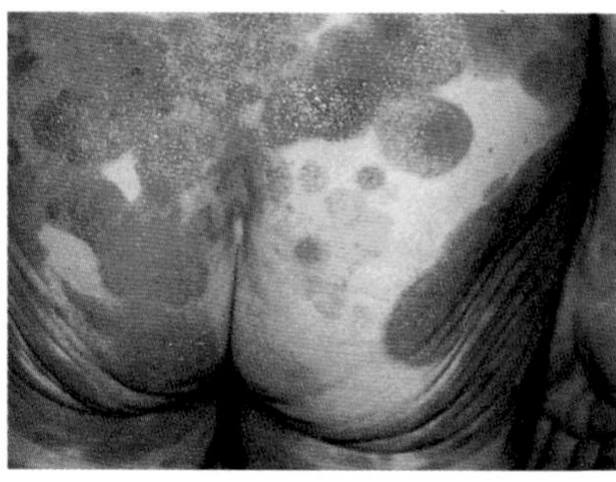

Geographic
Example: Mycosis fungoides

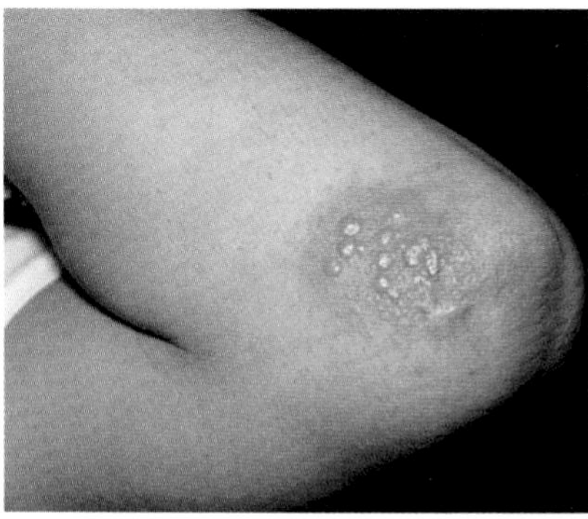

Clustered
Example: Grouped lesions of herpes simplex

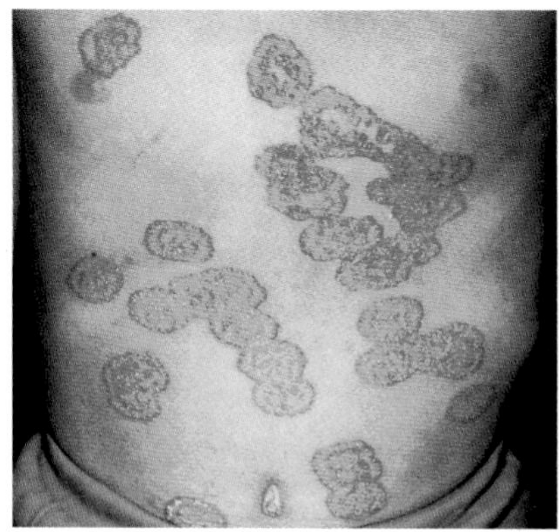

Serpiginous
Example: Tinea corporis

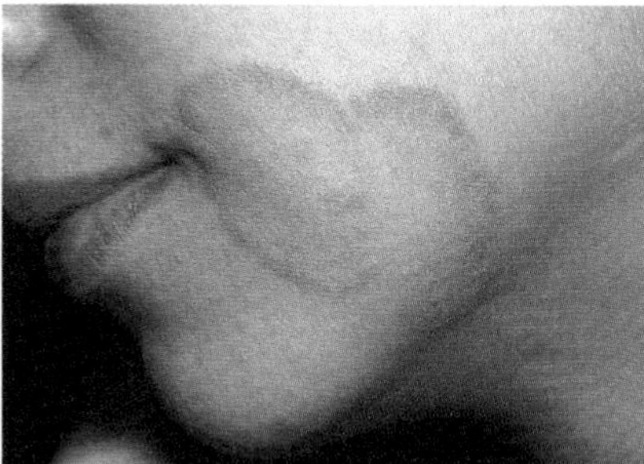

Annular, arciform
Example: Annular lesion of tinea faciale (ringworm)

(Sources of photos: *Linear Epidermal Nevus, Herpes Simplex, Tinea Faciale*—Goodheart HP. Goodheart's Photoguide of Common Skin Disorders: Diagnosis and Management, 2nd ed. Philadelphia, Lippincott Williams & Wilkins, 2003; *Mycosis Fungoides, Tinea Corporis*—Hall JC. Sauer's Manual of Skin Diseases, 8th ed. Philadelphia, Lippincott Williams & Wilkins, 2000)

TABLE 5-4 Elevated Skin Lesions

Primary Lesions

Flat, Nonpalpable Lesions With Changes in Skin Color

Macule—Small flat spot, up to 1.0 cm

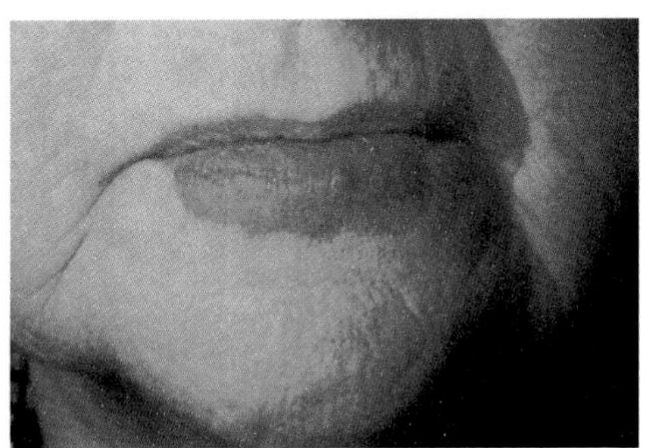

Hemangioma

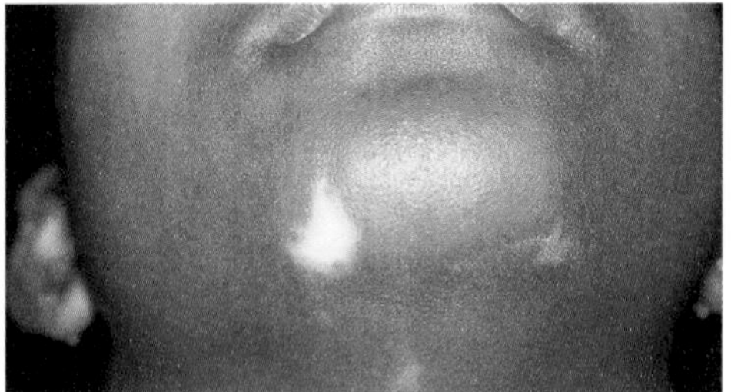

Vitiligo

Patch—Flat spot, 1.0 cm or larger

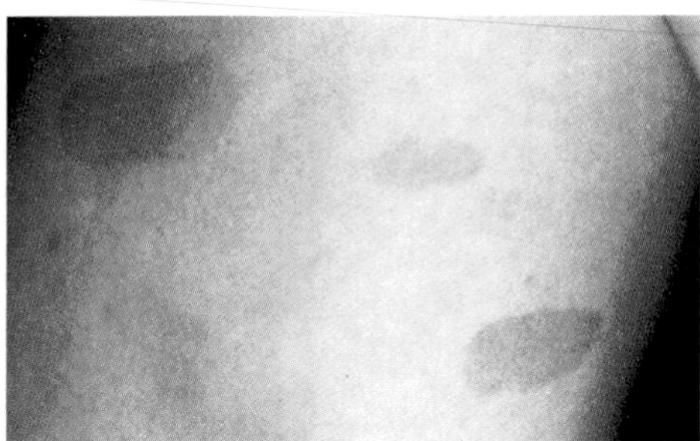

Café-au-lait spot

Palpable Elevations: Solid Masses

Plaque—Elevated superficial lesion 1.0 cm or larger, often formed by coalescence of papules

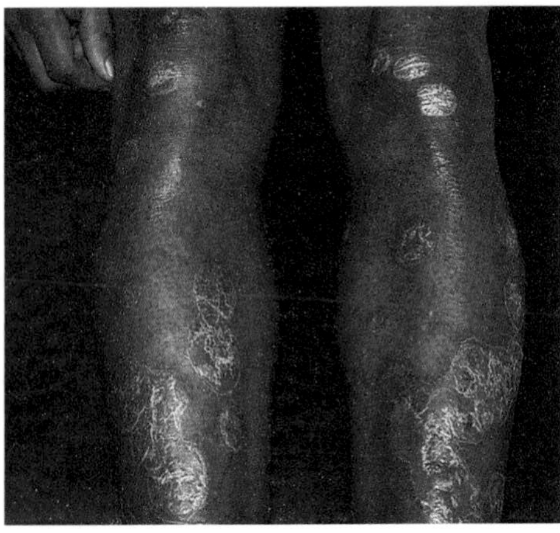

Psoriasis

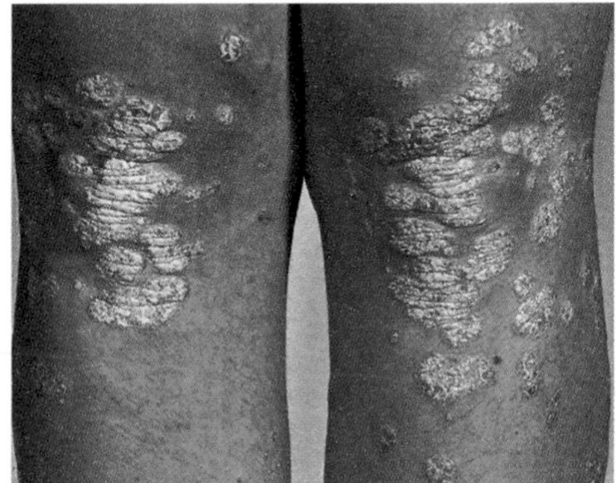

Psoriasis

(table continues next page)

Papule—Up to 1.0 cm

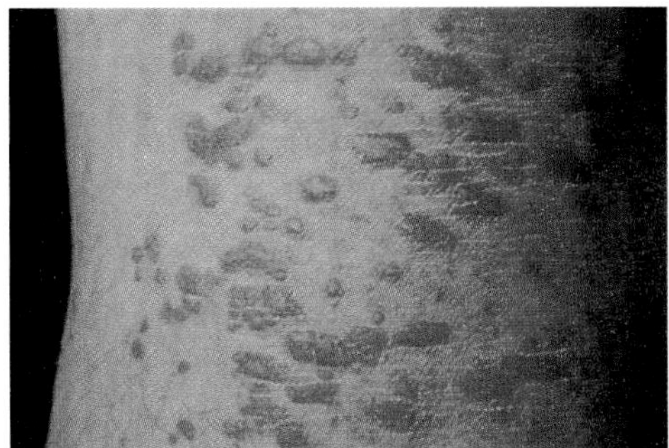

Psoriasis

Nodule—Marble-like lesion larger than 0.5 cm, often deeper and firmer than a papule

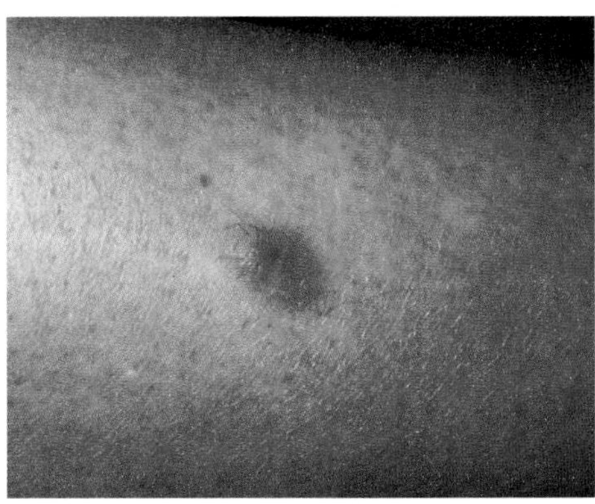

Dermatofibroma

Cyst—Nodule filled with expressible material, either liquid or semisolid

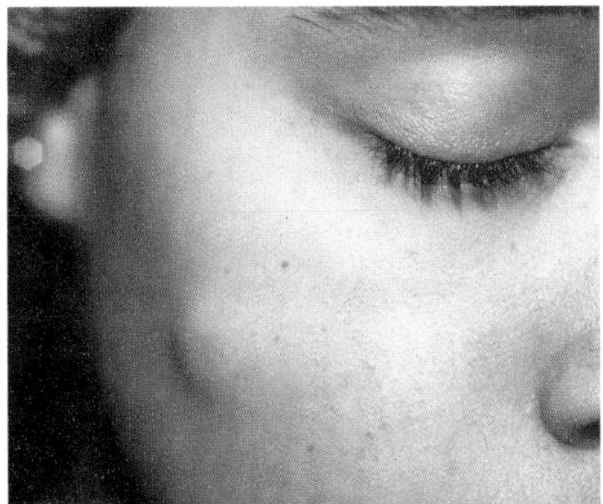

Epidermal inclusion cyst

Wheal—A somewhat irregular, relatively transient, superficial area of localized skin edema

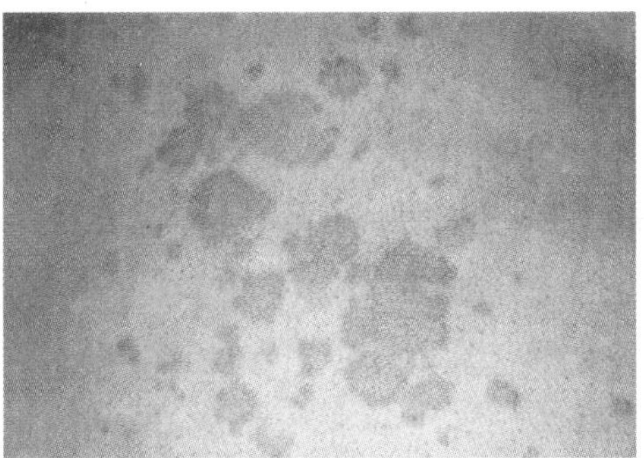

Urticaria

Palpable Elevations With Fluid-Filled Cavities

Vesicle—Up to 1.0 cm; filled with serous fluid

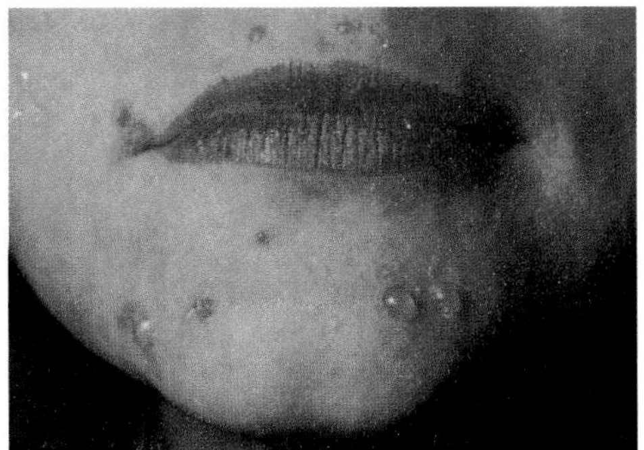

Herpes simplex

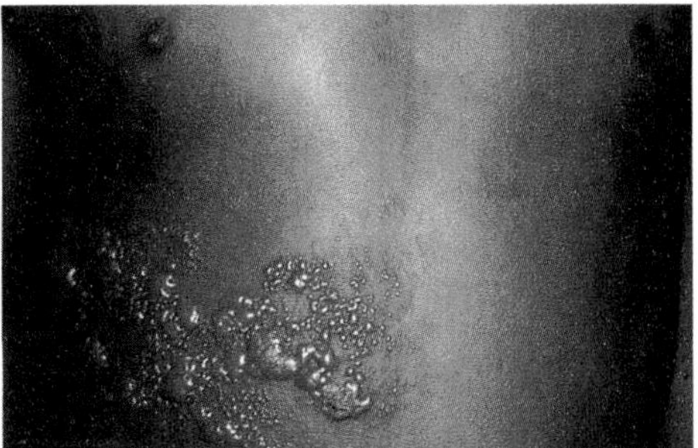

Herpes simplex

(table continues next page)

Bulla—1.0 cm or larger; filled with serous fluid

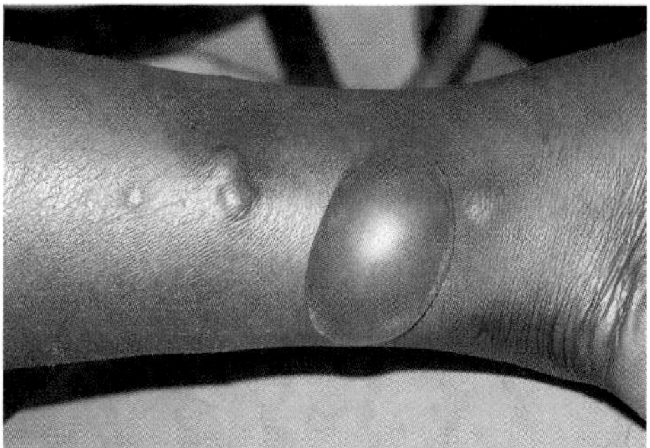

Insect bite

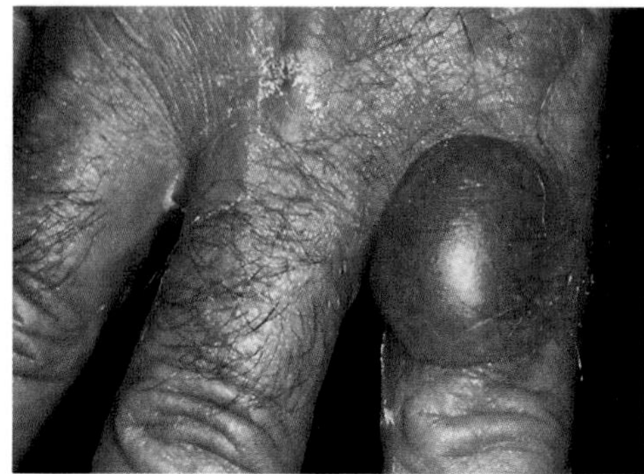

Insect bite

Pustule—Filled with pus

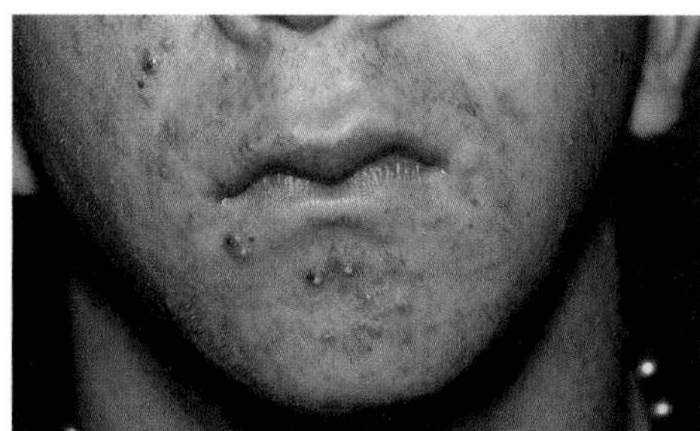

Acne

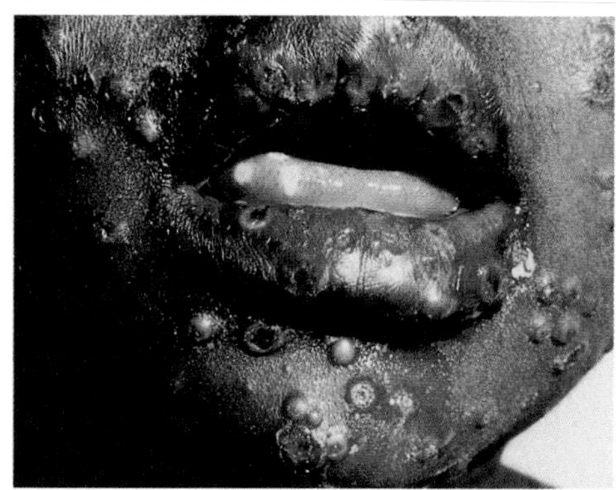

Small pox

Burrow (scabies)—A minute, slightly raised tunnel in the epidermis, commonly found on the finger webs and on the sides of the fingers. It looks like a short (5–15 mm), linear or curved gray line and may end in a tiny vesicle. Skin lesions include small papules, pustules, lichenified areas, and excoriations. With a magnifying lens, look for the *burrow* of the mite that causes scabies.

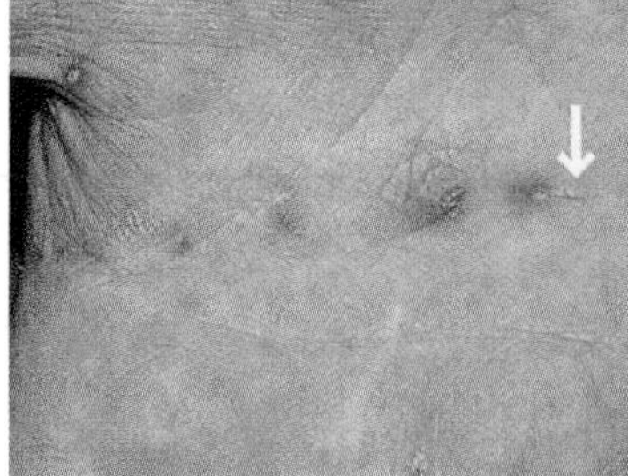

Scabies

(table continues next page)

Secondary Lesions (may arise from primary lesions)

Scale—A thin flake of dead exfoliated epidermis.

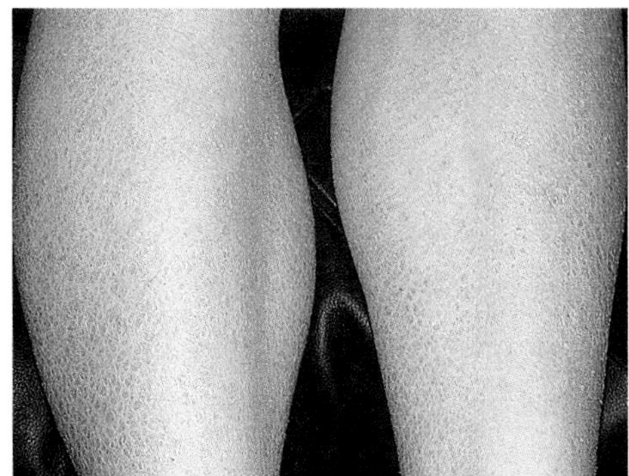

Ichthyosis vulgaris

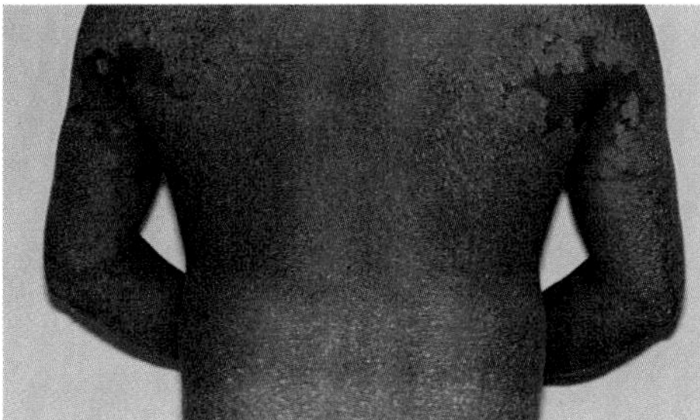

Dry skin

Crust—The dried residue of skin exudates such as serum, pus, or blood

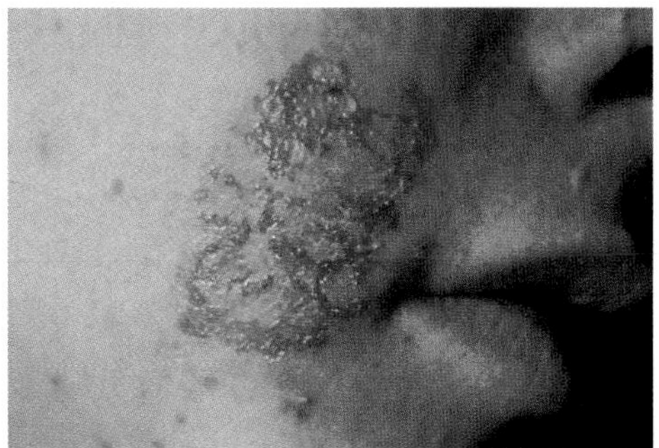

Impetigo

Lichenification—Visible and palpable thickening of the epidermis and roughening of the skin with increased visibility of the normal skin furrows (often from chronic rubbing)

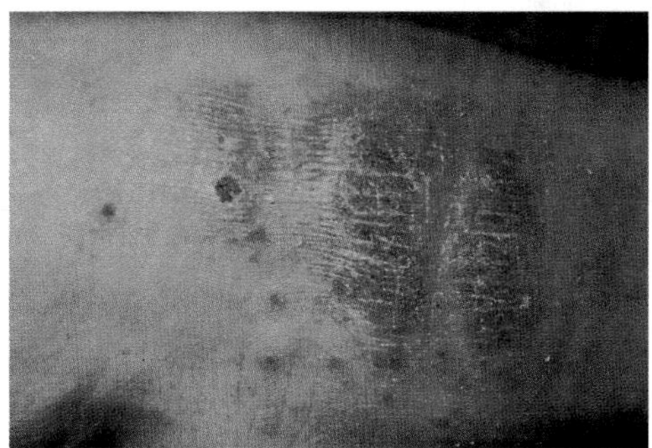

Neurodermatitis

Scars—Connective tissue that arises from injury or disease

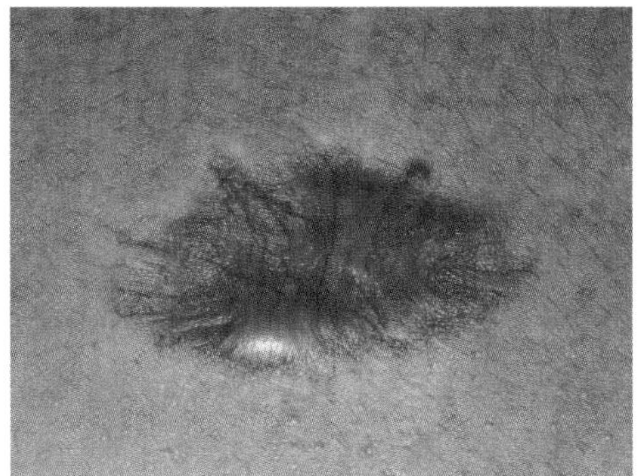

Hypertrophic scar from steroid injections

Keloids—Hypertrophic scarring that extends beyond the borders of the initiating injury

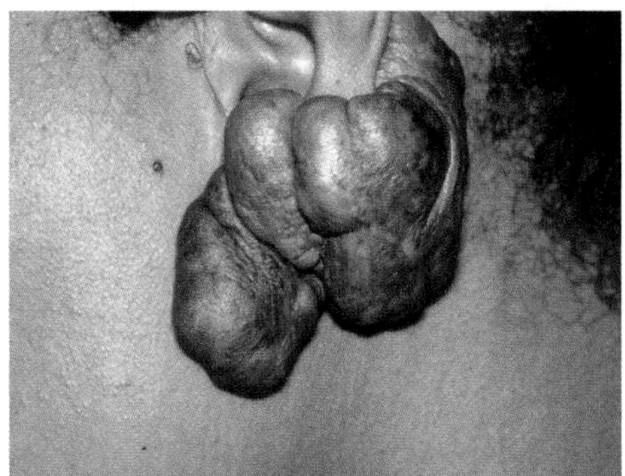

Keloid—ear lobe

Sources of photos: *Hemangioma, Café-au-Lait Spot, Elevated Nevus, Psoriasis (bottom), Dermatofibroma, Herpes Simplex, Insect Bite (bottom), Impetigo, Lichenification*—Hall JC. Sauer's Manual of Skin Diseases, 8th ed. Philadelphia, Lippincott Williams & Wilkins, 2000; *Vitiligo, Psoriasis (top), Epidermal Inclusion Cyst, Urticaria, Insect Bite (top), Acne, Ichthyosis, Psoriasis, Hypertrophic Scar, Keloids*—Goodheart HP. Goodheart's Photoguide of Common Skin Disorders: Diagnosis and Management, 2nd ed. Philadelphia, Lippincott Williams & Wilkins, 2003; *Small Pox*—Ostler HB, Mailbach HI, Hoke AW, Schwab IR. Diseases of the Eye and Skin: A Color Atlas. Philadelphia, Lippincott Williams & Wilkins, 2004)

TABLE 5-5 Depressed Skin Lesions*

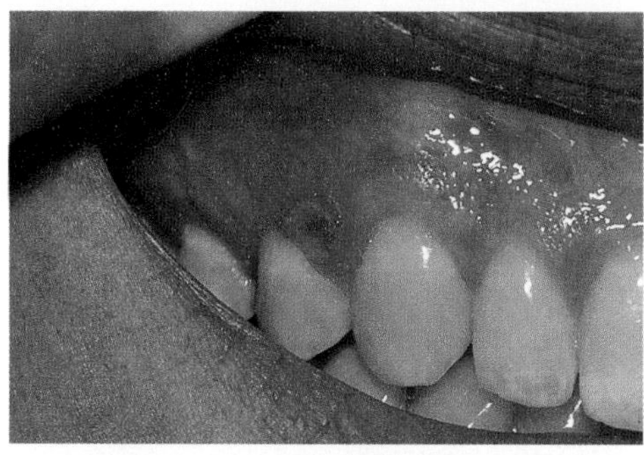

Erosion—Nonscarring loss of the superficial epidermis; surface is moist but does not bleed

Example: Aphthous stomatitis, moist area after the rupture of a vesicle, as in chickenpox

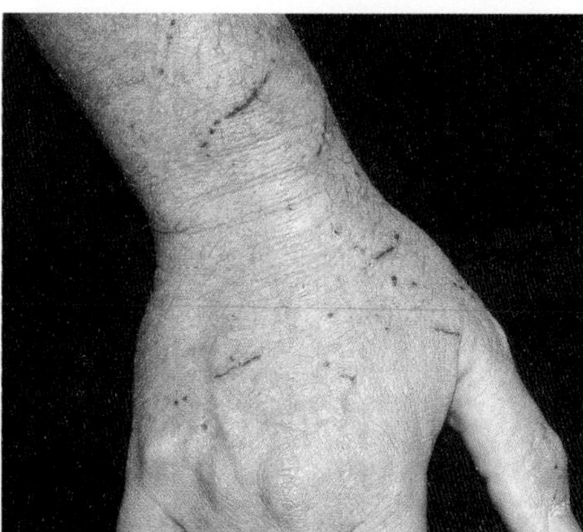

Excoriation—Linear or punctate erosions caused by scratching

Example: Cat scratches

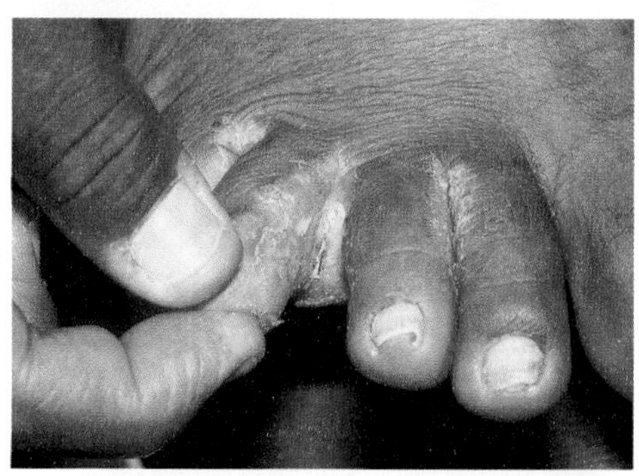

Fissure—A linear crack in the skin, often resulting from excessive dryness

Example: Athlete's foot

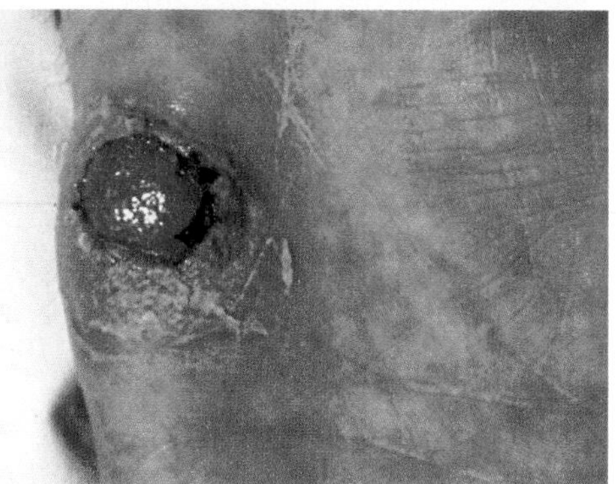

Ulcer—A deeper loss of epidermis and dermis; may bleed and scar

Examples: Stasis ulcer of venous insufficiency, syphilitic chancre

---

*These are secondary lesions (resulting from primary lesions).

(Sources of photos: *Erosion, Excoriation, Fissure*—Goodheart HP: Goodheart's Photoguide of Common Skin Disorders: Diagnosis and Management, 2nd ed. Philadelphia, Lippincott Williams & Wilkins, 2003; *Ulcer*—Hall JC: Sauer's Manual of Skin Diseases, 8th ed. Philadelphia, Lippincott Williams & Wilkins, 2000)

TABLE 5-6 Vascular and Purpuric Lesions of the Skin

Vascular Lesions

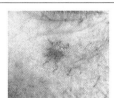

	*Spider Angioma**	*Spider Vein**	*Cherry Angioma*
		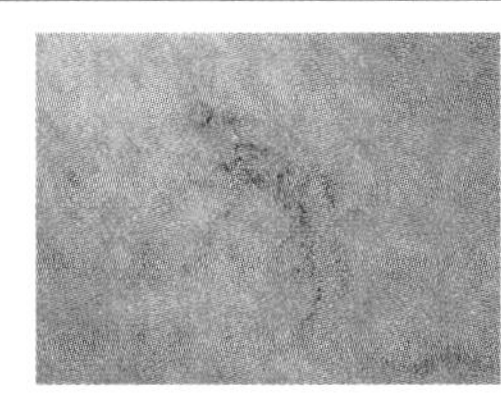	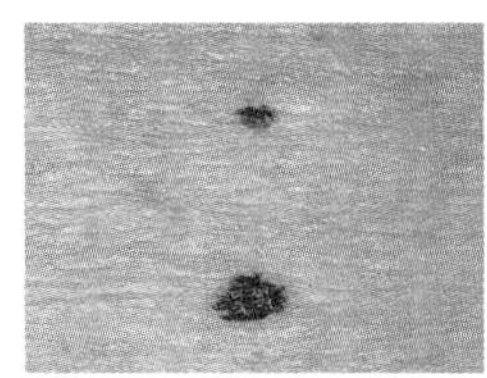
Color and Size	Fiery red. From very small to 2 cm	Bluish. Size variable, from very small to several inches	Bright or ruby red; may become brownish with age. 1–3 mm
Shape	Central body, sometimes raised, surrounded by erythema and radiating legs	Variable. May resemble a spider or be linear, irregular, cascading	Round, flat or sometimes raised, may be surrounded by a pale halo
Pulsatility and Effect of Pressure	Often seen in center of the spider, when pressure with a glass slide is applied. Pressure on the body causes blanching of the spider.	Absent. Pressure over the center does not cause blanching, but diffuse pressure blanches the veins.	Absent. May show partial blanching, especially if pressure applied with edge of a pinpoint
Distribution	Face, neck, arms, and upper trunk; almost never below the waist	Most often on the legs, near veins; also on the anterior chest	Trunk; also extremities
Significance	Liver disease, pregnancy, vitamin B deficiency; also occurs normally in some people	Often accompanies increased pressure in the superficial veins, as in varicose veins	None; increase in size and numbers with aging

Purpuric Lesions

	Petechia/Purpura	*Ecchymosis*
	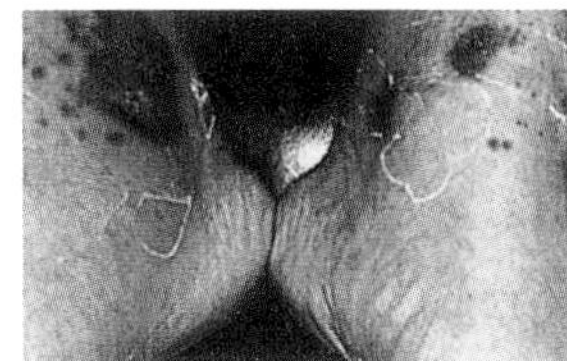	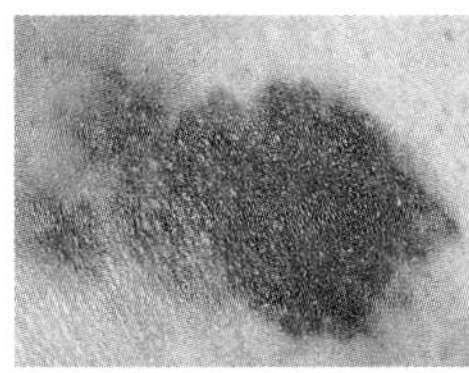
Color and Size	Deep red or reddish purple, fading away over time. Petechia, 1–3 mm; purpura, larger	Purple or purplish blue, fading to green, yellow, and brown with time. Variable size, larger than petechiae, >3 mm
Shape	Rounded, sometimes irregular; flat	Rounded, oval, or irregular; may have a central subcutaneous flat nodule (a hematoma)
Pulsatility and Effect of Pressure	Absent. No effect from pressure	Absent. No effect from pressure
Distribution	Variable	Variable
Significance	Blood outside the vessels; may suggest a bleeding disorder or, if petechiae, emboli to skin; palpable purpura in *vasculitis*	Blood outside the vessels; often secondary to bruising or trauma; also seen in bleeding disorders

*These are telangiectasias, or dilated small vessels that look red or bluish.

(Sources of photos: *Spider Angioma*—Marks R: Skin Disease in Old Age. Philadelphia, JB Lippincott, 1987; *Petechia/Purpura*—Kelley WN: Textbook of Internal Medicine. Philadelphia, JB Lippincott, 1989)

TABLE 5-7 Skin Tumors

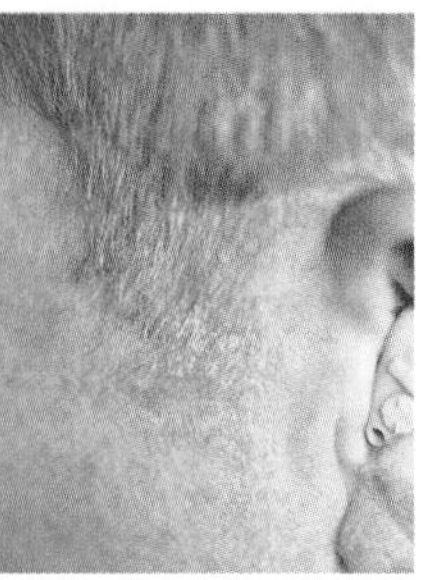
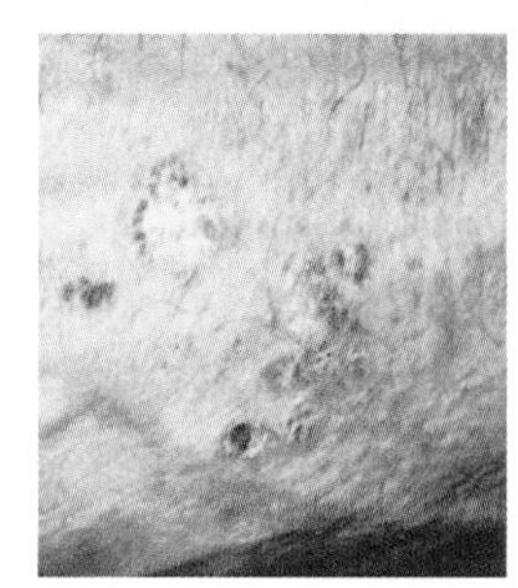

Actinic Keratosis

Superficial, flattened papules covered by a dry scale. Often multiple; can be round or irregular; pink, tan, or grayish. Appear on sun-exposed skin of older, fair-skinned persons. Though benign, 1 of every 1,000 per year develop into squamous cell carcinoma (suggested by rapid growth, induration, redness at the base, and ulceration). Keratoses on face and hand, typical locations, are shown.

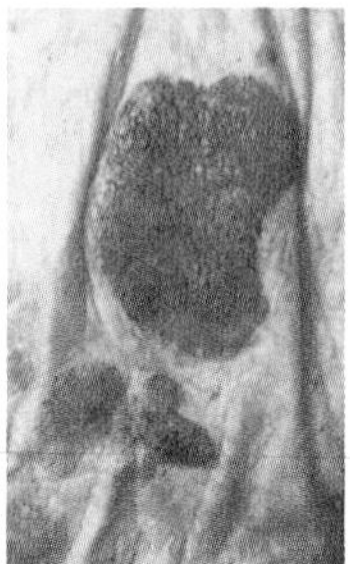
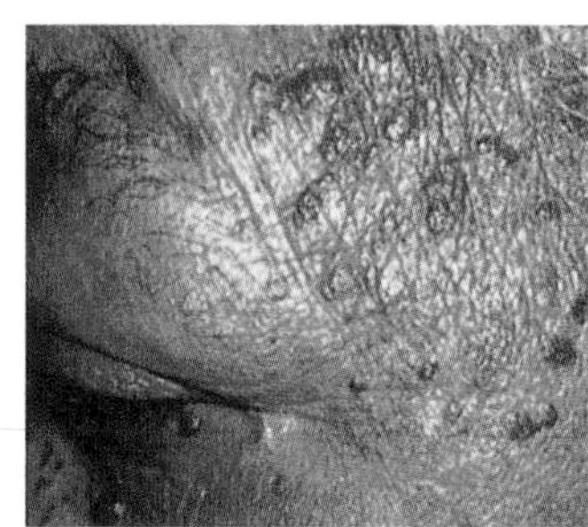

Seborrheic Keratosis

Common, benign, yellowish to brown raised lesions that feel slightly greasy and velvety or warty and have a "stuck on" appearance. Typically multiple and symmetrically distributed on the trunk of older people, but may also appear on the face and elsewhere. In black people, often younger women, may appear as small, deeply pigmented papules on the cheeks and temples (dermatosis papulosa nigra).

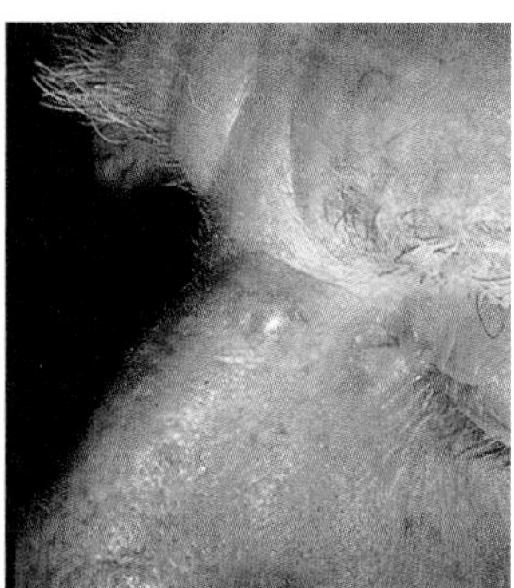

Basal Cell Carcinoma

A basal cell carcinoma, though malignant, grows slowly and seldom metastasizes. It is most common in fair-skinned adults over age 40, and usually appears on the face. An initial translucent nodule spreads, leaving a depressed center and a firm, elevated border. Telangiectatic vessels are often visible.

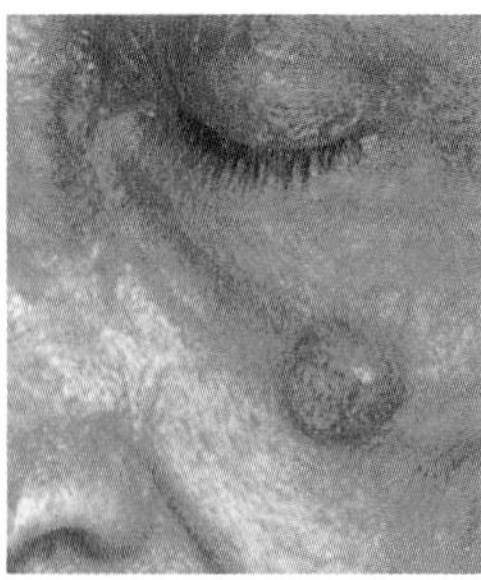
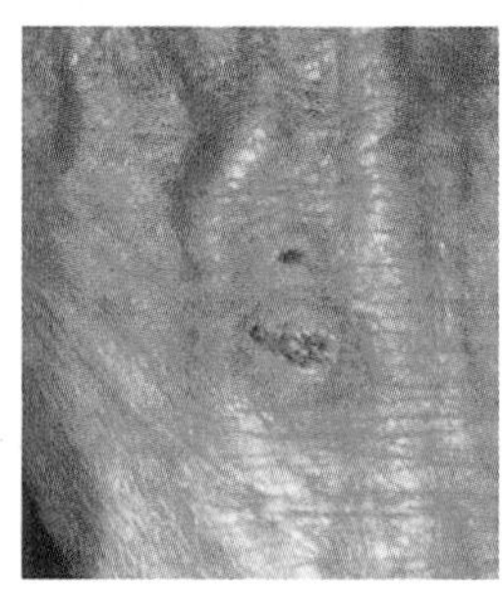

Squamous Cell Carcinoma

Usually appears on sun-exposed skin of fair-skinned adults older than 60. May develop in an actinic keratosis. Usually grows more quickly than a basal cell carcinoma, is firmer, and looks redder. The face and the back of the hand are often affected, as shown here.

(Sources of photos: *Basal Cell Carcinoma*—Rapini R. *Squamous Cell Carcinoma, Actinic Keratosis, Seborrheic Keratosis*—Sauer GC. Manual of Skin Diseases, 5th ed. Philadelphia, JB Lippincott, 1985)

TABLE 5-8 Benign and Malignant Nevi

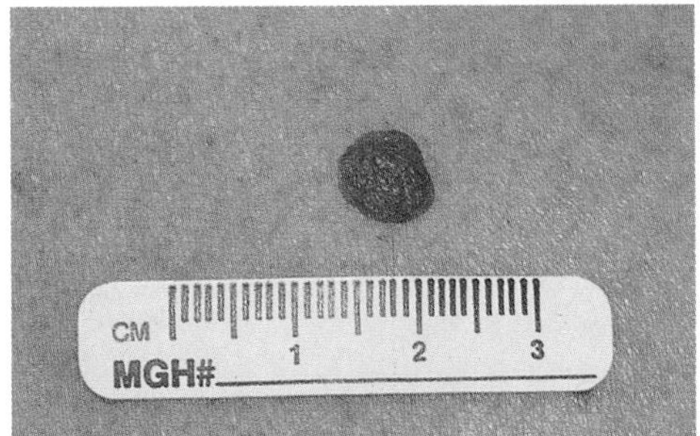

Benign Nevus

The *benign nevus*, or common mole, usually appears in the first few decades. Several nevi may arise at the same time, but their appearance usually remains unchanged. Note the following typical features and contrast them with those of atypical nevi and melanoma:

- Round or oval shape
- Sharply defined borders
- Uniform color, especially tan or brown
- Diameter <6 mm
- Flat or raised surface

Changes in these features raise the the spectre of *atypical (dysplastic) nevi,* or melanoma. Atypical nevi are varied in color but often dark and larger than 6 mm, with irregular borders that fade into the surrounding skin. Look for atypical nevi primarily on the trunk. They may number more than 50 to 100.

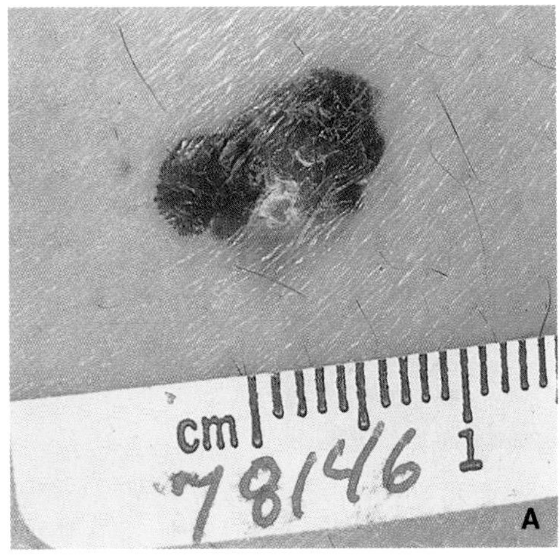

Malignant Melanoma

Learn the **ABCDEs** of melanoma from these reference standard photographs from the American Cancer Society:

- ***A**symmetry* (Fig. A)
- Irregular ***B**orders*, especially notching (Fig. B)
- Variation in ***C**olor*, especially mixtures of black, blue, and red (Figs. B, C)
- ***D**iameter* >6 mm (Fig. C)
- ***E**levation*, though also may be flat (Fig. C)

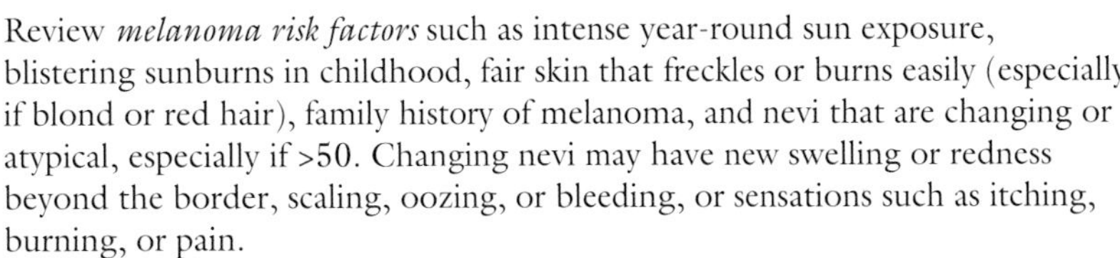

Review *melanoma risk factors* such as intense year-round sun exposure, blistering sunburns in childhood, fair skin that freckles or burns easily (especially if blond or red hair), family history of melanoma, and nevi that are changing or atypical, especially if >50. Changing nevi may have new swelling or redness beyond the border, scaling, oozing, or bleeding, or sensations such as itching, burning, or pain.

On darker skin, look for melanomas under the nails, on the hands, or on the soles of the feet.

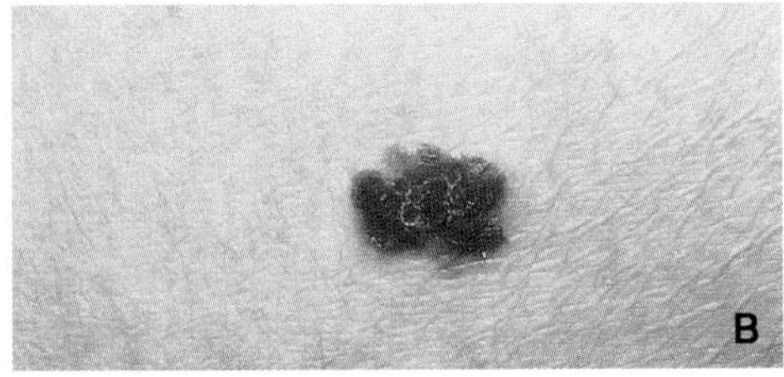

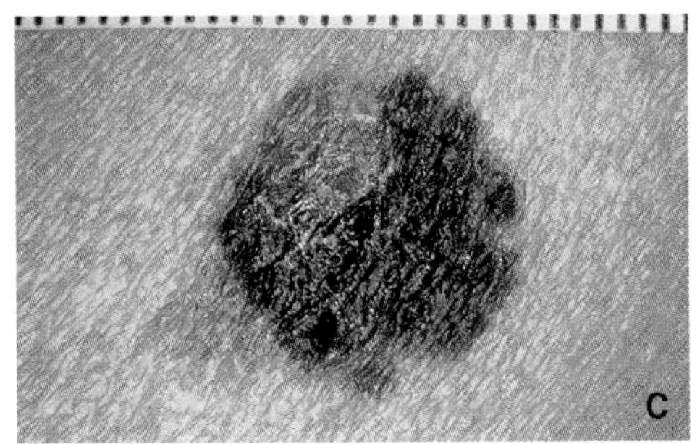

(Source: Courtesy of American Cancer Society; American Academy of Dermatology)

TABLE 5-9 Skin Lesions in Context

This table shows a variety of primary and secondary skin lesions. Try to identify them, including those indicated by letters, before reading the accompanying text.

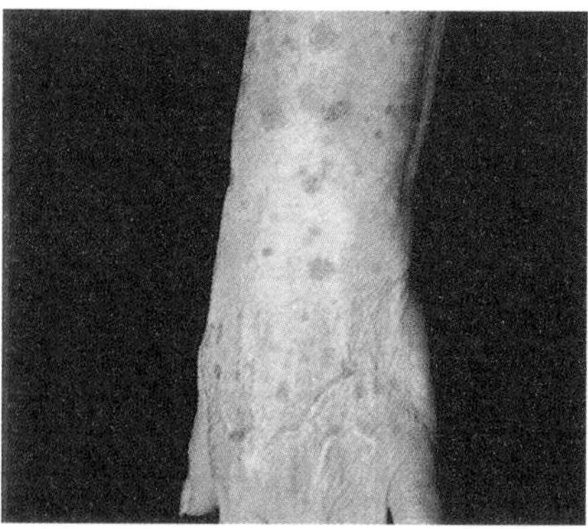

Macules on the dorsum of the hand, wrist, and forearm (*actinic lentigines*)

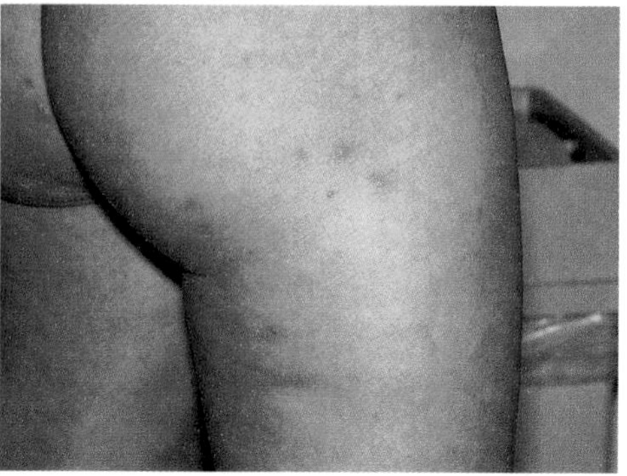

Papules and pustules (in hot tub folliculitis from *Pseudomonas*)

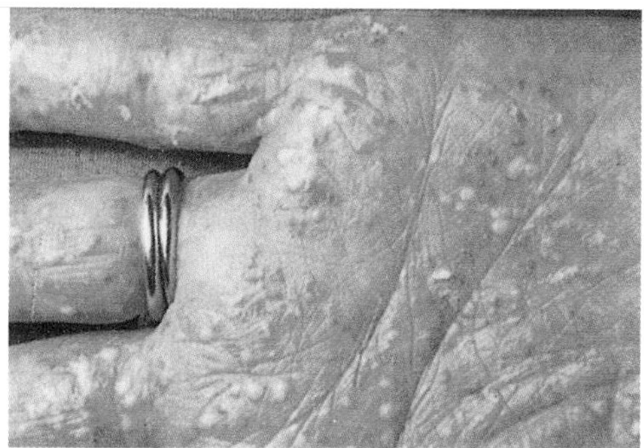

Pustules on the palm (in *pustular psoriasis*)

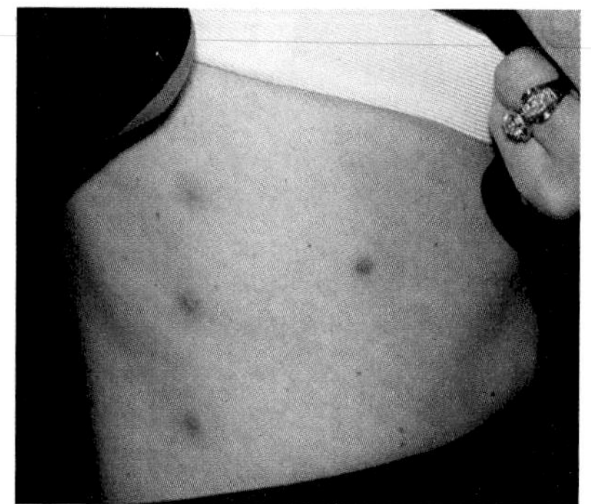

Vesicles (*chickenpox*)

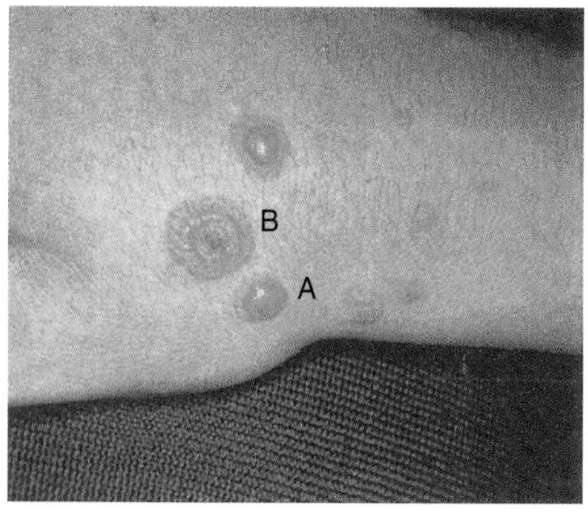

(A) Bulla, (B) target (or iris) lesion (in *erythema multiforme*)

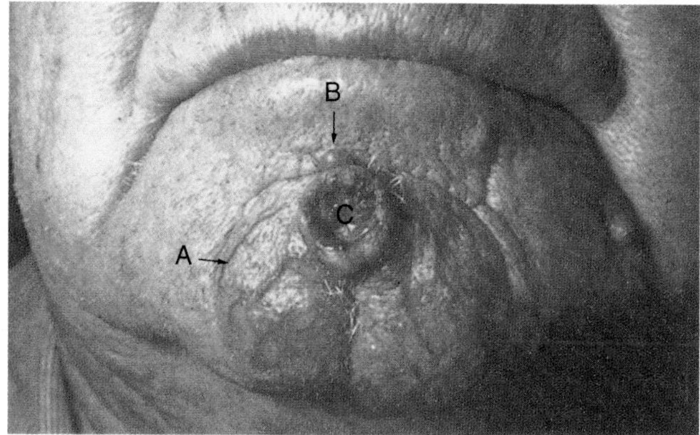

(A) Telangiectasia, (B) nodule, (C) ulcer (in *squamous cell carcinoma*)

(table continues next page)

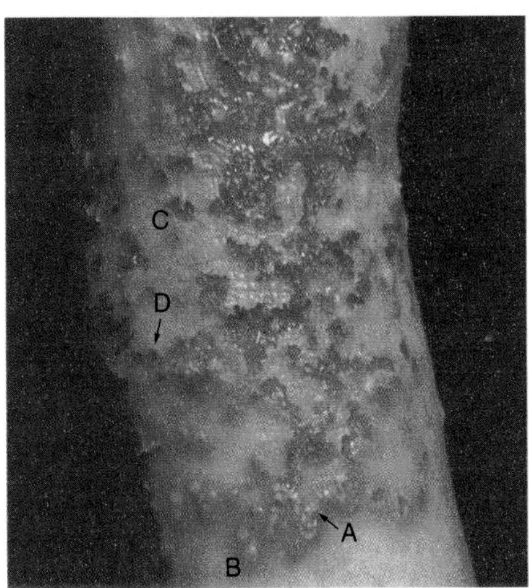

(A) Vesicle, (B) pustule, (C) erosions, (D) crust, on the back of a knee (in *infected atopic dermatitis*)

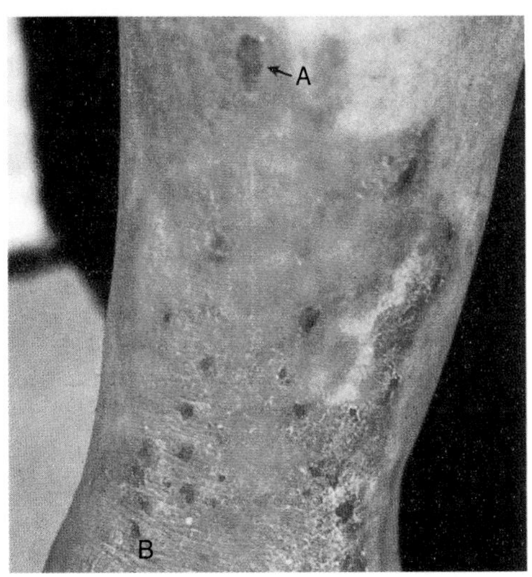

(A) Excoriation, (B) lichenification on the leg (in *atopic dermatitis*)

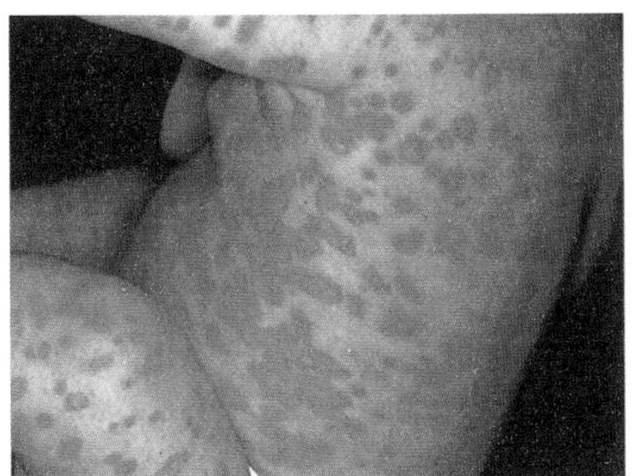

Wheals (*urticaria*) in a drug eruption in an infant

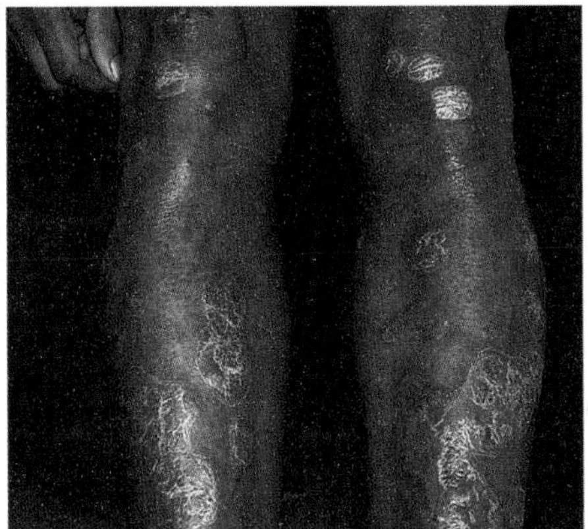

Plaques with scales on knee (*psoriasis*) and legs

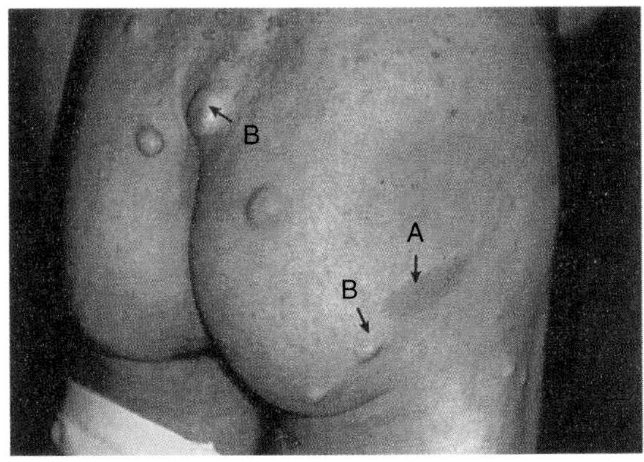

(A) Patch (café-au-lait spots), (B) nodules—a combination typical of neurofibromatosis.

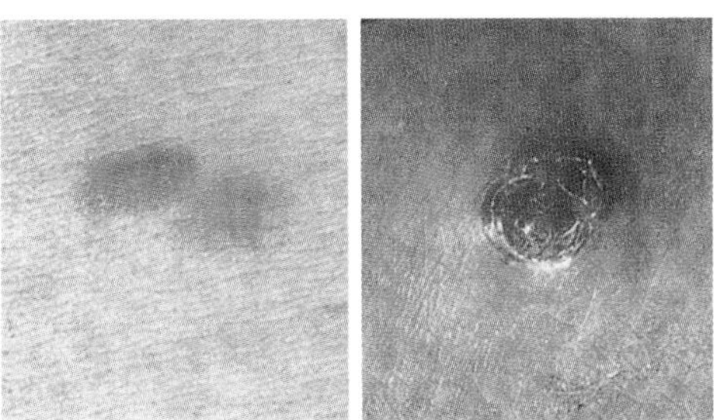

Kaposi's sarcoma in AIDS: This malignant tumor may appear in many forms: macules, papules, plaques, or nodules almost anywhere on the body. Lesions are often multiple and may involve internal structures. On left: ovoid, pinkish red plaques that typically lengthen along the skin line may become pigmented. On right: a purplish red nodule on the foot.

(Sources of photos: Sauer GC: Manual of Skin Diseases, 5th ed. Philadelphia, JB Lippincott, 1985; *Kaposi's Sarcoma in AIDS*—DeVita VT Jr, Hellman S, Rosenberg SA [eds]: AIDS: Etiology, Diagnosis, Treatment, and Prevention. Philadelphia, JB Lippincott, 1985; *Psoriasis, Papules, Vesicles (chickenpox)*—Goodheart HP. Goodheart's Photoguide of Common Skin Disorders: Diagnosis and Management, 2nd ed. Philadelphia, Lippincott Williams & Wilkins, 2003)

TABLE 5-10 Diseases and Related Skin Conditions

Addison's disease	Hyperpigmentation of skin and mucous membranes
AIDS	Hairy leukoplakia, Kaposi's sarcoma, herpes simplex virus (HSV), human papillomavirus (HPV), cytomegalovirus (CMV), molluscum contagiosum, mycobacterial skin infections, candidiasis and other cutaneous fungal infections, oral and anal squamous cell carcinoma, acquired ichthyosis, bacterial abscesses, psoriasis (often severe), erythroderma, seborrheic dermatitis (often severe)
Chronic renal disease	Pallor, xerosis, pruritus, hyperpigmentation, uremic frost, metastatic calcification in the skin, calciphylaxis, "half and half" nails, hemodialysis-related skin disease
CREST syndrome	Calcinosis, Raynaud's phenomenon, sclerodactyly, telangiectasias
Crohn's disease	Erythema nodosum, pyoderma gangrenosum, enterocutaneous fistulas, aphthous ulcers
Cushing's disease	Striae, skin atrophy, purpura, ecchymoses, telangiectasias, acne, moon facies, buffalo hump, hypertrichosis
Dermatomyositis	Heliotrope rash, Gottron's papules, periungual telangiectasias, alopecia, poikiloderma in sun-exposed areas, Raynaud's phenomenon
Diabetes	Necrobiosis lipoidica diabeticorum, diabetic bullae, diabetic dermopathy, granuloma annulare, acanthosis nigricans, candidiasis, neuropathic ulcers, eruptive xanthomas, peripheral vascular disease
Disseminated intravascular coagulation	Skin necrosis, petechiae, ecchymoses, hemorrhagic bullae, purpura fulminans
Dyslipidemias	Xanthomas (tendon, eruptive, and tuberous), xanthelasma (may occur in healthy people)
Gonococcemia	Erythematous macules to hemorrhagic pustules; lesions in acral distribution that can involve palms and soles
Hemochromatosis	Skin bronzing and hyperpigmentation
Hypothyroidism	Dry, rough, and pale skin; coarse and brittle hair; myxedema; alopecia (lateral third of the eyebrows to diffuse); skin cool to touch; thin and brittle nails
Hyperthyroidism	Warm, moist, soft, and velvety skin; thin and fine hair; alopecia; vitiligo; pretibial myxedema (in Graves' disease); hyperpigmentation (local or generalized)
Infective endocarditis	Janeway lesions, Osler nodes, splinter hemorrhages, petechiae
Kawasaki disease	Mucosal erythema (lips, tongue, and pharynx), strawberry tongue, cherry red lips, polymorphous rash (primarily on trunk), erythema of palms and soles with later desquamation of fingertips
Liver disease	Jaundice, spider angiomas and other telangiectasias, palmar erythema, Terry's nails, pruritus, purpura, caput medusae
Leukemia/lymphoma	Pallor, exfoliative erythroderma, nodules, petechiae, ecchymoses, pruritus, vasculitis, pyoderma gangrenosum, bullous diseases
Meningococcemia	Pink macules and papules, petechiae, hemorrhagic petechiae, hemorrhagic bullae, purpura fulminans
Neurofibromatoses 1 (von Recklinghausen's syndrome)	Neurofibromas, café au lait, freckling in the axillary and inguinal areas, plexiform neurofibroma
Pancreatitis (hemorrhagic)	Grey Turner sign, Cullen's sign, panniculitis
Pancreatic carcinoma	Panniculitis, migratory thrombophlebitis
Peripheral vascular disease	Dry, scaly, shiny atrophic skin; dystrophic, brittle toenails; cool skin; hairless shins; ulcers; pallor; cyanosis; gangrene
Pregnancy (physiologic changes)	Melasma, increased pigmentation of areolae, linea nigra, palmar erythema, varicose veins, striae, spider angiomas, hirsutism, pyogenic granuloma
Reiter's syndrome	Psoriasis-like skin and mucous membrane lesions, keratoderma blennorrhagicum, balanitis circinata

(table continues next page)

TABLE 5-10 Diseases and Related Skin Conditions *(Continued)*

Rheumatoid arthritis	Vasculitis, Raynaud's phenomenon, rheumatoid nodules, pyoderma gangrenosum, rheumatoid papules, erythematous to salmon-colored rashes
Rocky Mountain spotted fever	Erythematous rash that begins on wrists and ankles, then spreads to palms and soles; becomes more purpuric as it generalizes
Scleroderma	Thickened, taut, and shiny skin; ulcerations and pitted scars on fingertips; sclerodactyly; telangiectasias; Raynaud's phenomenon
Sickle cell	Jaundice, leg ulcers (malleolar regions), pallor
Syphilis	*1°:* Chancre (painless) *2°:* Rash ("the great imitator")—ham- to bronze-colored, generalized, maculopapular rash that involves the palms and soles, pustules, condylomata lata, alopecia ("moth-eaten"), white plaques on oral and genital mucosa *3°:* Gummas, granulomas
Systemic lupus erythematosus	Photosensitivity, malar (butterfly) rash, discoid rash, alopecia, vasculitis, oral ulcers, Raynaud's phenomenon
Thrombocytopenic purpura	Petechiae, ecchymoses
Tuberous sclerosis	Adenoma sebaceum (angiofibromas), ash-leaf spots, shagreen patch, perungual fibromas
Ulcerative colitis	Erythema nodosum, pyoderma gangrenosum
Viral exanthems	*Coxsackie A (hand, foot, and mouth):* Oral ulcers; macules, papules, and vesicles on hands, feet, and buttocks *Erythema infectiosum (fifth disease):* Erythema of cheeks ("slapped cheeks") followed by erythematous, pruritic, reticulated (net-like) rash that starts on trunk and proximal extremities (rash worsens with sun, fever, and temperature changes) *Roseola infantum (HSV 6):* Erythematous, maculopapular, discrete rash (often fever present) that begins on head and spreads to involve trunk and extremities, petechiae on soft palate *Rubella (German measles):* Erythematous, maculopapular, discrete rash (often fever present) that begins on head and spreads to involve trunk and extremities, petechiae on soft palate *Rubeola (measles):* Erythematous, maculopapular rash that begins on head and spreads to involve trunk and extremities (lesions become confluent on face and trunk, but are discrete on extremities), Koplik spots on buccal mucosa *Varicella (chickenpox):* Generalized, pruritic, vesicular (vesicles on an erythematous base, "dewdrop on a rose petal") rash begins on trunk and spreads peripherally, lesions appear in crops and are in different stages of healing *Herpes zoster (shingles):* Pruritic, vesicular rash (vesicles on an erythematous base) in a dermatomal distribution

TABLE 5-11 Pressure Ulcers

Pressure ulcers, also termed *decubitus* ulcers, usually develop over body prominences subject to unrelieved pressure, resulting in ischemic damage to underlying tissue. Prevention is important: inspect the skin thoroughly for *early warning signs* of erythema that blanches with pressure, especially in patients with risk factors.

Pressure ulcers form most commonly over the sacrum, ischial tuberosities, greater trochanters, and heels. A commonly applied staging system, based on depth of destroyed tissue, is illustrated below. Note that necrosis or eschar must be débrided before ulcers can be staged; and ulcers may not progress sequentially through the four stages.

Inspect ulcers for signs of infection (drainage, odor, cellulitis, or necrosis). Fever, chills, and pain suggest underlying osteomyelitis. Address the patient's overall health, including *comorbid conditions* such as vascular disease, diabetes, immune deficiencies, collagen vascular disease, malignancy, psychosis, or depression; nutritional status; pain and level of analgesia; risk for recurrence; psychosocial factors such as learning ability, social supports, and lifestyle; and evidence of polypharmacy, overmedication, or abuse of alcohol, tobacco, or illicit drugs.

Risk Factors for Pressure Ulcers

- Decreased mobility, especially if accompanied by increased pressure or movement causing friction or shear stress
- Decreased sensation, from brain or spinal cord lesions or peripheral nerve disease
- Decreased blood flow from hypotension or microvascular disease such as diabetes or atherosclerosis
- Fecal or urinary incontinence
- Presence of fracture
- Poor nutritional status or low albumin

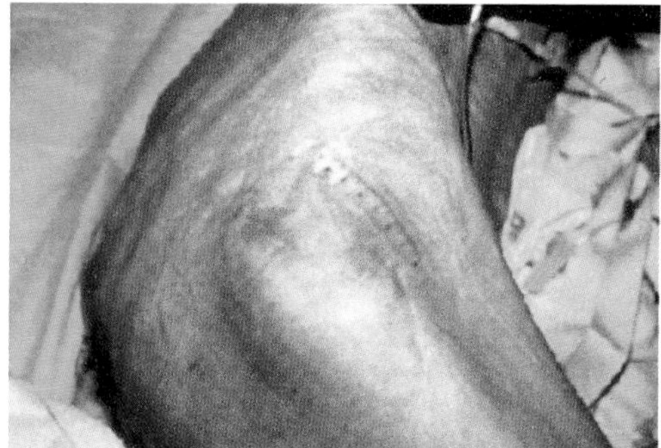

Stage I

Pressure-related alteration of intact skin, with changes in temperature (warmth or coolness), consistency (firm or boggy), sensation (pain or itching), or color (red, blue, or purple on darker skin; red on lighter skin)

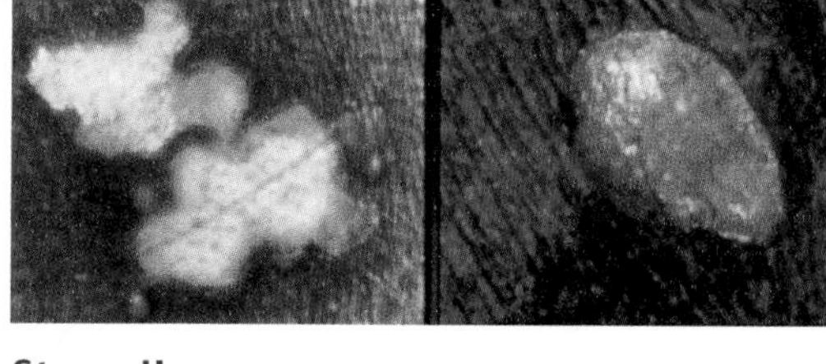

Stage II

Partial-thickness skin loss or ulceration involving the epidermis, dermis, or both

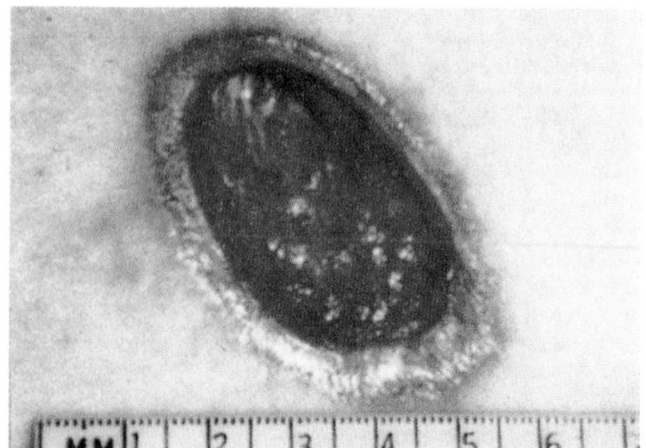

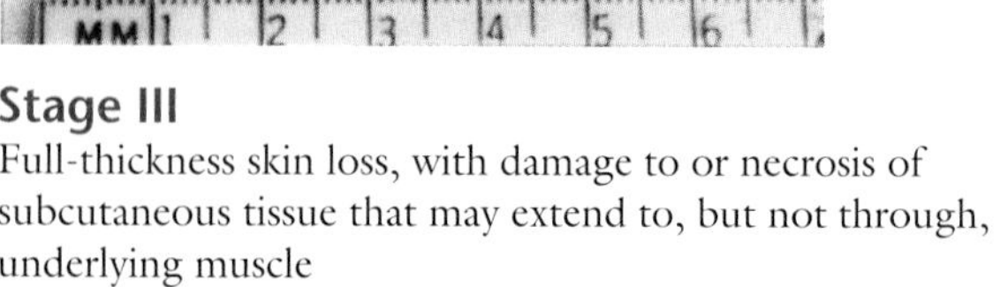

Stage III

Full-thickness skin loss, with damage to or necrosis of subcutaneous tissue that may extend to, but not through, underlying muscle

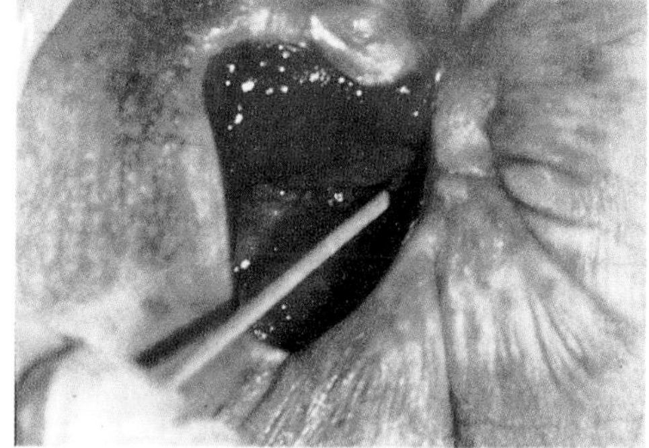

Stage IV

Full-thickness skin loss, with destruction, tissue necrosis, or damage to underlying muscle, bone, or supporting structures

(Source: National Pressure Ulcer Advisory Panel, Reston, VA)

TABLE 5-12 Hair Loss

Alopecia Areata

Clearly demarcated round or oval patches of hair loss, usually affecting young adults and children. There is no visible scaling or inflammation.

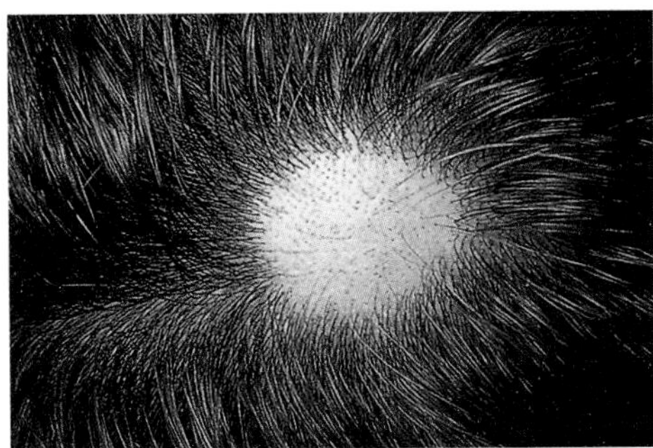

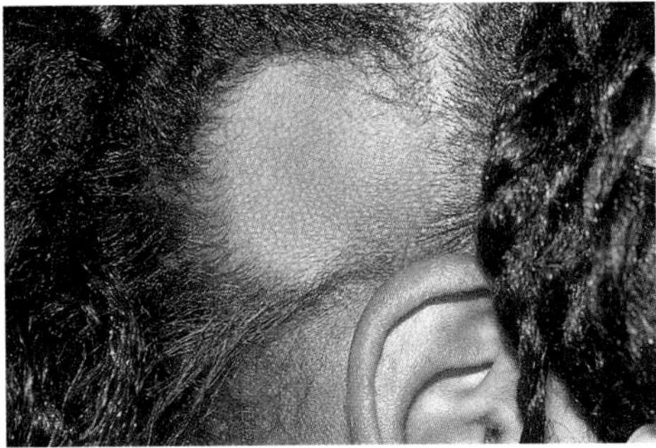

Trichotillomania

Hair loss from pulling, plucking, or twisting hair. Hair shafts are broken and of varying lengths. More common in children, often in settings of family or psychosocial stress.

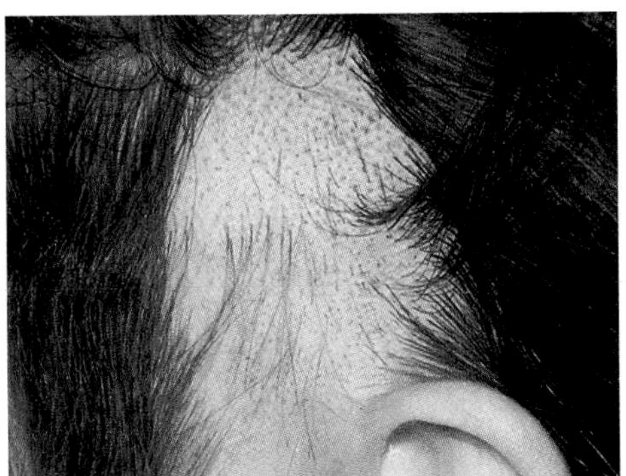

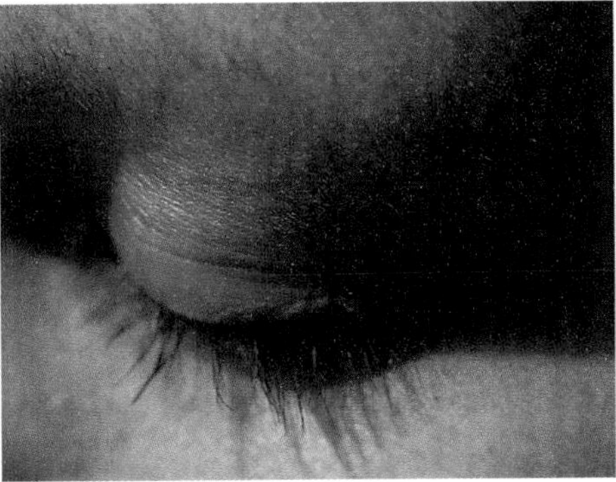

Tinea Capitis ("Ringworm")

Round scaling patches of alopecia. Hairs are broken off close to the surface of the scalp. Usually caused by fungal infection from *tinea tonsurans.* Mimics seborrheic dermatitis.

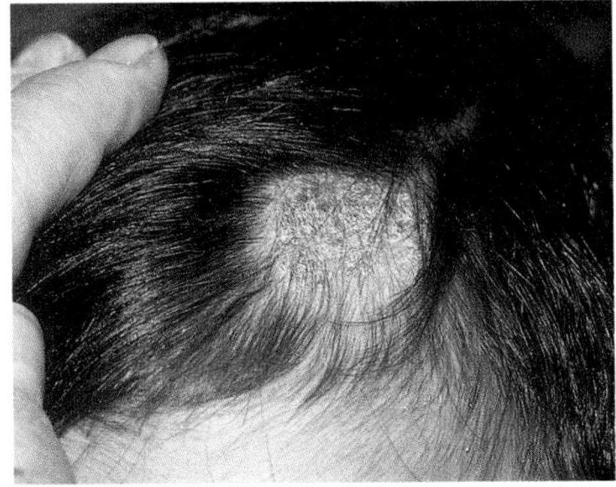

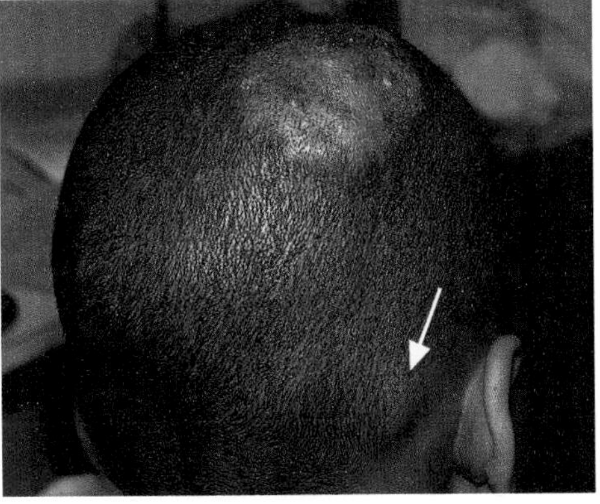

(Sources of photos: *Alopecia Areata (left), Trichotillomania (top)*—Hall JC. Sauer's Manual of Skin Diseases, 8th ed. Philadelphia, Lippincott Williams & Wilkins, 2000; *Alopecia Areata (bottom), Tinea Capitis*—Goodheart HP. Goodheart's Photoguide of Common Skin Disorders: Diagnosis and Management, 2nd ed. Philadelphia, Lippincott Williams & Wilkins, 2003; *Trichotillomania (bottom)*—Ostler HB, Mailbach HI, Hoke AW, Schwab IR. Diseases of the Eye and Skin: A Color Atlas. Philadelphia, Lippincott Williams & Wilkins, 2004)

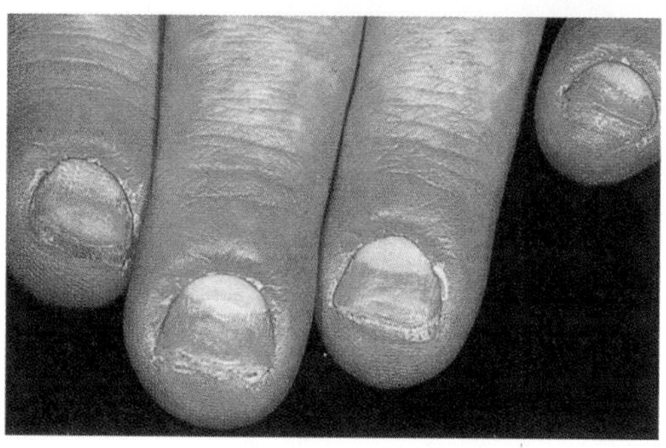

Paronychia

An inflammation of the proximal and lateral nail folds that may be acute or, as illustrated, chronic. The folds are red, swollen, and often tender. The cuticle may not be visible. People who frequently immerse their nails in water are especially susceptible. Multiple nails are often affected.

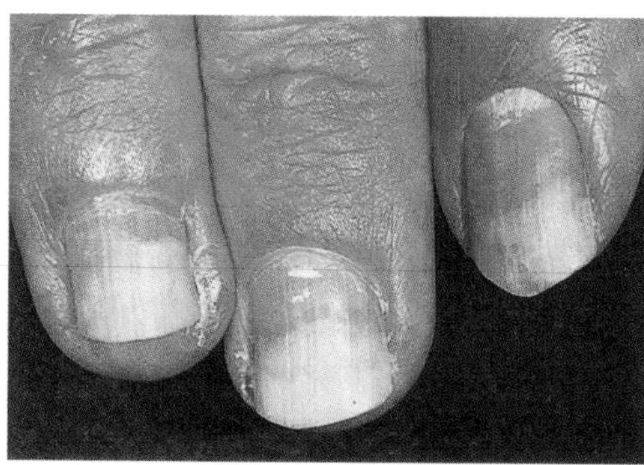

Onycholysis

A painless separation of the nail plate from the nail bed. It starts distally, enlarging the free edge of the nail to a varying degree. Several or all nails are usually affected. There are many causes.

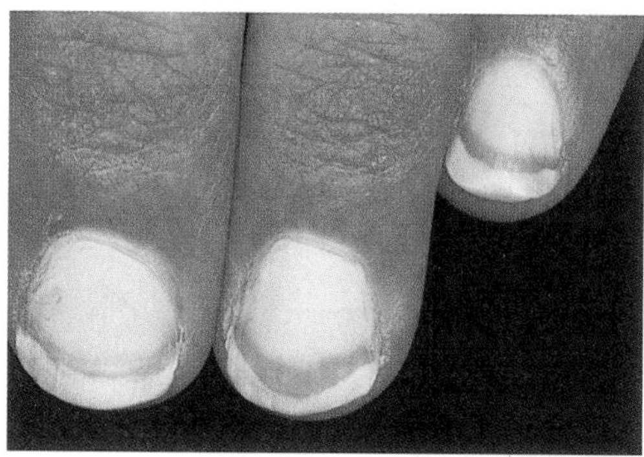

Terry's Nails

Nails are mostly whitish with a distal band of reddish brown. The lunulae of the nails may not be visible. Seen with aging and in people with chronic diseases such as cirrhosis of the liver, congestive heart failure, and non-insulin-dependent diabetes.

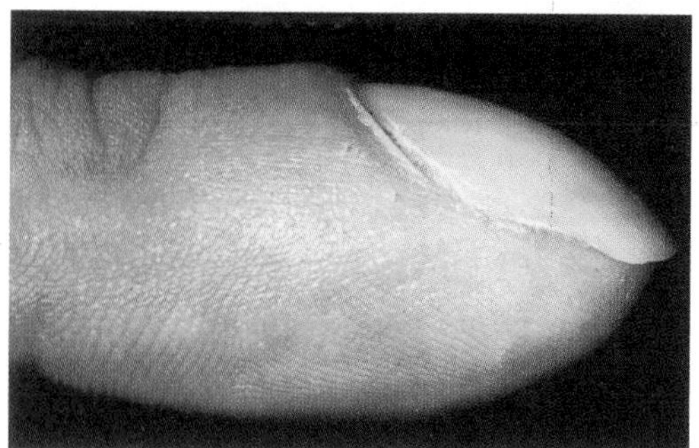

Clubbing of the Fingers

The distal phalanx of each finger is rounded and bulbous. The nail plate is more convex, and the angle between the plate and the proximal nail fold increases to 180° or more. The proximal nail fold, when palpated, feels spongy or floating. Causes are many, including chronic hypoxia from heart disease or lung cancer and hepatic cirrhosis.

(table continues next page)

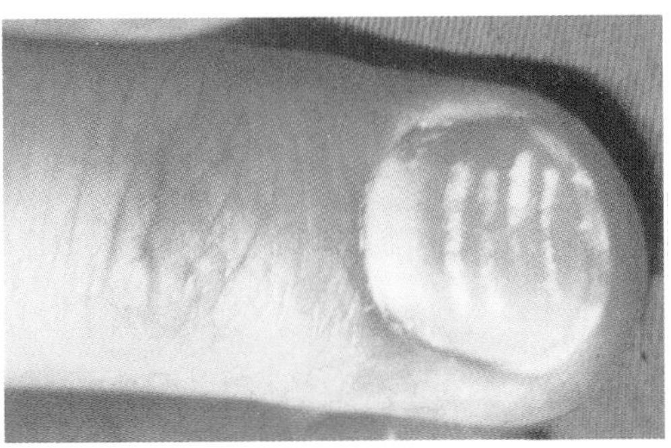

White Spots *(Leukonychia)*

Trauma to the nails is commonly followed by white spots that grow slowly out with the nail. Spots in the pattern illustrated are typical of overly vigorous and repeated manicuring. The curves in this example resemble the curve of the cuticle and proximal nail fold.

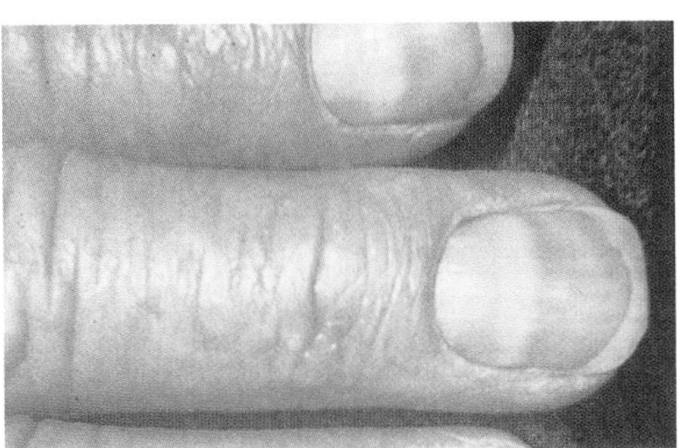

Transverse White Lines *(Mees' Lines)*

These are transverse lines, not spots, and their curves are similar to those of the lunula, not the cuticle. These uncommon lines may follow an acute or severe illness. They emerge from under the proximal nail folds and grow out with the nails.

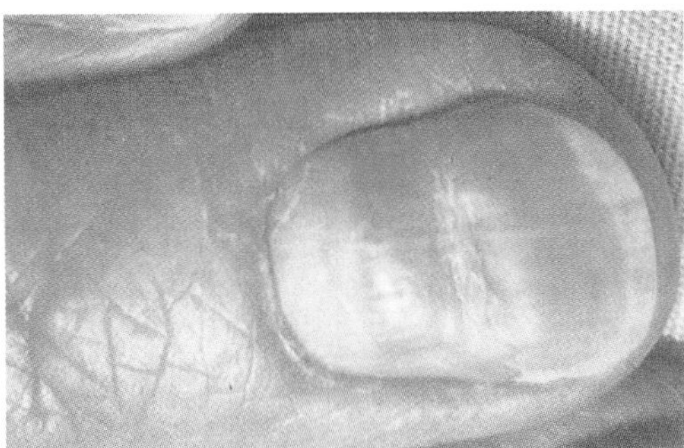

Beau's Lines

Beau's lines are transverse depressions in the nails associated with acute severe illness. The lines emerge from under the proximal nail folds weeks later and grow gradually out with the nails. As with Mees' lines, clinicians may be able to estimate the timing of a causal illness.

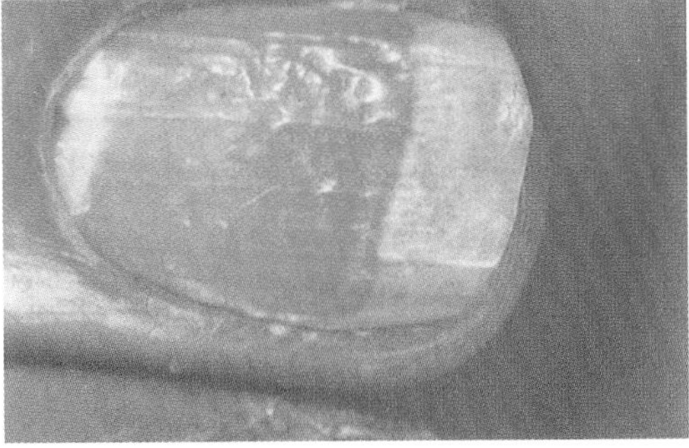

Psoriasis

Small pits in the nails may be early signs of psoriasis but are not specific for it. Additional findings, not shown here, include onycholysis and a circumscribed yellowish tan discoloration known as an "oil spot" lesion. Marked thickening of the nails may develop.

(Sources of photos: *Clubbing of the Fingers, Paronychia, Onycholysis, Terry's Nails*—Habif TP. Clinical Dermatology: A Color Guide to Diagnosis and Therapy, 2nd ed. St. Louis, CV Mosby, 1990; *White Spots, Transverse White Lines, Psoriasis, Beau's Lines*—Sams WM Jr, Lynch PJ. Principles and Practice of Dermatology. New York, Churchill Livingstone, 1990)

The Head and Neck

6

ANATOMY AND PHYSIOLOGY

THE HEAD

Regions of the head take their names from the underlying bones of the skull, for example, the frontal area. Knowing this anatomy helps to locate and describe physical findings.

Two paired salivary glands lie near the mandible: the *parotid gland,* superficial to and behind the mandible (both visible and palpable when enlarged), and the *submandibular gland,* located deep to the mandible. Feel for the latter as you bow and press your tongue against your lower incisors. Its lobular surface can often be felt against the tightened muscle. The openings of the parotid and submandibular ducts are visible within the oral cavity (see p. 167).

The *superficial temporal artery* passes upward just in front of the ear, where it is readily palpable. In many normal people, especially thin and elderly ones, the tortuous course of one of its branches can be traced across the forehead.

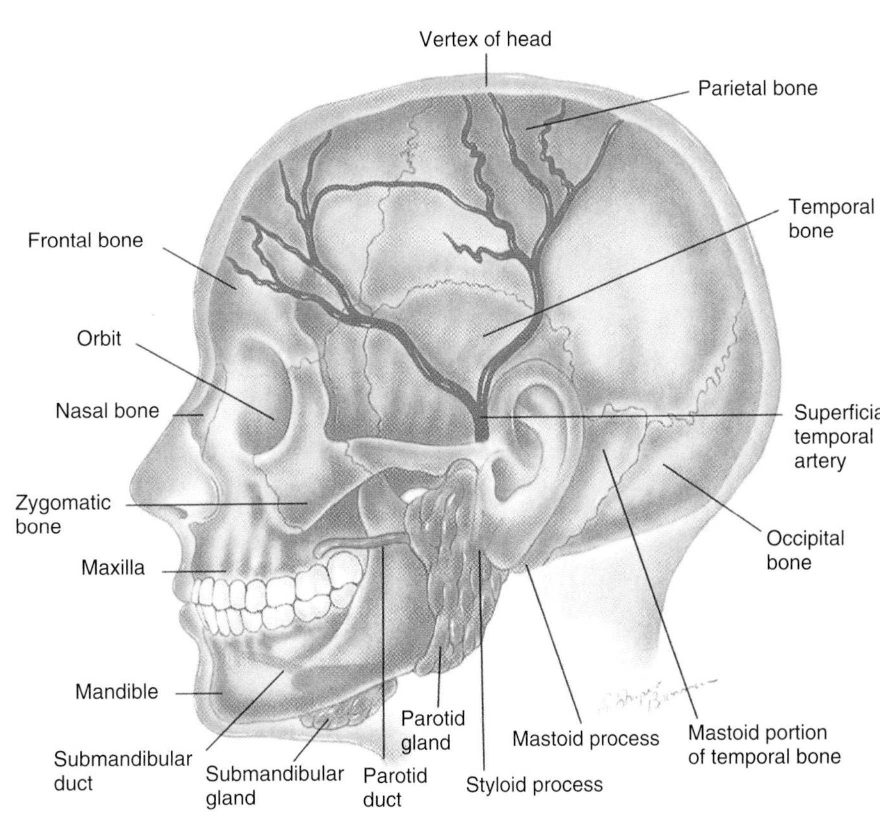

THE EYE

Anatomy. Begin by identifying the structures illustrated on this page. Note that the upper eyelid covers a portion of the iris but does not normally overlay the pupil. The opening between the eyelids is called the *palpebral fissure*. The white sclera may look somewhat buff colored at its periphery. Do not mistake this color for jaundice, which is a deeper yellow.

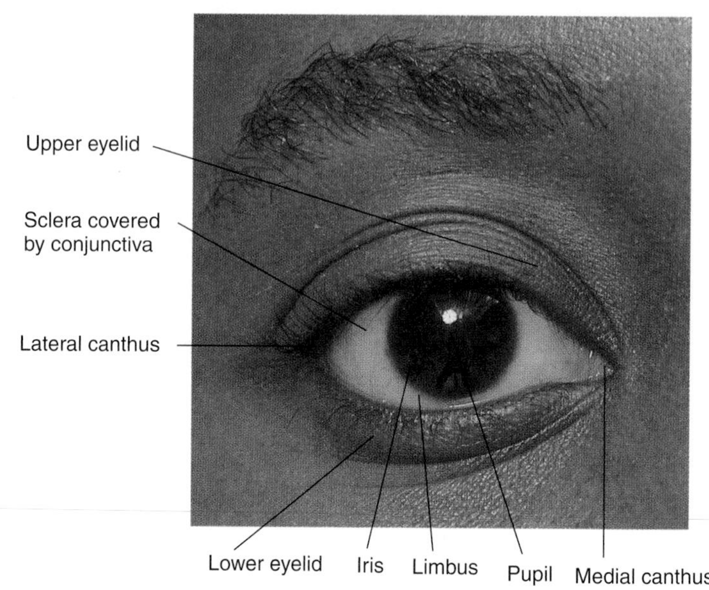

The *conjunctiva* is a clear mucous membrane with two easily visible components. The *bulbar conjunctiva* covers most of the anterior eyeball, adhering loosely to the underlying tissue. It meets the cornea at the *limbus*. The *palpebral conjunctiva* lines the eyelids. The two parts of the conjunctiva merge in a folded recess that permits movement of the eyeball.

Within the eyelids lie firm strips of connective tissue called *tarsal plates*. Each plate contains a parallel row of *meibomian glands*, which open on the lid margin. The *levator palpebrae* the muscle, which raises the upper eyelid, is innervated by the oculomotor nerve, Cranial Nerve III. Smooth muscle, innervated by the sympathetic nervous system, also contributes to lid elevation.

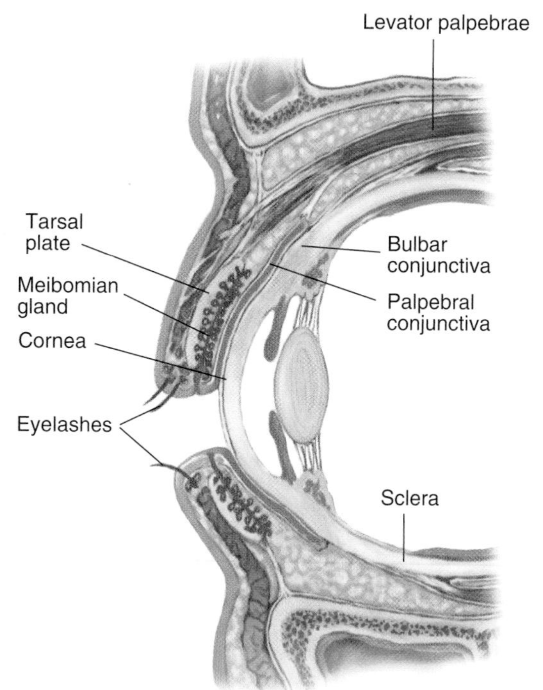

SAGITTAL SECTION OF ANTERIOR EYE WITH LIDS CLOSED

A film of tear fluid protects the conjunctiva and cornea from drying, inhibits microbial growth, and gives a smooth optical surface to the cornea. This fluid comes from the meibomian glands, conjunctival glands, and the lacrimal gland. The *lacrimal gland* lies mostly within the bony orbit, above and lateral to the eyeball. The tear fluid spreads across the eye and drains medially through two tiny holes called *lacrimal puncta*. The tears then pass into the *lacrimal sac* and on into the nose through the *nasolacrimal duct*. You can easily find a *punctum* atop the small elevation of the lower lid medially. The lacrimal sac rests in a small depression inside the bony orbit and is not visible.

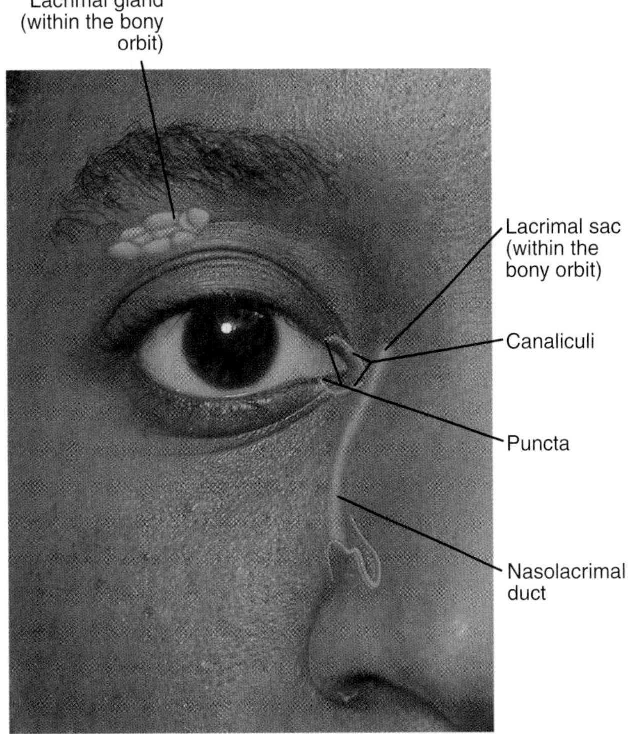

The eyeball is a spherical structure that focuses light on the neurosensory elements within the retina. The muscles of the iris control pupillary size. Muscles of the *ciliary body* control the thickness of the lens, allowing the eye to focus on near or distant objects.

A clear liquid called *aqueous humor* fills the anterior and posterior chambers of the eye. Aqueous humor is produced by the *ciliary body*, circulates from the posterior chamber through the pupil into the anterior chamber, and drains out through the *canal of Schlemm*. This circulatory system helps to control the pressure inside the eye.

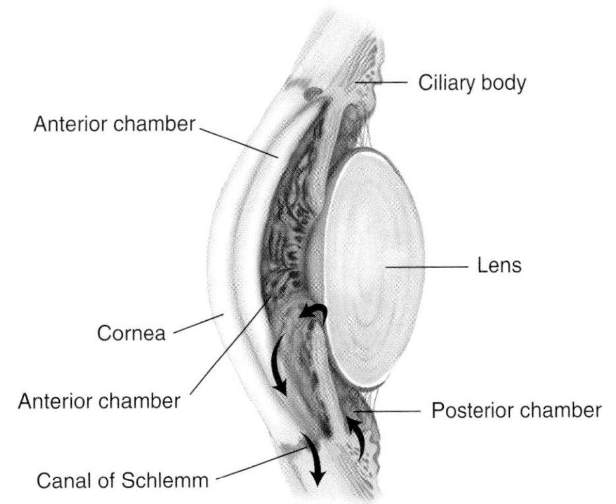

CIRCULATION OF AQUEOUS HUMOR

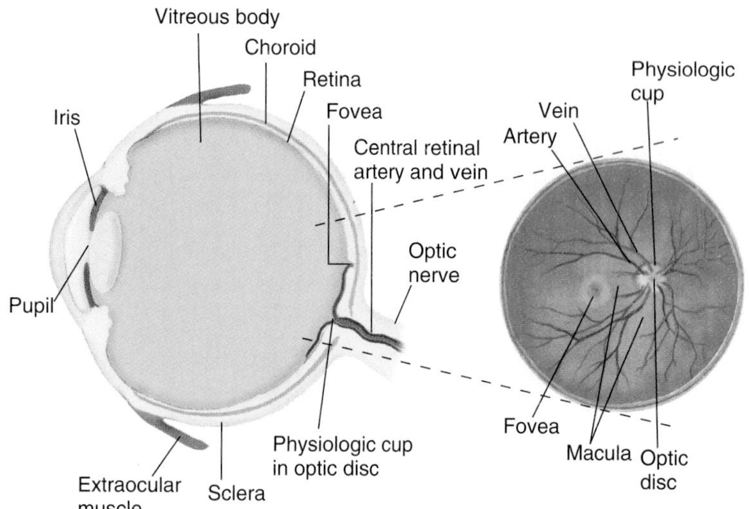

CROSS SECTION OF THE RIGHT EYE FROM ABOVE SHOWING A PORTION OF THE FUNDUS COMMONLY SEEN WITH THE OPHTHALMOSCOPE

The posterior part of the eye that is seen through an ophthalmoscope is often called the *fundus* of the eye. Structures here include the retina, choroid, fovea, macula, optic disc, and retinal vessels. The optic nerve with its retinal vessels enters the eyeball posteriorly. You can find it with an ophthalmoscope at the *optic disc.* Lateral and slightly inferior to the disc, there is a small depression in the retinal surface that marks the point of central vision. Around it is a darkened circular area called the *fovea.* The roughly circular *macula* (named for a microscopic yellow spot) surrounds the fovea but has no discernible margins. It does not quite reach the optic disc. You do not usually see the normal *vitreous body,* a transparent mass of gelatinous material that fills the eyeball behind the lens. It helps to maintain the shape of the eye.

Visual Fields. A *visual field* is the entire area seen by an eye when it looks at a central point. Fields are conventionally diagrammed on circles from the patient's point of view. The center of the circle represents the focus of gaze. The circumference is 90° from the line of gaze. Each visual field, shown by the white areas below, is divided into quadrants. Note that the fields extend farthest on the temporal sides. Visual fields are normally limited by the brows above, the cheeks below, and the nose medially. A lack of retinal receptors at the optic disc produces an oval blind spot in the normal field of each eye, 15° temporal to the line of gaze.

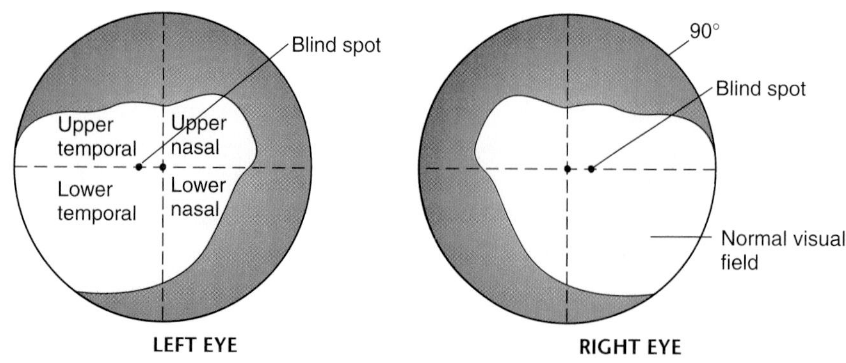

When a person is using both eyes, the two visual fields overlap in an area of binocular vision. Laterally, vision is monocular.

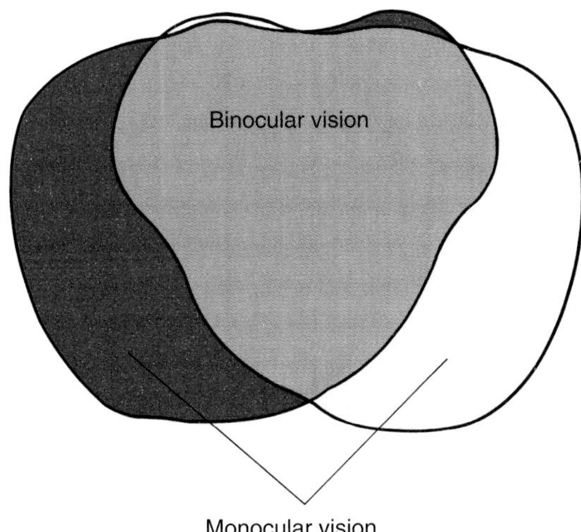

Visual Pathways. To see an image, light reflected from the image must pass through the pupil and be focused on sensory neurons in the retina. The image projected there is upside down and reversed right to left. An image from the upper nasal visual field thus strikes the lower temporal quadrant of the retina.

Nerve impulses, stimulated by light, are conducted through the retina, optic nerve, and optic tract on each side, then on through a curving tract called the *optic radiation*. This ends in the visual cortex, a part of the occipital lobe.

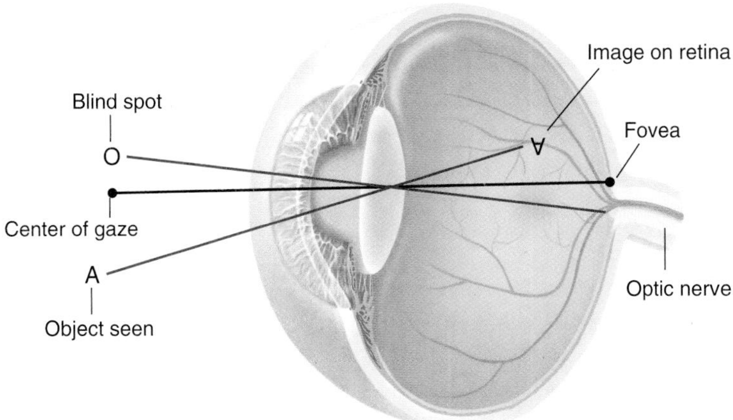

Pupillary Reactions. Pupillary size changes in response to light and to the effort of focusing on a near object.

The Light Reaction. A light beam shining onto one retina causes pupillary constriction in both that eye, termed the *direct reaction* to light, and in the opposite eye, the *consensual reaction*. The initial sensory pathways are similar to those described for vision: retina, optic nerve, and optic tract. The pathways diverge in the midbrain, however, and impulses are transmitted through the oculomotor nerve to the constrictor muscles of the iris of each eye.

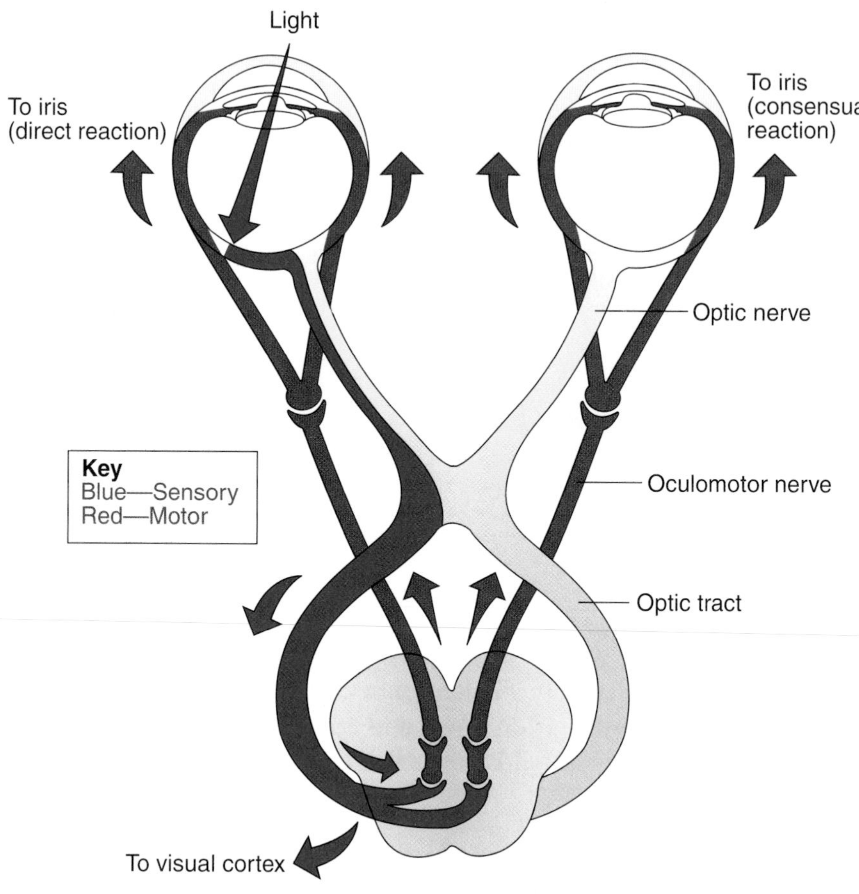

PATHWAYS OF THE LIGHT REACTION

The Near Reaction. When a person shifts gaze from a far object to a near one, the pupils constrict. This response, like the light reaction, is mediated by the oculomotor nerve. Coincident with this pupillary reaction, but not part of it, are (1) *convergence* of the eyes, an extraocular movement; and (2) *accommodation*, an increased convexity of the lenses caused by contraction of the ciliary muscles. This change in shape of the lenses brings near objects into focus but is not visible to the examiner.

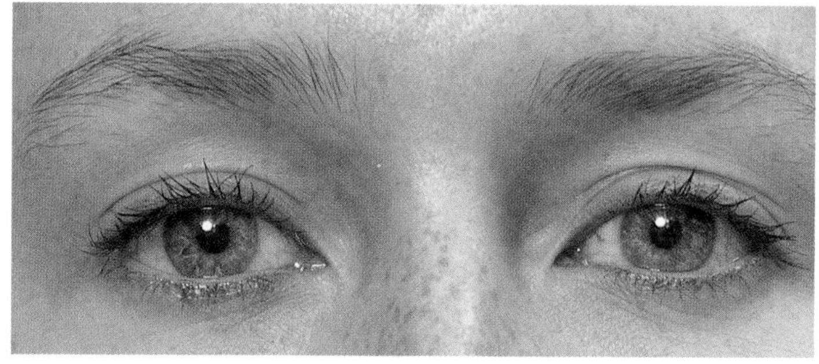

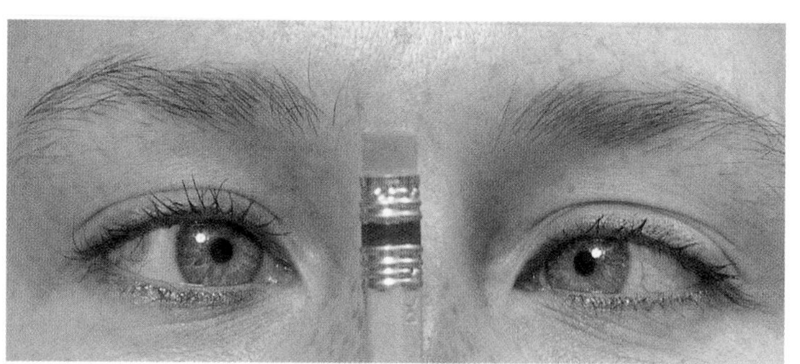

Autonomic Nerve Supply to the Eyes. Fibers travelling in the oculomotor nerve and producing pupillary constriction are part of the parasympathetic nervous system. The iris is also supplied by sympathetic fibers. When these are stimulated, the pupil dilates, and the upper eyelid rises a little, as if from fear. The sympathetic pathway starts in the hypothalamus and passes down through the brainstem and cervical cord into the neck. From there, it follows the carotid artery or its branches into the orbit. A lesion anywhere along this pathway may impair sympathetic effects on the pupil.

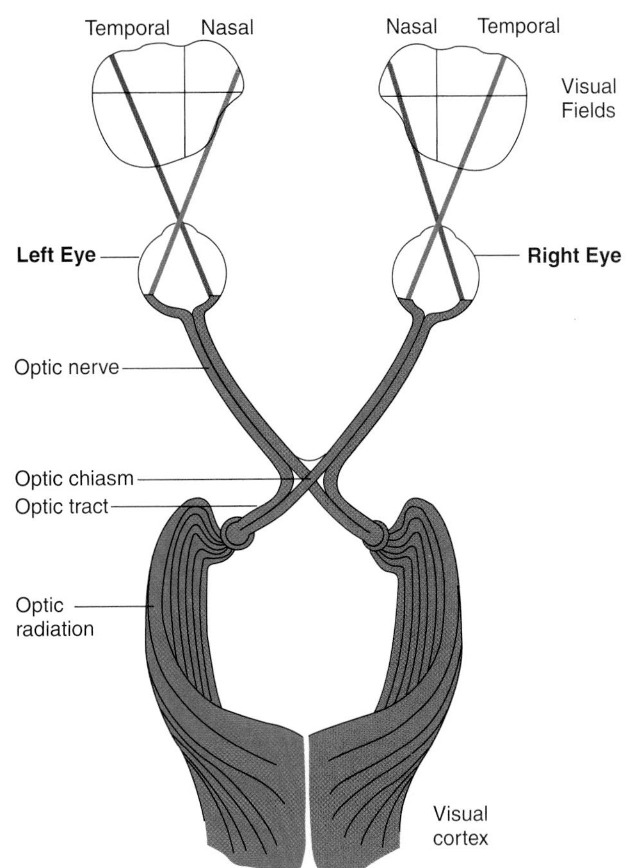

VISUAL PATHWAYS FROM THE RETINA TO THE VISUAL CORTEX

Extraocular Movements. The movement of each eye is controlled by the coordinated action of six muscles, the four rectus and two oblique muscles. You can test the function of each muscle and the nerve that supplies it by asking the patient to move the eye in the direction controlled by that muscle. There are six such *cardinal directions,* indicated by the lines on the figure below. When a person looks down and to the right, for example, the right inferior rectus (Cranial Nerve III) is principally responsible for moving the right eye, whereas the left superior oblique (Cranial Nerve IV) is principally responsible for moving the left. If one of these muscles is paralyzed, the eye will deviate from its normal position in that direction of gaze and the eyes will no longer appear conjugate, or parallel.

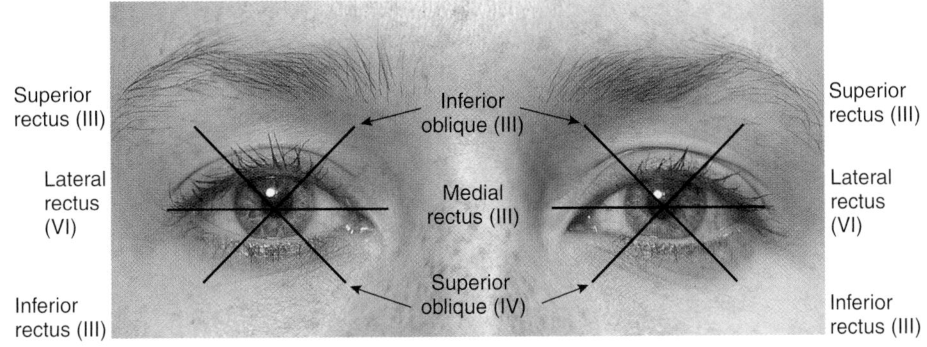

CARDINAL DIRECTIONS OF GAZE

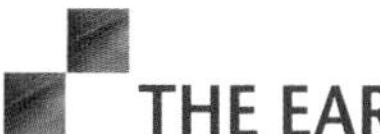

THE EAR

Anatomy. The ear has three compartments: the external ear, the middle ear, and the inner ear.

The *external ear* comprises the auricle and ear canal. The *auricle* consists chiefly of cartilage covered by skin and has a firm elastic consistency. Its prominent curved outer ridge is the *helix*. Parallel and anterior to the helix is another curved prominence, the *antihelix*. Inferiorly lies the fleshy projection of the earlobe, or *lobule*. The ear canal opens behind the *tragus,* a nodular eminence that points backward over the entrance to the canal.

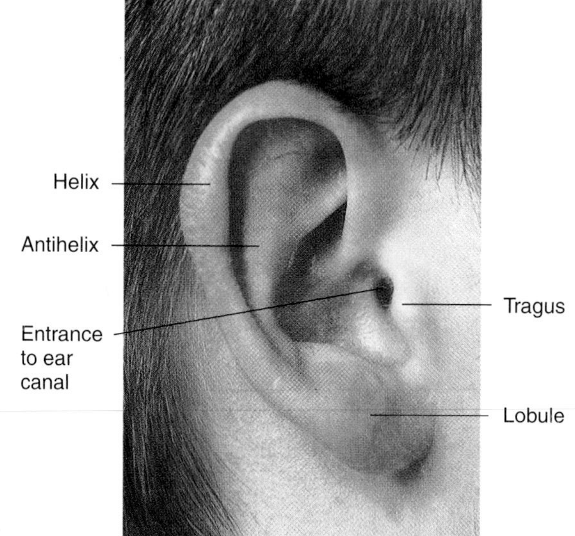

The *ear canal* curves inward approximately 24 mm. Cartilage surrounds its outer portion. The skin in this outer portion is hairy and contains glands that produce cerumen (wax). The inner portion of the canal is surrounded by bone and lined by thin, hairless skin. Pressure on this latter area causes pain—a point to remember when you examine the ear.

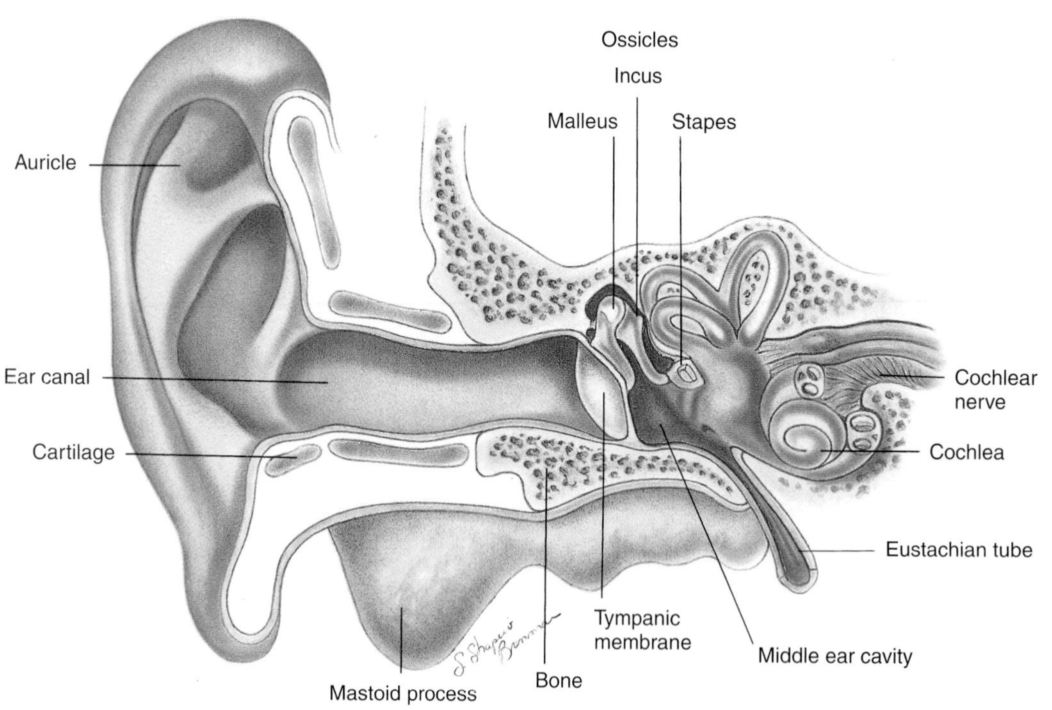

Behind and below the ear canal is the mastoid part of the temporal bone. The lowest portion of this bone, the *mastoid process*, is palpable behind the lobule.

At the end of the ear canal lies the *tympanic membrane*, or eardrum, marking the lateral limits of the middle ear. The *middle ear* is an air-filled cavity that transmits sound by way of three tiny bones, the *ossicles*. It is connected by the *eustachian tube* to the nasopharynx.

The eardrum is an oblique membrane held inward at its center by the *malleus*, one of its three ossicles. Find the *handle* and the *short process* of the malleus—the two chief landmarks. From the *umbo*, where the eardrum meets the tip of the malleus, a light reflection called the *cone of light* fans downward and anteriorly. Above the short process lies a small portion of the eardrum called the *pars flaccida*. The remainder of the drum is the *pars tensa*. Anterior and posterior malleolar folds, which extend obliquely upward from the short process, separate the pars flaccida from the pars tensa but are usually invisible unless the eardrum is retracted. A second ossicle, the *incus*, can sometimes be seen through the drum.

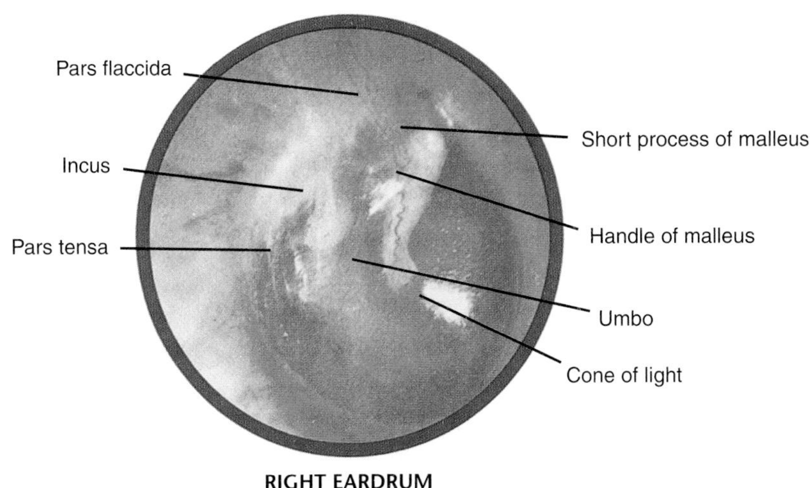

RIGHT EARDRUM

Much of the middle ear and all of the inner ear are inaccessible to direct examination. Some inferences concerning their condition can be made, however, by testing auditory function.

Pathways of Hearing. Vibrations of sound pass through the air of the external ear and are transmitted through the eardrum and ossicles of the middle ear to the *cochlea*, a part of the inner ear. The cochlea senses and codes the vibrations, and nerve impulses are sent to the brain through the cochlear nerve. The first part of this pathway—from the external ear through the middle ear—is known as the *conductive* phase, and a disorder here causes conductive hearing loss. The second part of the pathway, involving the cochlea and the cochlear nerve, is called the *sensorineural* phase; a disorder here causes sensorineural hearing loss.

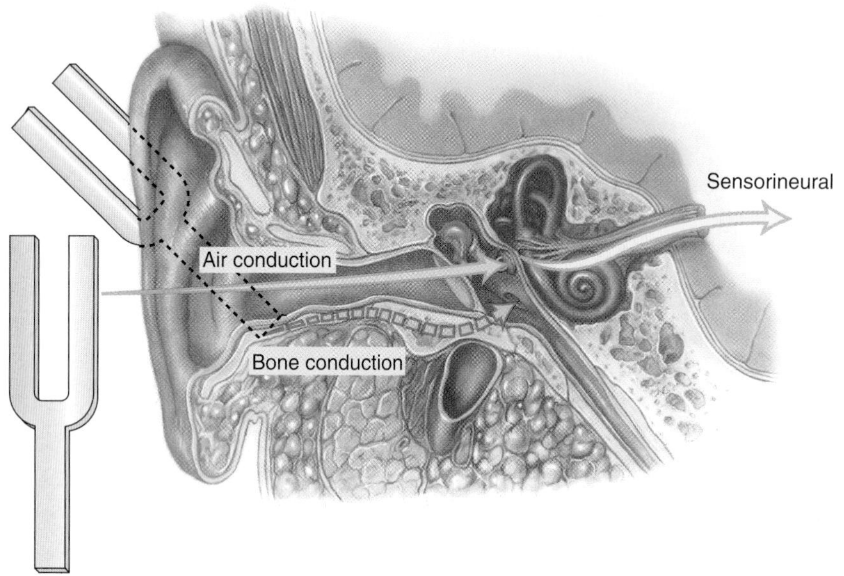

Air conduction describes the normal first phase in the hearing pathway. An alternate pathway, known as *bone conduction,* bypasses the external and the middle ear and is used for testing purposes. A vibrating tuning fork, placed on the head, sets the bone of the skull into vibration and stimulates the cochlea directly. In a normal person, air conduction is more sensitive.

Equilibrium. The labyrinth within the inner ear senses the position and movements of the head and helps to maintain balance.

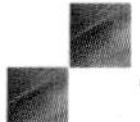

THE NOSE AND PARANASAL SINUSES

Review the terms used to describe the external anatomy of the nose.

Approximately the upper third of the nose is supported by bone, the lower two thirds by cartilage. Air enters the nasal cavity by way of the *anterior naris* on either side, then passes into a widened area known as the *vestibule* and on through the narrow nasal passage to the nasopharynx. The medial wall of each nasal cavity is formed by the *nasal septum,* which, like the external nose, is supported by both bone and cartilage. It is covered by a mucous membrane well supplied with blood. The vestibule, unlike the rest of the nasal cavity, is lined with hair-bearing skin, not mucosa.

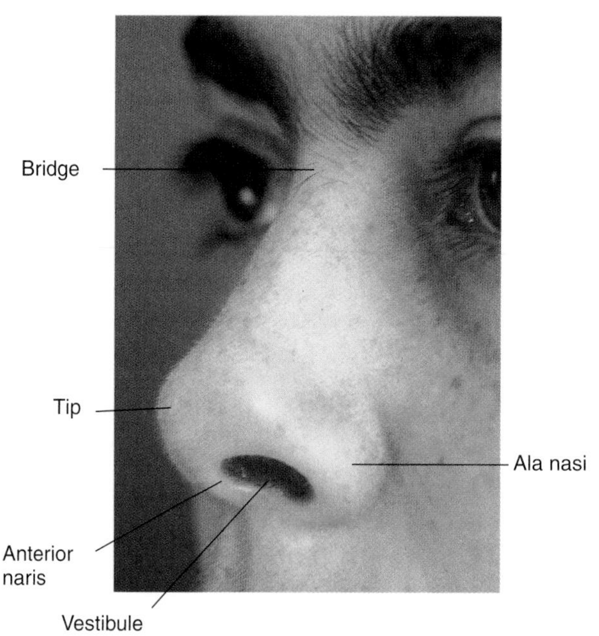

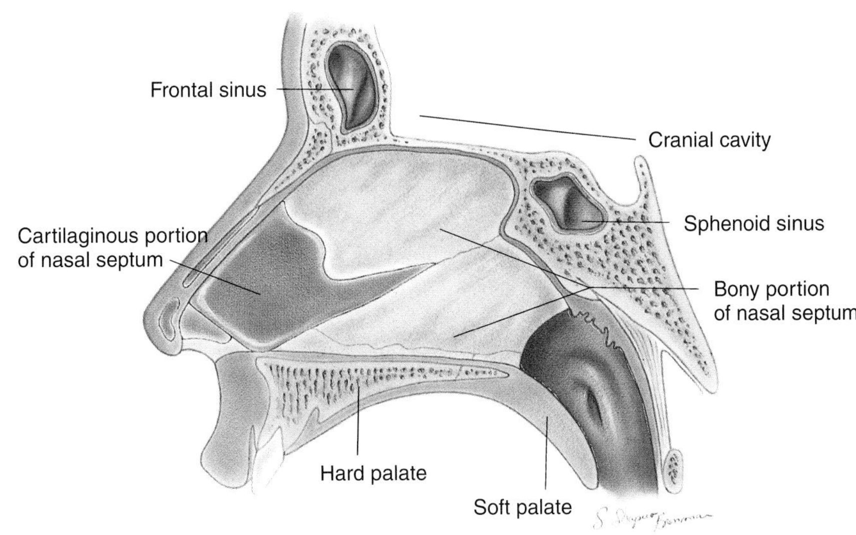

MEDIAL WALL—LEFT NASAL CAVITY (MUCOSA REMOVED)

Laterally, the anatomy is more complex. Curving bony structures, the *turbinates*, covered by a highly vascular mucous membrane, protrude into the nasal cavity. Below each turbinate is a groove, or meatus, each named according to the turbinate above it. Into the inferior meatus drains the nasolacrimal duct; into the middle meatus drain most of the paranasal sinuses. Their openings are not usually visible.

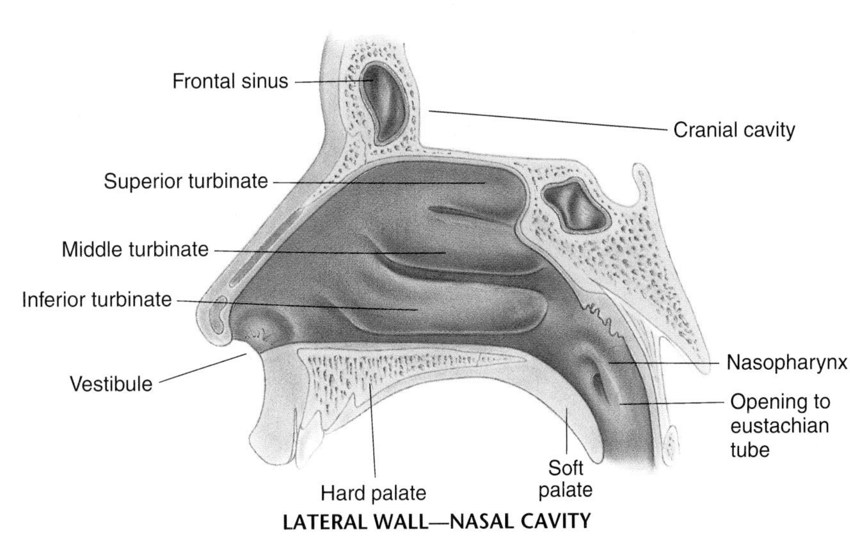

LATERAL WALL—NASAL CAVITY

The additional surface area provided by the turbinates and the mucosa covering them aids the nasal cavities in their principal functions: cleansing, humidification, and temperature control of inspired air.

Inspection of the nasal cavity through the anterior naris is usually limited to the vestibule, the anterior portion of the septum, and the lower and middle turbinates. Examination with a nasopharyngeal mirror is required for detection of posterior abnormalities. This technique is beyond the scope of this book.

The *paranasal sinuses* are air-filled cavities within the bones of the skull. Like the nasal cavities into which they drain, they are lined with mucous membrane. Their locations are diagrammed below. Only the frontal and maxillary sinuses are readily accessible to clinical examination.

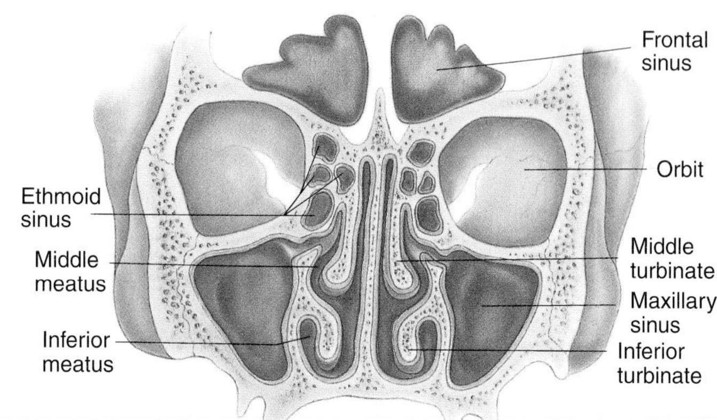

CROSS SECTION OF NASAL CAVITY—ANTERIOR VIEW

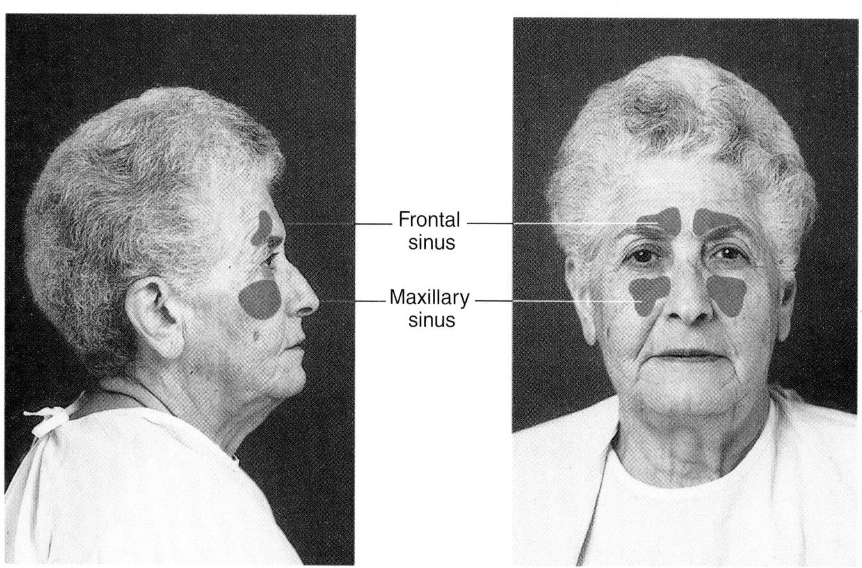

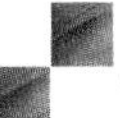

THE MOUTH AND PHARYNX

The *lips* are muscular folds that surround the entrance to the mouth. When opened, the gums (gingiva) and teeth are visible. Note the scalloped shape of the *gingival margins* and the pointed *interdental papillae*.

The *gingiva* is firmly attached to the teeth and to the maxilla or mandible in which they are seated. In lighter-skinned people, the gingiva is pale or coral pink and lightly stippled. In darker-skinned people, it may be diffusely or partly brown, as shown below. A midline mucosal fold, called a *labial frenulum*, connects each lip with the gingiva. A shallow *gingival sulcus* between the gum's thin margin and each tooth is not readily visible (but is probed and measured by dentists). Adjacent to the gingiva is the *alveolar mucosa*, which merges with the *labial mucosa* of the lip.

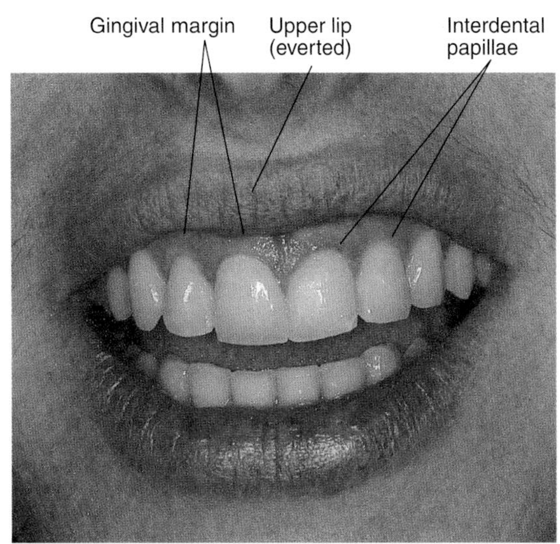

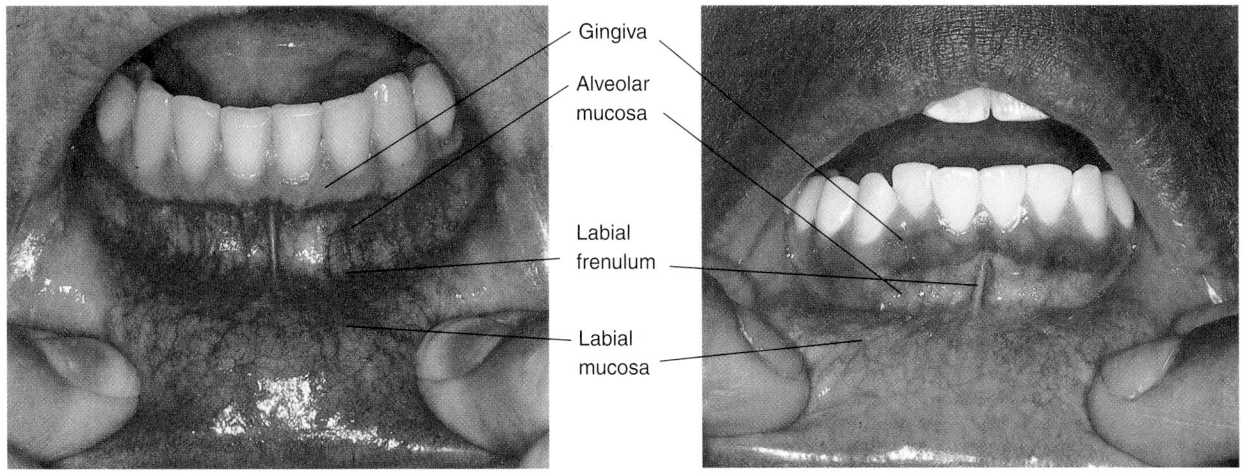

Each tooth, composed chiefly of dentin, lies rooted in a bony socket with only its enamel-covered crown exposed. Small blood vessels and nerves enter the tooth through its apex and pass into the pulp canal and pulp chamber.

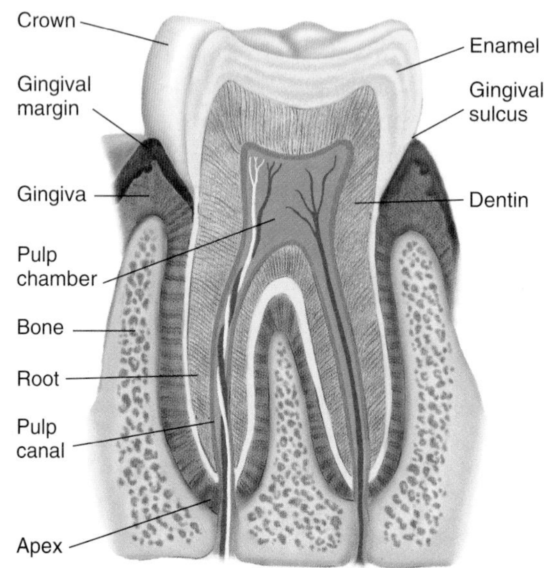

Note the terms designating the 32 adult teeth, 16 in each jaw.

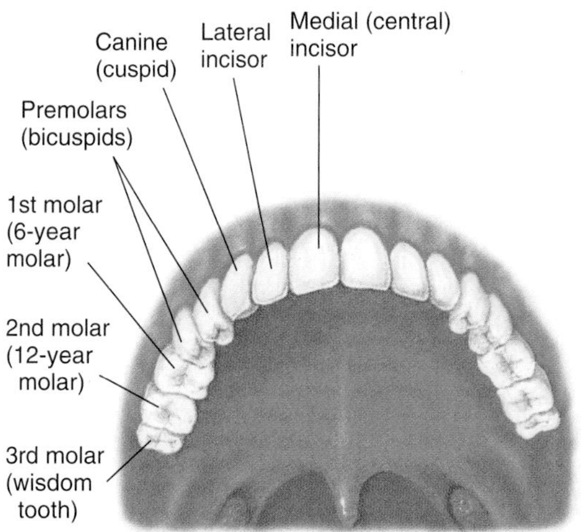

The dorsum of the *tongue* is covered with papillae, giving it a rough surface. Some of these papillae look like red dots, which contrast with the thin white coat that often covers the tongue. The undersurface of the tongue has no papillae. Note the midline *lingual frenulum* that connects the tongue to the floor of the mouth. At the base of the tongue the *ducts of the submandibular gland* (Wharton's ducts) pass forward and medially. They open on papillae that lie on each side of the lingual frenulum.

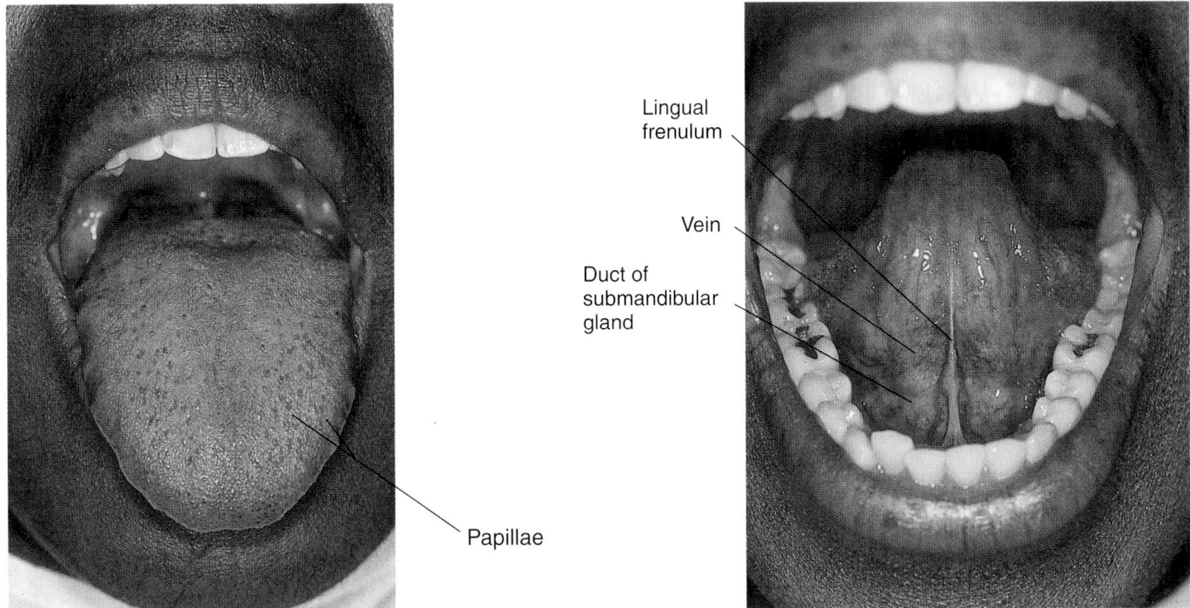

Above and behind the tongue rises an arch formed by the *anterior* and *posterior pillars,* the *soft palate,* and the *uvula.* A meshwork of small blood vessels may web the soft palate. The *pharynx* is visible in the recess behind the soft palate and tongue.

In the adjacent photograph, note the right tonsil protruding from the hollowed *tonsillar fossa,* or cavity, between the anterior and posterior pillars. In adults, tonsils are often small or absent, as in the empty left tonsillar fossa here.

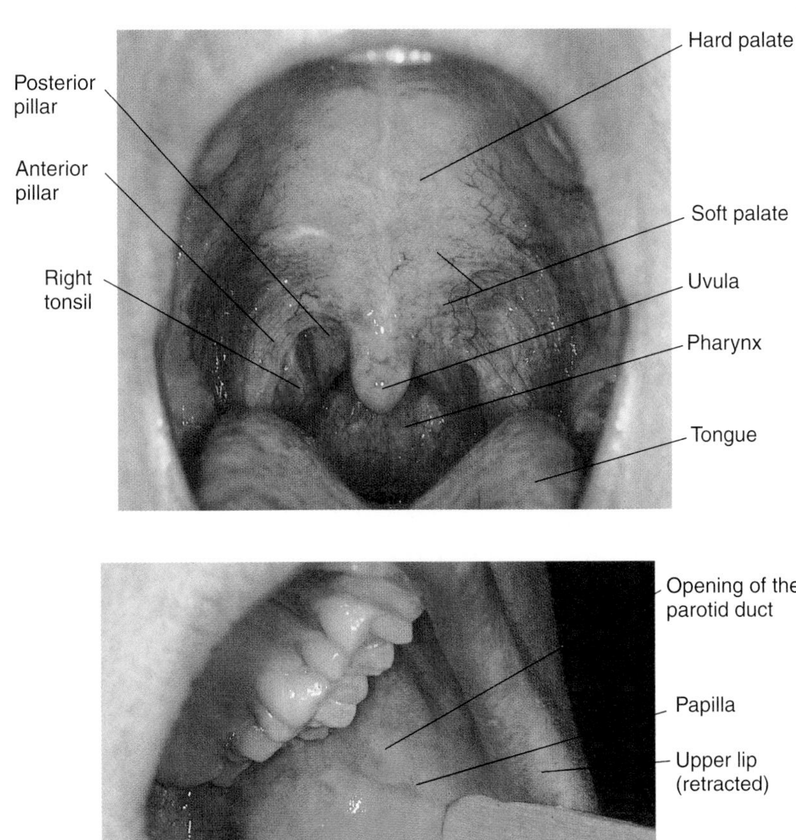

The *buccal mucosa* lines the cheeks. Each *parotid duct,* sometimes termed *Stenson's duct,* opens onto the buccal mucosa near the upper second molar. Its location is frequently marked by its own small papilla.

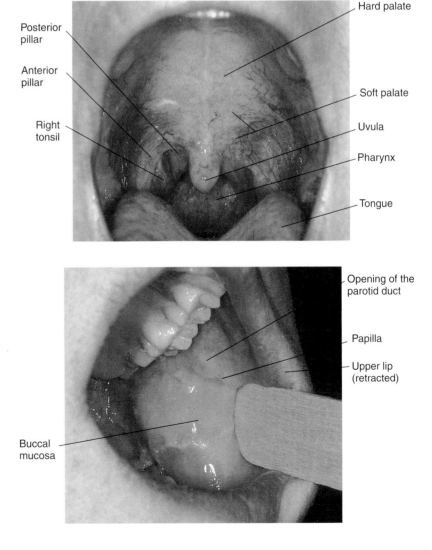

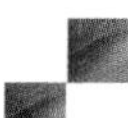

THE NECK

For descriptive purposes, divide each side of the neck into two triangles bounded by the sternomastoid muscle. Visualize the borders of the two triangles as follows:

- For the *anterior triangle:* the mandible above, the sternomastoid laterally, and the midline of the neck medially
- For the *posterior triangle:* the sternomastoid muscle, the trapezius, and the clavicle. Note that a portion of the omohyoid muscle crosses the lower portion of this triangle and can be mistaken for a lymph node or mass.

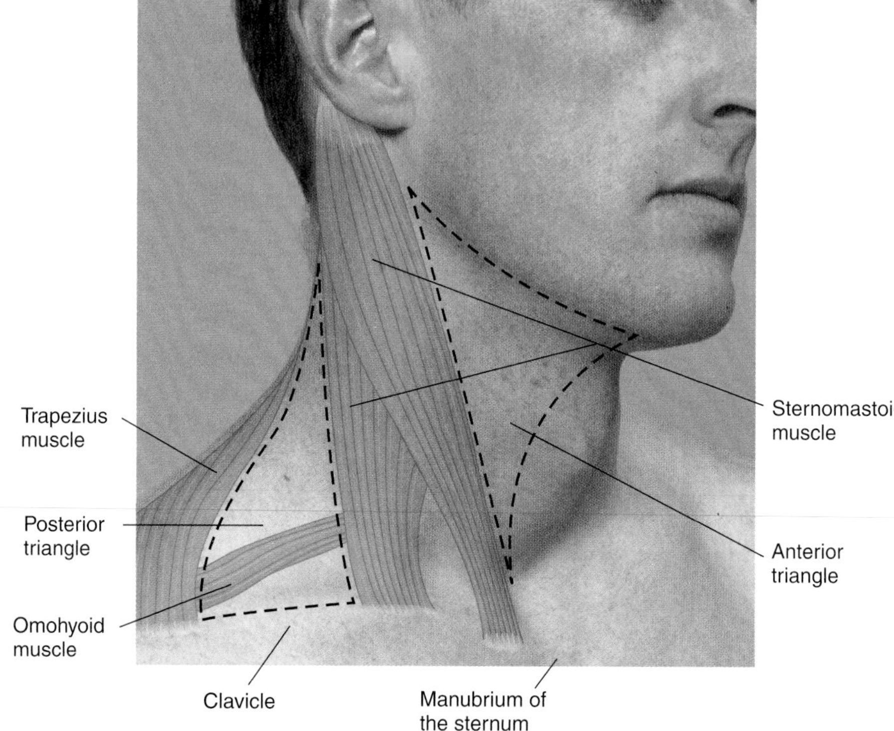

Great Vessels. Deep to the sternomastoids run the great vessels of the neck: the *carotid artery* and the *internal jugular vein*. The *external jugular vein* passes diagonally over the surface of the sternomastoid and may be helpful when trying to identify the jugular venous pressure (see p. 290).

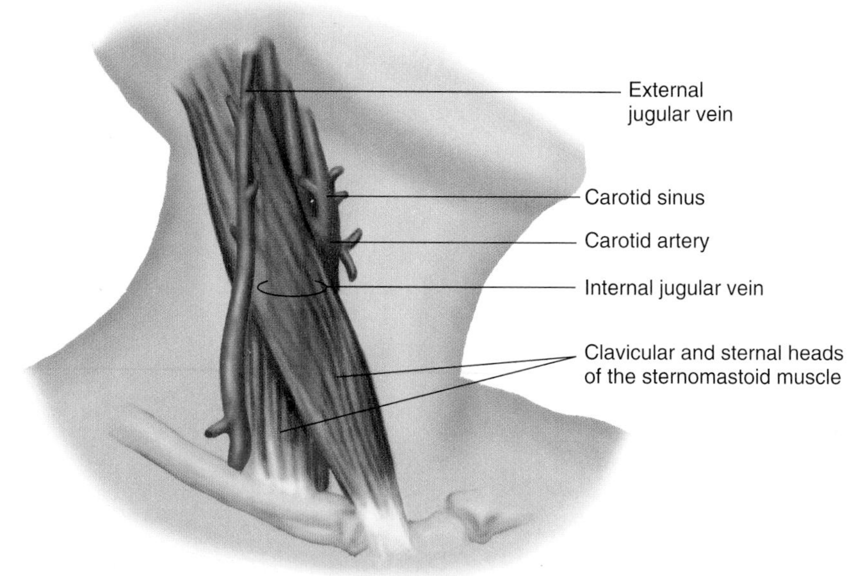

Midline Structures and Thyroid Gland. Now identify the following midline structures: (1) the mobile *hyoid bone* just below the mandible, (2) the *thyroid cartilage,* readily identified by the notch on its superior edge, (3) the *cricoid cartilage,* (4) the *tracheal rings,* and (5) the *thyroid gland.*

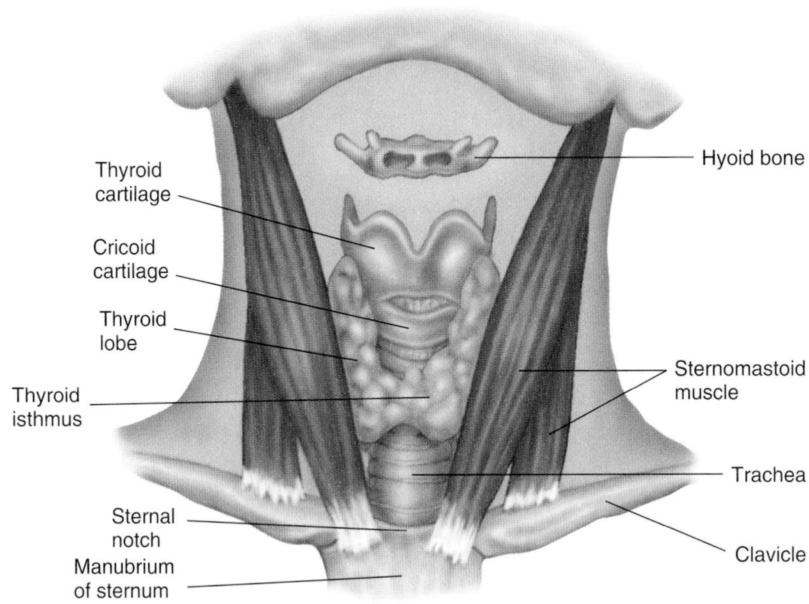

The isthmus of the thyroid gland lies across the trachea below the cricoid. The lateral lobes of this gland curve posteriorly around the sides of the trachea and the esophagus. Except in the midline, the thyroid gland is covered by thin straplike muscles, among which only the sternomastoids are visible. Women have larger and more easily palpable glands than men.

Lymph Nodes. The *lymph nodes* of the head and neck have been classified in a variety of ways. One classification is shown here, together with the directions of lymphatic drainage. The deep cervical chain is largely obscured by the overlying sternomastoid muscle, but at its two extremes, the tonsillar node and supraclavicular nodes may be palpable. The submandibular nodes lie superficial to the submandibular gland, from which they should be differentiated. Nodes are normally round or ovoid, smooth, and smaller than this gland. The gland is larger and has a lobulated, slightly irregular surface (see p. 153).

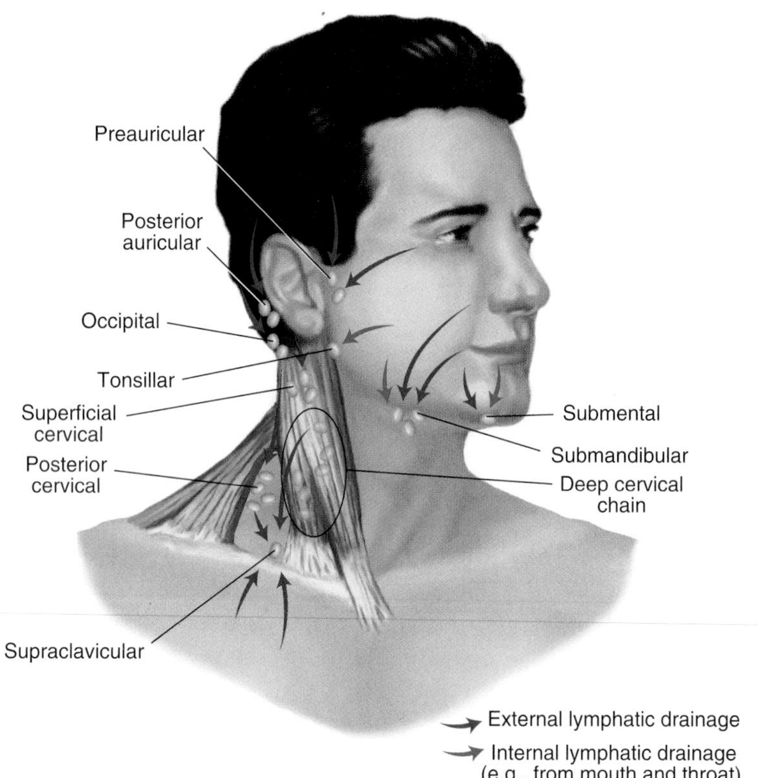

Note that the tonsillar, submandibular, and submental nodes drain portions of the mouth and throat as well as the face.

Knowledge of the lymphatic system is important to a sound clinical habit: whenever a malignant or inflammatory lesion is observed, look for involvement of the regional lymph nodes that drain it; whenever a node is enlarged or tender, look for a source such as infection in the area that it drains.

THE HEALTH HISTORY

Common or Concerning Symptoms

- Headache
- Change in vision: hyperopia, presbyopia, myopia, scotomas
- Double vision, or diplopia
- Hearing loss, earache; tinnitus
- Vertigo
- Nosebleed, or epistaxis
- Sore throat; hoarseness
- Swollen glands
- Goiter

THE HEAD

Headache is an extremely common symptom that always requires careful evaluation, because a small fraction of headaches arise from life-threatening conditions. It is important to elicit a full description of the headache and all seven attributes of the patient's pain (see p. 32). Is the headache one-sided or bilateral? Steady or throbbing? Continuous or comes and goes? After your usual open-ended approach, ask the patient to *point to the area of pain or discomfort.*

See Table 6-1, Headaches, pp. 206–209. *Tension* and *migraine headaches* are the most common kinds of recurring headaches.

Tension headaches often arise in the temporal areas; cluster headaches may be retro-orbital.

The most important attributes of headache are its *chronologic pattern* and *severity*. Is the problem new and acute? Chronic and recurring, with little change in pattern? Chronic and recurring, but with recent change in pattern or progressively severe? Does the pain recur at the same time every day?

Changing or progressively severe headaches increase the likelihood of *tumor, abscess,* or other *mass lesion.* Extremely severe headaches suggest *subarachnoid hemorrhage* or *meningitis.*

Ask about associated symptoms. Inquire specifically about associated nausea and vomiting and neurologic symptoms such as change in vision or motor-sensory deficits.

Visual aura or scintillating scotomas with *migraine.*[1] Nausea and vomiting common with migraine but also occur with brain tumors and subarachnoid hemorrhage.

Ask whether coughing, sneezing, or changing the position of the head have any effect (better, worse, or no effect) on the headache.

Such maneuvers may increase pain from brain tumor and acute sinusitis.

Ask about family history.

Family history may be positive in patients with migraine.

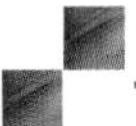

THE EYES

Start your inquiry about eye and vision problems with open-ended questions such as "How is your vision?" and "Have you had any trouble with your eyes?" If the patient reports a change in vision, pursue the related details:

Refractive errors most commonly explain gradual blurring. High blood glucose levels may cause blurring.[2]

- Is the onset sudden or gradual?

Sudden visual loss suggests *retinal detachment, vitreous hemorrhage,* or *occlusion of the central retinal artery.*

- Is the problem worse during close work or at distances?

Difficulty with close work suggests *hyperopia* (farsightedness) or *presbyopia* (aging vision); with distances, *myopia* (near-sightedness).

- Is there blurring of the entire field of vision or only parts of it? If the visual field defect is partial, is it central, peripheral, or only on one side?

Slow central loss in nuclear cataract (p. 216), *macular degeneration*[3] (p. 188); peripheral loss in advanced *open-angle glaucoma* (p. 181); one-sided loss in *hemianopsia* and *quadrantic defects* (p. 212).

- Are there specks in the vision or areas where the patient cannot see (*scotomas*)? If so, do they move around in the visual field with shifts in gaze or are they fixed?

Moving specks or strands suggest vitreous floaters; fixed defects (scotomas) suggest lesions in the retina or visual pathways.

- Has the patient seen lights flashing across the field of vision? Vitreous floaters may accompany this symptom.

Flashing lights or new vitreous floaters suggest detachment of vitreous from retina. Prompt eye consultation is indicated.

- Does the patient wear glasses?

Ask about ***pain*** in or around the eyes, *redness,* and *excessive tearing or watering* (see page 215).

Check for presence of ***diplopia,*** or double vision. If present, find out whether the images are side by side (horizontal diplopia) or on top of each other (vertical diplopia). Does diplopia persist with one eye closed? Which eye is affected?

One kind of horizontal diplopia is physiologic. Hold one finger upright about 6 inches in front of your face, a second at arm's length. When you focus on either finger, the image of the other is double. A patient who notices this phenomenon can be reassured.

Diplopia in adults may arise from a lesion in the brainstem or cerebellum, or from weakness or paralysis of one or more extraocular muscles, as in horizontal diplopia from palsy of CN III or VI, or vertical diplopia from palsy of CN III or IV. Diplopia in one eye, with the other closed, suggests a problem in the cornea or lens.

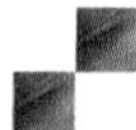

THE EARS

Opening questions are "How is your hearing?" and "Have you had any trouble with your ears?" If the patient has noticed a *hearing loss,* does it involve one or both ears? Did it start suddenly or gradually? What are the associated symptoms, if any? (See page 229.)

Try to distinguish between two basic types of hearing impairment: *conductive loss,* which results from problems in the external or middle ear, and *sensorineural loss,* from problems in the inner ear, the cochlear nerve, or its central connections in the brain. Two questions may be helpful . . . Does the patient have special difficulty understanding people as they talk? . . . What difference does a noisy environment make?

People with sensorineural loss have particular trouble understanding speech, often complaining that others mumble; noisy environments make hearing worse. In conductive loss, noisy environments may help.

Symptoms associated with hearing loss, such as earache or vertigo, help you to assess likely causes. In addition, inquire specifically about medications that might affect hearing and ask about sustained exposure to loud noise.

Medications that affect hearing include aminoglycosides, aspirin, NSAIDs, quinine, furosemide, and others.

Complaints of *earache,* or *pain in the ear,* are especially common. Ask about associated fever, sore throat, cough, and concurrent upper respiratory infection.

Pain suggests a problem in the external ear, such as *otitis externa,* or, if associated with symptoms of respiratory infection, in the inner ear, as in *otitis media.* It may also be referred from other structures in the mouth, throat, or neck.

Ask about *discharge from the ear,* especially if associated with earache or trauma.

Unusually soft wax, debris from inflammation or rash in the ear canal, or discharge through a perforated eardrum secondary to *acute* or *chronic otitis media*

Tinnitus is a perceived sound that has no external stimulus—commonly a musical ringing or a rushing or roaring noise. It can involve one or both ears. Tinnitus may accompany hearing loss and often remains unexplained. Occasionally, popping sounds originate in the temporomandibular joint, or vascular noises from the neck may be audible.

Tinnitus is a common symptom, increasing in frequency with age. When associated with hearing loss and vertigo, it suggests *Ménière's disease.*

Vertigo refers to the perception that the patient or the environment is rotating or spinning. These sensations point primarily to a problem in the labyrinths of the inner ear, peripheral lesions of CN VIII, or lesions in its central pathways or nuclei in the brain.

See Table 6-2, Vertigo, p. 210.

Vertigo is a challenging symptom for you as clinician, because patients differ widely in what they mean by the word "dizzy." "Are there times when you feel dizzy?" is an appropriate first question, but patients often find it difficult to be more specific. Ask "Do you feel unsteady, as if you are going to fall or black out? . . . Or do you feel the room is spinning (true vertigo)?" Get the story without biasing it. You may need to offer the patient several choices of wording. Ask if the patient feels pulled to the ground or off to one side. And if the dizziness is related to a change in body position. Pursue any associated feelings of clamminess or flushing, nausea, or vomiting. Check if any medications may be contributing.

Feeling unsteady, lightheaded, or "dizzy in the legs" sometimes suggests a cardiovascular etiology. A feeling of being pulled suggests true vertigo from an inner ear problem or a central or peripheral lesion of CN VIII.

THE NOSE AND SINUSES

Rhinorrhea refers to drainage from the nose and is often associated with *nasal congestion,* a sense of stuffiness or obstruction. These symptoms are frequently accompanied by *sneezing,* watery eyes, and throat discomfort, and also by *itching* in the eyes, nose, and throat.

Causes include viral infections, *allergic rhinitis* ("hay fever"), and *vasomotor rhinitis.* Itching favors an allergic cause.

Assess the chronology of the illness. Does it last for a week or so, especially when common colds and related syndromes are prevalent, or does it occur seasonally when pollens are in the air? Is it associated with specific contacts or environments? What remedies has the patient used? For how long? And how well do they work?

Relation to seasons or environmental contacts suggests allergy.

Excessive use of decongestants can worsen the symptoms, causing rhinitis medicamentosa.

Inquire about drugs that might cause stuffiness.

Oral contraceptives, reserpine, guanethidine, and alcohol

Are there symptoms in addition to rhinorrhea or congestion, such as pain and tenderness in the face or over the sinuses, local headache, or fever?

These together suggest *sinusitis.*[5-7]

Is the patient's nasal congestion limited to one side? If so, you may be dealing with a different problem that requires careful physical examination.

Consider a deviated nasal septum, foreign body, or tumor.

Epistaxis means bleeding from the nose. The blood usually originates from the nose itself, but may come from a paranasal sinus or the nasopharynx. The history is usually quite graphic! However, in patients who are lying down, or whose bleeding originates in posterior structures, blood may pass into the throat instead of out the nostrils. You must identify the source of the bleeding carefully—is it from the nose, or has it been coughed up or vomited? Assess the site of bleeding, its severity, and associated symptoms. Is it a recurrent problem? Has there been easy bruising or bleeding elsewhere in the body?

Local causes of epistaxis include trauma (especially nose picking), inflammation, drying and crusting of the nasal mucosa, tumors, and foreign bodies.

Bleeding disorders may contribute to epistaxis.

THE MOUTH, THROAT, AND NECK

Sore throat is a frequent complaint, usually associated with acute upper respiratory symptoms.

Fever, pharyngeal exudates, and anterior lymphadenopathy, especially in the absence of cough, suggest streptococcal pharyngitis, or *strep throat* (p. 232)

A *sore tongue* may be caused by local lesions as well as by systemic illness.

Aphthous ulcers (p. 238); sore smooth tongue of nutritional deficiency (p. 237)

Bleeding from the gums is a common symptom, especially when brushing teeth. Ask about local lesions and any tendency to bleed or bruise elsewhere.

Bleeding gums are most often caused by *gingivitis* (p. 235).

Hoarseness refers to an altered quality of the voice, often described as husky, rough, or harsh. The pitch may be lower than before. Hoarseness usually arises from disease of the larynx, but may also develop as extralaryngeal lesions press on the laryngeal nerves. Check for overuse of the voice, allergy, smoking or other inhaled irritants, and any associated symptoms. Is the problem acute or chronic? If hoarseness lasts more than 2 weeks, visual examination of the larynx by indirect or direct laryngoscopy is advisable.

Overuse of the voice (as in cheering) and acute infections are the most likely causes.

Causes of chronic hoarseness include smoking, allergy, voice abuse, hypothyroidism, chronic infections such as tuberculosis, and tumors.

Ask "Have you noticed any swollen glands or lumps in your neck?", since patients are more familiar with the lay terms than with "*lymph nodes.*"

Enlarged tender lymph nodes commonly accompany pharyngitis.

Assess thyroid function and ask about any evidence of an enlarged thyroid gland or *goiter*. To evaluate thyroid function, ask about *temperature intolerance* and *sweating*. Opening questions include "Do you prefer hot or cold weather?" "Do you dress more warmly or less warmly than other people?" "What about blankets . . . do you use more or fewer than others at home?" "Do you perspire more or less than others?" "Any new palpitations or change in weight?" Note that as people grow older, they sweat less, have less tolerance for cold, and tend to prefer warmer environments.

With goiter, thyroid function may be increased, decreased, or normal.

Intolerance to cold, preference for warm clothing and many blankets, and decreased sweating suggest *hypothyroidism*; the opposite symptoms, palpitations and involuntary weight loss, suggest *hyperthyroidism* (p. 239).

HEALTH PROMOTION AND COUNSELING

Important Topics for Health Promotion and Counseling

- Changes in vision: cataracts, macular degeneration, glaucoma
- Hearing loss
- Oral health

Vision and hearing, critical senses for experiencing the world around us, are two areas of special importance for health promotion and counseling. Oral health, often overlooked, also merits clinical attention.

Disorders of vision shift with age. Healthy young adults generally have refractive errors. Up to 25% of adults older than 65 have refractive errors; however, cataracts, macular degeneration, and glaucoma become more prevalent.[8] These disorders reduce awareness of the social and physical environment and contribute to falls and injuries. To improve detection of visual defects, test visual acuity with a Snellen chart or handheld card (p. 753). Examine the lens and fundi for clouding of the lens (*cataracts*); mottling of the *macula*, variations in the retinal pigmentation, subretinal hemorrhage or exudate (*macular degeneration*); and change in size and color of the optic cup (*glaucoma*). After diagnosis, review effective treatments—corrective lenses, cataract surgery, photocoagulation for choroidal neovascularization in macular degeneration, and topical medications for glaucoma.

Surveillance for glaucoma is especially important.[9] Glaucoma is the leading cause of blindness in African Americans and the second leading cause of blindness overall. There is gradual loss of vision with damage to the optic nerve, loss of visual fields beginning usually at the periphery, and pallor and increasing size of the optic cup (enlarging to more than half the diameter of the optic disc). Elevated intraocular pressure (IOP) is seen in up to 80% of cases and is linked to damage of the optic nerve. Risk factors include age older than 65, African American origin, diabetes mellitus, myopia, family history of glaucoma, and ocular hypertension (IOP ≥ 21 mm Hg). Screening tests include tonometry to measure IOP, ophthalmoscopy or slit-lamp examination of the optic nerve head, and perimetry to map the visual fields. In the hands of general clinicians, however, all three tests lack accuracy, so attention to risk factors and referral to eye specialists remain important tools for clinical care.

Hearing loss can also trouble the later years.[10] More than a third of adults older than age 65 have detectable hearing deficits, contributing to emotional isolation and social withdrawal. These losses may go undetected—unlike vision prerequisites for driving and vision, there is no mandate for widespread testing, and many seniors avoid use of hearing aids. Questionnaires and hand-held audioscopes work well for periodic screening. Less sensitive are the clinical "whisper test," rubbing fingers, or use of the tuning fork. Groups at risk are those with a history of congenital or familial hearing loss, syphilis, rubella, meningitis, or exposure to hazardous noise levels at work or on the battlefield.

Clinicians should play an active role in promoting oral health: up to half of all children ages 5 to 17 have from one to eight cavities, and the average U.S. adult has 10 to 17 teeth that are decayed, missing, or filled.[11] In adults, the prevalence of gingivitis and periodontal disease is 50% and 80%, respectively. In the United States, more than half of all adults older than age 65 have no teeth at all! Effective screening begins with careful examination of the mouth. Inspect the oral cavity for decayed or loose teeth, inflammation of the gingiva, and signs of periodontal disease (bleeding, pus, recession of the gums, and bad breath). Inspect the mucous membranes, the palate, the oral floor, and the surfaces of the tongue for ulcers and leukoplakia, warning signs for oral cancer and HIV disease.

To improve oral health, counsel patients to adopt daily hygiene measures. Use of fluoride-containing toothpastes reduces tooth decay, and brushing and flossing retard periodontal disease by removing bacterial plaques. Urge patients to seek dental care at least annually to receive the benefits of more specialized preventive care such as scaling, planing of roots, and topical fluorides.

Diet, tobacco and alcohol use, changes in salivary flow from medication, and proper use of dentures should also be addressed.[12] As with children, adults should avoid excessive intake of foods high in refined sugars, such as sucrose, which enhance attachment and colonization of cariogenic bacteria. Use of all tobacco products and excessive alcohol, the principal risk factors for oral cancers, should be avoided.

Saliva cleanses and lubricates the mouth. Many medications reduce salivary flow, increasing risk for tooth decay, mucositis, and gum disease from xerostomia, especially for the elderly. For those wearing dentures, be sure to counsel removal and cleaning each night to reduce bacterial plaque and risk of malodor. Regular massage of the gums relieves soreness and pressure from dentures on the underlying soft tissue.

TECHNIQUES OF EXAMINATION

THE HEAD

Because abnormalities covered by the hair are easily missed, ask if the patient has noticed anything wrong with the scalp or hair. If you detect a hairpiece or wig, ask the patient to remove it.

Examine:

The Hair. Note its quantity, distribution, texture, and pattern of loss, if any. You may see loose flakes of dandruff.

Fine hair in *hyperthyroidism;* coarse hair in *hypothyroidism.* Tiny white ovoid granules that adhere to hairs may be nits, or eggs of lice.

The Scalp. Part the hair in several places and look for scaliness, lumps, nevi, or other lesions.

Redness and scaling in *seborrheic dermatitis, psoriasis; soft lumps of pilar cysts* (wens)

The Skull. Observe the general size and contour of the skull. Note any deformities, depressions, lumps, or tenderness. Learn to recognize the irregularities in a normal skull, such as those near the suture lines between the parietal and occipital bones.

Enlarged skull in *hydrocephalus, Paget's disease* of bone. Tenderness after trauma

The Face. Note the patient's facial expression and contours. Observe for asymmetry, involuntary movements, edema, and masses.

See Table 6-3, Selected Facies (p. 211).

The Skin. Observe the skin, noting its color, pigmentation, texture, thickness, hair distribution, and any lesions.

Acne in many adolescents. *Hirsutism* (excessive facial hair) in some women with *polycystic ovary syndrome*

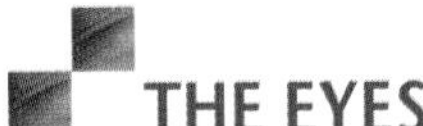

THE EYES

Important Areas of Examination

- Visual acuity
- Visual fields
- Conjunctiva and sclera
- Cornea, lens, and pupils
- Extraocular movements
- Fundi, including:
  Optic disc and cup
  Retina
  Retinal vessels

Visual Acuity. To test the acuity of central vision, use a Snellen eye chart, if possible, and light it well. Position the patient 20 feet from the chart.

Vision of 20/200 means that at 20 feet the patient can read print

Patients who use glasses other than for reading should put them on. Ask the patient to cover one eye with a card (to prevent peeking through the fingers) and to read the smallest line of print possible. Coaxing to attempt the next line may improve performance. A patient who cannot read the largest letter should be positioned closer to the chart; note the intervening distance. Determine the smallest line of print from which the patient can identify more than half the letters. Record the visual acuity designated at the side of this line, along with use of glasses, if any. Visual acuity is expressed as two numbers (e.g., 20/30): the first indicates the distance of patient from chart, and the second, the distance at which a normal eye can read the line of letters.

that a person with normal vision could read at 200 feet. The larger the second number, the worse the vision. "20/40 corrected" means the patient could read the 40 line with glasses (a correction).

Myopia is impaired far vision.

Testing near vision with a special hand-held card helps identify the need for reading glasses or bifocals in patients older than age 45. You can also use this card to test visual acuity at the bedside. Held 14 inches from the patient's eyes, the card simulates a Snellen chart. You may, however, let patients choose their own distance.

Presbyopia is the impaired near vision, found in middle-aged and older people. A presbyopic person often sees better when the card is farther away.

If you have no charts, screen visual acuity with any available print. If patients cannot read even the largest letters, test their ability to count your upraised fingers and distinguish light (such as your flashlight) from dark.

In the United States, a person is usually considered legally blind when vision in the better eye, corrected by glasses, is 20/200 or less. Legal blindness also results from a constricted field of vision: 20° or less in the better eye.

Visual Fields by Confrontation

Screening. Screening starts in the temporal fields because most defects involve these areas. Imagine the patient's visual fields projected onto a

Field defects that are all or partly temporal include:

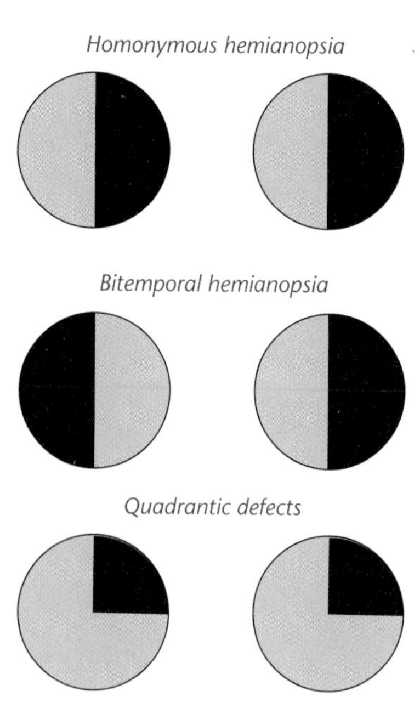

Review these patterns in Table 6-4, Visual Field Defects, p. 212.

glass bowl that encircles the front of the patient's head. Ask the patient to look with both eyes into your eyes. While you return the patient's gaze, place your hands about 2 feet apart, lateral to the patient's ears. Instruct the patient to point to your fingers as soon as they are seen. Then slowly move the wiggling fingers of both your hands along the imaginary bowl and toward the line of gaze until the patient identifies them. Repeat this pattern in the upper and lower temporal quadrants.

Usually a person sees both sets of fingers at the same time. If so, fields are usually normal.

Further Testing. If you find a defect, try to establish its boundaries. Test one eye at a time. If you suspect a temporal defect in the left visual field, for example, ask the patient to cover the right eye and, with the left one, to look into your eye directly opposite. Then slowly move your wiggling fingers from the defective area toward the better vision, noting where the patient first responds. Repeat this at several levels to define the border.

When the patient's left eye repeatedly does not see your fingers until they have crossed the line of gaze, a left temporal hemianopsia is present. It is diagrammed from the patient's viewpoint.

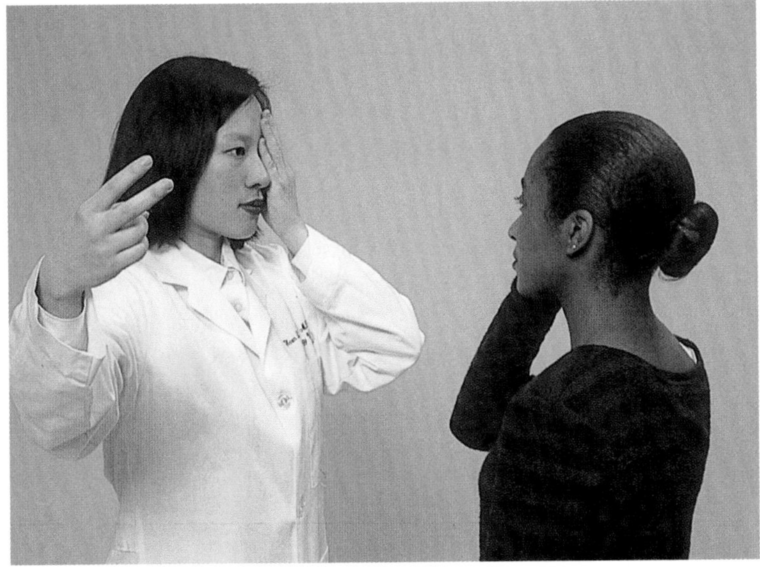

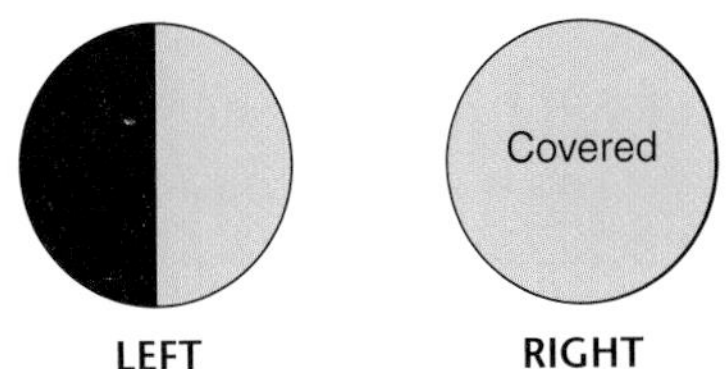

A left homonymous hemianopsia may thus be established.

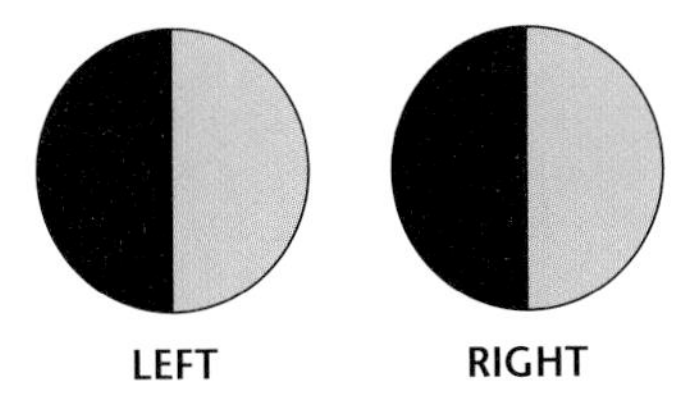

A temporal defect in the visual field of one eye suggests a nasal defect in the other eye. To test this hypothesis, examine the other eye in a similar way, again moving from the anticipated defect toward the better vision.

Small visual field defects and enlarged blind spots require a finer stimulus. Using a small red object such as a red-headed matchstick or the red eraser on a pencil, test one eye at a time. As the patient looks into your eye directly opposite, move the object about in the visual field. The normal blind spot can be found 15° temporal to the line of gaze—the small red object disappears. (Find your own blind spots for practice.)

An enlarged blind spot occurs in conditions affecting the optic nerve, e.g., *glaucoma, optic neuritis,* and *papilledema.*

Position and Alignment of the Eyes. Stand in front of the patient and survey the eyes for position and alignment with each other. If one or both eyes seem to protrude, assess them from above (see p. 200).

Inward or outward deviation of the eyes; abnormal protrusion in *Graves' disease* or ocular tumors

Eyebrows. Inspect the eyebrows, noting their quantity and distribution and any scaliness of the underlying skin.

Scaliness in *seborrheic dermatitis;* lateral sparseness in hypothyroidism

Eyelids. Note the position of the lids in relation to the eyeballs. Inspect for the following:

See Table 6-5, Variations and Abnormalities of the Eyelids (p. 213).

- Width of the palpebral fissures
- Edema of the lids
- Color of the lids

Red inflamed lid margins in blepharitis, often with crusting

- Lesions
- Condition and direction of the eyelashes
- Adequacy with which the eyelids close. Look for this especially when the eyes are unusually prominent, when there is facial paralysis, or when the patient is unconscious.

Failure of the eyelids to close exposes the corneas to serious damage.

Lacrimal Apparatus. Briefly inspect the regions of the lacrimal gland and lacrimal sac for swelling.

See Table 6-6, Lumps and Swellings in and Around the Eyes (p. 214).

Look for excessive tearing or dryness of the eyes. Assessment of dryness may require special testing by an ophthalmologist. To test for nasolacrimal duct obstruction, see p. 201.

Excessive tearing may be due to increased production or impaired drainage of tears. In the first group, causes include conjunctival inflammation and corneal irritation; in the second, ectropion (p. 213 and nasolacrimal duct obstruction.

Conjunctiva and Sclera. Ask the patient to look up as you depress both lower lids with your thumbs, exposing the sclera and conjunctiva. Inspect the sclera and palpebral conjunctiva for color, and note the vascular pattern against the white scleral background. Look for any nodules or swelling.

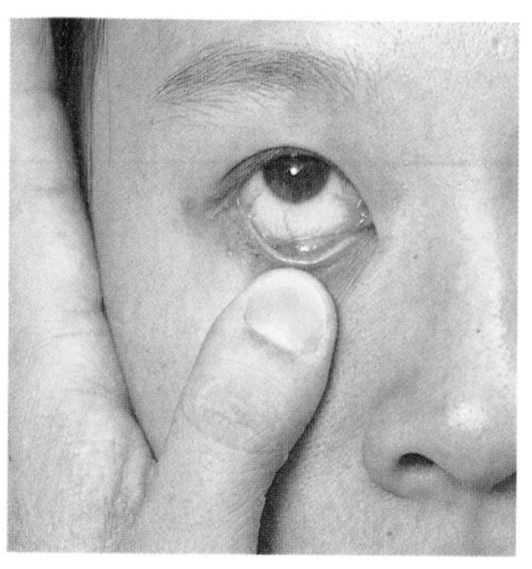

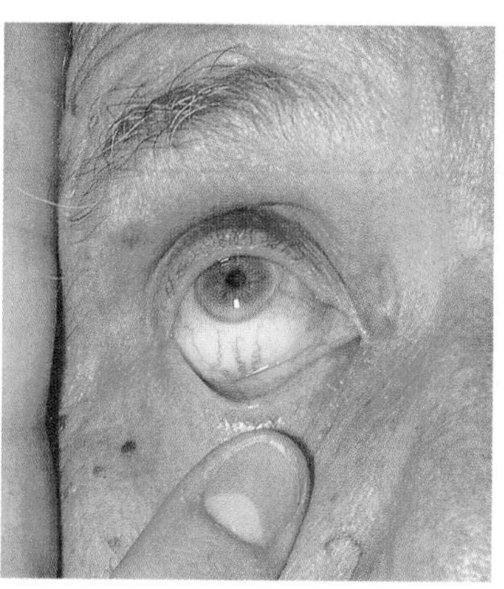

A yellow sclera indicates jaundice.

If you need a fuller view of the eye, rest your thumb and finger on the bones of the cheek and brow, respectively, and spread the lids.

Ask the patient to look to each side and down. This technique gives you a good view of the sclera and bulbar conjunctiva, but not of the palpebral conjunctiva of the upper lid. For this purpose, you need to evert the lid (see p. 201).

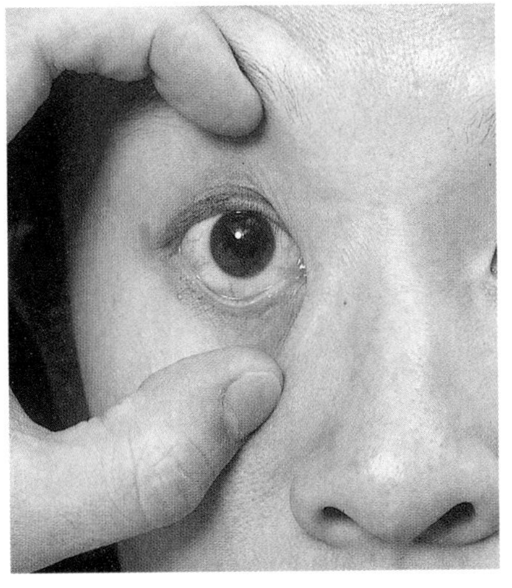

The local redness below is due to *nodular episcleritis:*

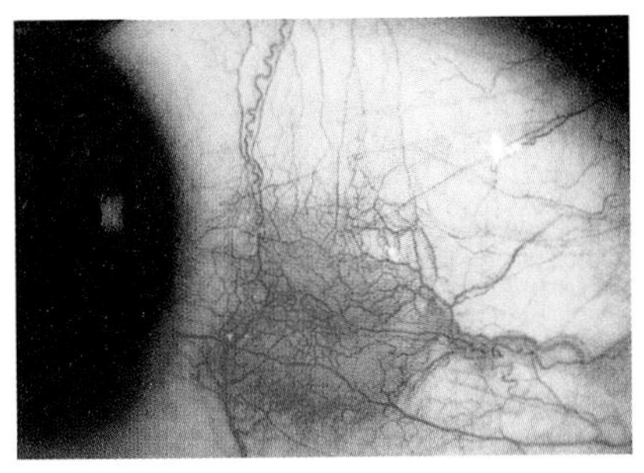

For comparisons, see Table 6-7, Red Eyes (p. 215).

Cornea and Lens. With oblique lighting, inspect the cornea of each eye for opacities and note any opacities in the lens that may be visible through the pupil.

See Table 6-8, Opacities of the Cornea and Lens (p. 216).

Iris. At the same time, inspect each iris. The markings should be clearly defined. With your light shining directly from the temporal side, look for a crescentic shadow on the medial side of the iris. Because the iris is normally fairly flat and forms a relatively open angle with the cornea, this lighting casts no shadow.

Occasionally the iris bows abnormally far forward, forming a very narrow angle with the cornea. The light then casts a crescentic shadow.

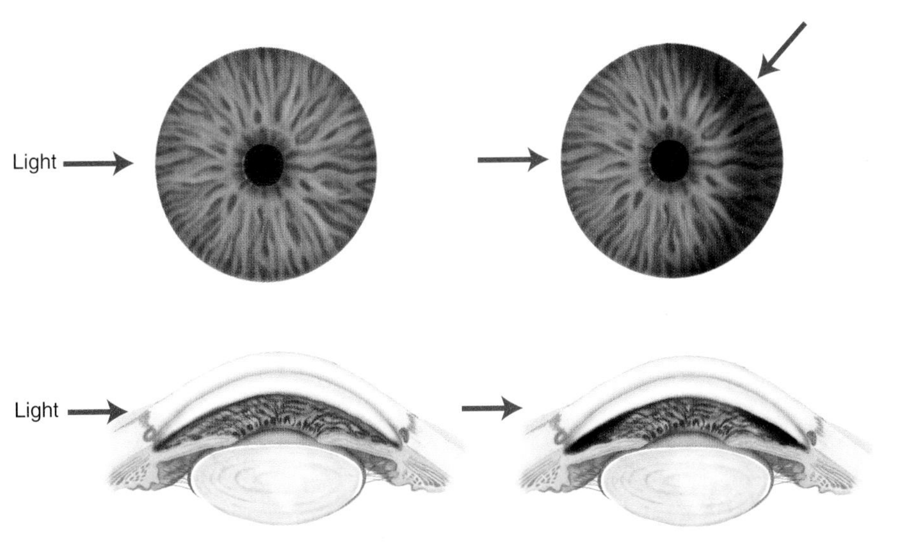

This narrow angle increases the risk for acute *narrow-angle glaucoma*—a sudden increase in intraocular pressure when drainage of the aqueous humor is blocked.

In *open-angle glaucoma*—the common form of glaucoma—the normal spatial relation between iris and cornea is preserved and the iris is fully lit.

Pupils. Inspect the *size, shape,* and *symmetry* of the pupils. If the pupils are large (>5 mm), small (<3 mm), or unequal, measure them. A card with black circles of varying sizes facilitates measurement.

Miosis refers to constriction of the pupils, *mydriasis* to dilation.

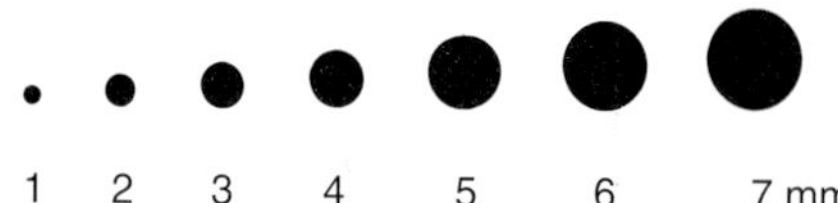

Pupillary inequality of less than 0.5 mm (*anisocoria*) is visible in about 20% of normal people. If pupillary reactions are normal, anisocoria is considered benign.

Compare benign anisocoria with *Horner's syndrome, oculomotor nerve paralysis,* and *tonic pupil.* See Table 6-9, Pupillary Abnormalities (p. 217).

Test the *pupillary reaction to light.* Ask the patient to look into the distance, and shine a bright light obliquely into each pupil in turn. (Both the distant gaze and the oblique lighting help to prevent a near reaction.) Look for:

- The *direct reaction* (pupillary constriction in the same eye)
- The *consensual reaction* (pupillary constriction in the opposite eye)

Always darken the room and use a bright light before deciding that a light reaction is absent.

If the reaction to light is impaired or questionable, test the *near reaction* in normal room light. Testing one eye at a time makes it easier to concentrate on pupillary responses, without the distraction of extraocular movement. Hold your finger or pencil about 10 cm from the patient's eye. Ask the patient to look alternately at it and into the distance directly behind it. Watch for pupillary constriction with near effort.

Testing the near reaction is helpful in diagnosing *Argyll Robertson* and *tonic (Adie's) pupils* (see p. 217).

Extraocular Muscles. From about 2 feet directly in front of the patient, shine a light onto the patient's eyes and ask the patient to look at it. *Inspect the reflections in the corneas.* They should be visible slightly nasal to the center of the pupils.

Asymmetry of the corneal reflections indicates a deviation from normal ocular alignment. A temporal light reflection on one cornea, for example, indicates a nasal deviation of that eye. See Table 6-10, Dysconjugate Gaze (p. 218).

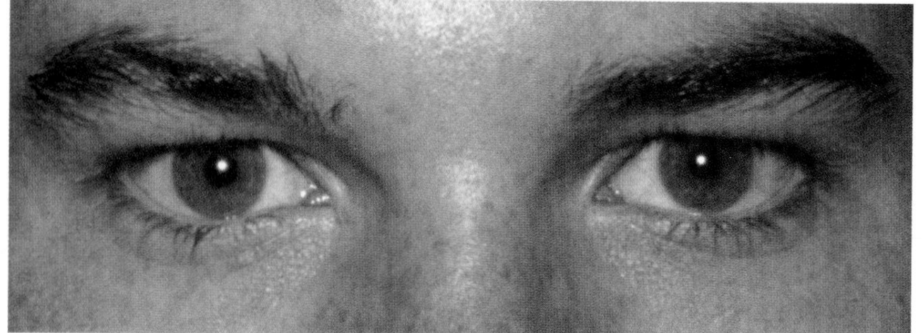

A *cover–uncover test* may reveal a slight or latent muscle imbalance not otherwise seen (see p. 218).

Now *assess the extraocular movements,* looking for:

- The normal *conjugate movements* of the eyes in each direction, or any *deviation* from normal

See Table 6-10, Dysconjugate Gaze (p. 218).

- *Nystagmus,* a fine rhythmic oscillation of the eyes. A few beats of nystagmus on extreme lateral gaze are normal. If you see it, bring your finger in to within the field of binocular vision and look again.

Sustained nystagmus within the binocular field of gaze is seen in a variety of neurologic conditions. See Table 17-4, Nystagmus (pp. 655–656).

- *Lid lag* as the eyes move from up to down.

Lid lag of *hyperthyroidism*

To make these observations, *ask the patient to follow your finger or pencil* as you sweep through the six cardinal directions of gaze. Making a wide H in the air, lead the patient's gaze (1) to the patient's extreme right, (2) to the right and upward, and (3) down on the right; then (4) without pausing in the middle, to the extreme left, (5) to the left and upward, and (6) down on the left. Pause during upward and lateral gaze to detect nystagmus. Move your finger or pencil at a comfortable distance from the patient. Because middle-aged or older people may have difficulty focusing on near objects, make this distance greater for them than for young people. Some patients move their heads to follow your finger. If necessary, hold the head in the proper midline position.

In paralysis of the CN VI, illustrated below, the eyes are conjugate in right lateral gaze but not in left lateral gaze, *left infranuclear ophthalmoplegia*

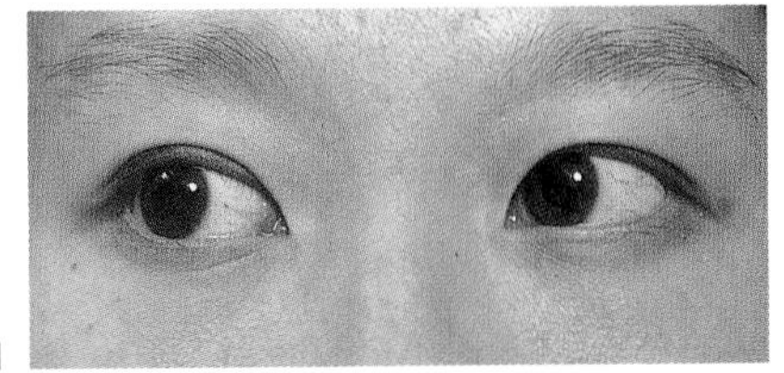

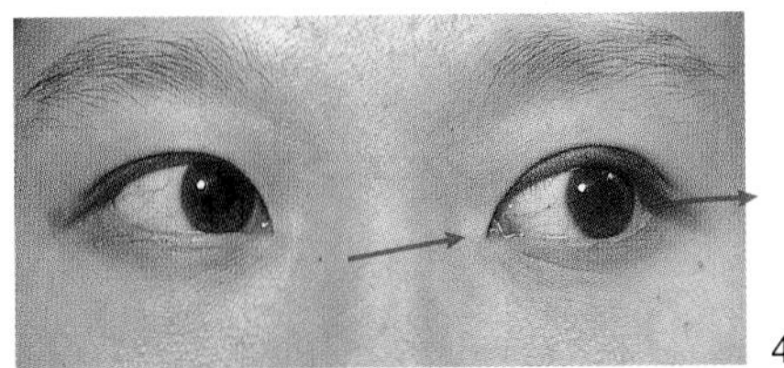

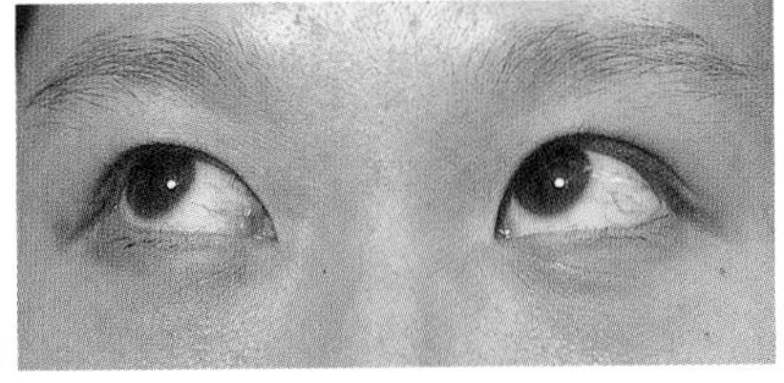

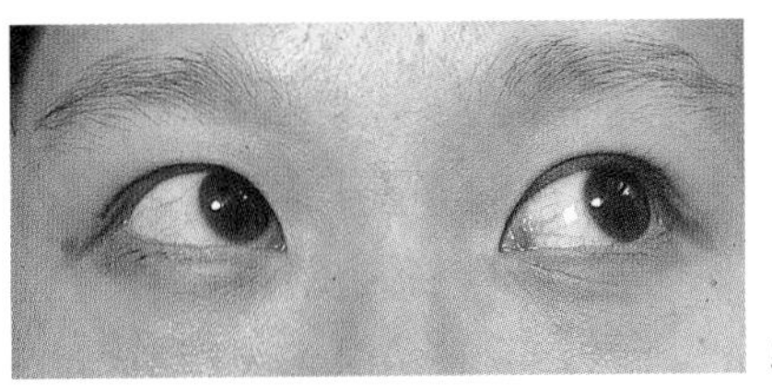

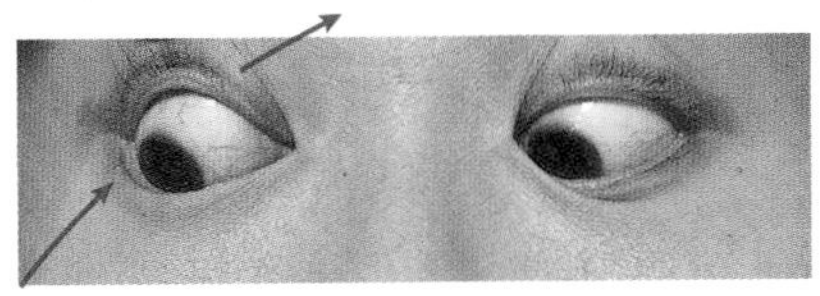

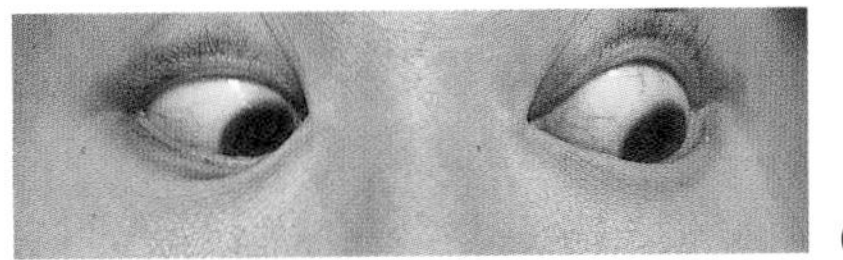

LOOKING RIGHT

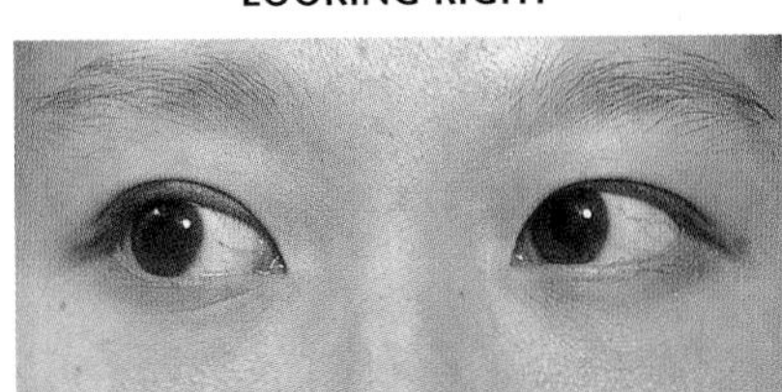

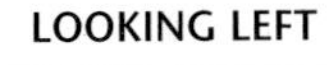

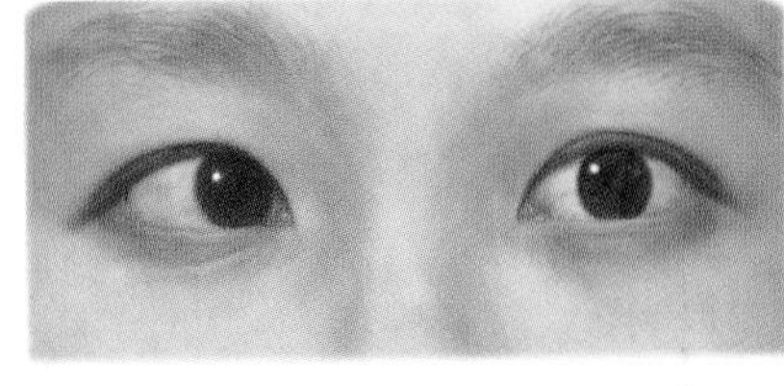

If you suspect a lid lag or hyperthyroidism, ask the patient to follow your finger again as you move it slowly from up to down in the midline. The lid should overlap the iris slightly throughout this movement.

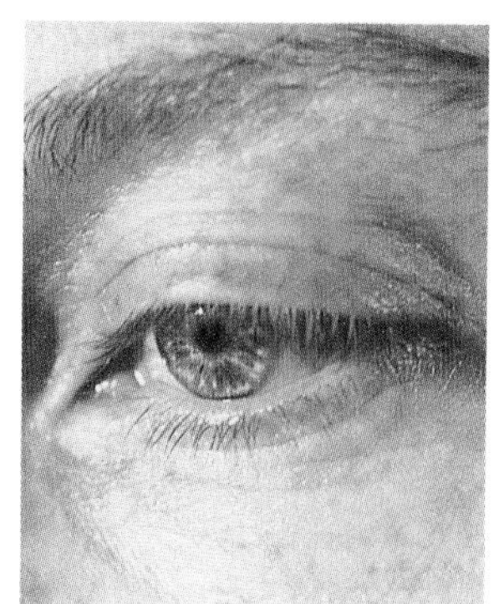

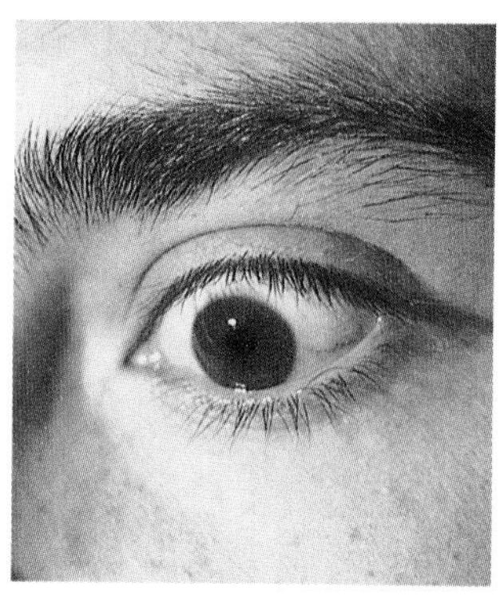

In the lid lag of hyperthyroidism, a rim of sclera is seen between the upper lid and iris; the lid seems to lag behind the eyeball.

Finally, test for *convergence*. Ask the patient to follow your finger or pencil as you move it in toward the bridge of the nose. The converging eyes normally follow the object to within 5 cm to 8 cm of the nose.

Poor convergence in *hyperthyroidism*

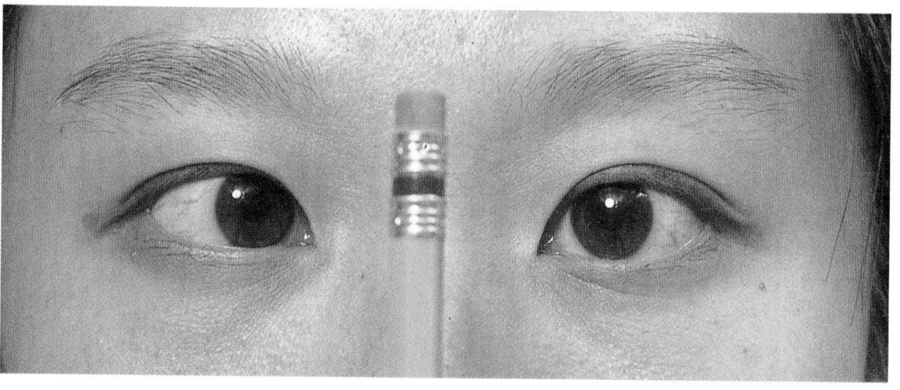

CONVERGENCE

Ophthalmoscopic Examination. In general health care, you should usually examine your patients' eyes *without dilating their pupils*. Your view is therefore limited to the posterior structures of the retina. To see more peripheral structures, to evaluate the macula well, or to investigate unexplained visual loss, ophthalmologists dilate the pupils with mydriatic drops unless this is contraindicated.

Contraindications for mydriatic drops include (1) head injury and coma, in which continuing observations of pupillary reactions are essential, and (2) any suspicion of narrow-angle glaucoma.

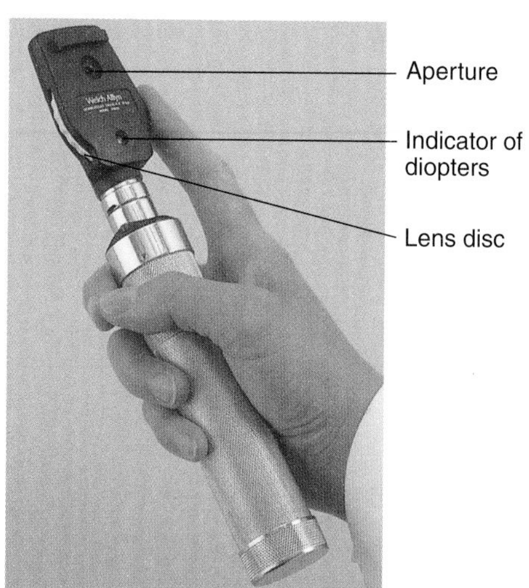

At first, using the ophthalmoscope may seem awkward, and it may be difficult to visualize the fundus. With patience and practice of proper technique, the fundus will come into view, and you will be able to assess important structures such as the optic disc and the retinal vessels. Remove your glasses unless you have marked nearsightedness or severe astigmatism. (However, if the patient's refractive errors make it difficult to focus on the fundi, it may be easier to keep your glasses on.)

Review the components of the ophthalmoscope pictured on the previous page. Then follow the steps for using the ophthalmoscope, and your examination skills will improve over time.

STEPS FOR USING THE OPHTHALMOSCOPE

- Darken the room. Switch on the ophthalmoscope light and turn the lens disc until you see the large round beam of white light.* Shine the light on the back of your hand to check the type of light, its desired brightness, and the electrical charge of the ophthalmoscope.
- Turn the lens disc to the 0 diopter (a diopter is a unit that measures the power of a lens to converge or diverge light). At this diopter, the lens neither converges nor diverges light. Keep your finger on the edge of the lens disc so you can turn the disc to focus the lens when you examine the fundus.
- Remember, hold the ophthalmoscope *in your right hand* to examine *the patient's right eye;* hold it *in your left hand* to examine *the patient's left eye.* This keeps you from bumping the patient's nose and gives you more mobility and closer range for visualizing the fundus. At first, you may have difficulty using the nondominant eye, but this will abate with practice.
- Hold the ophthalmoscope firmly braced against the medial aspect of your bony orbit, with the handle tilted laterally at about a 20° slant from the vertical. Check to make sure you can see clearly through the aperture. Instruct the patient to look slightly up and over your shoulder at a point directly ahead on the wall.
- Place yourself about 15 inches away from the patient and at an angle 15° lateral to the patient's line of vision. Shine the light beam on the pupil and look for the orange glow in the pupil—the *red reflex*. Note any opacities interrupting the red reflex.
- Now, place the thumb of your other hand across the patient's eyebrow (this technique helps keep you steady but is not essential). Keeping the light beam focused on the red reflex, move in with the ophthalmoscope on the 15° angle toward the pupil until you are very close to it, almost touching the patient's eyelashes.

Try to keep both eyes open and relaxed, as if gazing into the distance, to help minimize any fluctuating blurriness as your eyes attempt to accommodate.

You may need to lower the brightness of the light beam to make the examination more comfortable for the patient, avoid *hippus* (spasm of the pupil), and improve your observations.

Absence of a *red reflex* suggests an opacity of the lens (cataract) or possibly of the vitreous. Less commonly, a *detached retina* or, in children, a *retinoblastoma* may obscure this reflex. Do not be fooled by an artificial eye, which has no red reflex.

* Some clinicians like to use the large round beam for large pupils, the small round beam for small pupils. The other beams are rarely helpful. The slitlike beam is sometimes used to assess elevations or concavities in the retina, the green (or red-free) beam to detect small red lesions, and the grid to make measurements. Ignore the last three lights and practice with the large round white beam.

Now you are ready to inspect the *optic disc* and the *retina*. You should be seeing the optic disc—a yellowish orange to creamy pink oval or round structure that may fill your field of gaze or even exceed it. Of interest, the ophthalmoscope magnifies the normal retina about 15 times and the normal iris about 4 times. The optic disc actually measures about 1.5 mm. Follow the steps below for this important segment of the physical examination:

When the lens has been removed surgically, its magnifying effect is lost. Retinal structures then look much smaller than usual, and you can see a much larger expanse of fundus.

STEPS FOR EXAMINING THE OPTIC DISC AND THE RETINA

The Optic Disc

- First, *locate the optic disc.* Look for the round yellowish orange structure described above. If you do not see it at first, follow a blood vessel centrally until you do. You can tell which direction is central by noting the angles at which vessels branch—the vessel size becomes progressively larger at each junction as you approach the disc.

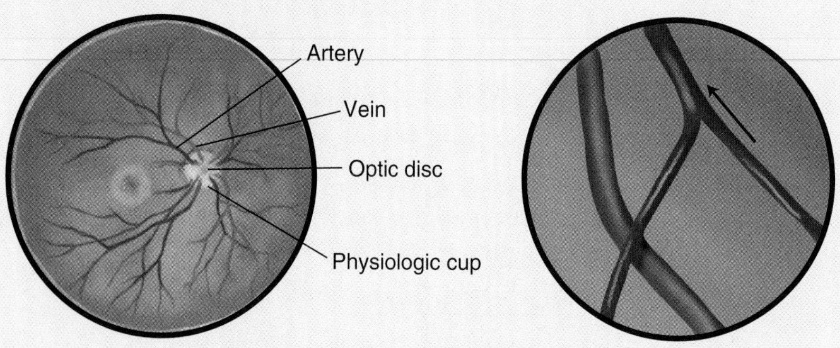

- Now, *bring the optic disc into sharp focus* by adjusting the lens of your ophthalmoscope. If both you and the patient have no refractive errors, the retina should be in focus at 0 diopters. If structures are blurred, rotate the lens disc until you find the sharpest focus.
  For example, if the patient is myopic (nearsighted), rotate the lens disc counterclockwise to the minus diopters; in a hyperopic (farsighted) patient, move the disc clockwise to the plus diopters. You can correct your own refractive error in the same way.
- *Inspect the optic disc.* Note the following features:
  - *The sharpness or clarity of the disc outline.* The nasal portion of the disc margin may be somewhat blurred, a normal finding.
  - *The color of the disc,* normally yellowish orange to creamy pink. White or pigmented crescents may ring the disc, a normal finding.
  - *The size of the central physiologic cup,* if present. It is usually yellowish white. The horizontal diameter is usually less than half the horizontal diameter of the disc.
  - *The comparative symmetry* of the eyes and findings in the fundi

(continued)

In a refractive error, light rays from a distance do not focus on the retina. In myopia, they focus anterior to it; in hyperopia, posterior to it. Retinal structures in a myopic eye look larger than normal.

See Table 6-11, Normal Variations of the Optic Disc (p. 219), and Table 6-12, Abnormalities of the Optic Disc (p. 220).

An enlarged cup suggests chronic open-angle glaucoma.

STEPS FOR EXAMINING THE OPTIC DISC AND THE RETINA (Continued)

Detecting Papilledema. *Papilledema* describes swelling of the optic disc and anterior bulging of the physiologic cup. Increased intracranial pressure is transmitted to the optic nerve, causing stasis of axoplasmic flow, intra-axonal edema, and swelling of the optic nerve head. Papilledema often signals serious disorders of the brain, such as meningitis, subarachnoid hemorrhage, trauma, and mass lesions, so searching for this important disorder is a priority during all your fundoscopic examinations.

If you detect papilledema, measure elevation of the optic disc by subtracting the difference in the diopters of the two lenses needed to focus clearly on the elevated disc and on the uninvolved retina. *Note that at the retina, 3 diopters = 1 mm.*

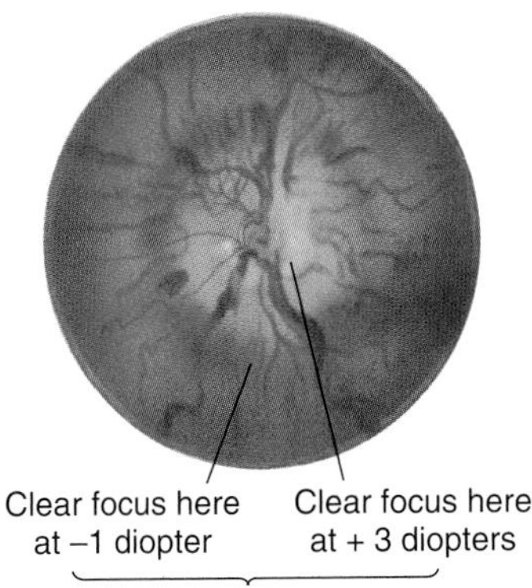

PAPILLEDEMA

Photo from Tasman W, Jaeger E (eds.). The Wills Eye Hospital Atlas of Clinical Ophthalmology, 2nd ed. Philadelphia, Lippincott Williams & Wilkins, 2001.

Venous pulsations, seen in many but not all normal eyegrounds, may also be obliterated.

Loss of venous pulsations in pathologic conditions like head trauma, meningitis, or mass lesions may be an early sign of elevated intracranial pressure.

The Retina—Arteries, Veins, Fovea, and Macula

- *Inspect the retina,* including arteries and veins as they extend to the periphery, arteriovenous crossings, the fovea, and the macula. Distinguish arteries from veins based on the features listed below.

	Arteries	Veins
Color	Light red	Dark red
Size	Smaller (⅔ to ⅘ the diameter of veins)	Larger
Light Reflex (*reflection*)	Bright	Inconspicuous or absent

- *Follow the vessels peripherally in each of four directions,* noting their relative sizes and the character of the arteriovenous crossings.

  Identify any lesions of the surrounding *retina* and note their size, shape, color, and distribution. As you search the retina, *move your head and instrument as a unit,* using the patient's pupil as an imaginary fulcrum. At first, you may repeatedly lose your view of the retina because your light falls out of the pupil. You will improve with practice.

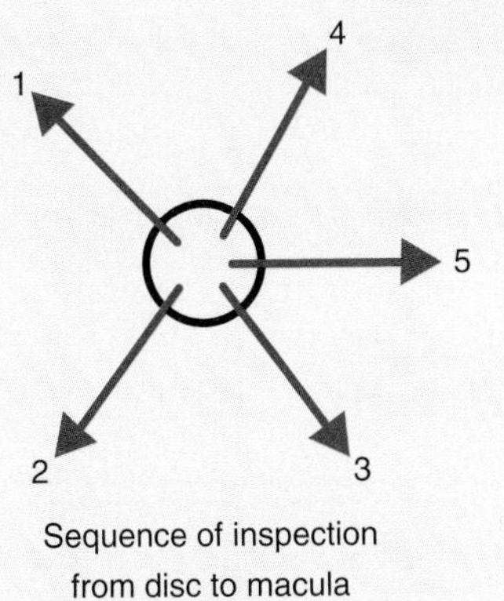

Sequence of inspection from disc to macula
LEFT EYE

See Table 6-13, Retinal Arteries and Arteriovenous Crossings: Normal and Hypertensive (p. 221); Table 6-14, Red Spots and Streaks in the Fundi (p. 222); Table 6-15, Ocular Fundi (pp. 223–224); Table 6-16, Light-Colored Spots in the Fundi (p. 225).

(continued)

STEPS FOR EXAMINING THE OPTIC DISC AND THE RETINA (Continued)

Lesions of the retina can be measured in terms of "disc diameters" from the optic disc. For example, among the cotton-wool patches illustrated on the right, note the irregular patches between 11 and 12 o'clock, 1 to 2 disc diameters from the disc. Each measures about one-half by one-half disc diameters.

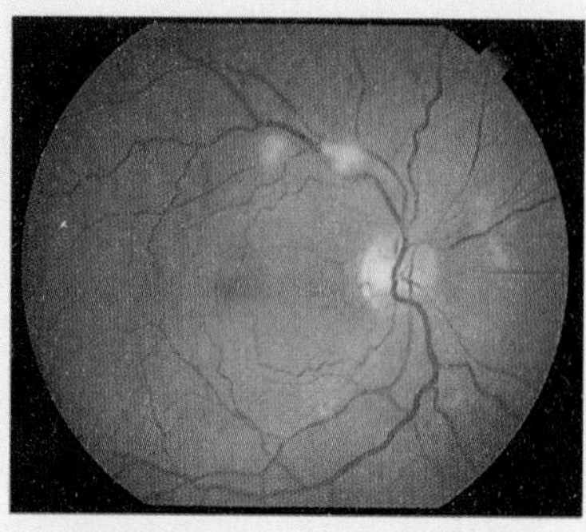

COTTON-WOOL PATCHES

- Inspect the *fovea* and surrounding *macula.* Direct your light beam laterally or by asking the patient to look directly into the light. Except in older people, the tiny bright reflection at the center of the fovea helps to orient you. Shimmering light reflections in the macular area are common in young people.

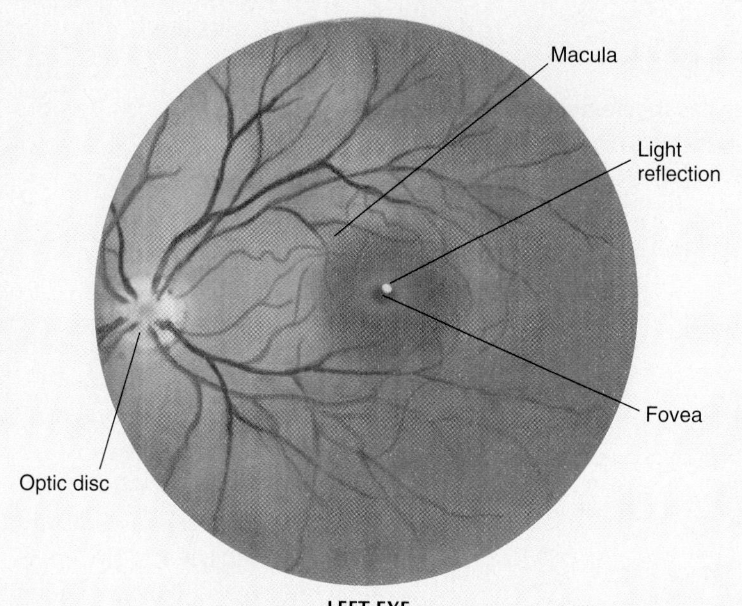

LEFT EYE

- *Inspect the anterior structures.* Look for opacities in the *vitreous* or *lens* by rotating the lens disc progressively to diopters of around +10 or +12. This technique allows you to focus on the more anterior structures in the eye.

Macular degeneration is an important cause of poor central vision in the elderly. Types include *dry atrophic* (more common but less severe) and *wet exudative,* or neovascular. Undigested cellular debris, called *drusen,* may be hard and sharply defined, as seen below, or soft and confluent with altered pigmentation (see p. 216).

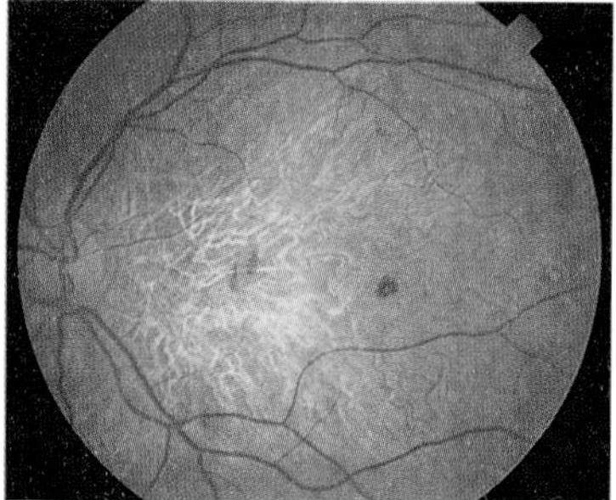

Photo from Tasman W, Jaeger E (eds). The Wills Eye Hospital Atlas of Clinical Ophthalmology, 2nd ed. Philadelphia, Lippincott Williams & Wilkins, 2001.

Vitreous floaters may be seen as dark specks or strands between the fundus and the lens. Cataracts are densities in the lens (see p. 216).

THE EARS

The Auricle. Inspect each auricle and surrounding tissues for deformities, lumps, or skin lesions.

See Table 6-17, Lumps On or Near the Ear (p. 226).

If ear pain, discharge, or inflammation is present, move the auricle up and down, press the tragus, and press firmly just behind the ear.

Movement of the auricle and tragus (the "tug test") is painful in acute *otitis externa* (inflammation of the ear canal), but not in *otitis media* (inflammation of the middle ear). Tenderness behind the ear may be present in otitis media.

Ear Canal and Drum. To see the ear canal and drum, use an otoscope with the largest ear speculum that the canal will accommodate. Position the patient's head so that you can see comfortably through the instrument. To straighten the ear canal, grasp the auricle firmly but gently and pull it upward, backward, and slightly away from the head.

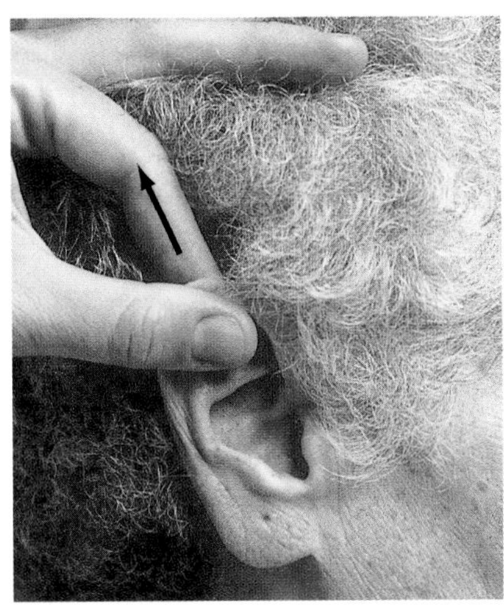

Holding the otoscope handle between your thumb and fingers, brace your hand against the patient's face. Your hand and instrument thus follow unexpected movements by the patient. (If you are uncomfortable switching hands for the left ear, as shown below, you may reach over that ear to pull it up and back with your left hand and rest your otoscope-holding right hand on the head behind the ear.)

Insert the speculum gently into the ear canal, directing it somewhat down and forward and through the hairs, if any.

Nontender nodular swellings covered by normal skin deep in the ear canals suggest *exostoses.* These are nonmalignant overgrowths, which may obscure the drum.

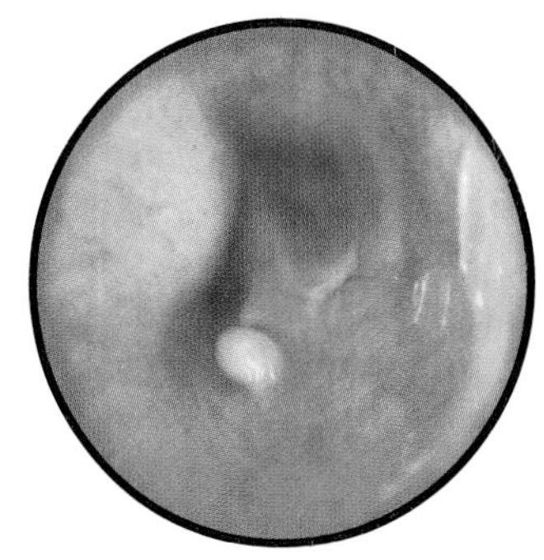

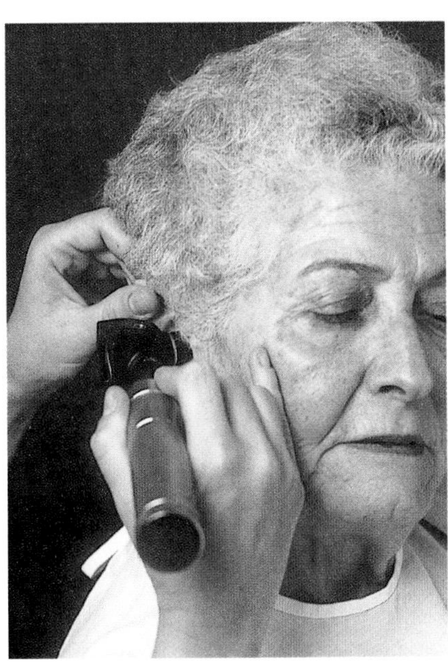

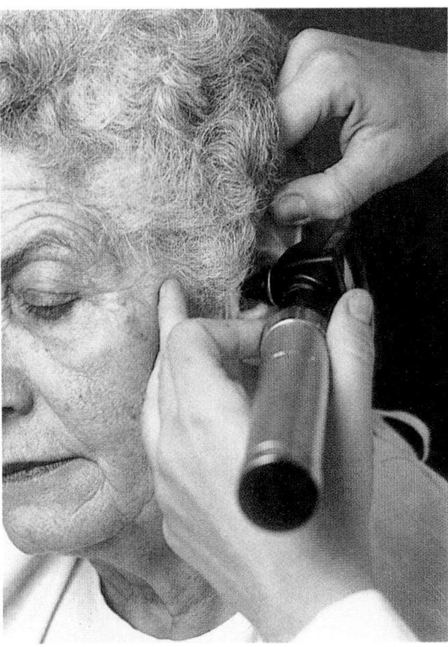

Inspect the ear canal, noting any discharge, foreign bodies, redness of the skin, or swelling. Cerumen, which varies in color and consistency from yellow and flaky to brown and sticky or even to dark and hard, may wholly or partly obscure your view.

In acute *otitis externa*, shown below, the canal is often swollen, narrowed, moist, pale, and tender. It may be reddened.

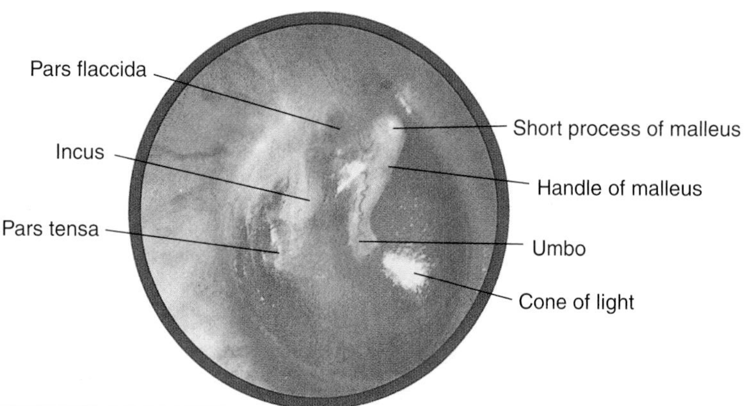

RIGHT EARDRUM

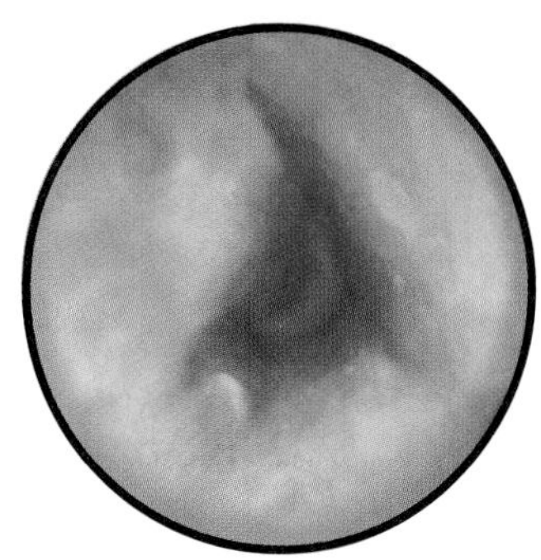

In *chronic otitis externa*, the skin of the canal is often thickened, red, and itchy.

Inspect the eardrum, noting its color and contour. The cone of light—usually easy to see—helps to orient you.

Red bulging drum of acute purulent otitis media, amber drum of a serous effusion

Identify the *handle of the malleus,* noting its position, and inspect the *short process of the malleus.*

An unusually prominent short process and a prominent handle that looks more horizontal suggest a retracted drum.

Gently move the speculum so that you can see as much of the drum as possible, including the *pars flaccida* superiorly and the margins of the *pars tensa.* Look for any perforations. The anterior and inferior margins of the drum may be obscured by the curving wall of the ear canal.

See Table 6-18, Abnormalities of the Eardrum (pp. 227–228).

Mobility of the eardrum can be evaluated with a pneumatic otoscope.

A serous effusion, a thickened drum, or purulent otitis media may decrease mobility.

Auditory Acuity. To estimate hearing, test one ear at a time. Ask the patient to occlude one ear with a finger, or better still, occlude it yourself. When auditory acuity on the two sides is different, move your finger rapidly, but gently, in the occluded canal. The noise so produced helps prevent the occluded ear from doing the work of the ear you wish to test. Then, standing 1 or 2 feet away, exhale fully (so as to minimize the intensity of your voice) and whisper softly toward the unoccluded ear. Choose numbers or other words with two equally accented syllables, such as "nine-four," or "baseball." If necessary, increase the intensity of your voice to a medium whisper, a loud whisper, and then a soft, medium, and loud voice. To make sure the patient does not read your lips, cover your mouth or obstruct the patient's vision.

Air and Bone Conduction. If hearing is diminished, *try to distinguish between conductive and sensorineural hearing loss.* You need a quiet room and a tuning fork, preferably of 512 Hz or possibly 1024 Hz. These frequencies fall within the range of human speech (300 Hz to 3000 Hz)—functionally the most important range. Forks with lower pitches may lead to overestimating bone conduction and can also be felt as vibration.

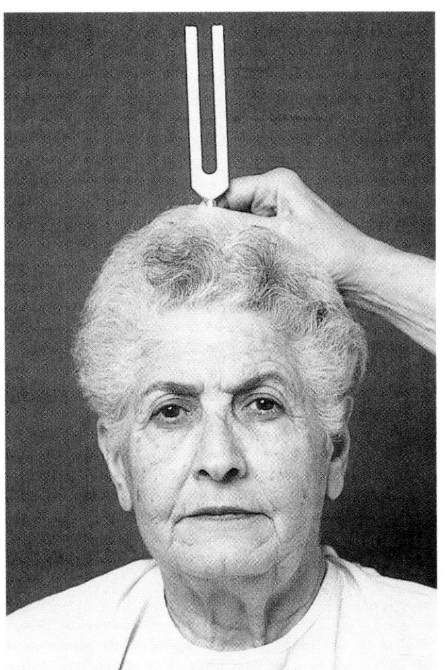

Set the fork into light vibration by briskly stroking it between the thumb and index finger or by tapping it on your knuckles.

- *Test for lateralization* (Weber test). Place the base of the lightly vibrating tuning fork firmly on top of the patient's head or on the midforehead.

In unilateral *conductive hearing loss,* sound is heard in (lateralized to) the impaired ear. Visible explanations include acute otitis media, perforation of the eardrum, and obstruction of the ear canal, as by cerumen.

Ask where the patient hears it: on one or both sides. Normally the sound is heard in the midline or equally in both ears. If nothing is heard, try again, pressing the fork more firmly on the head.

In unilateral *sensorineural hearing loss,* sound is heard in the good ear.

- *Compare air conduction (AC) and bone conduction (BC)* (Rinne test). Place the base of a lightly vibrating tuning fork on the mastoid bone, behind the ear and level with the canal. When the patient can no longer hear the sound, quickly place the fork close to the ear canal and ascertain whether the sound can be heard again. Here the "U" of the fork should face forward, thus maximizing its sound for the patient. Normally the sound is heard longer through air than through bone (AC > BC).

In conductive hearing loss, sound is heard through bone as long as or longer than it is through air (BC = AC or BC > AC). In sensorineural hearing loss, sound is heard longer through air (AC > BC). See Table 6-19, Patterns of Hearing Loss (p. 229).

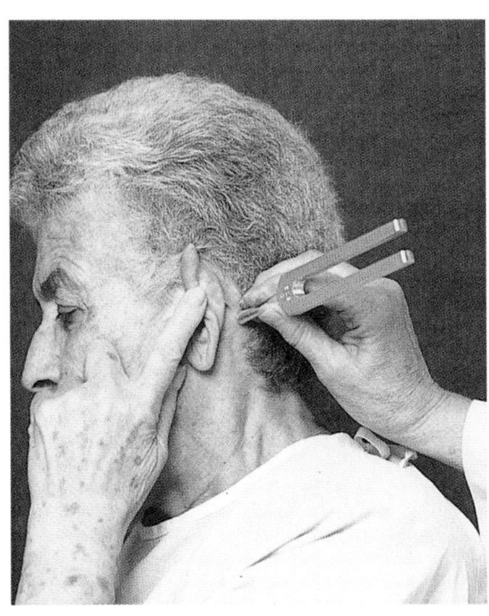

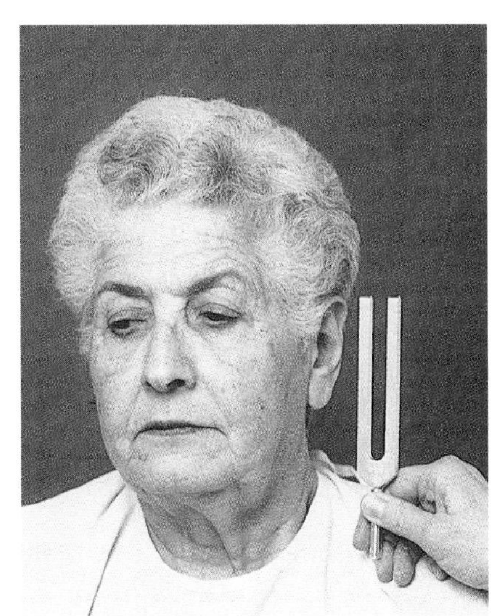

THE NOSE AND PARANASAL SINUSES

Inspect the anterior and inferior surfaces of the nose. Gentle pressure on the tip of the nose with your thumb usually widens the nostrils and, with the aid of a penlight or otoscope light, you can get a partial view of each nasal *vestibule.* If the tip is tender, be particularly gentle and manipulate the nose as little as possible.

Tenderness of the nasal tip or alae suggests local infection such as a furuncle.

Note any asymmetry or deformity of the nose.

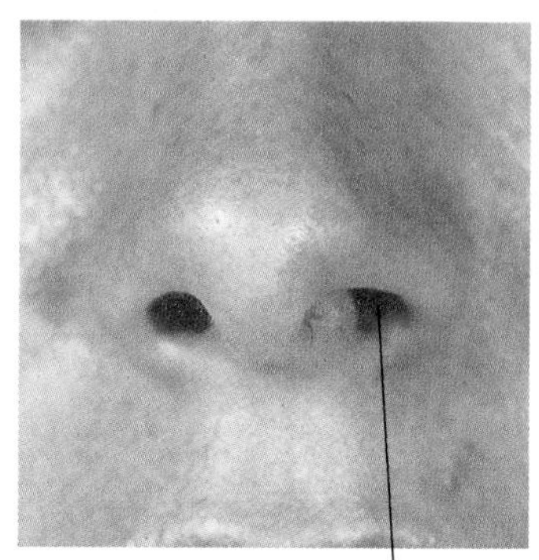

Test for nasal obstruction, if indicated, by pressing on each ala nasi in turn and asking the patient to breathe in.

Inspect the inside of the nose with an otoscope and the largest ear speculum available.[‡] Tilt the patient's head back a bit and insert the speculum gently into the vestibule of each nostril, avoiding contact with the sensitive nasal septum. Hold the otoscope handle to one side to avoid the patient's chin and improve your mobility. By directing the speculum posteriorly, then upward in small steps, try to see the inferior and middle turbinates, the nasal septum, and the narrow nasal passage between them. Some asymmetry of the two sides is normal.

Deviation of the lower septum is common and may be easily visible, as illustrated above. Deviation seldom obstructs air flow.

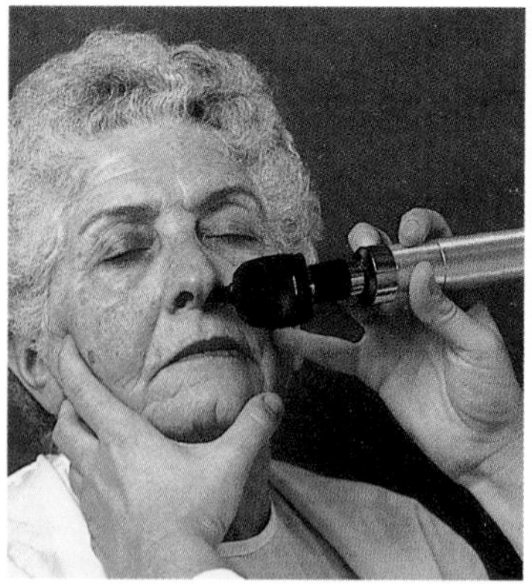

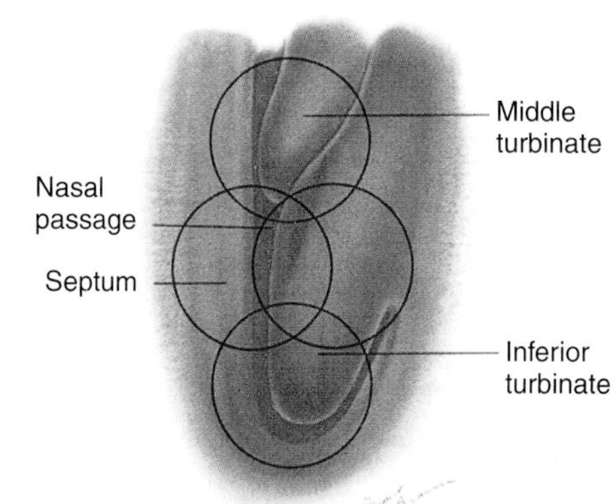

Observe the nasal mucosa, the nasal septum, and any abnormalities.

- The *nasal mucosa* that covers the septum and turbinates. Note its color and any swelling, bleeding, or exudate. If exudate is present, note its character: clear, mucopurulent, or purulent. The nasal mucosa is normally somewhat redder than the oral mucosa.

In *viral rhinitis* the mucosa is reddened and swollen; in *allergic rhinitis* it may be pale, bluish, or red.

[‡]A nasal illuminator, equipped with a short wide nasal speculum but lacking an otoscope's magnification, may also be used, but structures look much smaller. Otolaryngologists use special equipment not widely available to others.

- The *nasal septum*. Note any deviation, inflammation, or perforation of the septum. The lower anterior portion of the septum (where the patient's finger can reach) is a common source of *epistaxis* (nosebleed).

Fresh blood or crusting may be seen. Causes of septal perforation include trauma, surgery, and the intranasal use of cocaine or amphetamines.

- Any *abnormalities* such as ulcers or polyps.

Polyps are pale, semitranslucent masses that usually come from the middle meatus. Ulcers may result from nasal use of cocaine.

Make it a habit to place all nasal and ear specula outside your instrument case after use. Then discard them or clean and disinfect them appropriately. (Check the policies of your institution.)

Palpate for sinus tenderness. Press up on the *frontal sinuses* from under the bony brows, avoiding pressure on the eyes. Then press up on the *maxillary sinuses.*

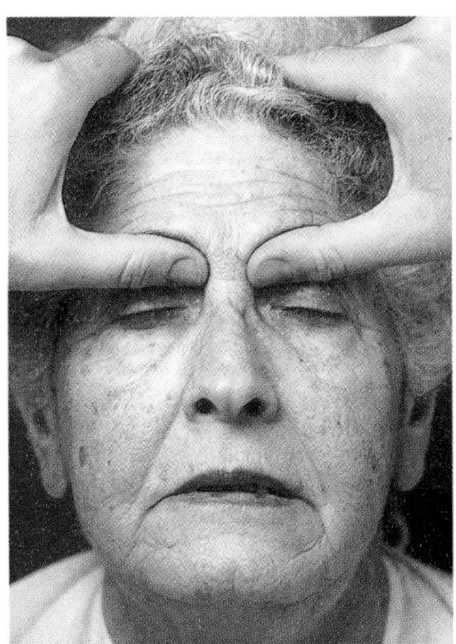

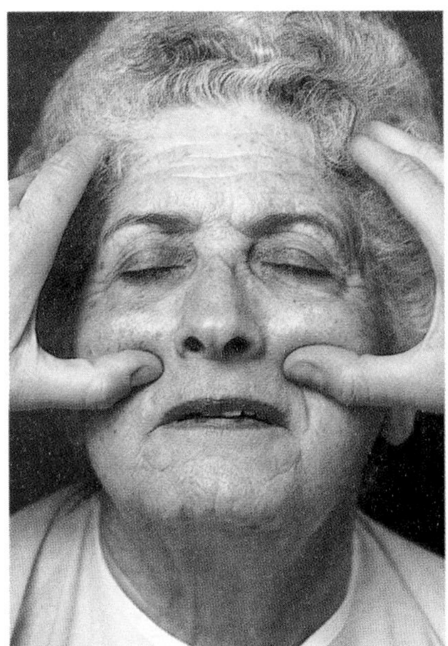

Local tenderness, together with symptoms such as pain, fever, and nasal discharge, suggest *acute sinusitis* involving the frontal or maxillary sinuses.[5–7] Transillumination may be diagnostically useful. For this technique, see p. 202.

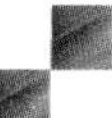

THE MOUTH AND PHARYNX

If the patient wears dentures, offer a paper towel and ask the patient to remove them so that you can see the mucosa underneath. If you detect any suspicious ulcers or nodules, put on a glove and palpate any lesions, noting especially any thickening or infiltration of the tissues that might suggest malignancy.

Bright red edematous mucosa underneath a denture suggests denture sore mouth. There may be ulcers or papillary granulation tissue.

Inspect the following:

The Lips. Observe their color and moisture, and note any lumps, ulcers, cracking, or scaliness.

Cyanosis, pallor. See Table 6-20, Abnormalities of the Lips (pp. 230–231).

The Oral Mucosa. Look into the patient's mouth and, with a good light and the help of a tongue blade, inspect the oral mucosa for color, ulcers, white patches, and nodules. The wavy white line on this buccal mucosa developed where the upper and lower teeth meet. Irritation from sucking or chewing may cause or intensify it.

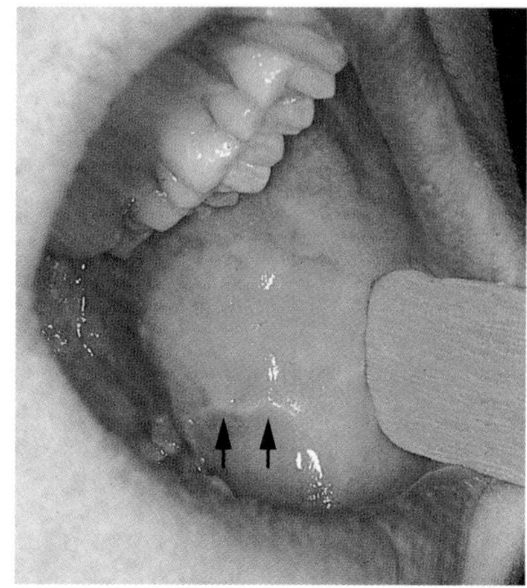

An *aphthous ulcer* on the labial mucosa is shown by the patient.

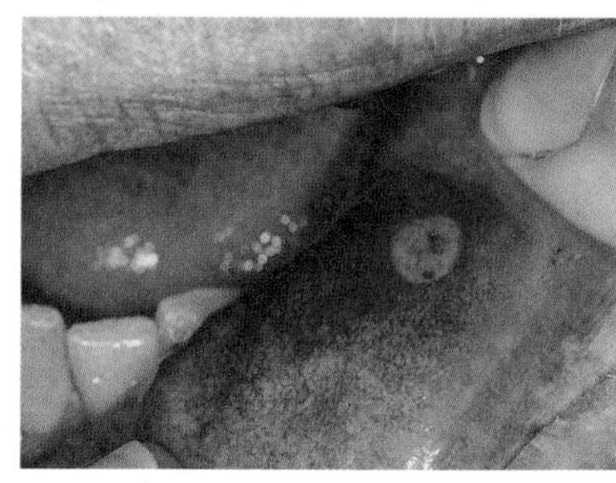

See Table 6-21, Findings in the Pharynx, Palate, and Oral Mucosa (pp. 232–234).

The Gums and Teeth. Note the color of the gums, normally pink. Patchy brownness may be present, especially but not exclusively in black people.

Redness of *gingivitis,* black line of *lead poisoning*

Inspect the gum margins and the interdental papillae for swelling or ulceration.

Swollen interdental papillae in *gingivitis.* See Table 6-22, Findings in the Gums and Teeth (pp. 235–236).

Inspect the teeth. Are any of them missing, discolored, misshapen, or abnormally positioned? You can check for looseness with your gloved thumb and index finger.

The Roof of the Mouth. Inspect the color and architecture of the hard palate.

Torus palatinus, a midline lump (see p. 233)

The Tongue and the Floor of the Mouth. Ask the patient to put out his or her tongue. Inspect it for symmetry—a test of the hypoglossal nerve (Cranial Nerve XII).

Note the color and texture of the dorsum of the tongue.

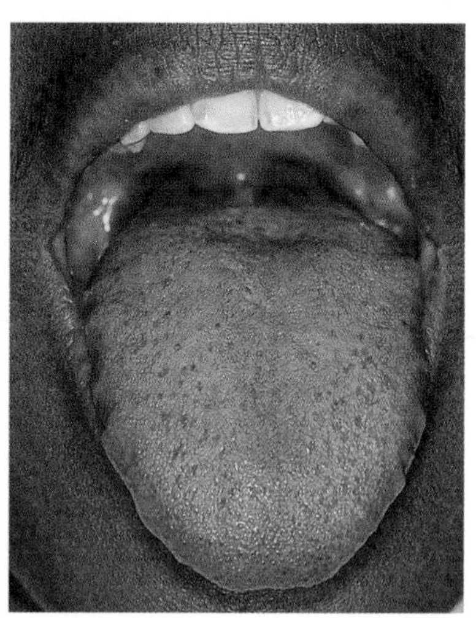

Asymmetric protrusion suggests a lesion of Cranial Nerve XII, as shown below.

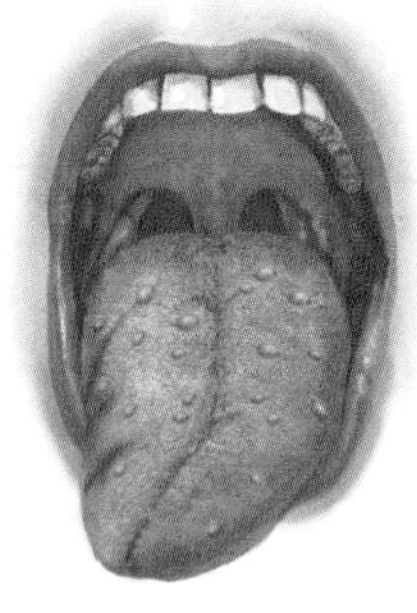

Inspect the sides and undersurface of the tongue and the floor of the mouth. These are the areas where cancer most often develops. Note any white or reddened areas, nodules, or ulcerations. Because cancer of the tongue is more

Cancer of the tongue is the second most common cancer of the mouth, second only to cancer of common in men over age 50, especially in smokers and drinkers of alcohol, palpation is indicated. Explain what you plan to do and put on gloves. Ask the patient to protrude his tongue. With your right hand, grasp the tip of the tongue with a square of gauze and gently pull it to the patient's left. Inspect the side of the tongue, and then palpate it with your gloved left hand, feeling for any induration (hardness). Reverse the procedure for the other side.

the lip. Any persistent nodule or ulcer, red or white, must be suspect. Induration of the lesion further increases the possibility of malignancy. Cancer occurs most often on the side of the tongue, next most often at its base.

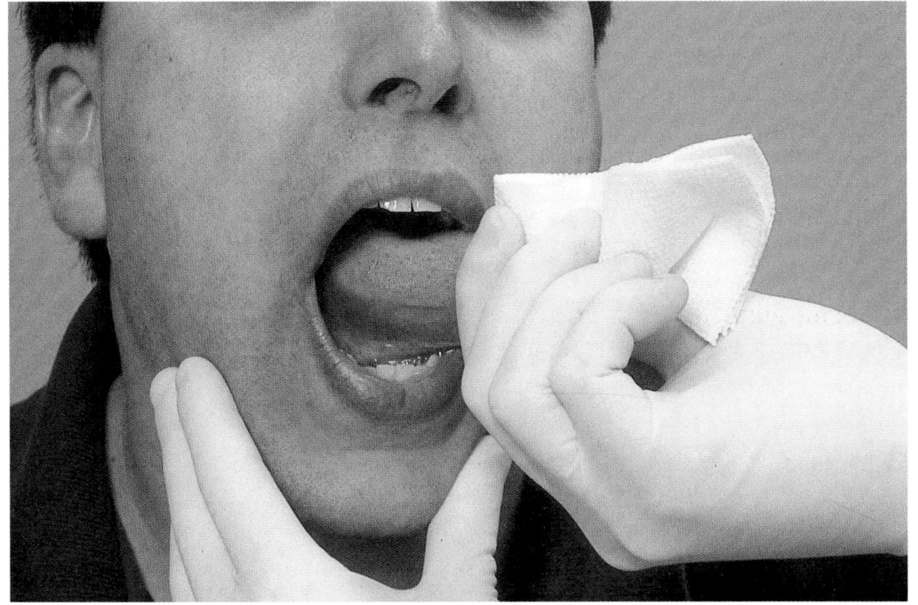

A carcinoma on the left side of a tongue:

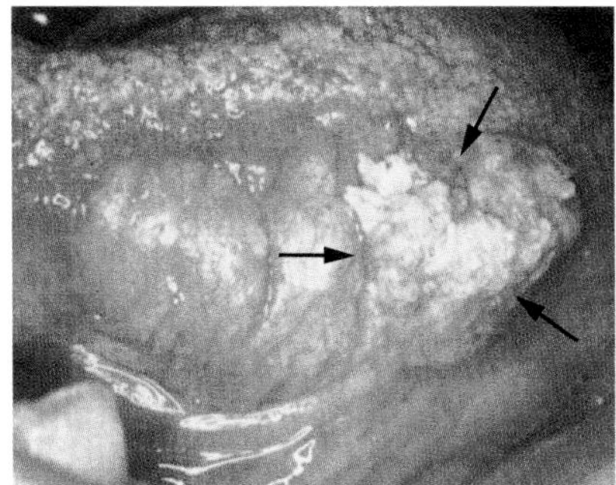

(Photo reprinted by permission of the New England Journal of Medicine, 328: 186, 1993—arrows added)

See Table 6-23, Findings In or Under the Tongue (pp. 237–238).

The Pharynx. Now, with the patient's mouth open but the tongue not protruded, ask the patient to say "ah" or yawn. This action may let you see the pharynx well. If not, press a tongue blade firmly down upon the midpoint of the arched tongue—far enough back to get good visualization of the pharynx but not so far that you cause gagging. Simultaneously, ask for an "ah" or a yawn. Note the rise of the soft palate—a test of Cranial Nerve X (the vagal nerve).

In CN X paralysis, the soft palate fails to rise and the uvula deviates to the opposite side.

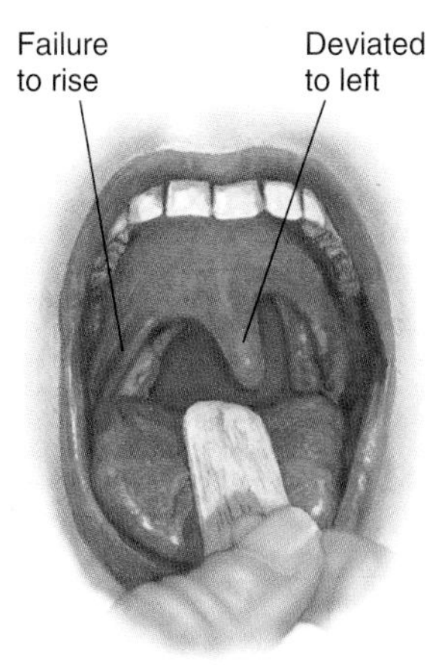

Inspect the soft palate, anterior and posterior pillars, uvula, tonsils, and pharynx. Note their color and symmetry and look for exudate, swelling, ulceration, or tonsillar enlargement. If possible, palpate any suspicious area for induration or tenderness. Tonsils have crypts, or deep infoldings of squamous epithelium. Whitish spots of normal exfoliating epithelium may sometimes be seen in these crypts.

See Table 6-21, Findings in the Pharynx, Palate, and Oral Mucosa (pp. 232–234).

Discard your tongue blade after use.

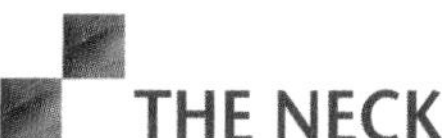

THE NECK

Inspect the neck, noting its symmetry and any masses or scars. Look for enlargement of the parotid or submandibular glands, and note any visible lymph nodes.

A scar of past thyroid surgery is often a clue to unsuspected thyroid disease.

The Lymph Nodes. *Palpate the lymph nodes.* Using the pads of your index and middle fingers, move the skin over the underlying tissues in each area. The patient should be relaxed, with neck flexed slightly forward and, if needed, slightly toward the side being examined. You can usually examine both sides at once. For the submental node, however, it is helpful to feel with one hand while bracing the top of the head with the other.

Feel in sequence for the following nodes:

1. *Preauricular*—in front of the ear
2. *Posterior auricular*—superficial to the mastoid process
3. *Occipital*—at the base of the skull posteriorly
4. *Tonsillar*—at the angle of the mandible
5. *Submandibular*—midway between the angle and the tip of the mandible. These nodes are usually smaller and smoother than the lobulated submandibular gland against which they lie.
6. *Submental*—in the midline a few centimeters behind the tip of the mandible
7. *Superficial cervical*—superficial to the sternomastoid
8. *Posterior cervical*—along the anterior edge of the trapezius
9. *Deep cervical chain*—deep to the sternomastoid and often inaccessible to examination. Hook your thumb and fingers around either side of the sternomastoid muscle to find them.
10. *Supraclavicular*—deep in the angle formed by the clavicle and the sternomastoid

A "tonsillar node" that pulsates is really the carotid artery. A small, hard, tender "tonsillar node" high and deep between the mandible and the sternomastoid is probably a styloid process.

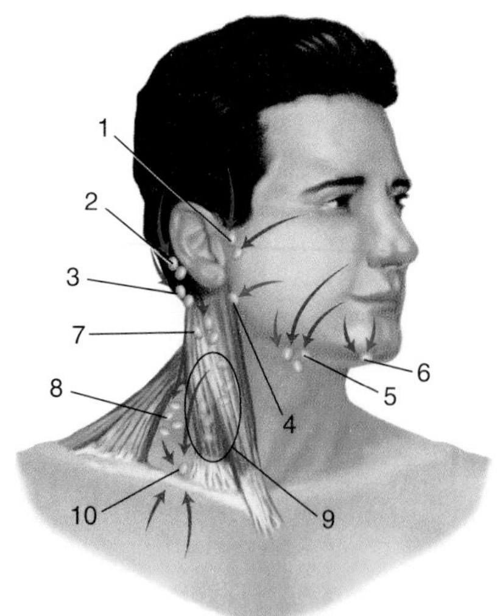

Enlargement of a supraclavicular node, especially on the left, suggests possible metastasis from a thoracic or an abdominal malignancy.

Note their size, shape, delimitation (discrete or matted together), mobility, consistency, and any tenderness. Small, mobile, discrete, nontender nodes, sometimes termed "shotty," are frequently found in normal persons.

Tender nodes suggest inflammation; hard or fixed nodes suggest malignancy.

- Using the pads of the 2nd and 3rd fingers, palpate the preauricular nodes with a gentle rotary motion. Then examine the posterior auricular and occipital lymph nodes.

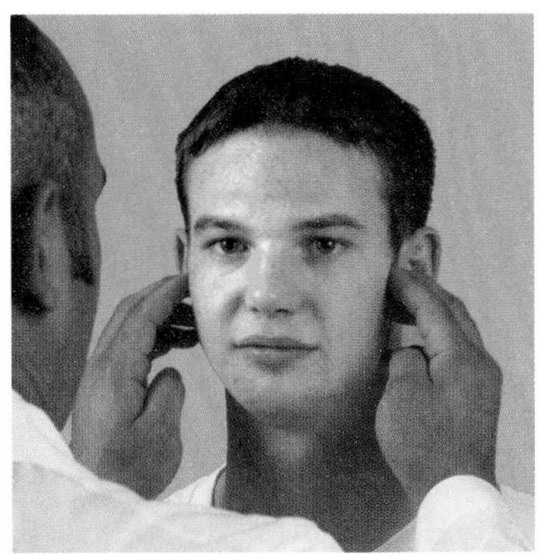

- Palpate the anterior cervical chain, located anterior and superficial to the sternomastoid. Then palpate the posterior cervical chain along the trapezius (anterior edge) and along the sternomastoid (posterior edge). Flex the patient's neck slightly forward toward the side being examined. Examine the supraclavicular nodes in the angle between the clavicle and the sternomastoid.

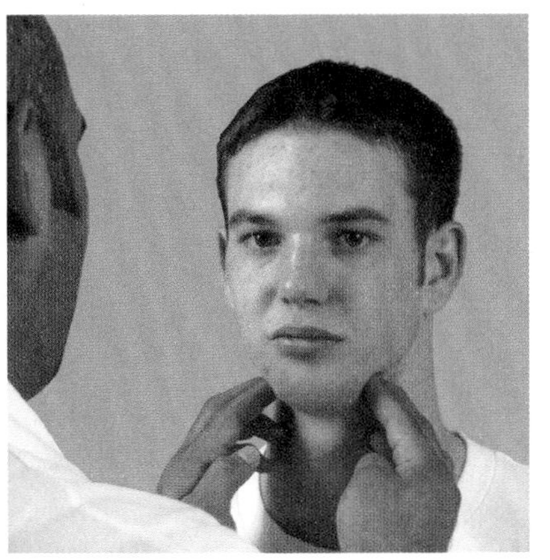

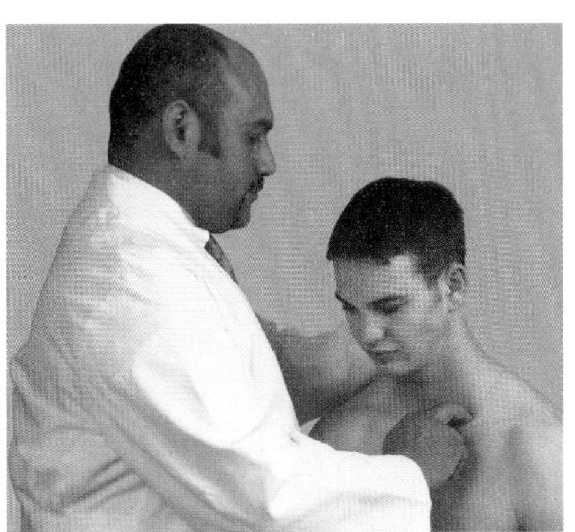

Enlarged or tender nodes, if unexplained, call for (1) reexamination of the regions they drain, and (2) careful assessment of lymph nodes elsewhere so that you can distinguish between regional and generalized lymphadenopathy.

Occasionally you may mistake a band of muscle or an artery for a lymph node. You should be able to roll a node in two directions: up and down, and side to side. Neither a muscle nor an artery will pass this test.

Diffuse lymphadenopathy raises the suspicion of HIV or AIDS.

The Trachea and the Thyroid Gland. To orient yourself to the neck, identify the thyroid and cricoid cartilages and the trachea below them.

- *Inspect the trachea* for any deviation from its usual midline position. Then *feel for any deviation.* Place your finger along one side of the trachea and note the space between it and the sternomastoid. Compare it with the other side. The spaces should be symmetric.

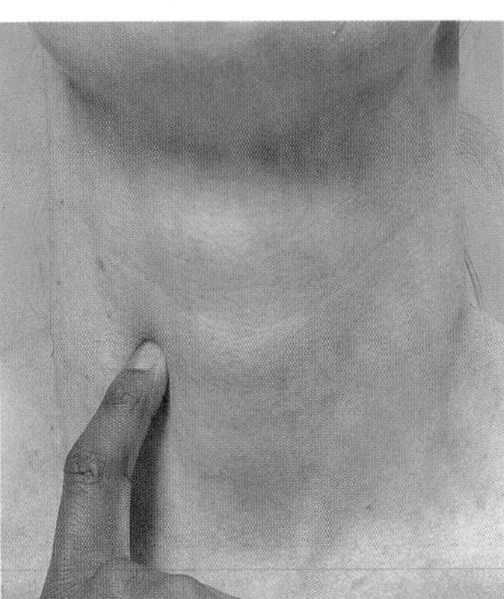

Masses in the neck may push the trachea to one side. Tracheal deviation may also signify important problems in the thorax, such as a mediastinal mass, atelectasis, or a large pneumothorax (see pp. 276–277).

- *Inspect the neck for the thyroid gland.* Tip the patient's head back a bit. Using tangential lighting directed downward from the tip of the patient's chin, *inspect the region below the cricoid cartilage* for the gland. The lower, shadowed border of each thyroid gland shown here is outlined by arrows.

The lower border of this large thyroid gland is outlined by tangential lighting. *Goiter* is a general term for an enlarged thyroid gland.[13,14]

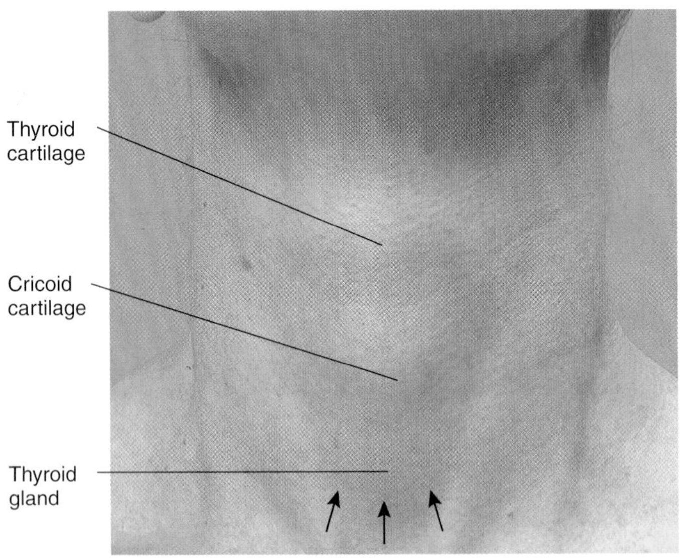

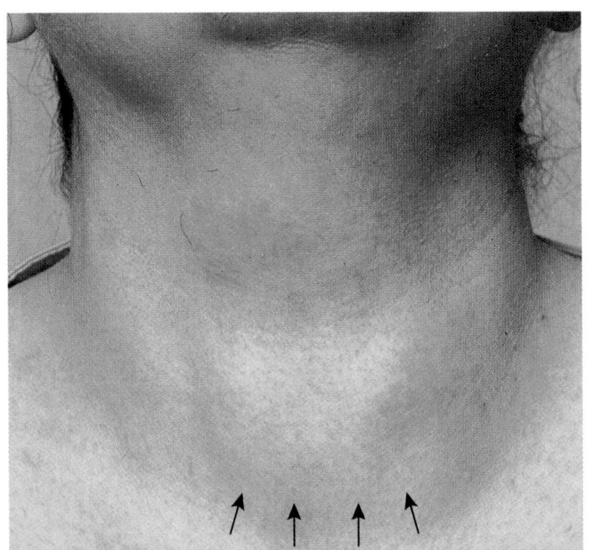

AT REST

Ask the patient to sip some water and to extend the neck again and swallow. Watch for upward movement of the thyroid gland, noting its contour and symmetry. The thyroid cartilage, the cricoid cartilage, and the thyroid gland all rise with swallowing and then fall to their resting positions.

With swallowing, the lower border of this large gland rises and looks less symmetric.

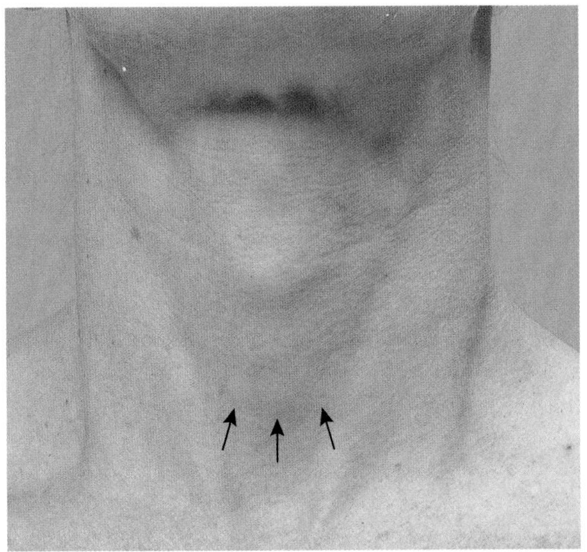

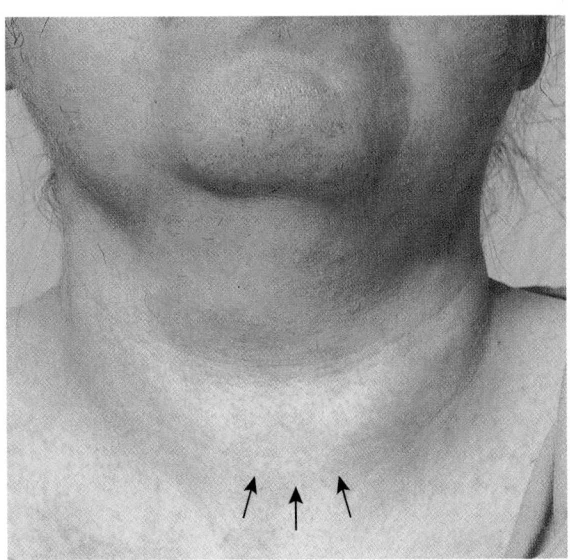

SWALLOWING

Until you become familiar with this examination, check your visual observations with your fingers from in front of the patient. This will orient you to the next step.

You are now ready to *palpate the thyroid gland*. This may seem difficult at first. Use the cues from visual inspection. Find your landmarks—the notched thyroid cartilage and the cricoid cartilage below it. Locate the *thyroid isthmus,* usually overlying the second, third, and fourth tracheal rings.

Adopt good technique, and follow the steps on the next page, which outline the posterior approach (technique for the anterior approach is similar). With experience you will become more adept. The thyroid gland is usually easier to feel in a long slender neck than in a short stocky one. In shorter necks, added extension of the neck may help. In some people, however, the thyroid gland is partially or wholly substernal and not amenable to physical examination.

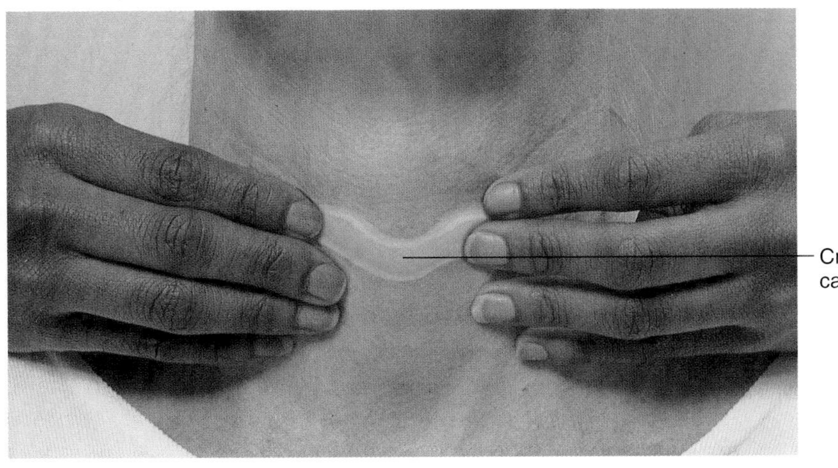

STEPS FOR PALPATING THE THYROID GLAND

- Ask the patient to flex the neck slightly forward to relax the sternomastoid muscles.
- Place the fingers of both hands on the patient's neck so that your index fingers are just below the cricoid cartilage.
- Ask the patient to sip and swallow water as before. Feel for the thyroid isthmus rising up under your finger pads. It is often but not always palpable.
- Displace the trachea to the right with the fingers of the left hand; with the right-hand fingers, palpate laterally for the right lobe of the thyroid in the space between the displaced trachea and the relaxed sternomastoid. Find the lateral margin. In similar fashion, examine the left lobe.

  The lobes are somewhat harder to feel than the isthmus, so practice is needed. The anterior surface of a lateral lobe is approximately the size of the distal phalanx of the thumb and feels somewhat rubbery.
- Note the *size, shape,* and *consistency* of the gland and identify any *nodules* or *tenderness.*

If the thyroid gland is enlarged, listen over the lateral lobes with a stethoscope to detect a *bruit,* a sound similar to a cardiac murmur but of noncardiac origin.

Although physical characteristics of the thyroid gland, such as size, shape, and consistency, are diagnostically important, assessment of thyroid function depends upon symptoms, signs elsewhere in the body, and laboratory tests.[15,16] See Table 6-24, Thyroid Enlargement and Function (p. 239).

Soft in Graves' disease; firm in Hashimoto's thyroiditis, malignancy. Benign and malignant nodules,[17] tenderness in thyroiditis

A localized systolic or continuous bruit may be heard in hyperthyroidism.

The Carotid Arteries and Jugular Veins. Defer a detailed examination of these vessels until the patient lies down for the cardiovascular examination. Jugular venous distention, however, may be visible in the sitting position and should not be overlooked. You should also be alert to unusually prominent arterial pulsations. See Chapter 8 for further discussion.

Note: Many clinicians would complete examination of the cranial nerves (see pp. 611–616) at this point.

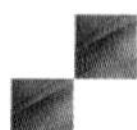

SPECIAL TECHNIQUES

For Assessing Protruding Eyes (Proptosis or Exophthalmos). For eyes that seem unusually prominent, stand behind the seated patient and inspect from above. Draw the upper lids gently upward, then compare the protrusion of the eyes and the relationship of the corneas to the lower lids. For objective measurement, use an exophthalmometer. This instrument measures the distance between the lateral angle of the orbit and an imaginary line across the most anterior point of the cornea. The upper limits of normal are 20 mm in whites and 22 mm in blacks.[18,19]

Exophthalmos is an abnormal protrusion of the eye.

When protrusion exceeds normal, further evaluation by ultrasound or computerized tomography scan often follows.[20]

For Nasolacrimal Duct Obstruction. This test helps identify the cause of excessive tearing. Ask the patient to look up. Press on the lower lid close to the medial canthus, just inside the rim of the bony orbit—this compresses the lacrimal sac. Look for fluid regurgitated out of the puncta into the eye. Avoid this test if the area is inflamed and tender.

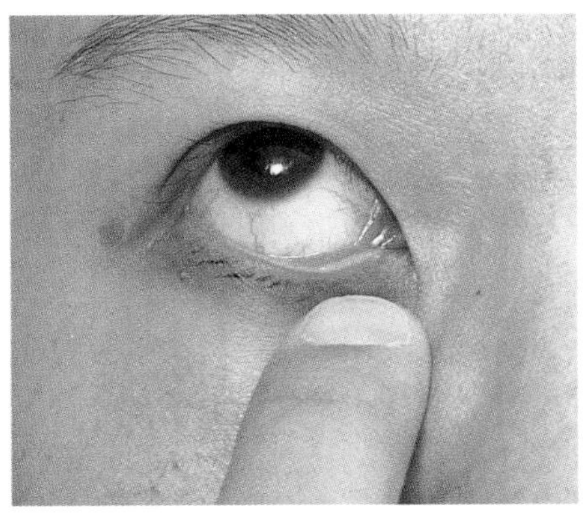

Discharge of mucopurulent fluid from the puncta suggests an obstructed nasolacrimal duct.

For Inspection of the Upper Palpebral Conjunctiva. Adequate examination of the eye in search of a foreign body requires eversion of the upper eyelid. Follow these steps:

- Instruct the patient to look down. Get the patient to relax the eyes—by reassurance and by gentle, assured, and deliberate movements. Raise the upper eyelid slightly so that the eyelashes protrude, and then grasp the upper eyelashes and pull them gently down and forward.

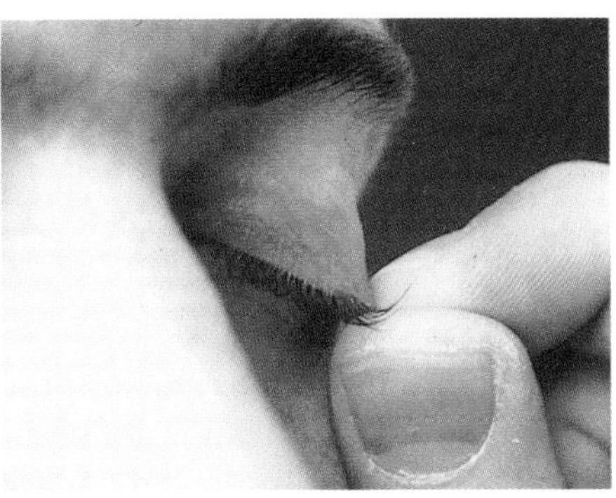

- Place a small stick such as an applicator or a tongue blade at least 1 cm above the lid margin (and therefore at the upper border of the tarsal plate). Push down on the stick as you raise the edge of the lid, thus everting the eyelid or turning it "inside out." Do not press on the eyeball itself.

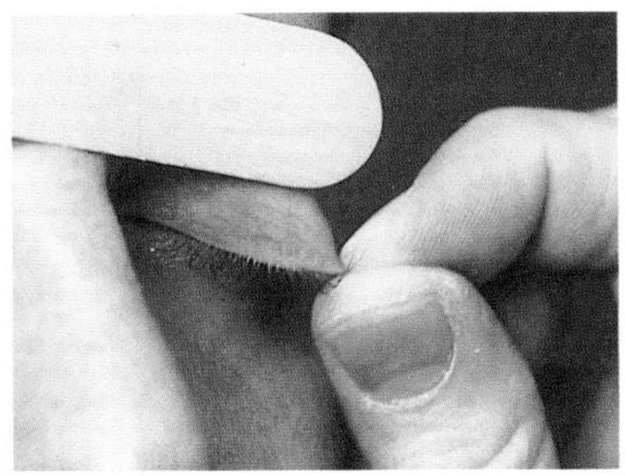

- Secure the upper lashes against the eyebrow with your thumb and inspect the palpebral conjunctiva. After your inspection, grasp the upper eyelashes and pull them gently forward. Ask the patient to look up. The eyelid will return to its normal position.

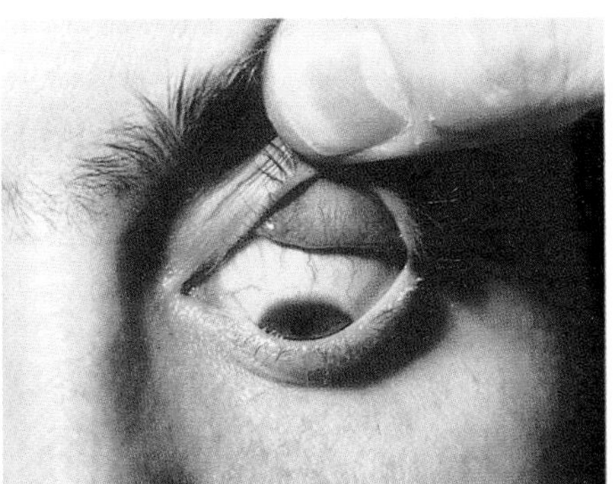

This view allows you to see the upper palpebral conjunctiva and look for a foreign body that might be lodged there.

Swinging Flashlight Test. The swinging flashlight test is a clinical test for functional impairment in the optic nerves. In dim light, note the size of the pupils. After asking the patient to gaze into the distance, swing the beam of a penlight first into one pupil, then into the other. Normally, each illuminated eye looks or promptly becomes constricted. The opposite eye also constricts consensually.

When the optic nerve is damaged, as in the left eye below, the sensory or afferent stimulus sent to the brainstem is reduced. The pupil dilates instead of constricting when the light moves from the good right eye into the left eye. This response is an *afferent pupillary defect,* sometimes termed a *Marcus Gunn pupil.* The opposite eye responds consensually.

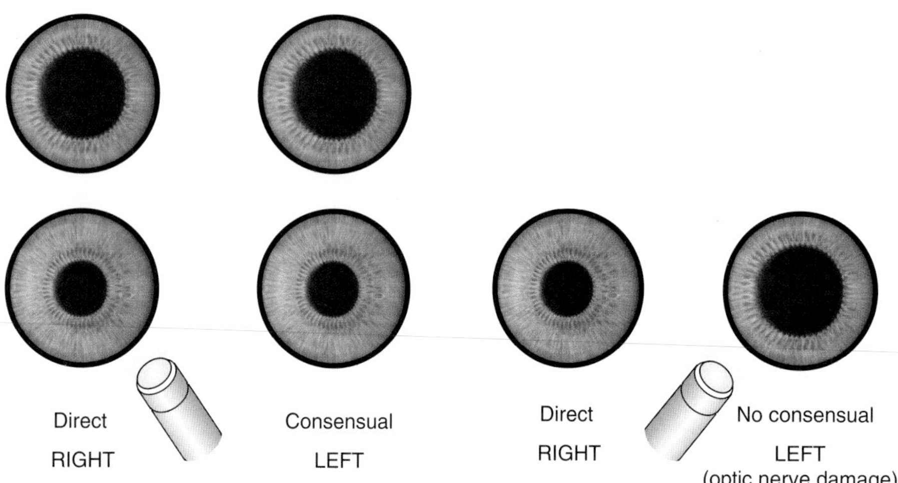

Transillumination of the Sinuses. When sinus tenderness or other symptoms suggest sinusitis, this test can at times be helpful but is not highly sensitive or specific for diagnosis. The room should be thoroughly darkened. Using a strong, narrow light source, place the light snugly deep under each brow, close to the nose. Shield the light with your hand. Look for a dim red glow as light is transmitted through the air-filled frontal sinus to the forehead.

Absence of glow on one or both sides suggests a thickened mucosa or secretions in the frontal sinus, but it may also result from developmental absence of one or both sinuses.

Ask the patient to tilt his or her head back with mouth opened wide. (An upper denture should first be removed.) Shine the light downward from just below the inner aspect of each eye. Look through the open mouth at the hard palate. A reddish glow indicates a normal air-filled maxillary sinus.

Absence of glow suggests thickened mucosa or secretions in the maxillary sinus. See p. 756 for an alternative method of transilluminating the maxillary sinuses.

RECORDING YOUR FINDINGS

Note that initially you may use sentences to describe your findings; later you will use phrases. The style below contains phrases appropriate for most write-ups.

Recording the Physical Examination— The Head, Eyes, Ears, Nose, and Throat (HEENT)

HEENT: Head—The skull is normocephalic/atraumatic (NC/AT). Hair with average texture. *Eyes*—Visual acuity 20/20 bilaterally. Sclera white, conjunctiva pink. Pupils are 4 mm constricting to 2 mm, equally round and reactive to light and accommodations. Disc margins sharp; no hemorrhages or exudates, no arteriolar narrowing. *Ears*—Acuity good to whispered voice. Tympanic membranes (TMs) with good cone of light. Weber midline. AC > BC. *Nose*—Nasal mucosa pink, septum midline; no sinus tenderness. *Throat (or Mouth)*—Oral mucosa pink, dentition good, pharynx without exudates.

Neck—Trachea midline. Neck supple; thyroid isthmus palpable, lobes not felt.

Lymph Nodes—No cervical, axillary, epitrochlear, inguinal adenopathy.

OR

Head—The skull is normocephalic/atraumatic. Frontal balding. *Eyes*—Visual acuity 20/100 bilaterally. Sclera white; conjunctiva injected. Pupils constrict 3 mm to 2 mm, equally round and reactive to light and accommodation. Disc margins sharp; no hemorrhages or exudates. Arteriolar-to-venous ratio (AV ratio) 2:4; no A-V nicking. *Ears*—Acuity diminished to whispered voice; intact to spoken voice. TMs clear. *Nose*—Mucosa swollen with erythema and clear drainage. Septum midline. Tender over maxillary sinuses. *Throat*—Oral mucosa pink, dental caries in lower molars, pharynx erythematous, no exudates.

Neck—Trachea midline. Neck supple; thyroid isthmus midline, lobes palpable but not enlarged.

Lymph Nodes—Submandibular and anterior cervical lymph nodes tender, 1 × 1 cm, rubbery and mobile; no posterior cervical, epitrochlear, axillary, or inguinal lymphadenopathy.

Suggests myopia and mild arteriolar narrowing. Also upper respiratory infection.

Bibliography

CITATIONS

1. Goadsby PJ, Lipton RB, Ferrari MD. Migraine: current understanding and treatment. N Engl J Med 346(4):257–270, 2002.
2. Shingleton BJ, O'Donoghue MW. Blurred vision. N Engl J Med 343(8):556–562, 2000.
3. Fine SL, Berger JW, Macguire MG, et al. Age-related macular degeneration. N Engl J Med 342(7):483–492, 2000.
4. Coleman AC. Glaucoma. Lancet 20:1803–1810, 1999.
5. Piccirillo JF. Acute bacterial sinusitis. N Engl J Med 351(9): 902–910, 2004.
6. Spector SL, Bernstein IL, Li JT, et al. Parameters for the diagnosis and management of sinusitis. J Allergy Clin Immunol 102(6, part 2):S107–S144, 1998.
7. Williams JW, Simel DL, Roberts L, et al. Clinical evaluation for sinusitis: making the diagnosis by history and physical examination. Ann Intern Med 117:705–710, 1992.
8. U.S. Preventive Services Task Force. Screening for visual impairment. In Guide to Clinical Preventive Services, 2nd ed, pp. 373–382. Baltimore, Williams & Wilkins, 1996.
9. U.S. Preventive Services Task Force. Screening for glaucoma. In Guide to Clinical Preventive Services, 2nd ed., pp. 383–391. Baltimore, Williams & Wilkins, 1996.
10. U.S. Preventive Services Task Force. Screening for hearing impairment. In Guide to Clinical Preventive Services, 2nd ed., pp. 393–405. Baltimore, Williams & Wilkins, 1996.
11. U.S. Preventive Services Task Force. Counseling to prevent dental and periodontal disease. In Guide to Clinical Preventive Services, 2nd ed., pp. 711–721. Baltimore, Williams & Wilkins, 1996.
12. Greene JC, Greene AR. Oral health. In Woolf SH, Jonas S, Lawrence RS (eds). Health Promotion and Disease Prevention in Clinical Practice, pp. 315–334. Baltimore, Williams & Wilkins, 1996.
13. McGuirt WF. The neck mass. Med Clin N Am 83:219–234, 1989.
14. Siminoski K. Does this patient have a goiter? JAMA 273(10): 813–817, 1995.
15. U.S. Preventive Services Task Force. Screening for thyroid disease: recommendation statement. Ann Intern Med 140(2): 125–127, 2004.
16. Surks MI, Ortiz E, Daniels GH, et al. Subclinical thyroid disease: scientific review and guidelines for diagnosis and management. JAMA 291(2):228–238, 2004.
17. Hegedus L. The thyroid nodule. N Engl J Med 351(17): 1764–1771, 2004.
18. Gladstone GJ. Ophthalmologic aspects of thyroid-related orbitopathy. Endocrinol Metab Clin North Am 27:91–100, 1998.
19. Bartley GB, et al. Clinical features of Graves' ophthalmopathy in an incidence cohort. Am J Ophthalmol 121:284–290, 1996.
20. Hallin ES, Feldon SE. Graves' ophthalmopathy. II. Correlation of clinical signs with measures derived from computed tomography. Br J Ophthalmol 72:678–682, 1988.
21. Headache Classification Subcommittee of the International Headache Society. The international headache classification. Cephalalgia 24(Suppl 1):1–160, 2004.
22. Rollnik JD, Karst M, Fink M, et al. Botulinum toxin type A and EMG: a key to the understanding of chronic tension-type headaches? Headache 41(10):985–989, 2001.
23. Smetana GW, Shmerling RH. Does this patient have temporal arteritis? JAMA 287(1):92–101, 2002.
24. Haas DC. Chronic post-traumatic headaches classified and compared with natural headaches. Cephalalgia 16(7):486–493, 1996.
25. Kroenke K, Lucas CA, Rosengerg ML, et al. Causes of persistent dizziness: a prospective study of 100 patients in ambulatory care. Ann Intern Med 117(11):898–904, 1992.
26. Kroenke K, Hoffman RM, Einstadter D. How common are various causes of dizziness? A critical review. South Med J 93(2):160–167, quiz 168, 2000.
27. Tusa RJ. Vertigo. Neurol Clin 19(1):23–55, 2001.
28. Branch W. Approach to the patient with dizziness. Available at: www.utdol.com. Accessed February 26, 2005.
29. Lockwood AH, Salvi RJ, Burkard RF. Tinnitus. N Engl J Med 347(12):904–910, 2002.
30. Matthies C, Samii M. Management of 1000 vestibular schwannomas (acoustic neuromas): clinical presentation. Neurosurgery 1:1–10, 1997.
31. Leibowitz HM. The red eye. N Engl J Med 342(5):345–351, 2000.
32. Wong TY, Mitchell P. Hypertensive retinopathy. N Engl J Med 351(22):2310–2317, 2004.

ADDITIONAL REFERENCES

Bahra A, May A. Cluster headache: a prospective clinical study with diagnostic implications. Neurology 58(3):354–361, 2002.

The Eye

Albert DM, Jakobiec FA. Principles and Practice of Ophthalmology, 2nd ed. Philadelphia, WB Saunders, 2000.

Congdon N, O'Colmain, Klaver CC, et al. Causes and prevalence of visual impairment among adults in the United States. Arch Ophthalmol 122(4):477–485, 2004.

Fong DS, Aiello LP, Ferris FL, et al. Diabetic retinopathy. Diabetes Care 27(10):2540–2553, 2004.

Gold DH, Weingeist TA. Color Atlas of the Eye in Systemic Disease. Philadelphia, Lippincott Williams & Wilkins, 2001.

McCluskey PJ, Towler HM, Lightman S. Management of chronic uveitis. BMJ 320(7234):555–558, 2000.

Ostler HB, Maibach HI, Hoke AW, Schwab IR. Diseases of the Eye and Skin. A Color Atlas. Philadelphia, Lippincott Williams & Wilkins, 2004.

Sheilds SR. Managing eye disease in primary care. Part 1. How to screen for occult disease. Postgrad Med 108(5):69–72, 75–78, 2000.

Spoor TC (ed). Atlas of Neuro-ophthalmology. New York, Taylor & Francis, 2004.

Tasman W, Jaeger EA. The Wills Eye Hospital Atlas of Clinical Ophthalmology, 2nd ed. Philadelphia, Lippincott Williams & Wilkins, 2001.

Yanoff M, Duker JS. Ophthalmology, 2nd ed. St. Louis, Mosby, 2004.

BIBLIOGRAPHY

The Ears, Nose, and Throat

Bevan Y, Shapiro N, MacLean CH, et al. Screening and management of adult hearing loss in primary care: scientific review. JAMA 289(15):1976–1985, 2003.

Bull TR. Color Atlas of ENT Diagnosis, 4th ed. New York, Thieme, 2003.

Doty RL (ed). Handbook of Olfaction and Gustation, 2nd ed. (Neurological Disease and Therapy, Vol 57). New York, Marcel Dekker, 2003.

Ebell MH, Smith MA, Barry HC, et al. Does this patient have strep throat? JAMA 284(22):2912–2918, 2000.

Hendley JO. Otitis media. N Engl J Med 347(15):1169–1174, 2002.

Kennedy DW. A 48-year-old man with recurrent sinusitis. JAMA 283(16):2143–2150, 2000.

O'Donoghue GM, Narula AA, Bates GJ. Clinical ENT: An Illustrated Textbook, 2nd ed. San Diego, Singular Pub Group, 2000.

Young T, Skatrud J, Peppard PE. Risk factors for obstructive sleep apnea in adults. JAMA 291(16):2013–2016, 2004.

The Mouth

Eisen D, Lynch DP. The Mouth: Diagnosis and Treatment. St. Louis, Mosby, 1998.

Field EA, Longman L, Tyldesley WR, et al. Tyldesley's Oral Medicine, 5th ed. New York, Oxford University Press, 2003.

Langlais RP, Miller CS. Color Atlas of Common Oral Diseases, 3rd ed. Philadelphia, Lippincott Williams & Wilkins, 2003.

Neville BW, Damm DD, White DK. Color Atlas of Clinical Oral Pathology, 2nd ed. Baltimore, Williams & Wilkins, 1999.

Newman MF, Carranza FA, Takei H. Carranza's Clinical Periodontology, 9th ed. Philadelphia, WB Saunders, 2002.

Regezi JA, Sciubba JJ, Jordan RCK. Oral Pathology: Clinical Pathologic Correlations, 4th ed. St. Louis, WB Saunders, 2003.

The Neck

Bliss SJ, Flanders SA, Saint S. A pain in the neck. N Engl J Med 350(10):1037–1042, 2004.

Henry PH, Long DL. Enlargement of the lymph nodes and spleen. In Kasper DL, Fauci AS, Longo DL, et al (eds). Harrison's Principles of Internal Medicine, 16th ed. New York, McGraw-Hill, 2005.

Prisco MK. Evaluating neck masses. Nurse Pract 25(4):30–32, 35–36, 38, 2000.

Schwetschenau E, Kelley DJ. The adult neck mass. Am Fam Physician 67(6):1190, 1192, 1195, 2003.

TABLE 6-1 Headaches[21]

Type	Process	Location	Quality and Severity
Primary Headaches			
Tension	Unclear—muscle contraction or vasoconstriction unlikely[22]	Usually bilateral; may be generalized or localized to the back of the head and upper neck or to the frontotemporal area	Pressing or tightening pain; mild to moderate intensity
Migraines ▪ With aura ▪ Without aura ▪ Variants	Primary neuronal dysfunction, possibly of brainstem origin, causing imbalance of excitatory and inhibitory neurotransmitters and affecting craniovascular modulation[1]	Unilateral in ~70%; bifrontal or global in ~30%	Throbbing or aching, variable in severity
Cluster	Unclear—possibly extracranial vasodilation from neural dysfunction with trigeminovascular pain	Unilateral, usually behind or around the eye	Deep, continuous, severe
Secondary Headaches			
Analgesic Rebound	Withdrawal of medication	Previous headache pattern	Variable
Headaches From Eye Disorders			
Errors of Refraction (farsightedness and astigmatism, but not nearsightedness)	Probably the sustained contraction of the extraocular muscles, and possibly of the frontal, temporal, and occipital muscles	Around and over the eyes, may radiate to the occipital area	Steady, aching, dull
Acute Glaucoma	Sudden increase in intraocular pressure (see p. 181)	In and around one eye	Steady, aching, often severe
Headache From Sinusitis	Mucosal inflammation of the paranasal sinuses	Usually above the eye (frontal sinus) or over the maxillary sinus	Aching or throbbing, variable in severity; consider possible migraine
Meningitis	Infection of the meninges surrounding the brain	Generalized	Steady or throbbing, very severe

Timing			Associated Factors	Factors That Aggravate or Provoke	Factors That Relieve
Onset	*Duration*	*Course*			
Gradual	Minutes to days	Often recurrent or persistent over long periods; annual prevalence ~40%	Sometimes photophobia, phonophobia; nausea absent	Sustained muscle tension, as in driving or typing	Possible massage, relaxation
Fairly rapid, reaching a peak in 1–2 hours	4–72 hours	Peak incidence early to mid-adolescence; prevalence is ~6% in men and ~15% in women. Recurrent—usually monthly but weekly in ~10%	Nausea, vomiting, photophobia, phonophobia, visual auras (flickering zig-zagging lines), motor auras affecting hand or arm, sensory auras (numbness, tingling usually precede headache)	May be provoked by alcohol, certain foods, or tension. More common premenstrually. Aggravated by noise and bright light.	Quiet, dark room; sleep; sometimes transient relief from pressure on the involved artery, if early in the course
Abrupt, peaks within minutes	Up to 3 hours	Episodic, clustered in time with several each day for 4–8 weeks and then relief for 6–12 months; prevalence <1%, more common in men	Lacrimation, rhinorrhea, miosis, ptosis, eyelid edema, conjunctival infection	During attack, sensitivity to alcohol may increase	
Variable	Depends on prior headache pattern	Depends on frequency of "mini-withdrawals"	Depends on prior headache pattern	Fever, carbon monoxide, hypoxia, withdrawal of caffeine, other headache triggers	Depends on cause
Gradual	Variable	Variable	Eye fatigue, "sandy" sensations in the eyes, redness of the conjunctiva	Prolonged use of the eyes, particularly for close work	Rest of the eyes
Often rapid	Variable, may depend on treatment	Variable, may depend on treatment	Diminished vision, sometimes nausea and vomiting	Sometimes provoked by drops that dilate the pupils	
Variable	Often several hours at a time, recurring over days or longer	Often recurrent in a repetitive daily pattern	Local tenderness, nasal congestion, discharge, and fever	May be aggravated by coughing, sneezing, or jarring the head	Nasal decongestants, antibiotics
Fairly rapid	Variable, usually days	A persistent headache in an acute illness	Fever, stiff neck		

(table continues next page)

TABLE 6-1 Headaches[21] *(Continued)*

Type	Process	Location	Quality and Severity
Giant Cell (Temporal) Arteritis[23]	Vasculitis from cell-mediated immune response to elastic lamina of artery	Localized near the involved artery, most often the temporal, also the occipital; age related	Throbbing, generalized, persistent; often severe
Posttraumatic Headache	Mechanism unclear; episodes similar to tension-type and migraine without aura headaches[24]	May be localized to the injured area, but not necessarily	Generalized, dull, aching, constant
Subarachnoid Hemorrhage	Bleeding, most often from a ruptured intracranial aneurysm	Generalized	Very severe, "the worst of my life"
Brain Tumor	Displacement of or traction on pain-sensitive arteries and veins or pressure on nerves	Varies with the location of the tumor	Aching, steady, variable in intensity
Cranial Neuralgias			
Trigeminal Neuralgia (CNV)	Compression of CN V, often by aberrant loop or artery of vein	Cheek, jaws, lips, or gums; trigeminal nerve divisions 2 and 3 > 1	Shocklike, stabbing, burning; severe

Note: Blanks appear in these tables when the categories are not applicable or not usually helpful in assessing the problem.

Timing			Associated Factors	Factors That Aggravate or Provoke	Factors That Relieve
Onset	*Duration*	*Course*			
Gradual or rapid	Variable	Recurrent or persistent over weeks to months	Tenderness of the adjacent scalp; fever (in ~50%), fatigue, weight loss; new headache (~60%), jaw claudication (~50%), visual loss or blindness (~15%–20%), polymyalgia rheumatica (~50%)	Movement of neck and shoulders	
Within hours to 1–2 days of the injury	Weeks, months, or even years	Tends to diminish over time	Poor concentration, problems with memory, vertigo, irritability, restlessness, fatigue	Mental and physical exertion, straining, stooping, emotional excitement, alcohol	Rest
Usually abrupt, severe; prodromal symptoms may occur	Variable, usually days	A persistent headache in an acute illness	Nausea, vomiting, possibly loss of consciousness, neck pain		
Variable	Often brief	Often intermittent but progressive	May be aggravated by coughing, sneezing, or sudden movements of the head		
Abrupt, paroxysmal	Each jab lasts seconds but recurs at intervals of seconds or minutes	May last for months, then disappear for months, but often recurs. It is uncommon at night.	Exhaustion from recurrent pain	Touching certain areas of the lower face or mouth; chewing, talking, brushing teeth	

TABLE 6-2 Dizziness and Vertigo

"Dizziness" is a nonspecific term used by patients encompassing several disorders that clinicians must carefully sort out. A detailed history usually identifies the primary etiology.[25–30] It is important to learn the specific meanings of the following terms or conditions:

- *Vertigo*—a spinning sensation accompanied by nystagmus and ataxia; usually from *peripheral vestibular dysfunction* (~40% of "dizzy" patients) but may be from a *central brainstem lesion* (~10%; causes include atherosclerosis, multiple sclerosis, vertebrobasilar migraine, or TIA)
- *Presyncope*—a near faint from "feeling faint or lightheaded"; causes include orthostatic hypotension, especially from medication, arrhythmias, and vasovagal attacks (~5%)
- *Dysequilibrium*—unsteadiness or imbalance when walking, especially in older patients (see p. 858); causes include fear of walking, visual loss, weakness from musculoskeletal problems, and peripheral neuropathy (up to 15%)
- *Psychiatric*—causes include anxiety, panic disorder, hyperventilation, depression, somatization disorder, alcohol, and substance abuse (~10%)
- *Multifactorial or unknown*—(up to 20%)

Peripheral and Central Vertigo

	Onset	*Duration and Course*	*Hearing*	*Tinnitus*	*Additional Features*
Peripheral Vertigo					
▪ *Benign Positional Vertigo*	Sudden, on rolling onto affected side or tilting head up	Onset a few seconds to <1 minute Lasts a few weeks, may recur	Not affected	Absent	Sometimes nausea, vomiting Nystagmus
▪ *Vestibular Neuronitis (acute labyrinthitis)*	Sudden	Onset hours to up to 2 weeks May recur over 12–18 months	Not affected	Absent	Nausea, vomiting, nystagmus
▪ *Ménière's Disease*	Sudden	Onset several hours to ≥1 day Recurrent	Sensorineural hearing loss—recurs, eventually progresses	Present, fluctuating	Pressure or fullness in affected ear; nausea, vomiting, nystagmus
▪ *Drug Toxicity*	Insidious or acute—linked to loop diuretics, aminoglycosides, salicylates, alcohol	May or may not be reversible Partial adaptation occurs	May be impaired	May be present	Nausea, vomiting
▪ *Acoustic Neuroma*	Insidious from CN VIII compression, vestibular branch	Variable	Impaired, one side	Present	May involve CN V and VII
Central Vertigo	Often sudden (see causes above)	Variable but rarely continuous	Not affected	Absent	Usually with other brainstem deficits—dysarthria, ataxia, crossed motor and sensory deficits

TABLE 6-3 Selected Facies

Facial Swelling

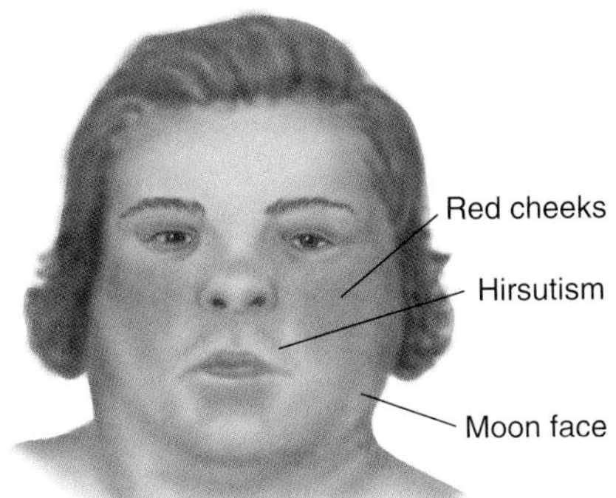

Cushing's Syndrome

The increased adrenal hormone production of Cushing's syndrome produces a round or "moon" face with red cheeks. Excessive hair growth may be present in the mustache and sideburn areas and on the chin.

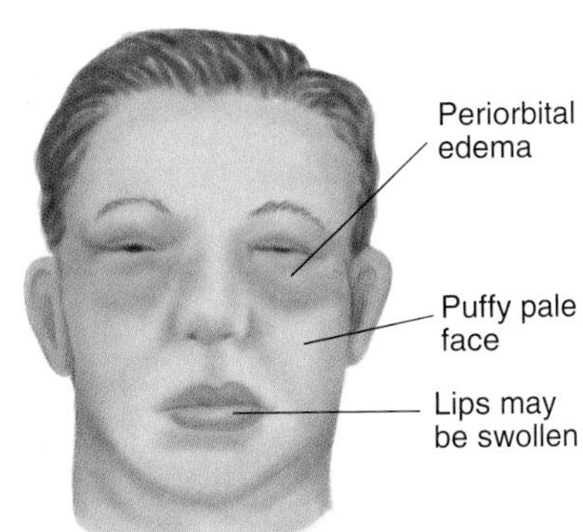

Nephrotic Syndrome

The face is edematous and often pale. Swelling usually appears first around the eyes and in the morning. The eyes may become slitlike when edema is severe.

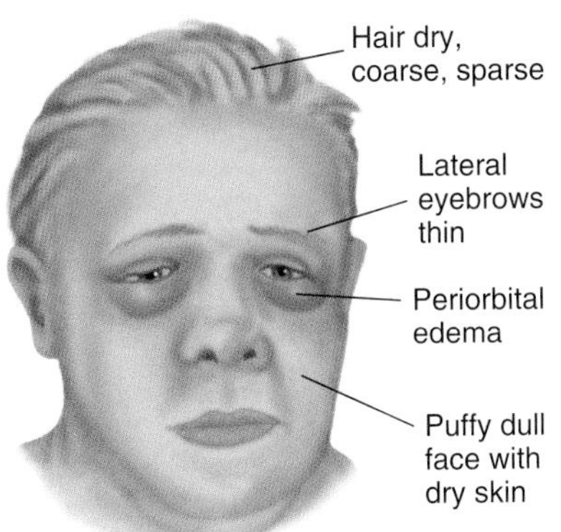

Myxedema

The patient with severe hypothyroidism (*myxedema*) has a dull, puffy facies. The edema, often particularly pronounced around the eyes, does not pit with pressure. The hair and eyebrows are dry, coarse, and thinned. The skin is dry.

Other Facies

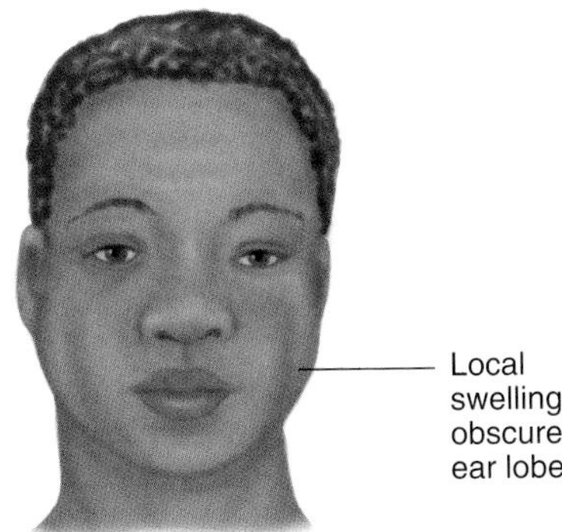

Parotid Gland Enlargement

Chronic bilateral asymptomatic parotid gland enlargement may be associated with obesity, diabetes, cirrhosis, and other conditions. Note the swellings anterior to the ear lobes and above the angles of the jaw. Gradual unilateral enlargement suggests neoplasm. Acute enlargement is seen in mumps.

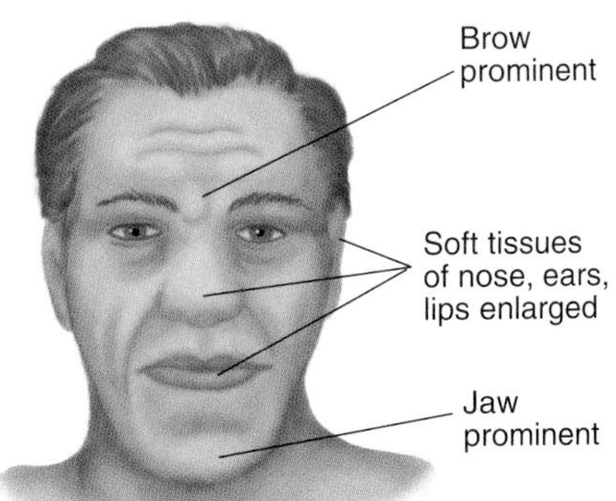

Acromegaly

The increased growth hormone of acromegaly produces enlargement of both bone and soft tissues. The head is elongated, with bony prominence of the forehead, nose, and lower jaw. Soft tissues of the nose, lips, and ears also enlarge. The facial features appear generally coarsened.

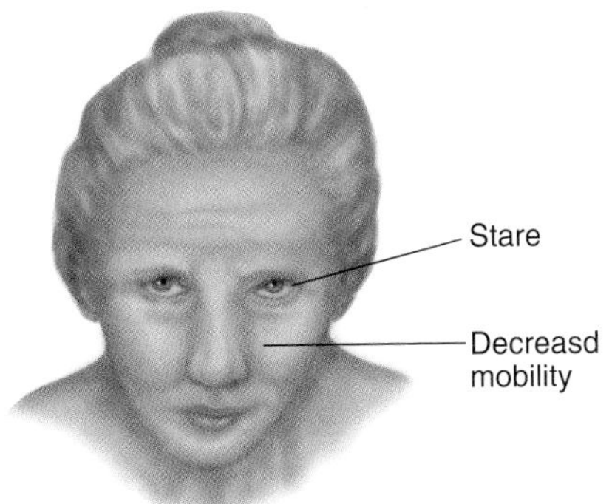

Parkinson's Disease

Decreased facial mobility blunts expression. A masklike face may result, with decreased blinking and a characteristic stare. Since the neck and upper trunk tend to flex forward, the patient seems to peer upward toward the observer. Facial skin becomes oily, and drooling may occur.

Visual Field Defects

1 Horizontal Defect Occlusion of a branch of the central retinal artery may cause a horizontal (altitudinal) defect. Shown is the lower field defect associated with occlusion of the superior branch of this artery.

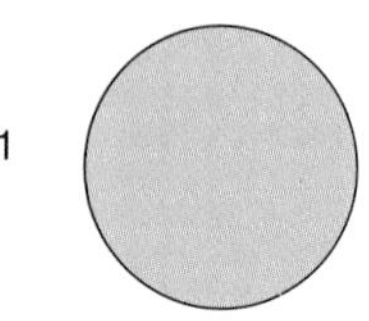

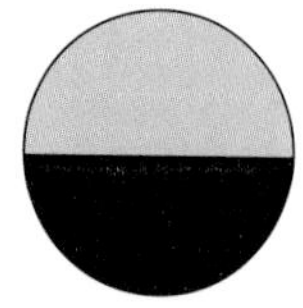

2 Blind Right Eye (right optic nerve) A lesion of the optic nerve, and of course of the eye itself, produces unilateral blindness.

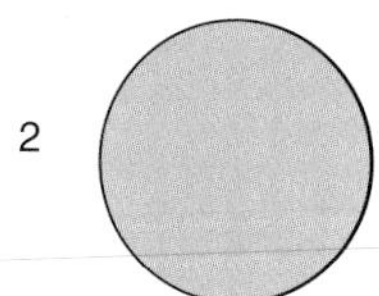

3 Bitemporal Hemianopsia (optic chiasm) A lesion at the optic chiasm may involve only fibers crossing over to the opposite side. Since these fibers originate in the nasal half of each retina, visual loss involves the temporal half of each field.

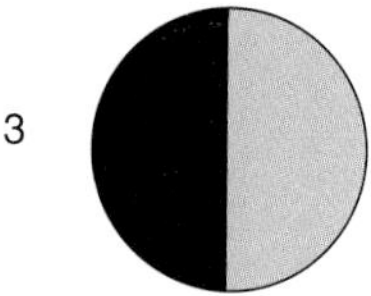

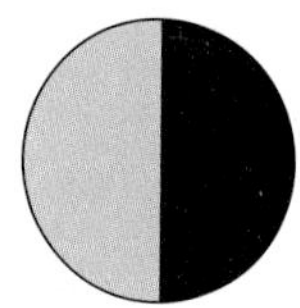

4 Left Homonymous Hemianopsia (right optic tract) A lesion of the optic tract interrupts fibers originating on the same side of both eyes. Visual loss in the eyes is therefore similar (homonymous) and involves half of each field (hemianopsia).

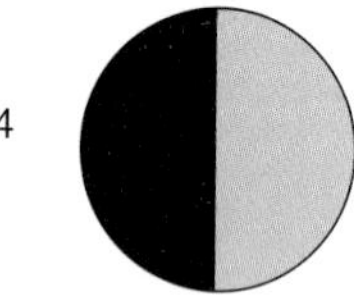

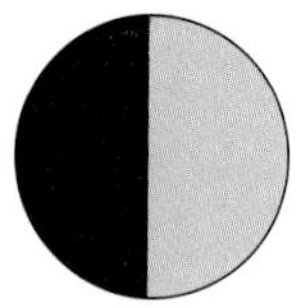

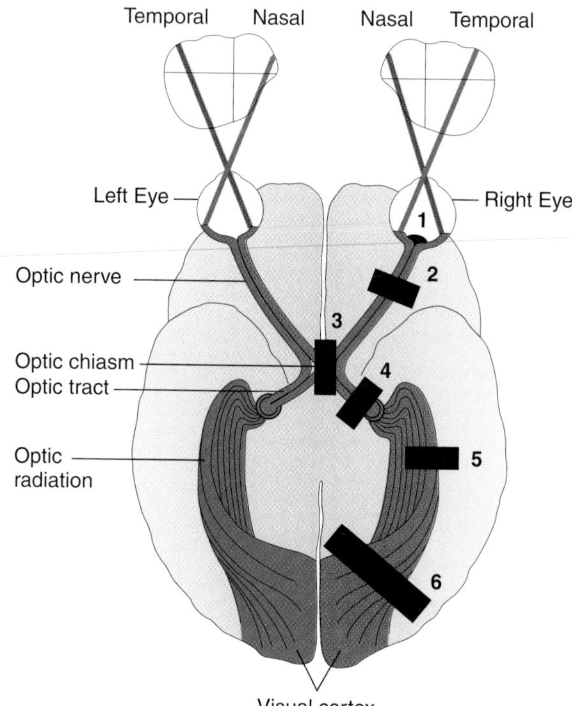

5 Homonymous Left Superior Quadrantic Defect (right optic radiation, partial) A partial lesion of the optic radiation in the temporal lobe may involve only a portion of the nerve fibers, producing, for example, a homonymous quadrantic defect.

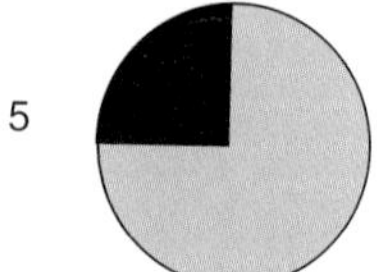

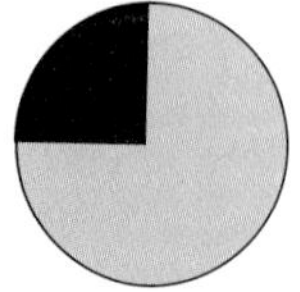

6 Left Homonymous Hemianopsia (right optic radiation) A complete interruption of fibers in the optic radiation produces a visual defect similar to that produced by a lesion of the optic tract.

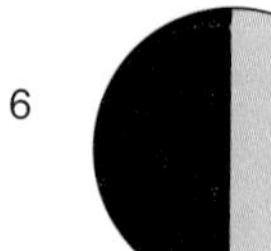

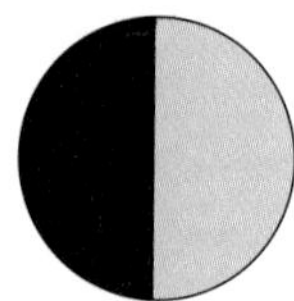

TABLE 6-5 Variations and Abnormalities of the Eyelids

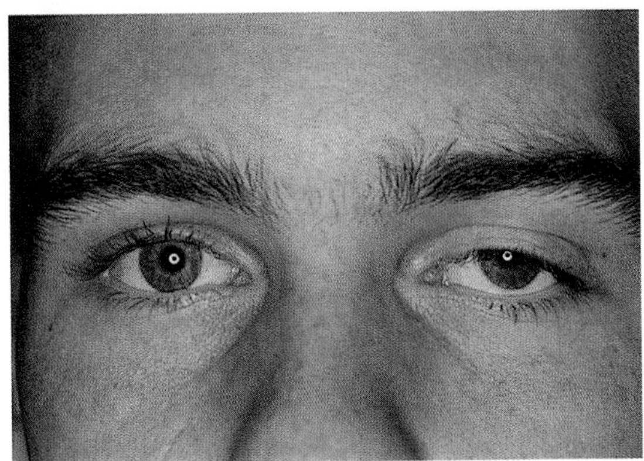

Ptosis

Ptosis is a drooping of the upper lid. Causes include myasthenia gravis, damage to the oculomotor nerve, and damage to the sympathetic nerve supply (*Horner's syndrome*). A weakened muscle, relaxed tissues, and the weight of herniated fat may cause senile ptosis. Ptosis may also be congenital.

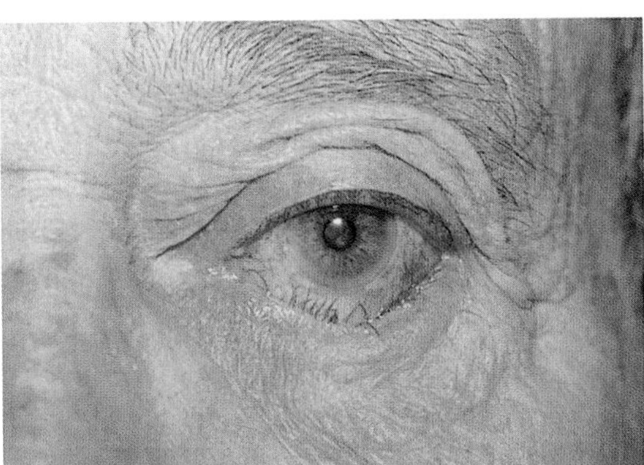

Entropion

Entropion, more common in the elderly, is an inward turning of the lid margin. The lower lashes, which are often invisible when turned inward, irritate the conjunctiva and lower cornea. Asking the patient to squeeze the lids together and then open them may reveal an entropion that is not obvious.

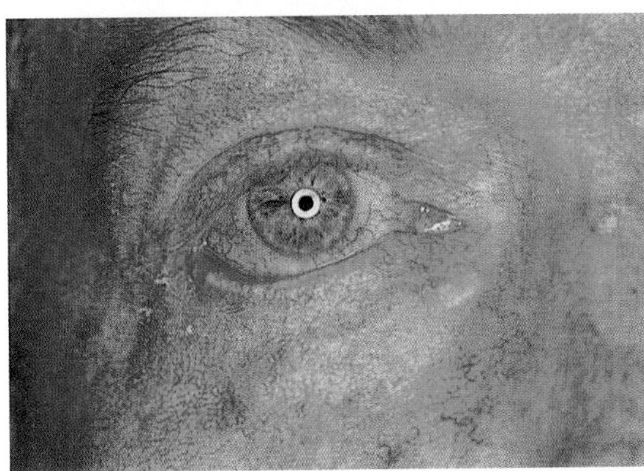

Ectropion

In ectropion the margin of the lower lid is turned outward, exposing the palpebral conjunctiva. When the punctum of the lower lid turns outward, the eye no longer drains satisfactorily, and tearing occurs. Ectropion is more common in the elderly.

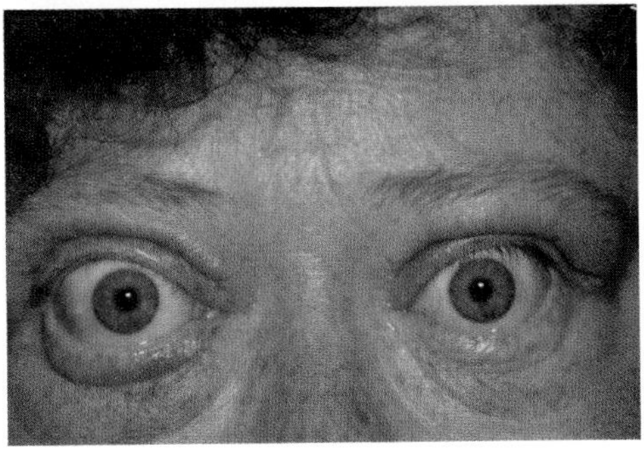

Lid Retraction and Exophthalmos

A wide-eyed stare suggests retracted eyelids. Note the rim of sclera between the upper lid and the iris. Retracted lids and a lid lag (p. 183) are often due to hyperthyroidism.

In exophthalmos the eyeball protrudes forward. When bilateral, it suggests the infiltrative ophthalmopathy of Graves' hyperthyroidism. Edema of the eyelids and conjunctival injection may be associated. Unilateral exophthalmos seen in Graves' disease or a tumor or inflammation in the orbit.

(Source of photos: *Ptosis, Ectropion, Entropion*—Tasman W, Jaeger E (eds). The Wills Eye Hospital Atlas of Clinical Ophthalmology, 2nd ed. Philadelphia, Lippincott Williams & Wilkins, 2001.)

TABLE 6-6 Lumps and Swellings in and Around the Eyes

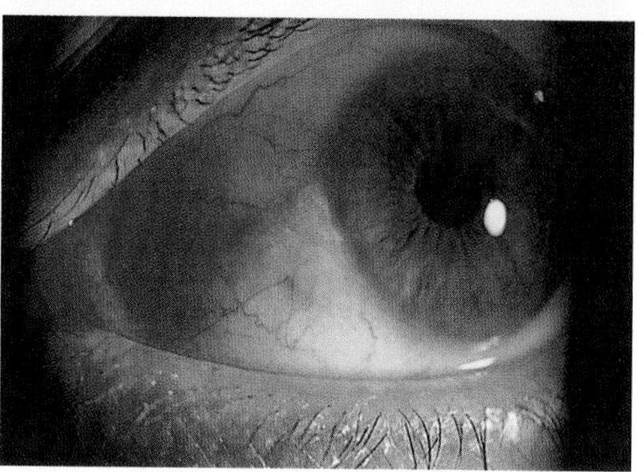

Pinguecula

A harmless yellowish triangular nodule in the bulbar conjunctiva on either side of the iris. Appears frequently with aging, first on the nasal and then on the temporal side.

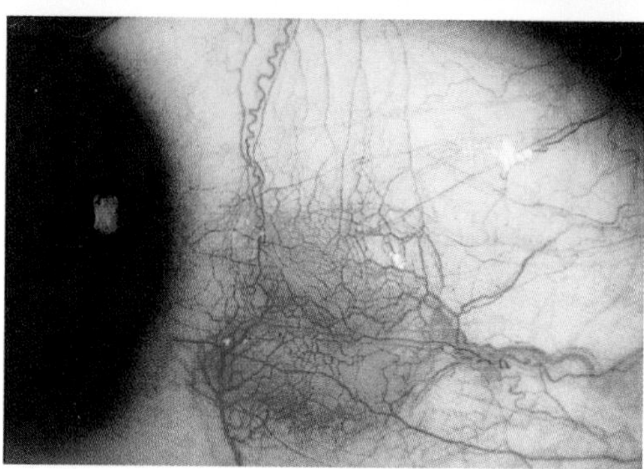

Episcleritis

A localized ocular redness from inflammation of the episcleral vessels. Vessels appear salmon pink and are movable over the scleral surface. May be nodular, as shown, or may show only redness and dilated vessels.

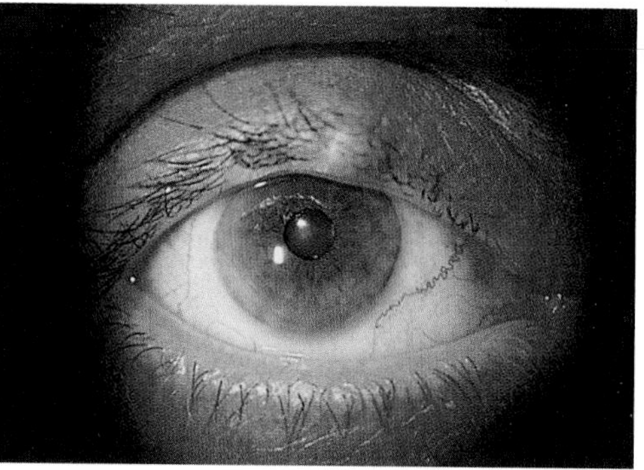

Sty

A painful, tender red infection in a gland at the margin of the eyelid.

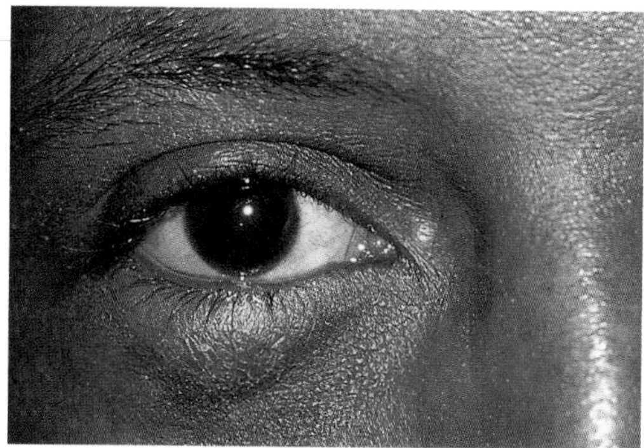

Chalazion

A subacute nontender and usually painless nodule involving a meibomian gland. May become acutely inflamed but, unlike a sty, usually points inside the lid rather than on the lid margin.

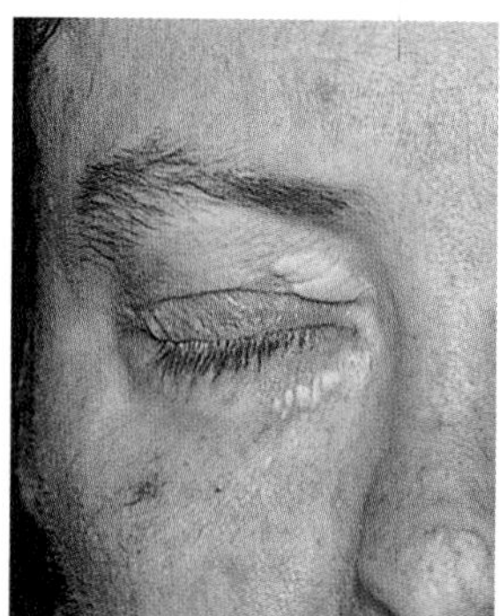

Xanthelasma

Slightly raised, yellowish, well-circumscribed plaques that appear along the nasal portions of one or both eyelids. May accompany lipid disorders.

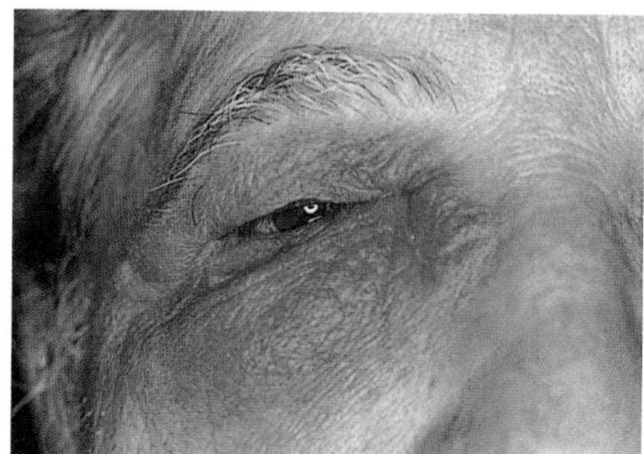

Inflammation of the Lacrimal Sac (Dacryocystitis)

A swelling between the lower eyelid and nose. An *acute* inflammation (illustrated) is painful, red, and tender. *Chronic* inflammation is associated with obstruction of the nasolacrimal duct. Tearing is prominent, and pressure on the sac produces regurgitation of material through the puncta of the eyelids.

(Source of photos: Tasman W, Jaeger E (eds). The Wills Eye Hospital Atlas of Clinical Ophthalmology, 2nd ed. Philadelphia, Lippincott Williams & Wilkins, 2001.)

TABLE 6-7 Red Eyes

	Conjunctivitis	Subconjunctival Hemorrhage
	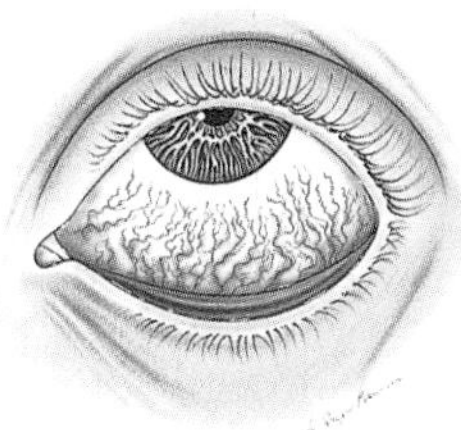	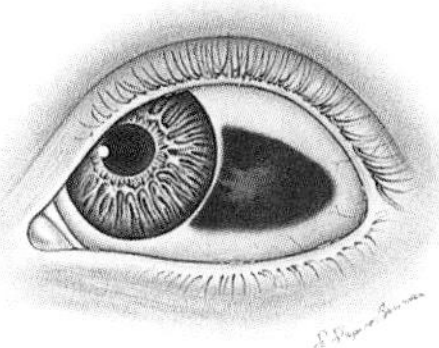
Pattern of Redness	Conjunctival injection: diffuse dilatation of conjunctival vessels with redness that tends to be maximal peripherally	Leakage of blood outside of the vessels, producing a homogeneous, sharply demarcated, red area that fades over days to yellow and then disappears
Pain	Mild discomfort rather than pain	Absent
Vision	Not affected except for temporary mild blurring due to discharge	Not affected
Ocular Discharge	Watery, mucoid, or mucopurulent	Absent
Pupil	Not affected	Not affected
Cornea	Clear	Clear
Significance	Bacterial, viral, and other infections; allergy; irritation	Often none. May result from trauma, bleeding disorders, or a sudden increase in venous pressure, as from cough

	Corneal Injury or Infection	Acute Iritis	Glaucoma
	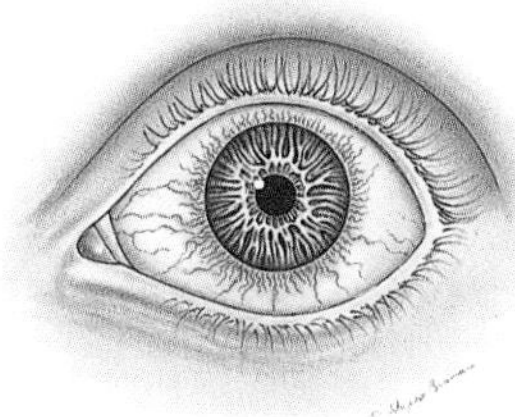	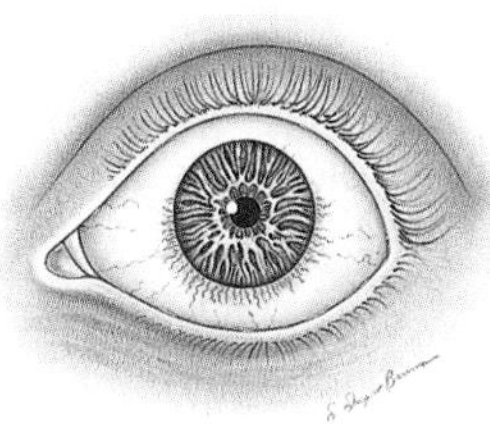	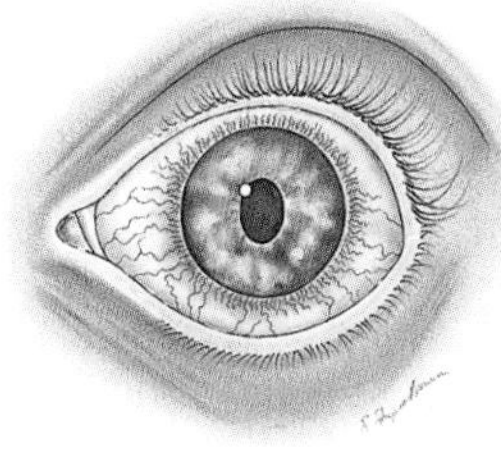
Pattern of Redness	Ciliary injection: dilation of deeper vessels that are visible as radiating vessels or a reddish violet flush around the limbus. Ciliary injection is an important sign of these three conditions but may not be apparent. The eye may be diffusely red instead. Other clues of these more serious disorders are pain, decreased vision, unequal pupils, and a less than perfectly clear cornea.		
Pain	Moderate to severe, superficial	Moderate, aching, deep	Severe, aching, deep
Vision	Usually decreased	Decreased	Decreased
Ocular Discharge	Watery or purulent	Absent	Absent
Pupil	Not affected unless iritis develops	May be small and, with time, irregular	Dilated, fixed
Cornea	Changes depending on cause	Clear or slightly clouded	Steamy, cloudy
Significance	Abrasions, and other injuries; viral and bacterial infections	Associated with many ocular and systemic disorders	Acute increase in intraocular pressure—an emergency

TABLE 6-8 Opacities of the Cornea and Lens

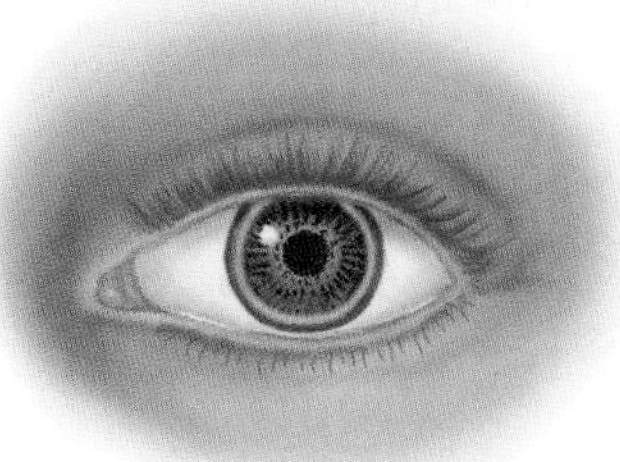

Corneal Arcus. A thin grayish white arc or circle not quite at the edge of the cornea. Accompanies normal aging but also seen in younger people, especially African Americans. In young people, suggests possible hyperlipoproteinemia. Usually benign.

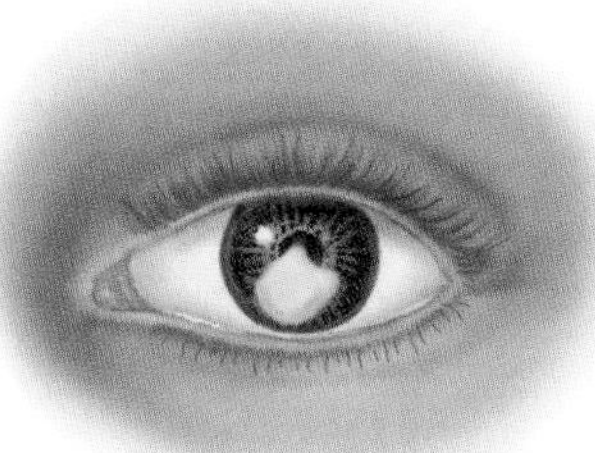

Corneal Scar. A superficial grayish white opacity in the cornea, secondary to an old injury or to inflammation. Size and shape are variable. Do not confuse with the opaque lens of a cataract, visible on a deeper plane and only through the pupil.

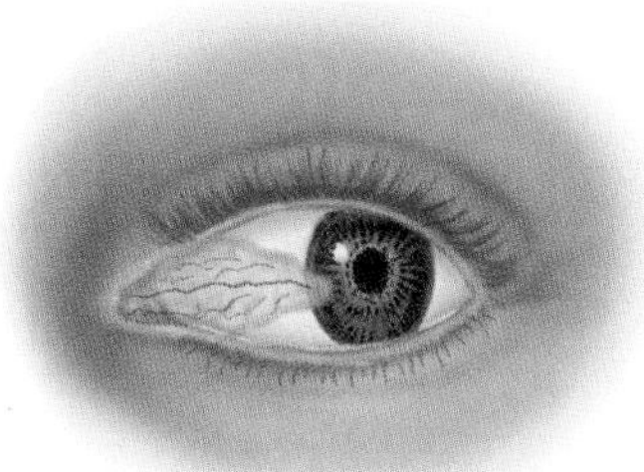

Pterygium. A triangular thickening of the bulbar conjunctiva that grows slowly across the outer surface of the cornea, usually from the nasal side. Reddening may occur. May interfere with vision as it encroaches on the pupil.

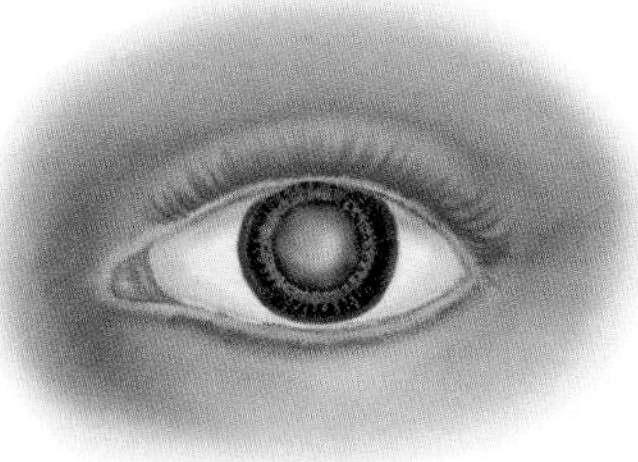

Cataracts. Opacities of the lenses visible through the pupil; most common in old age.

Nuclear cataract. A nuclear cataract looks gray when seen by a flashlight. If the pupil is widely dilated, the gray opacity is surrounded by a black rim. Through an ophthalmoscope, the cataract looks black against the red reflex.

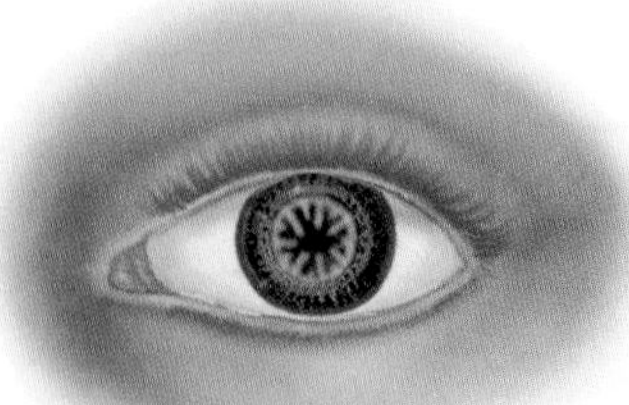

Peripheral cataract. Produces spokelike shadows that point inward—gray against black as seen with a flashlight, or black against red with an ophthalmoscope. A dilated pupil, as shown here, facilitates this observation.

TABLE 6-9 Pupillary Abnormalities

Unequal Pupils (*Anisocoria*)—When anisocoria is greater in bright light than in dim light, the larger pupil cannot constrict properly. Causes include blunt trauma to the eye, open-angle glaucoma (p. 181), and impaired parasympathetic nerve supply to the iris, as in tonic pupil and oculomotor nerve paralysis. When anisocoria is greater in dim light, the smaller pupil cannot dilate properly, as in Horner's syndrome, caused by an interruption of the sympathetic nerve supply. See also Table 17-10, Pupils in Comatose Patients, p. 666.

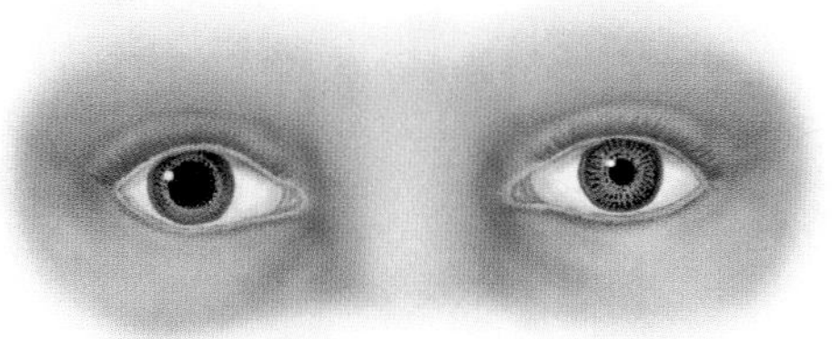

Tonic Pupil (*Adie's Pupil*). Pupil is large, regular, and usually unilateral. Reaction to light is severely reduced and slowed, or even absent. Near reaction, although very slow, is present. Slow accommodation causes blurred vision. Deep tendon reflexes are often decreased.

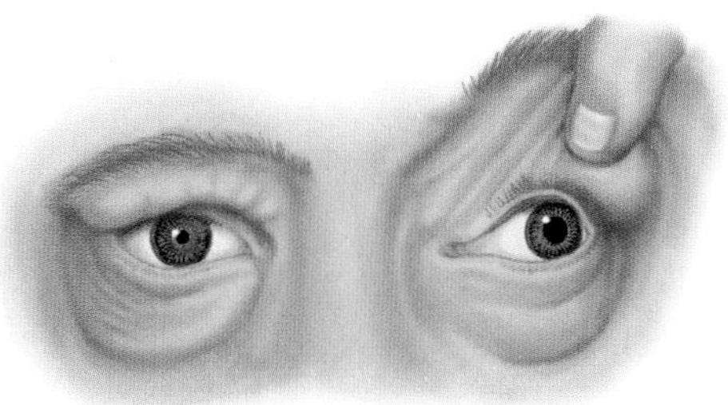

Oculomotor Nerve (CN III) Paralysis. The dilated pupil (6–7 mm) is fixed to light and near effort. Ptosis of the upper eyelid and lateral deviation of the eye are often, but not always, present. An even more dilated (8–9 mm) and fixed pupil may result from atropine-like eyedrops.

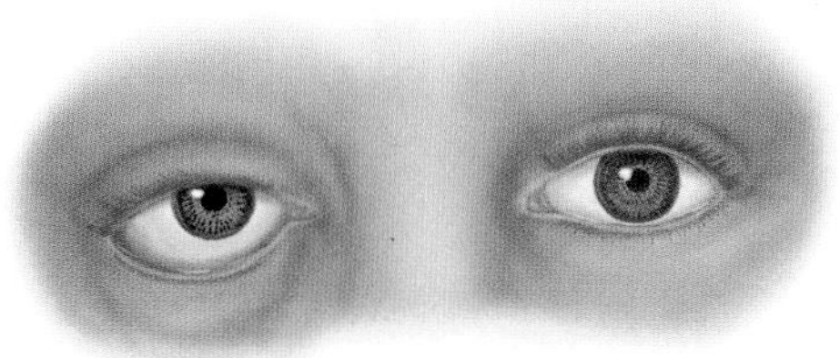

Horner's Syndrome. The affected pupil, though small, reacts briskly to light and near effort. Ptosis of the eyelid is present, perhaps with loss of sweating on the forehead. In congenital Horner's syndrome, the involved iris is lighter in color than its fellow (*heterochromia*).

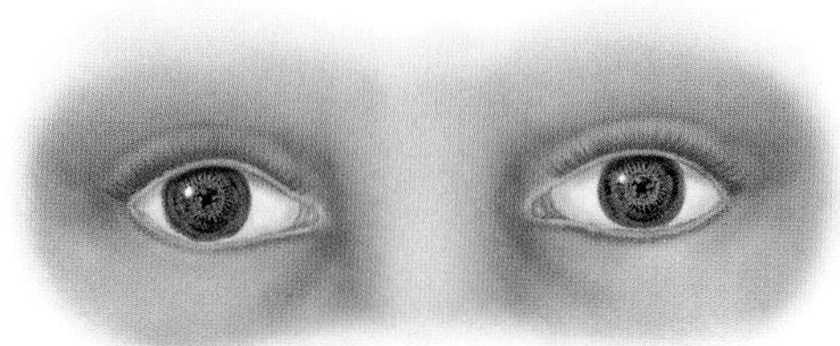

Small Irregular Pupils. Small, irregular pupils that accommodate but do not react to light indicate *Argyll Robertson pupils.* Seen in central nervous system syphilis.

Equal Pupils and One Blind Eye. Unilateral blindness does not cause anisocoria as long as the sympathetic and parasympathetic innervation to both irises is normal. A light directed into the seeing eye produces a direct reaction in that eye and a consensual reaction in the blind eye. A light directed into the blind eye, however, causes no response in either eye.

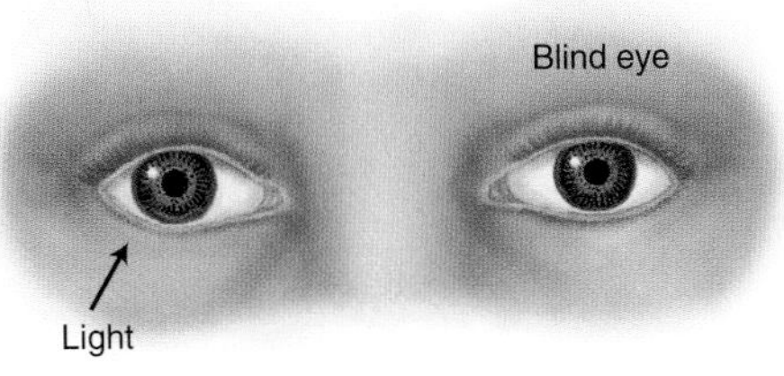

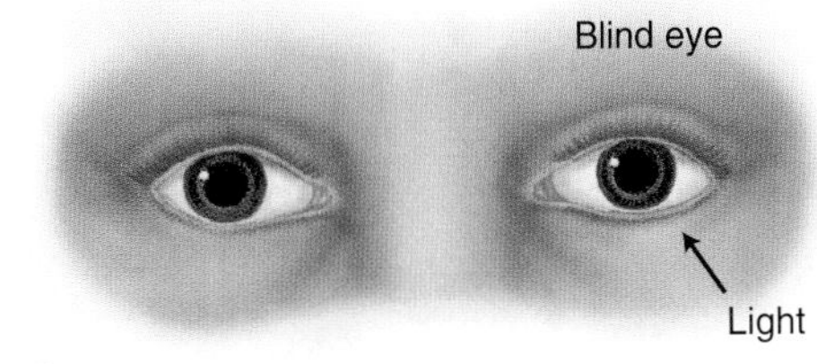

TABLE 6-10 Dysconjugate Gaze

There are a variety of gaze abnormality patterns that give clinicians clues about brainstem developmental disorders and cranial nerve abnormalities.

Developmental Disorders

Developmental dysconjugate gaze is caused by an imbalance in ocular muscle tone. This imbalance has many causes, may be hereditary, and usually appears in early childhood. These gaze deviations are classified according to direction:

Esotropia

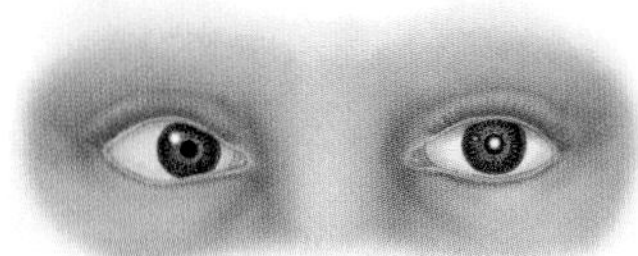

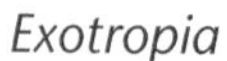

Exotropia

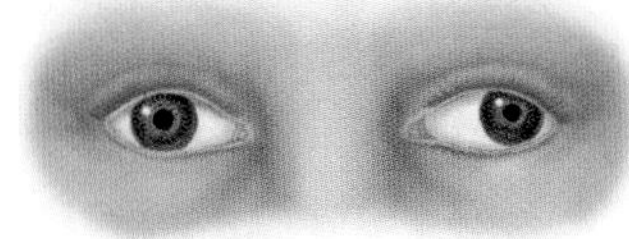

Cover–Uncover Test

A cover–uncover test may be helpful. Here is what you would see in the right monocular esotropia illustrated above.

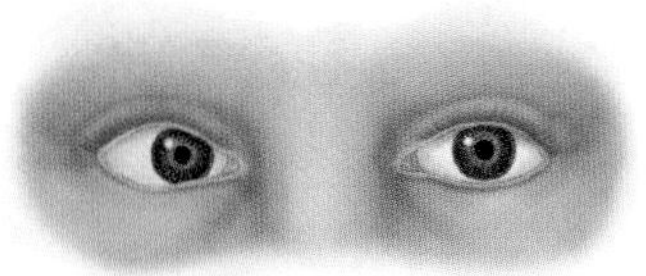

Corneal reflections are asymmetric.

COVER

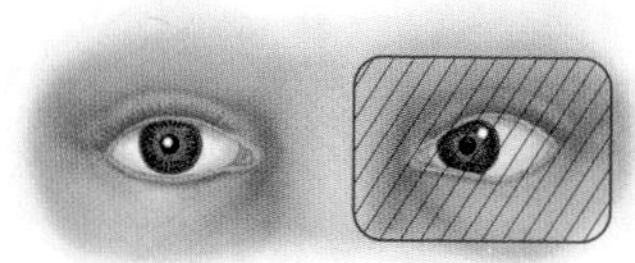

The right eye moves outward to fix on the light. (The left eye is not seen but moves inward to the same degree.)

UNCOVER

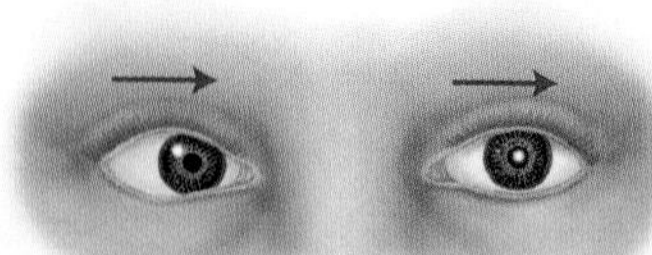

The left eye moves outward to fix on the light. The right eye deviates inward again.

Disorders of Cranial Nerves

New onset of dysconjugate gaze in adult life is usually the result of cranial nerve injuries, lesions, or abnormalities from such causes as trauma, multiple sclerosis, syphilis, and others.

A Left Cranial Nerve VI Paralysis

LOOKING TO THE RIGHT

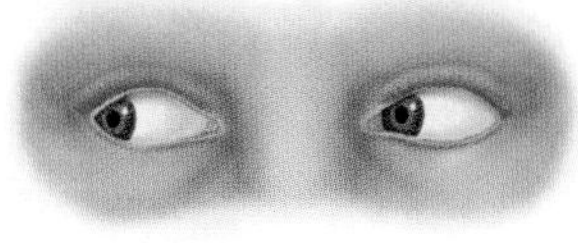

Eyes are conjugate.

LOOKING STRAIGHT AHEAD

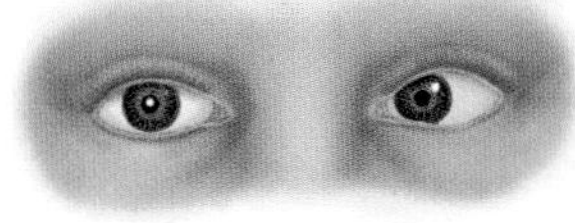

Esotropia appears.

LOOKING TO THE LEFT

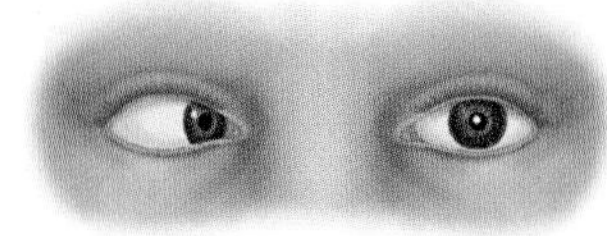

Esotropia is maximum.

A Left Cranial Nerve IV Paralysis

LOOKING DOWN AND TO THE RIGHT

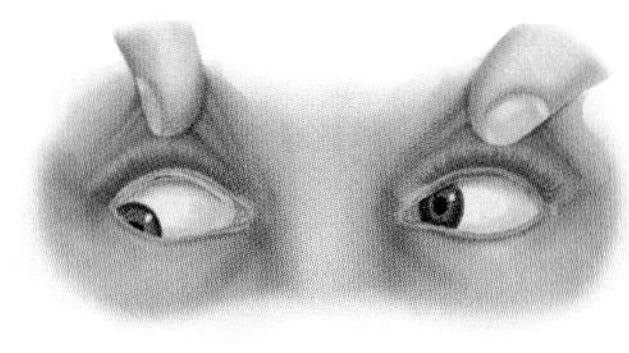

The left eye cannot look down when turned inward. Deviation is maximum in this direction.

A Left Cranial Nerve III Paralysis

LOOKING STRAIGHT AHEAD

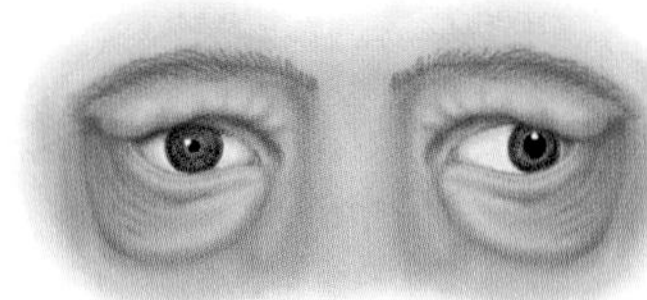

The eye is pulled outward by action of the 6th nerve. Upward, downward, and inward movements are impaired or lost. Ptosis and pupillary dilation may be associated.

TABLE 6-11 Normal Variations of the Optic Disc

Physiologic Cupping

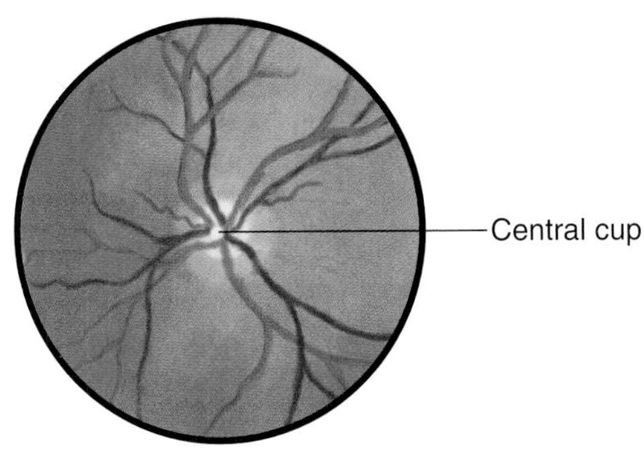

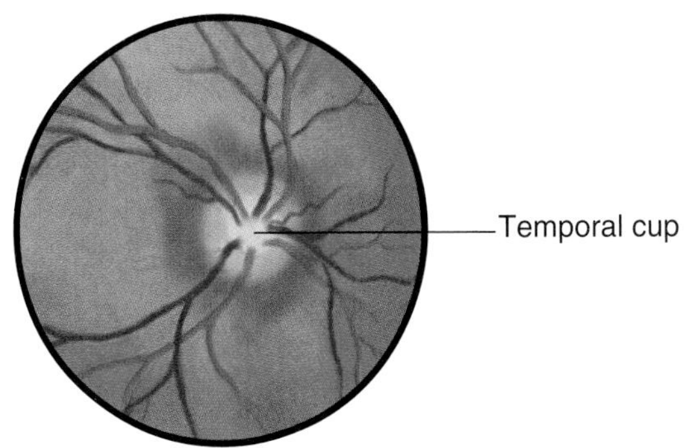

The physiologic cup is a small whitish depression in the optic disc from which the retinal vessels appear to emerge. Although sometimes absent, the cup is usually visible either centrally or toward the temporal side of the disc. Grayish spots are often seen at its base.

Rings and Crescents

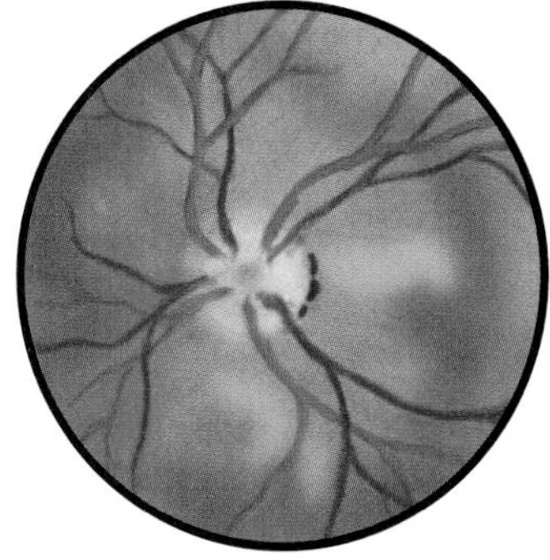

Rings and crescents are often seen around the optic disc. These are developmental variations in which you can glimpse either white sclera, black retinal pigment, or both, especially along the temporal border of the disc. Rings and crescents are not part of the disc itself and should not be included in your estimates of disc diameters.

Medullated Nerve Fibers

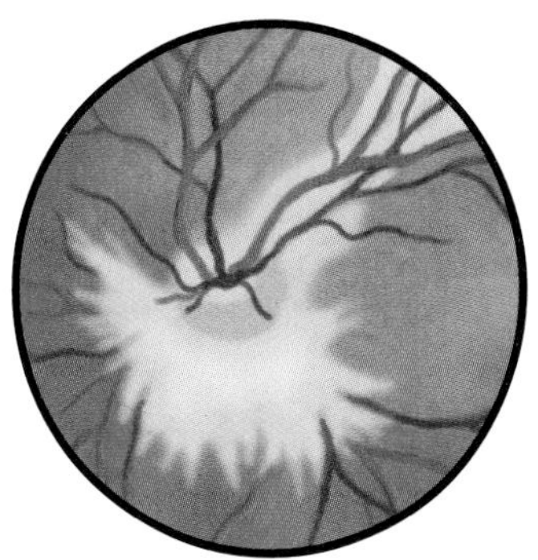

Medullated nerve fibers are a much less common but dramatic finding. Appearing as irregular white patches with feathered margins, they obscure the disc edge and retinal vessels. They have no pathologic significance.

TABLE 6-12 Abnormalities of the Optic Disc

	Process	Appearance
Normal		
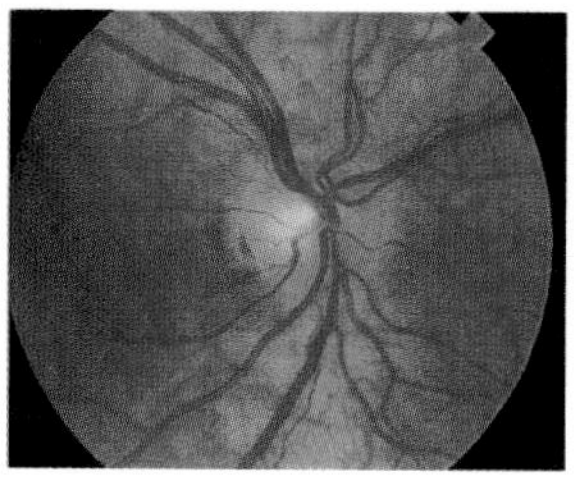	Tiny disc vessels give normal color to the disc.	Color yellowish orange to creamy pink Disc vessels tiny Disc margins sharp (except perhaps nasally) The physiologic cup is located centrally or somewhat temporally. It may be conspicuous or absent. Its diameter from side to side is usually less than half that of the disc.
Papilledema		
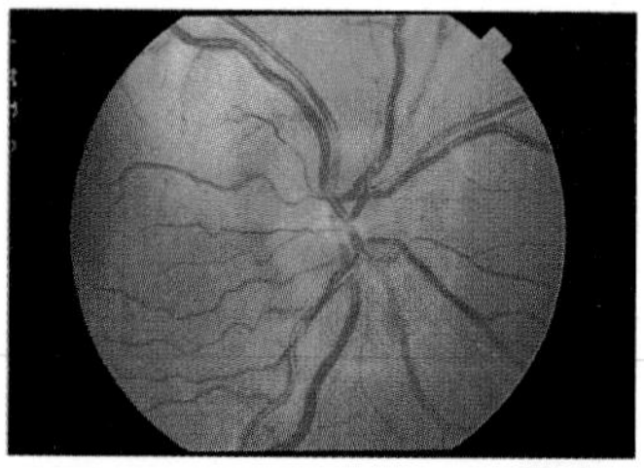	Venous stasis leads to engorgement and swelling.	Color pink, hyperemic Disc vessels more visible, more numerous, curve over the borders of the disc Disc swollen with margins blurred The physiologic cup is not visible.
Glaucomatous Cupping		
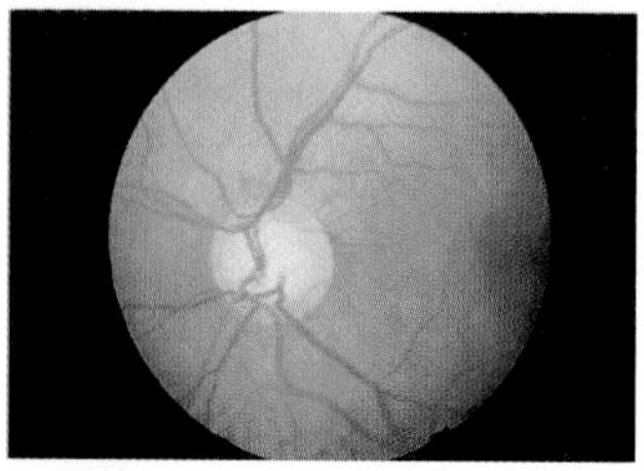	Increased pressure within the eye leads to increased cupping (backward depression of the disc) and atrophy. The base of the enlarged cup is pale.	The physiologic cup is enlarged, occupying more than half of the disc's diameter, at times extending to the edge of the disc. Retinal vessels sink in and under it, and may be displaced nasally.
Optic Atrophy		
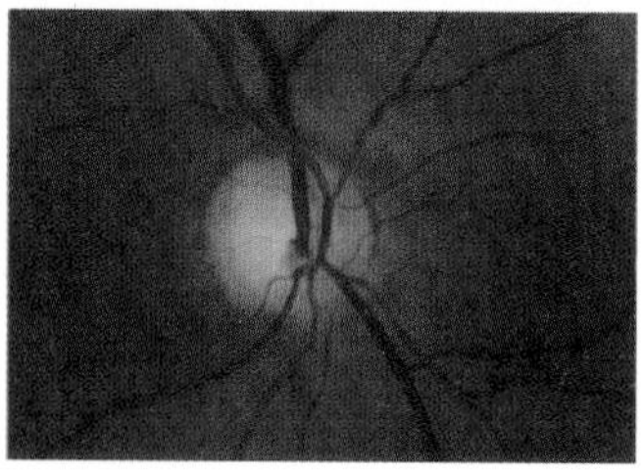	Death of optic nerve fibers leads to loss of the tiny disc vessels.	Color white Disc vessels absent

(Source of photos: Tasman W, Jaeger E (eds). The Wills Eye Hospital Atlas of Clinical Ophthalmology, 2nd ed. Philadelphia, Lippincott Williams & Wilkins, 2001.)

TABLE 6-13 Retinal Arteries and Arteriovenous Crossings: Normal and Hypertensive

Normal Retinal Artery and Arteriovenous (A-V) Crossing

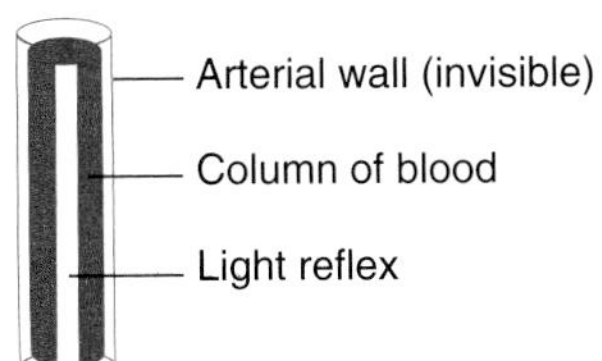

The normal arterial wall is transparent. Only the column of blood within it can usually be seen. The normal light reflex is *narrow—about one fourth the diameter of the blood column.* Because the arterial wall is transparent, a vein crossing beneath the artery can be seen right up to the column of blood on either side.

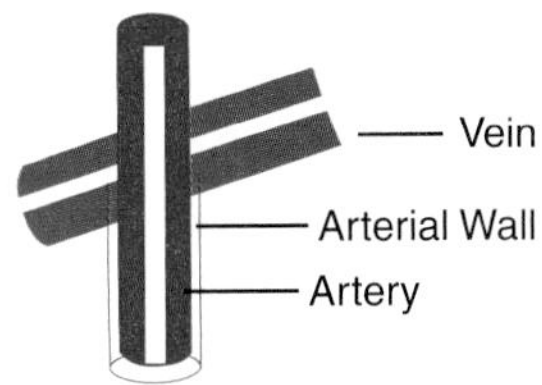

Retinal Arteries in Hypertension

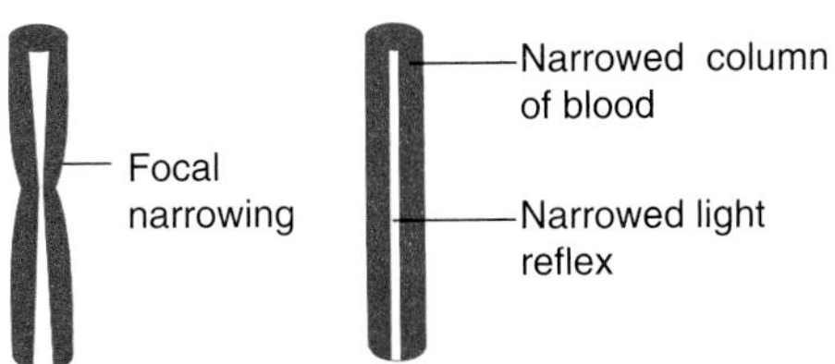

In hypertension, the arteries may show areas of focal or generalized narrowing. The light reflex is also narrowed. The arterial wall thickens and becomes less transparent.

Copper Wiring

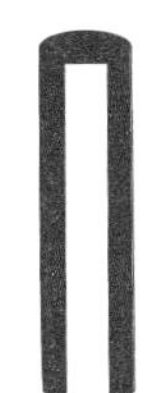

Sometimes the arteries, especially those close to the disc, become full and somewhat tortuous and develop an increased light reflex with a bright coppery luster.

Silver Wiring

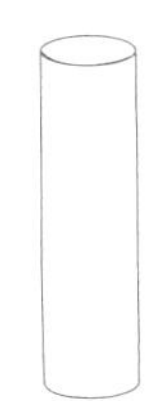

Occasionally a portion of a narrowed artery develops such an opaque wall that no blood is visible within it. It is then called a silver wire artery.

Arteriovenous Crossing

When the arterial walls lose their transparency, changes appear in the arteriovenous crossings. Decreased transparency of the retina probably also contributes to the first two changes shown below.

CONCEALMENT OR A-V NICKING

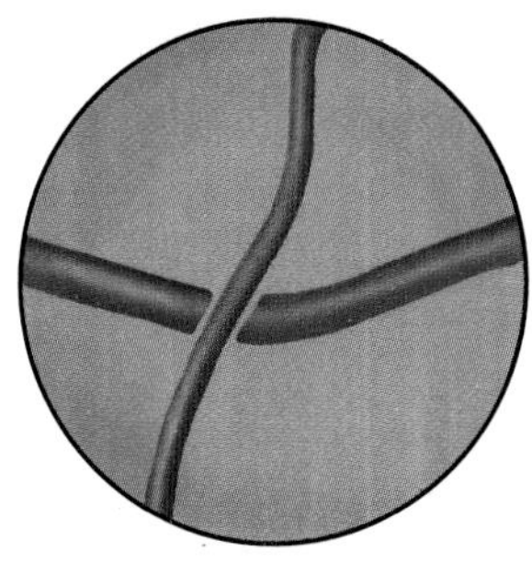

The vein appears to stop abruptly on either side of the artery.

TAPERING AND BANKING

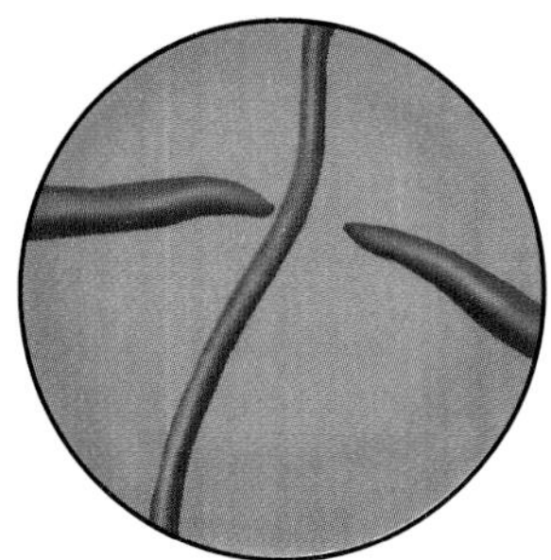

Tapering. The vein appears to taper down on either side of the artery.

BANKING

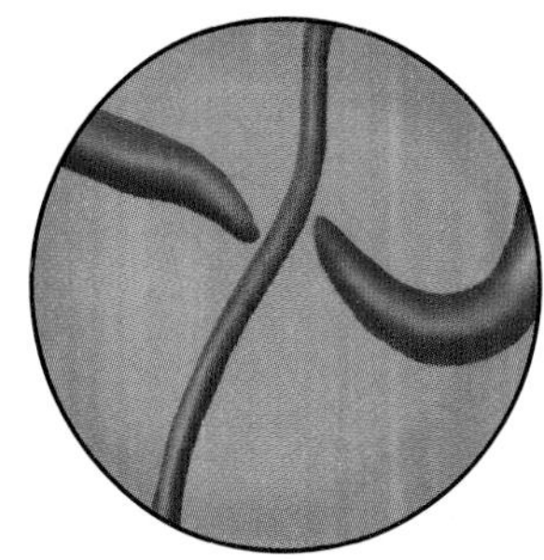

Banking. The vein is twisted on the distal side of the artery and forms a dark, wide knuckle.

TABLE 6-14 Red Spots and Streaks in the Fundi

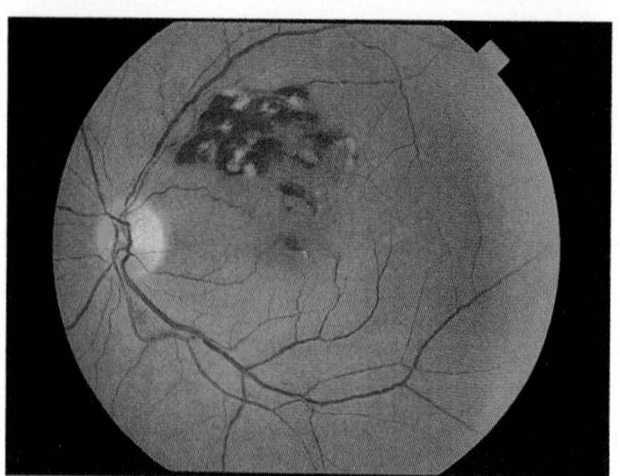

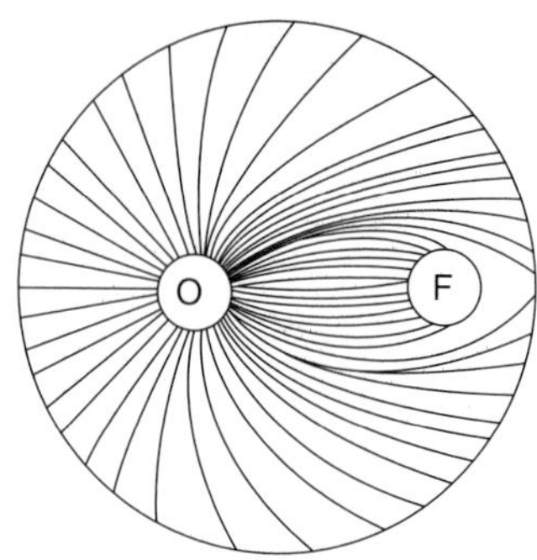

Superficial Retinal Hemorrhages—Small, linear, flame-shaped, red streaks in the fundi, shaped by the superficial bundles of nerve fibers that radiate from the optic disc in the pattern illustrated (O = optic disc; F = fovea). Sometimes the hemorrhages occur in clusters and look like a larger hemorrhage, but can be identified by the linear streaking at the edges. Superficial hemorrhages are seen in severe hypertension, papilledema, and occlusion of the retinal vein, among other conditions. An occasional superficial hemorrhage has a white center consisting of fibrin. White-centered retinal hemorrhages have many causes.

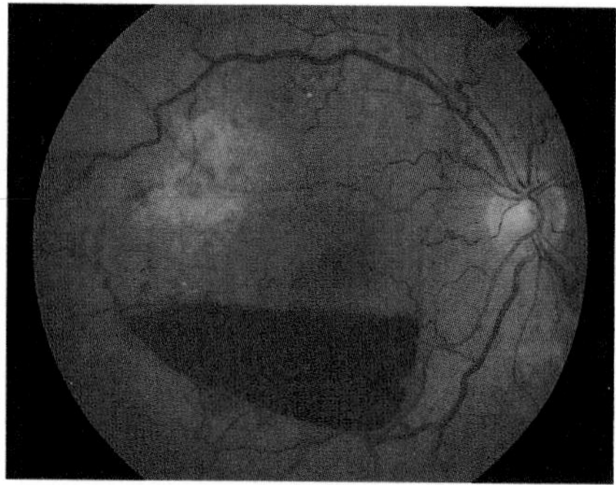

Preretinal Hemorrhage—Develops when blood escapes into the potential space between retina and vitreous. This hemorrhage is typically larger than retinal hemorrhages. Because it is anterior to the retina, it obscures any underlying retinal vessels. In an erect patient, red cells settle, creating a horizontal line of demarcation between plasma above and cells below. Causes include a sudden increase in intracranial pressure.

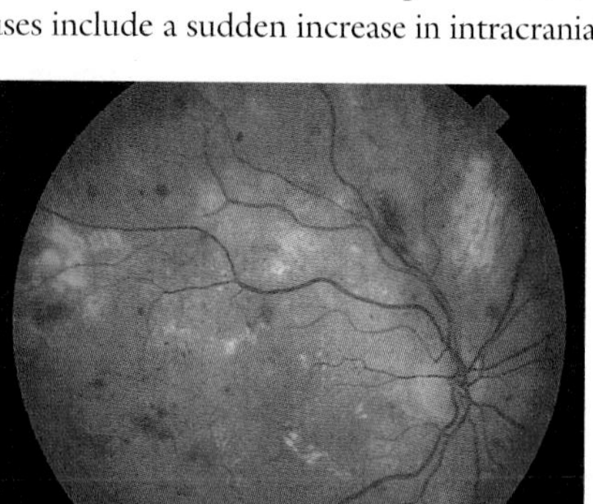

Deep Retinal Hemorrhages—Small, rounded, slightly irregular red spots that are sometimes called dot or blot hemorrhages. They occur in a deeper layer of the retina than flame-shaped hemorrhages. Diabetes is a common cause.

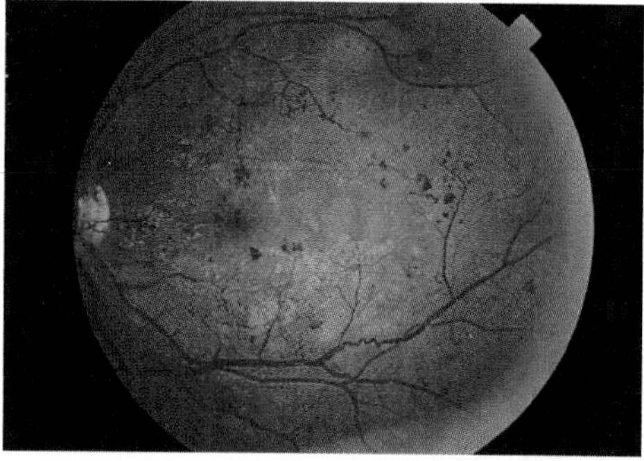

Microaneurysms—Tiny, round, red spots seen commonly but not exclusively in and around the macular area. They are minute dilatations of very small retinal vessels, but the vascular connections are too small to be seen ophthalmoscopically. They arise from diabetic retinopathy but have other causes.

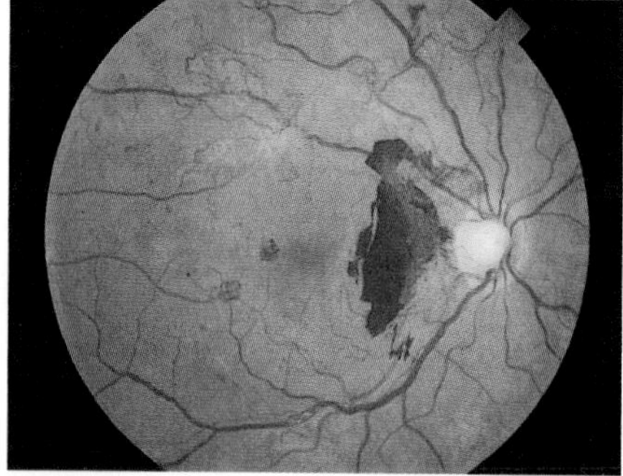

Neovascularization—Refers to the formation of new blood vessels. They are more numerous, more tortuous, and narrower than other blood vessels in the area and form disorderly looking red arcades. A common cause is the late, proliferative stage of diabetic retinopathy. The vessels may grow into the vitreous, where retinal detachment or hemorrhage may cause loss of vision.

(Source of photos: Tasman W, Jaeger E (eds). The Wills Eye Hospital Atlas of Clinical Ophthalmology, 2nd ed. Philadelphia, Lippincott Williams & Wilkins, 2001.)

TABLE 6-15 Ocular Fundi

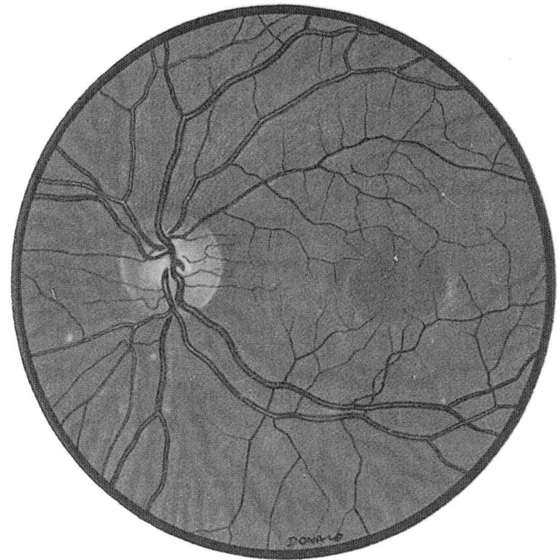

Normal Fundus of a Fair-Skinned Person

Inspect the optic disc. Follow the major vessels in four directions, noting their relative sizes and any arteriovenous crossings—both normal here. Inspect the macular area. The slightly darker fovea is just discernible; no light reflex is visible in this subject. Look for any lesions in the retina. Note the striped, or tessellated, character of the fundus, especially in the lower field that comes from normal underlying choroidal vessels.

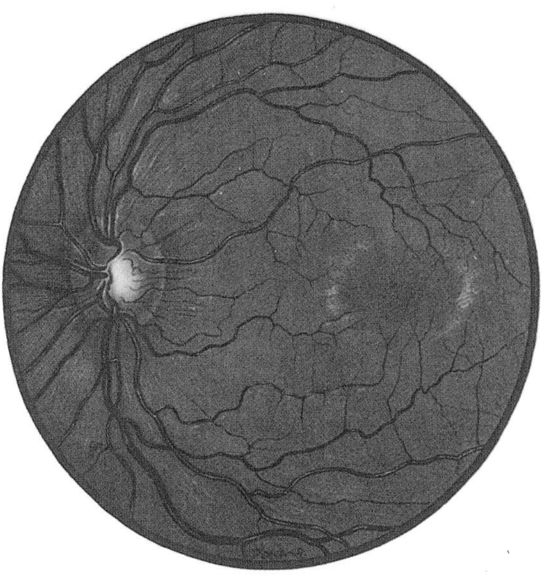

Normal Fundus of a Dark-Skinned Person

Again, inspect the disc, vessels, macula, and retina. The ring around the fovea is a normal light reflection. The color of the fundus has a grayish brown, almost purplish cast, which comes from pigment in the retina and the choroid, that characteristically obscures the choroidal vessels; no tessellation is visible. The fundus of a light-skinned person with brunette coloring is redder.

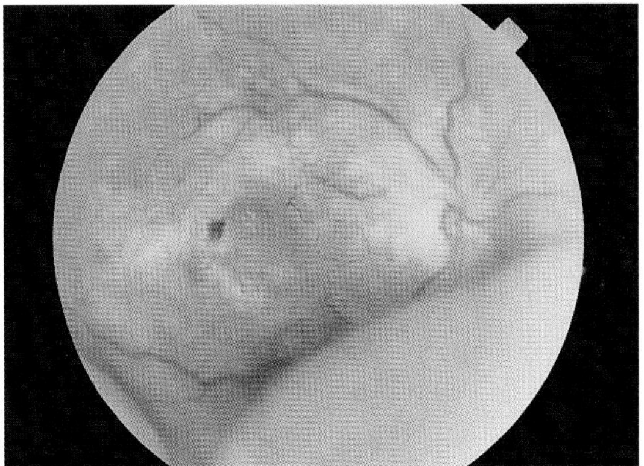

Hypertensive Retinopathy[32]

Inspect the fundus. The nasal border of the optic disc is blurred. The light reflexes from the arteries just above and below the disc are increased. Note venous tapering—at the A-V crossing, about 1 disc diameter above the disc.

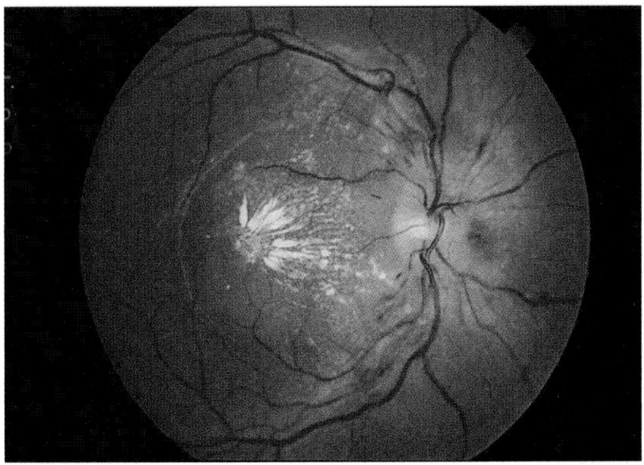

Hypertensive Retinopathy With Macular Star

Punctate exudates are readily visible: some are scattered; others radiate from the fovea to form a macular star. Note the two small, soft exudates about 1 disc diameter from the disc. Find the flame-shaped hemorrhages sweeping toward 7 o'clock and 8 o'clock; a few more may be seen toward 10 o'clock. These fundi show changes typical of accelerated (malignant) hypertension and are often accompanied by a papilledema (p. 220).

(Source of photos: *Hypertensive Retinopathy, Hypertensive Retinopathy With Macular Star*—Tasman W, Jaeger E (eds). The Wills Eye Hospital Atlas of Clinical Ophthalmology, 2nd ed. Philadelphia, Lippincott Williams & Wilkins, 2001.)

(table continues next page)

Diabetic Retinopathy

Study carefully the fundi in the series of photographs below. They represent a national standard used by ophthalmologists to assess diabetic retinopathy.

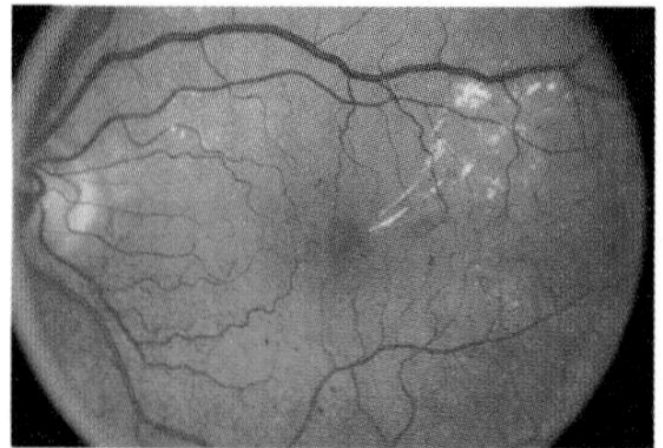

Nonproliferative Retinopathy, Moderately Severe

Note tiny red dots or microaneurysms. Note also the ring of hard exudates (white spots) located superotemporally. Retinal thickening or edema in the area of the hard exudates can impair visual acuity if it extends into the center of the macula (detection requires specialized stereoscopic examination).

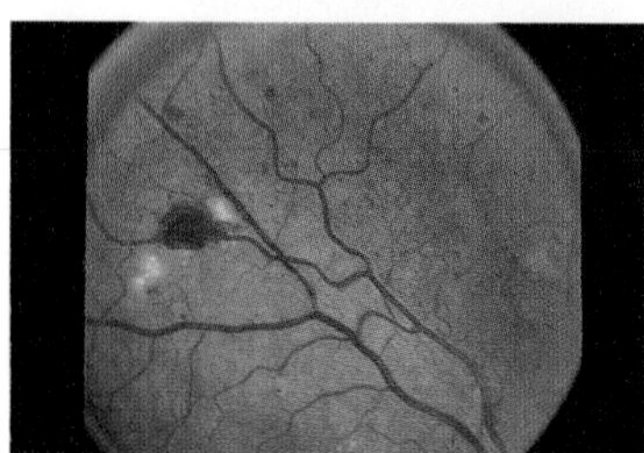

Nonproliferative Retinopathy, Severe

In the superior temporal quadrant, note the large retinal hemorrhage between two cotton-wool patches, beading of the retinal vein just above them, and tiny tortuous retinal vessels above the superior temporal artery.

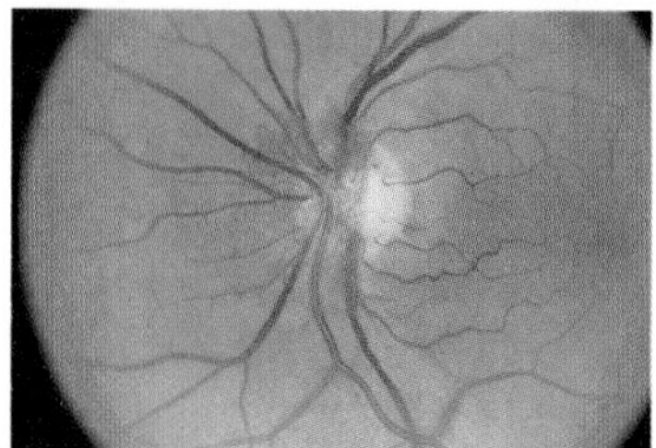

Proliferative Retinopathy, With Neovascularization

Note new preretinal vessels arising on the disc and extending across the disc margins. Visual acuity is still normal, but the risk for visual loss is high (photocoagulation reduces this risk by > 50%).

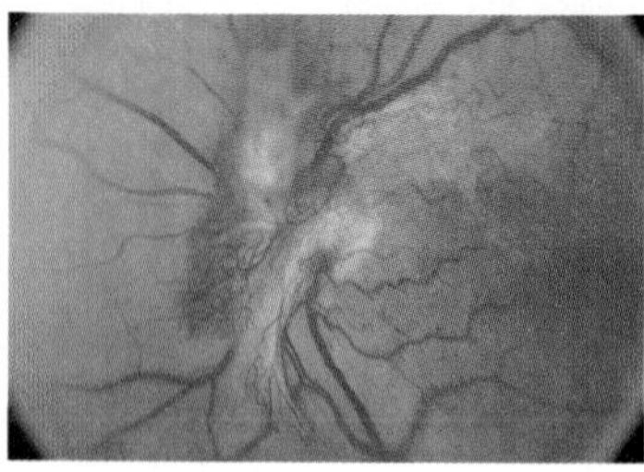

Proliferative Retinopathy, Advanced

This is the same eye, but 2 years later and without treatment. Neovascularization has increased, now with fibrous proliferations, distortion of the macula, and reduced visual acuity.

(Source of photos: *Nonproliferative Retinopathy, Moderately Severe; Proliferative Retinopathy, With Neovascularization; Nonproliferative Retinopathy, Severe; Proliferative Retinopathy, Advanced*—Early Treatment Diabetic Retinopathy Study Research Group. Courtesy of MF Davis, MD, University of Wisconsin, Madison.)

TABLE 6-16 Light-Colored Spots in the Fundi

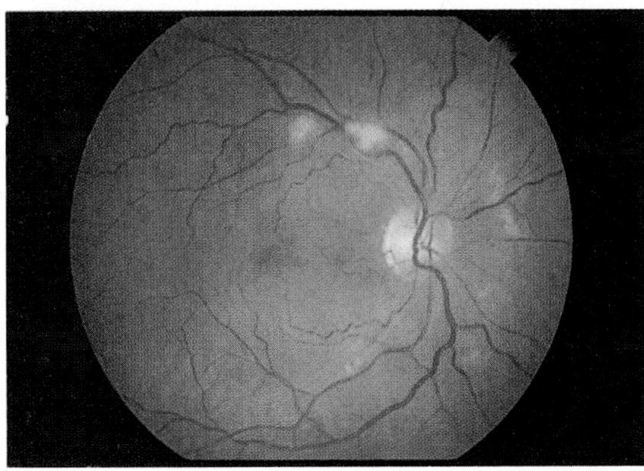

Cotton-Wool Patches (*Soft Exudates*)

Cotton-wool patches are white or grayish, ovoid lesions with irregular "soft" borders. They are moderate in size but usually smaller than the disc. They result from infarcted nerve fibers and are seen in hypertension and many other conditions.

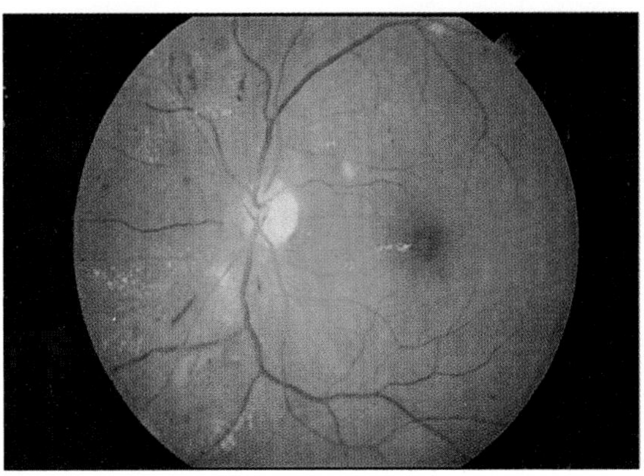

Hard Exudates

Hard exudates are creamy or yellowish, often bright lesions with well-defined "hard" borders. They are small and round (as shown in the lower group of exudates) but may coalesce into larger irregular spots (as shown in the upper group). They often occur in clusters or in circular, linear, or star-shaped patterns. Causes include diabetes and hypertension.

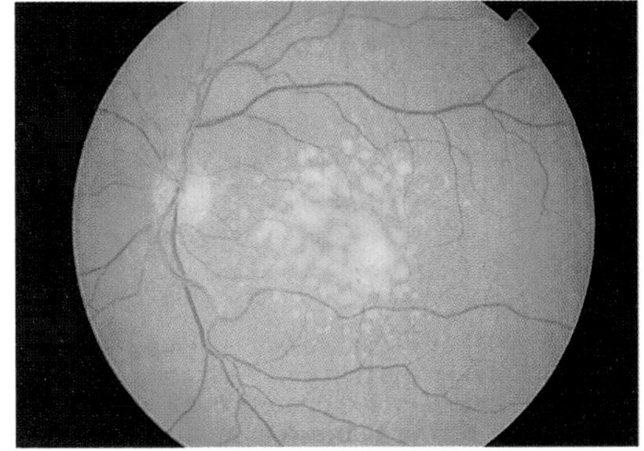

Drusen

Drusen are yellowish round spots that vary from tiny to small. The edges may be soft, as here, or hard (p. 188). They are haphazardly distributed but may concentrate at the posterior pole. Drusen appear with normal aging but may also accompany various conditions, including age-related macular degeneration.

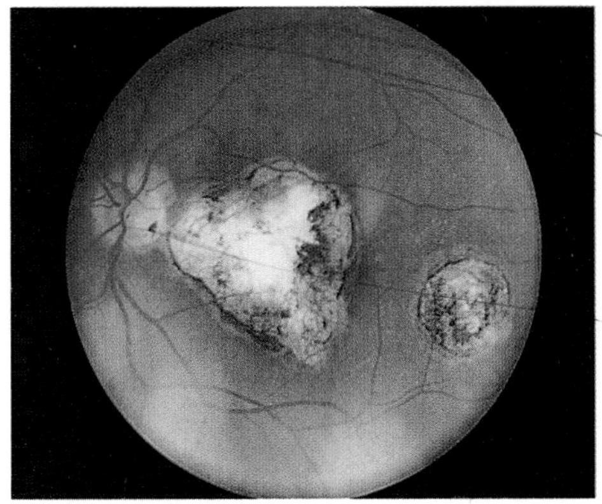

Healed Chorioretinitis

Here inflammation has destroyed the superficial tissues to reveal a well-defined, irregular patch of white sclera marked with dark pigment. Size varies from small to very large. *Toxoplasmosis* is illustrated. Multiple, small, somewhat similar-looking areas may be due to laser treatments. Here there is also a temporal scar near the macula.

(Source of photos: *Cotton-Wool Patches, Hard Exudates; Drusen, Healed Chorioretinitis*—Tasman W, Jaeger E (eds). The Wills Eye Hospital Atlas of Clinical Ophthalmology, 2nd ed. Philadelphia, Lippincott Williams & Wilkins, 2001.)

TABLE 6-17 Lumps on or Near the Ear

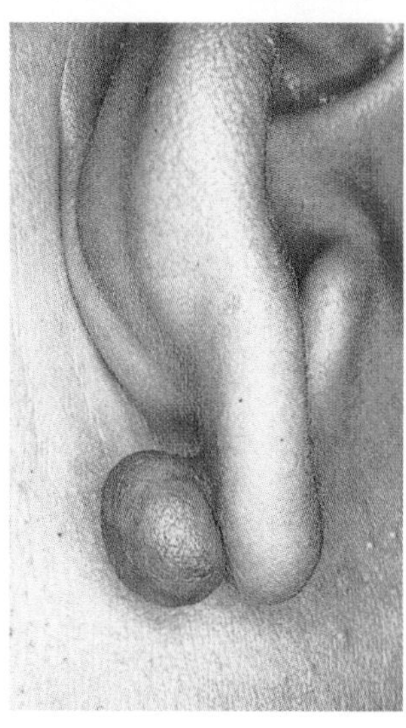

Keloid. A firm, nodular, hypertrophic mass of scar tissue extending beyond the area of injury. It may develop in any scarred area but is most common on the shoulders and upper chest. A keloid on a pierced earlobe may have troublesome cosmetic effects. Keloids are more common in darker-skinned people. Recurrence may follow treatment.

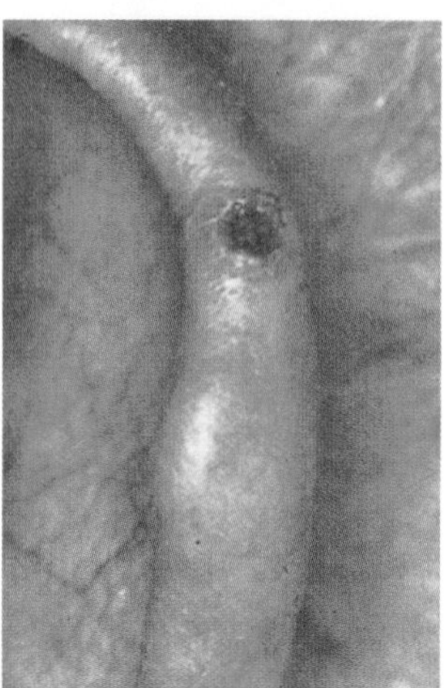

Chondrodermatitis Helicis. This chronic inflammatory lesion starts as a painful, tender papule on the helix or antihelix. Here the upper lesion is at a later stage of ulceration and crusting. Reddening may occur. Biopsy is needed to rule out carcinoma.

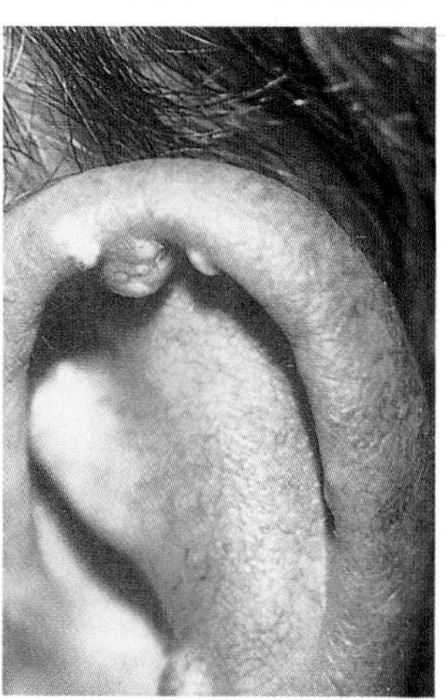

Tophi. A deposit of uric acid crystals characteristic of chronic tophaceous gout. It appears as hard nodules in the helix or antihelix and may discharge chalky white crystals through the skin. It also may appear near the joints: hands (p. 567), feet, and other areas. It usually develops after chronic sustained high blood levels of uric acid.

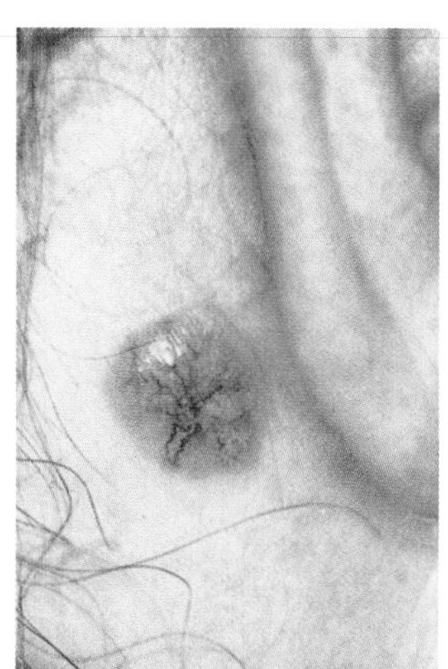

Basal Cell Carcinoma. This raised nodule shows the lustrous surface and telangiectatic vessels of basal cell carcinoma, a common slow-growing malignancy that rarely metastasizes. Growth and ulceration may occur. These are more frequent in fair-skinned people overexposed to sunlight.

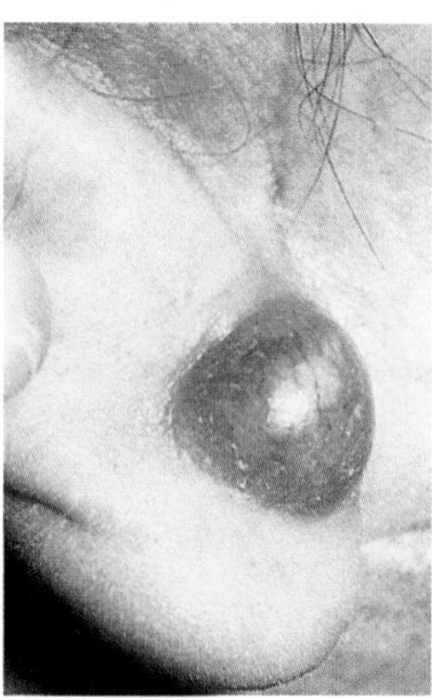

Cutaneous Cyst. Formerly called a *sebaceous cyst,* a dome-shaped lump in the dermis forms a benign closed firm sac attached to the epidermis. A dark dot (blackhead) may be visible on its surface. Histologically, it is usually either (1) an *epidermoid* cyst, common on the face and neck, or (2) a *pilar (trichilemmal)* cyst, common in the scalp. Both may become inflamed.

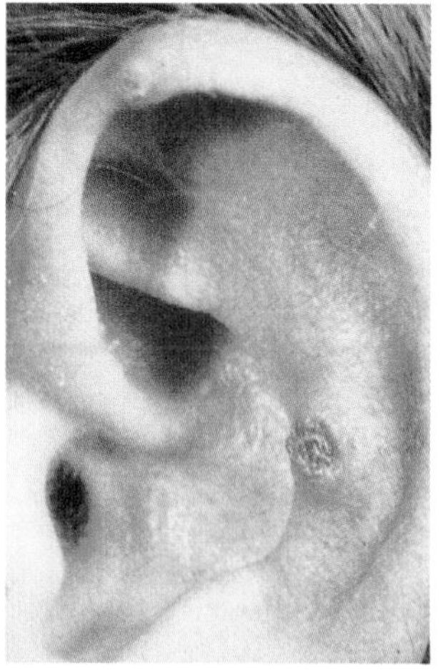

Rheumatoid Nodules. In chronic rheumatoid arthritis, look for small lumps on the helix or antihelix and additional nodules elsewhere on the hands, along the surface of the ulna distal to the elbow (p. 567), and on the knees and heels. Ulceration may result from repeated injuries. Such nodules may antedate the arthritis.

(Sources of photos: *Keloid*—Sams WM Jr, Lynch PJ (eds). Principles and Practice of Dermatology. Edinburgh, Churchill Livingstone, 1990; *Tophi*—du Vivier A. Atlas of Clinical Dermatology, 2nd ed. London, UK: Gower Medical Publishing, 1993; *Cutaneous Cyst, Chondrodermatitis Helicis*—Young EM, Newcomer VD, Kligman AM. Geriatric Dermatology: Color Atlas and Practitioner's Guide. Philadelphia, Lea & Febiger, 1993; *Basal Cell Carcinoma*—N Engl J Med, 326:169–170, 1992; *Rheumatoid Nodules*—Champion RH, Burton JL, Ebling FJG (eds). Rook/Wilkinson/Ebling Textbook of Dermatology, 5th ed. Oxford, UK: Blackwell Scientific, 1992.)

TABLE 6-18 Abnormalities of the Eardrum

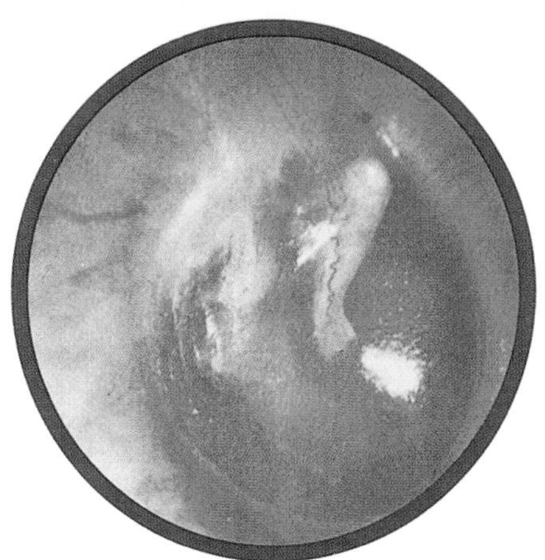

Normal Eardrum

This normal right eardrum (tympanic membrane) is pinkish gray. Note the malleus lying behind the upper part of the drum. Above the short process lies the *pars flaccida*. The remainder of the drum is the *pars tensa*. From the umbo, the bright cone of light fans anteriorly and downward. Posterior to the malleus, part of the incus is visible behind the drum. The small blood vessels along the handle of the malleus are normal.

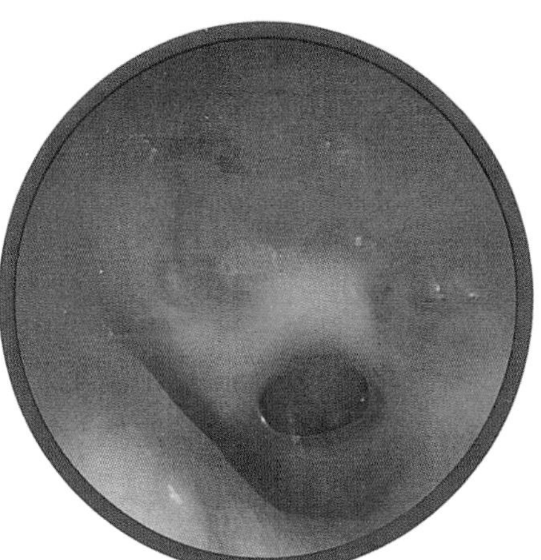

Perforation of the Drum

Perforations are holes in the eardrum that usually result from purulent infections of the middle ear. They are classified as *central* perforations, which do not extend to the margin of the drum, and *marginal* perforations, which do involve the margin.

The more common central perforation is illustrated here. A reddened ring of granulation tissue surrounds the perforation, indicating chronic infection. The eardrum itself is scarred, and no landmarks are visible. Discharge from the infected middle ear may drain out through such a perforation. A perforation often closes in the healing process, as in the next photo. The membrane covering the hole may be exceedingly thin and transparent.

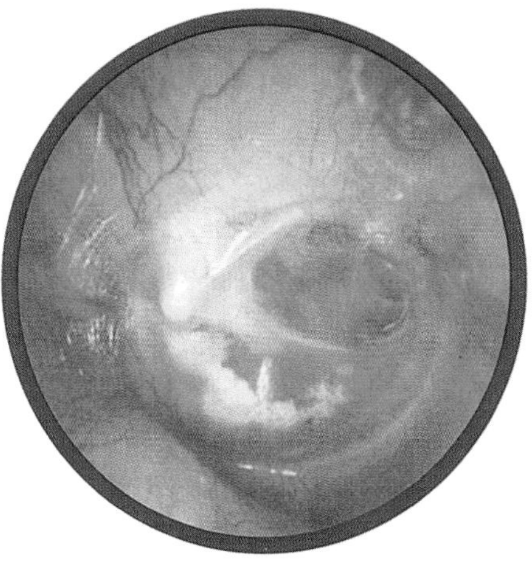

Tympanosclerosis

In the inferior portion of this left eardrum, there is a large, chalky white patch with irregular margins. It is typical of tympanosclerosis: a deposition of hyaline material within the layers of the tympanic membrane that sometimes follows a severe episode of otitis media. It does not usually impair hearing and is seldom clinically significant.

Other abnormalities in this eardrum include a *healed perforation* (the large oval area in the upper posterior drum) and signs of a *retracted drum*. A retracted drum is pulled medially, away from the examiner's eye, and the malleolar folds are tightened into sharp outlines. The short process often protrudes sharply, and the handle of the malleus, pulled inward at the umbo, looks foreshortened and more horizontal.

(Sources of photos: *Normal Eardrum*—Hawke M, Keene M, Alberti PW. Clinical Otoscopy: A Text and Colour Atlas. Edinburgh, Churchill Livingstone, 1984; *Perforation of the Drum, Tympanosclerosis*—Courtesy of Michael Hawke, MD, Toronto, Canada.)

(table continues next page)

TABLE 6-18 Abnormalities of the Eardrum *(Continued)*

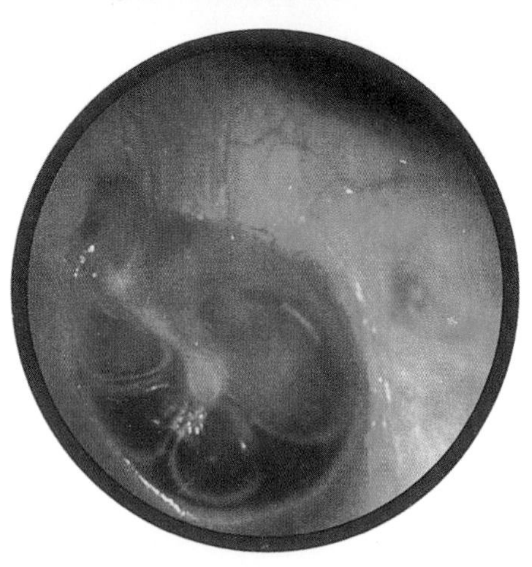

Serous Effusion

Serous effusions are usually caused by viral upper respiratory infections (*otitis media with serous effusion*) or by sudden changes in atmospheric pressure as from flying or diving (*otitic barotrauma*). The eustachian tube cannot equalize the air pressure in the middle ear with that of the outside air. Air is partly or completely absorbed from the middle ear into the bloodstream, and serous fluid accumulates there instead. Symptoms include fullness and popping sensations in the ear, mild conduction hearing loss, and perhaps some pain.

Amber fluid behind the eardrum is characteristic, as in this patient with otitic barotrauma. A fluid level, a line between air above and amber fluid below, can be seen on either side of the short process. Air bubbles (not always present) can be seen here within the amber fluid.

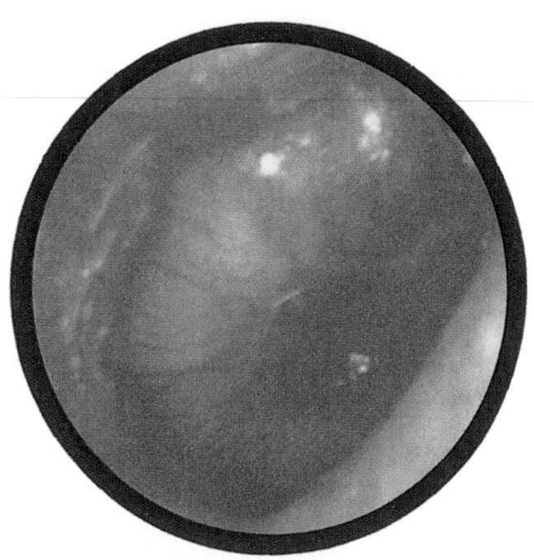

Acute Otitis Media With Purulent Effusion

Acute otitis media with purulent effusion is caused by bacterial infection. Symptoms include earache, fever, and hearing loss. The eardrum reddens, loses its landmarks, and bulges laterally, toward the examiner's eye.

Here the eardrum is bulging, and most landmarks are obscured. Redness is most obvious near the umbo, but dilated vessels can be seen in all segments of the drum. A diffuse redness of the entire drum often develops. Spontaneous rupture (perforation) of the drum may follow, with discharge of purulent material into the ear canal.

Hearing loss is of the conductive type. Acute purulent otitis media is much more common in children than in adults.

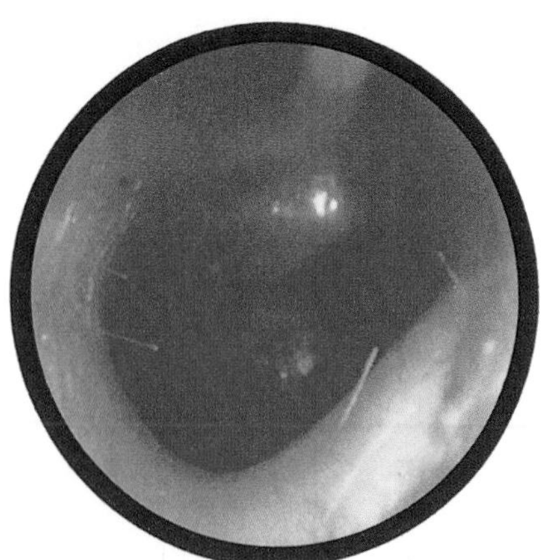

Bullous Myringitis

Bullous myringitis is a viral infection characterized by painful hemorrhagic vesicles that appear on the tympanic membrane, the ear canal, or both. Symptoms include earache, blood-tinged discharge from the ear, and hearing loss of the conductive type.

In this right ear, at least two large vesicles (bullae) are discernible on the drum. The drum is reddened, and its landmarks are obscured.

Several different viruses may cause this condition, including mycoplasma.

(Sources of photos: *Serous Effusion*—Hawke M, Keene M, Alberti PW. Clinical Otoscopy: A Text and Colour Atlas. Edinburgh, Churchill Livingstone, 1984; *Acute Otitis Media, Bullous Myringitis*—The Wellcome Trust, National Medical Slide Bank, London, UK.)

TABLE 6-19 Patterns of Hearing Loss

	Conductive Loss	Sensorineural Loss
	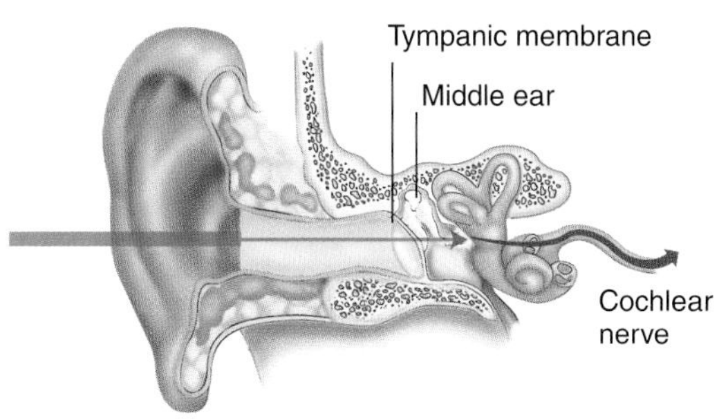	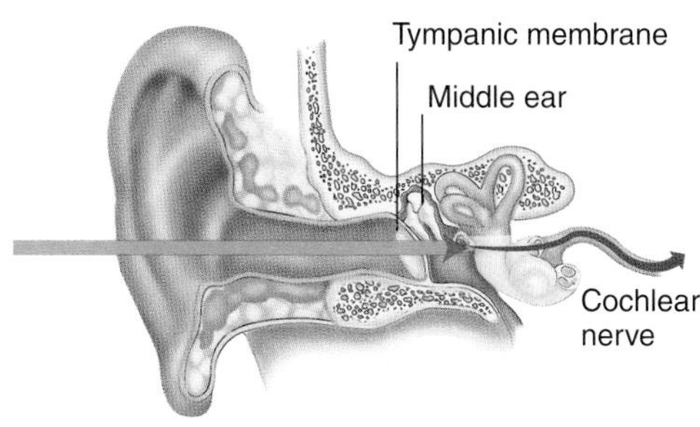
Pathophysiology	External or middle ear disorder impairs sound conduction to inner ear. Causes include foreign body, *otitis media,* perforated eardrum, and otosclerosis of ossicles.	Inner ear disorder involves cochlear nerve and neuronal impulse transmission to the brain. Causes include loud noise exposure, inner ear infections, trauma, tremors, congenital and familial disorders, and aging.
Usual Age of Onset	Childhood and young adulthood, up to age 40	Middle or later years
Ear Canal and Drum	Abnormality usually visible, except in otosclerosis	Problem not visible
Effects	▪ Little effect on sound ▪ Hearing seems to improve in noisy environment ▪ Voice becomes soft because inner ear and cochlear nerve are intact	▪ Higher registers are lost, so sound may be distorted. ▪ Hearing worsens in noisy environment ▪ Voice may be loud because hearing is difficult.
Weber Test ***(in unilateral hearing loss)***	▪ Tuning fork at vertex ▪ Sound lateralizes to *impaired ear*—room noise not well heard, so detection of vibrations *improves.*	▪ Tuning fork at vertex ▪ Sound lateralizes to *good ear*—inner ear or cochlear nerve damage impairs transmission to affected ear
Rinne Test	▪ Tuning fork at external auditory meatus then on mastoid bone ▪ Bone conduction longer than or equal to air conduction (BC ≥ AC). While air conduction through the external or middle ear is impaired, vibrations through bone bypass the problem to reach the cochlea.	▪ Tuning fork at external auditory meatus then on mastoid bone ▪ Air conduction longer than bone conduction (AC > BC). The inner ear or cochlear nerve is less able to transmit impulses regardless of how the vibrations reach the cochlea. The normal pattern prevails.

TABLE 6-20 Abnormalities of the Lips

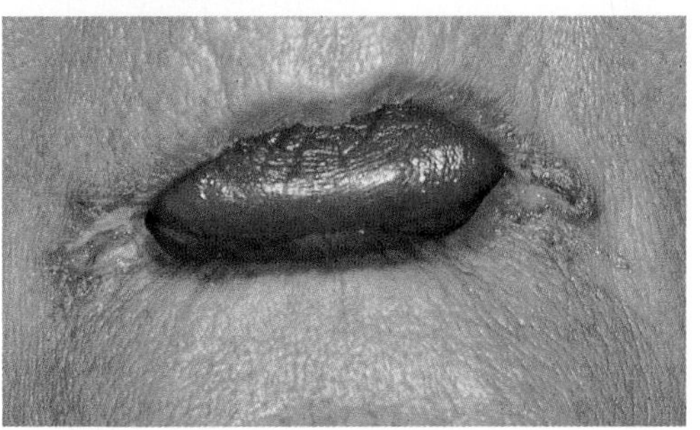

Angular Cheilitis

Angular cheilitis starts with softening of the skin at the angles of the mouth, followed by fissuring. It may be due to nutritional deficiency or, more commonly, to overclosure of the mouth, as in people with no teeth or with ill-fitting dentures. Saliva wets and macerates the infolded skin, often leading to secondary infection with *Candida*, as in this example.

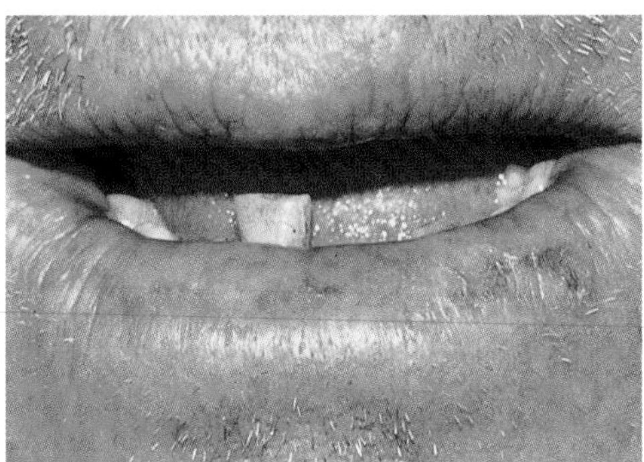

Actinic Cheilitis

Actinic cheilitis results from excessive exposure to sunlight and affects primarily the lower lip. Fair-skinned men who work outdoors are most often affected. The lip loses its normal redness and may become scaly, somewhat thickened, and slightly everted. Because solar damage also predisposes to carcinoma of the lip, be alert to this possibility.

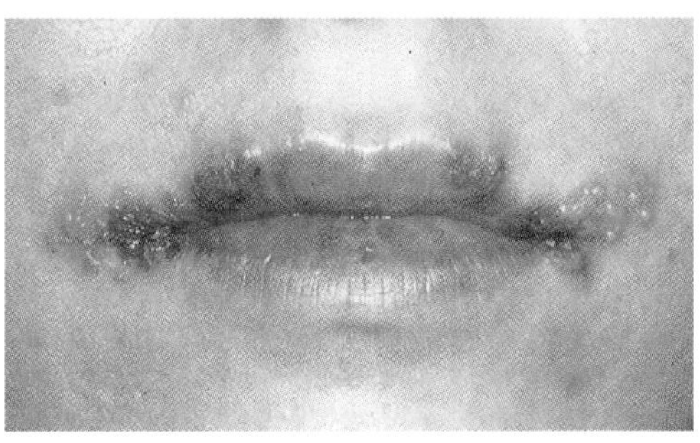

Herpes Simplex *(Cold Sore, Fever Blister)*

The herpes simplex virus (HSV) produces recurrent and painful vesicular eruptions of the lips and surrounding skin. A small cluster of vesicles first develops. As these break, yellow-brown crusts form, and healing ensues within 10 to 14 days. Both of these stages are visible here.

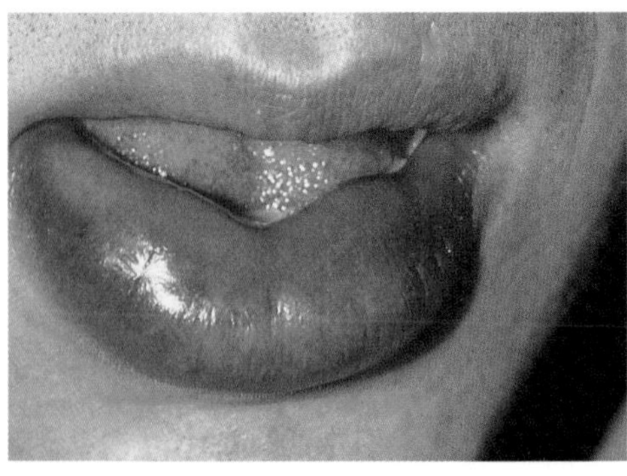

Angioedema

Angioedema is a diffuse, nonpitting, tense swelling of the dermis and subcutaneous tissue. It develops rapidly, and typically disappears over subsequent hours or days. Although usually allergic in nature and sometimes associated with hives, angioedema does not itch.

(Sources of photos: *Angular Cheilitis, Herpes Simplex, Angioedema*—Neville B, et al. Color Atlas of Clinical Oral Pathology. Philadelphia, Lea & Febiger, 1991; Used with permission; *Actinic Cheilitis*—Langlais RP, Miller CS. Color Atlas of Common Oral Diseases. Philadelphia, Lea & Febiger, 1992. Used with permission.)

(table continues next page)

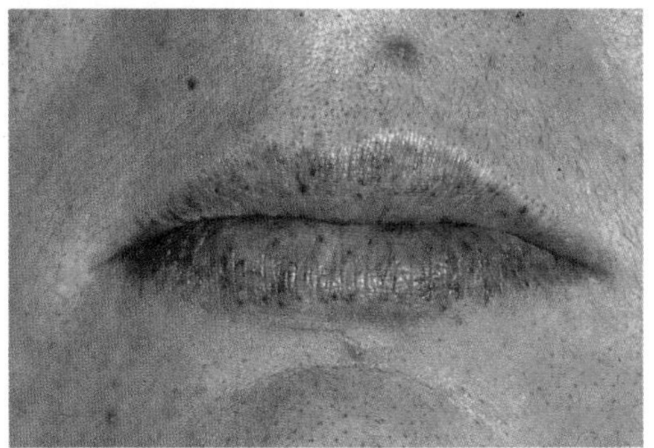

Hereditary Hemorrhagic Telangiectasia

Multiple small red spots on the lips strongly suggest hereditary hemorrhagic telangiectasia. Spots may also be visible on the face and hands and in the mouth. The spots are dilated capillaries and may bleed when traumatized. Affected people often have nosebleeds and gastrointestinal bleeding.

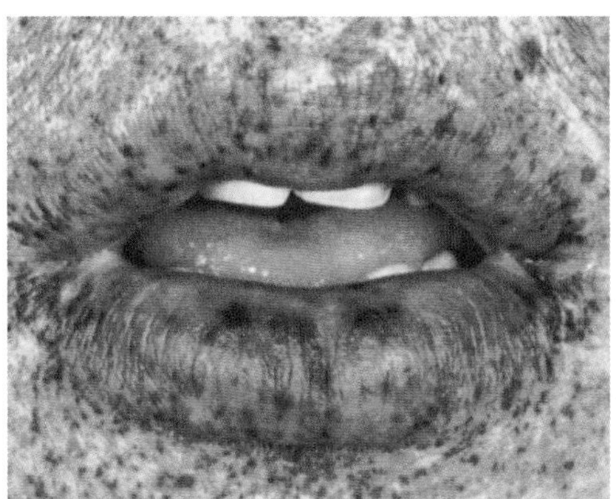

Peutz-Jeghers Syndrome

When pigmented spots on the lips are more prominent than freckling of the surrounding skin, suspect this syndrome. Pigment in the buccal mucosa helps to confirm the diagnosis. Pigmented spots may also be found on the face and hands. Multiple intestinal polyps are often associated.

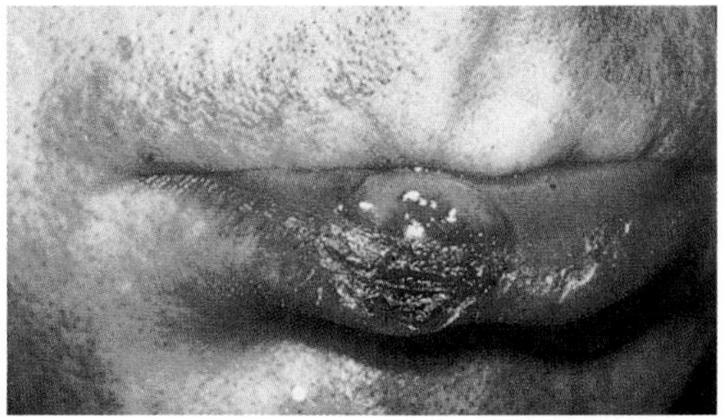

Chancre of Syphilis

This lesion of primary syphilis may appear on the lip rather than on the genitalia. It is a firm, buttonlike lesion that ulcerates and may become crusted. A chancre may resemble a carcinoma or a crusted cold sore. Because it is infectious, use gloves to feel any suspicious lesion.

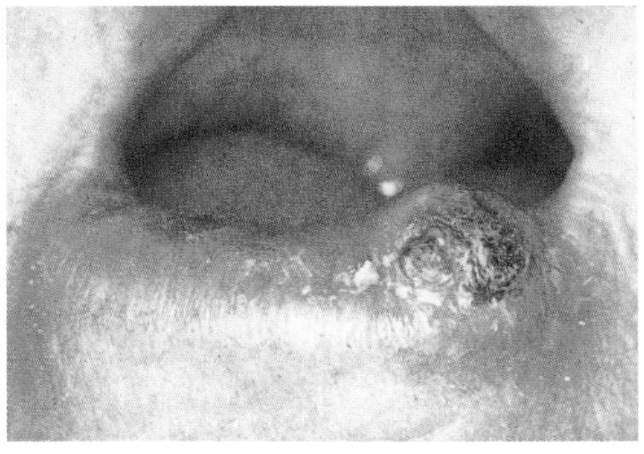

Carcinoma of the Lip

Like actinic cheilitis, carcinoma usually affects the lower lip. It may appear as a scaly plaque, as an ulcer with or without a crust, or as a nodular lesion, illustrated here. Fair skin and prolonged exposure to the sun are common risk factors.

(Sources of photos: *Hereditary Hemorrhagic Telangiectasia*—Langlais RP, Miller CS. Color Atlas of Common Oral Diseases. Philadelphia, Lea & Febiger, 1992; Used with permission; *Peutz-Jeghers Syndrome*—Robinson HBG, Miller AS. Colby, Kerr, and Robinson's Color Atlas of Oral Pathology. Philadelphia, JB Lippincott, 1990; *Chancre of Syphilis*—Wisdom A. A Colour Atlas of Sexually Transmitted Diseases, 2nd ed. London, Wolfe Medical Publications, 1989; *Carcinoma of the Lip*—Tyldesley WR. A Colour Atlas of Orofacial Diseases, 2nd ed. London, Wolfe Medical Publications, 1991.)

TABLE 6-21 Findings in the Pharynx, Palate, and Oral Mucosa

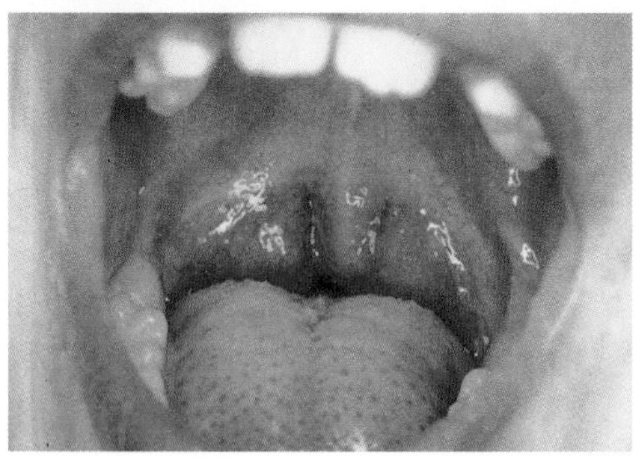

Large Normal Tonsils

Normal tonsils may be large without being infected, especially in children. They may protrude medially beyond the pillars and even to the midline. Here they touch the sides of the uvula and obscure the pharynx. Their color is within normal limits. The white marks are light reflections, not exudate.

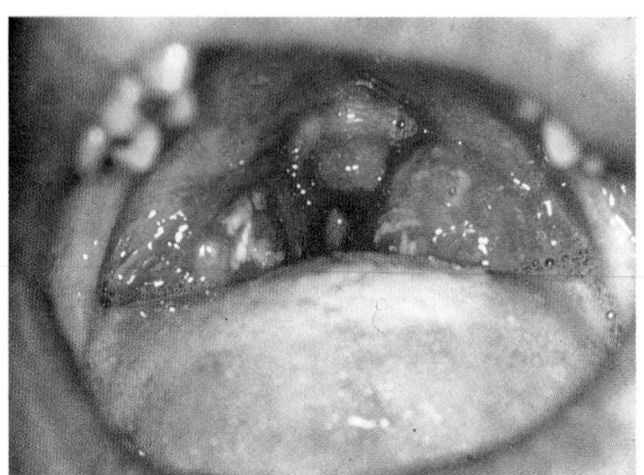

Exudative Tonsillitis

This red throat has a white exudate on the tonsils. This, together with fever and enlarged cervical nodes, increases the probability of *group A streptococcal infection*, or infectious mononucleosis. Some anterior cervical lymph nodes are usually enlarged in the former, posterior nodes in the latter.

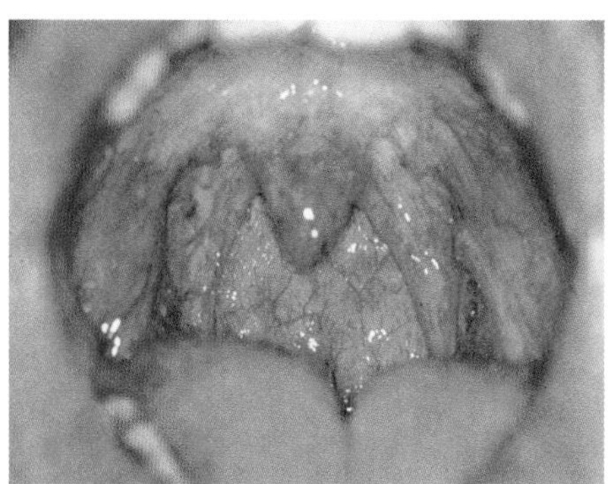

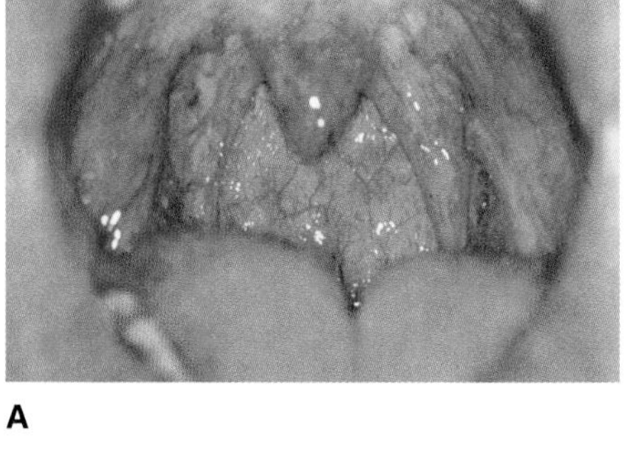

A

Pharyngitis

These two photos show reddened throats without exudate.

In **A**, redness and vascularity of the pillars and uvula are mild to moderate.

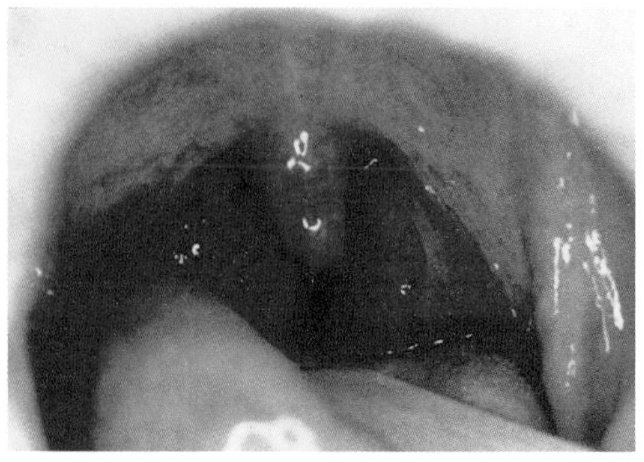

B

In **B**, redness is diffuse and intense. Each patient would probably complain of a sore throat, or at least a scratchy one. Possible causes include several kinds of viruses and bacteria. If the patient has no fever, exudate, or enlargement of cervical lymph node, the chances of infection by either of two common causes—*group A streptococci* and *Epstein-Barr virus* (infectious mononucleosis)—are very small.

(Sources of photos: *Large Normal Tonsils, Exudative Tonsillitis, Pharyngitis [**A and B**]*—The Wellcome Trust, National Medical Slide Bank, London, UK.)

(table continues next page)

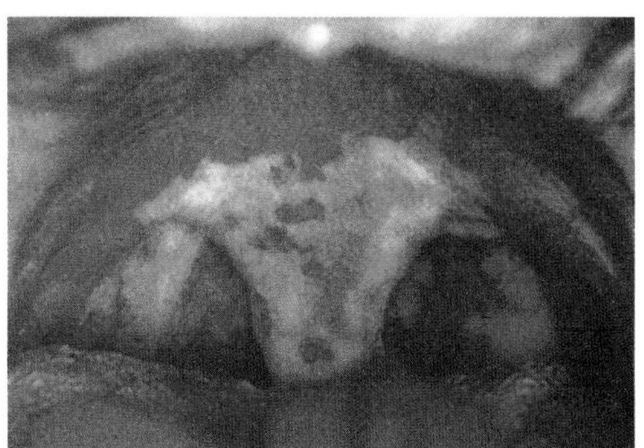

Diphtheria

Diphtheria (an acute infection caused by *Corynebacterium diphtheriae*) is now rare but still important. Prompt diagnosis may lead to life-saving treatment. The throat is dull red, and a gray exudate (pseudomembrane) is present on the uvula, pharynx, and tongue. The airway may become obstructed.

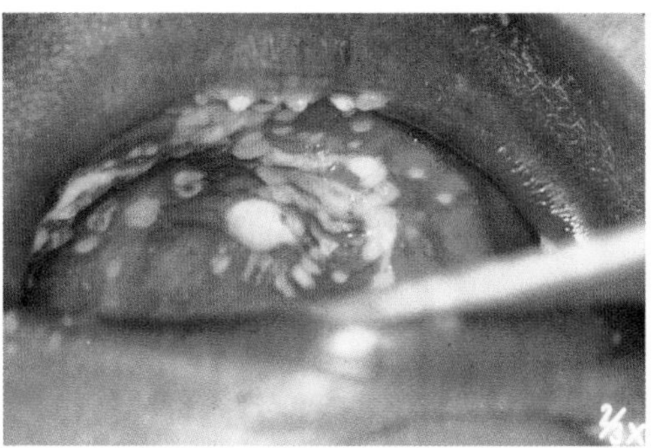

Thrush on the Palate (Candidiasis)

Thrush is a yeast infection due to *Candida*. Shown here on the palate, it may appear elsewhere in the mouth (see p. 237). Thick, white plaques are somewhat adherent to the underlying mucosa. Predisposing factors include (1) prolonged treatment with antibiotics or corticosteroids, and (2) AIDS.

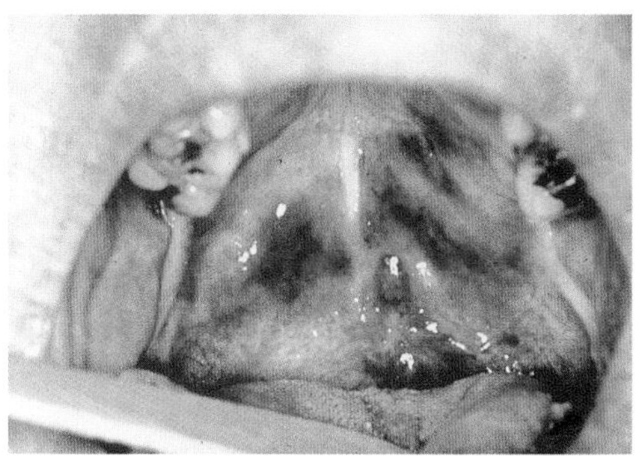

Kaposi's Sarcoma in AIDS

The deep purple color of these lesions, although not necessarily present, strongly suggests Kaposi's sarcoma. The lesions may be raised or flat. Among people with AIDS, the palate, as illustrated here, is a common site for this tumor.

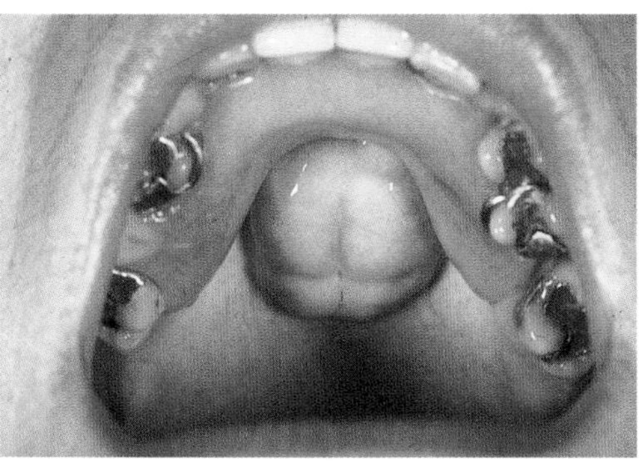

Torus Palatinus

A torus palatinus is a midline bony growth in the hard palate that is fairly common in adults. Its size and lobulation vary. Although alarming at first glance, it is harmless. In this example, an upper denture has been fitted around the torus.

(Sources of photos: *Diphtheria*—Harnisch JP, et al. Diphtheria among alcoholic urban adults. Ann Intern Med 1989;111:77; *Thrush on the Palate*—The Wellcome Trust, National Medical Slide Bank, London, UK; *Kaposi's Sarcoma in AIDS*—Ioachim HL. Textbook and Atlas of Disease Associated With Acquired Immune Deficiency Syndrome. London, UK, Gower Medical Publishing, 1989.)

(table continues next page)

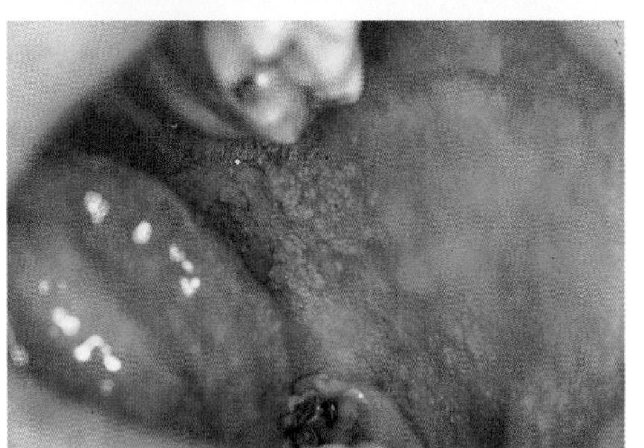

Fordyce Spots *(Fordyce Granules)*

Fordyce spots are normal sebaceous glands that appear as small yellowish spots in the buccal mucosa or on the lips. A worried person who has suddenly noticed them may be reassured. Here they are seen best anterior to the tongue and lower jaw. These spots are usually not so numerous.

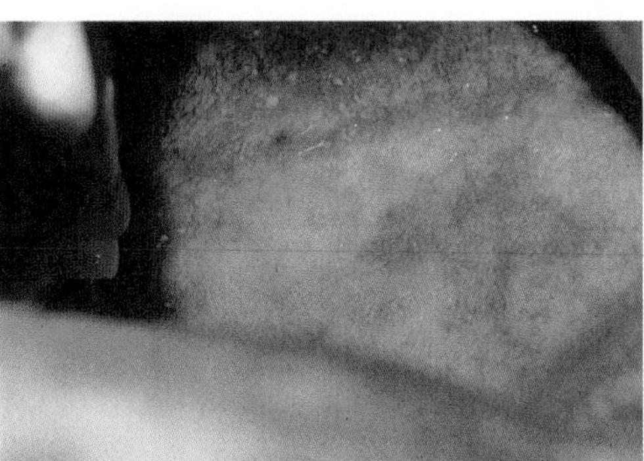

Koplik's Spots

Koplik's spots are an early sign of measles (rubeola). Search for small white specks that resemble grains of salt on a red background. They usually appear on the buccal mucosa near the first and second molars. In this photo, look also in the upper third of the mucosa. The rash of measles appears within a day.

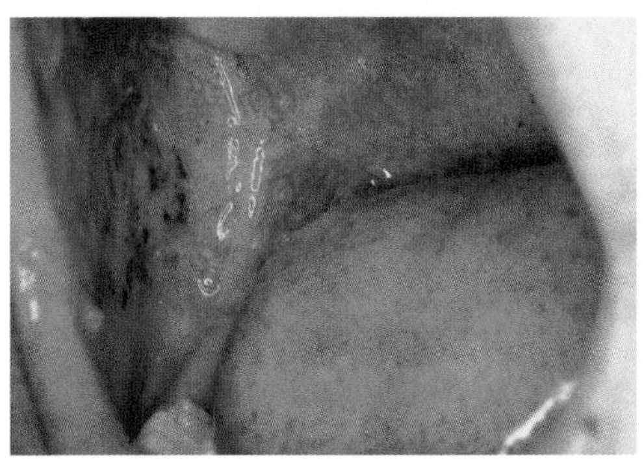

Petechiae

Petechiae are small red spots that result when blood escapes from capillaries into the tissues. Petechiae in the buccal mucosa, as shown, are often caused by accidentally biting the cheek. Oral petechiae may be due to infection or decreased platelets, as well as to trauma.

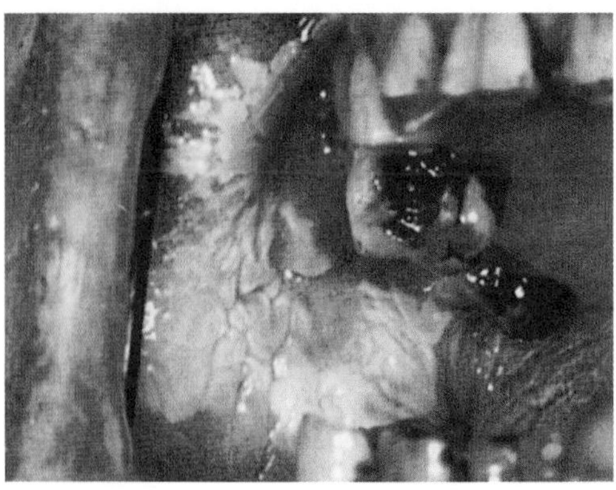

Leukoplakia

A thickened white patch (*leukoplakia*) may occur anywhere in the oral mucosa. The extensive example shown on this buccal mucosa resulted from frequent chewing of tobacco, a local irritant. This kind of irritation may lead to cancer.

(Sources of photos: *Fordyce Spots*—Neville B, et al. Color Atlas of Clinical Oral Pathology. Philadelphia, Lea & Febiger, 1991; Used with permission; *Koplik's Spots, Petechiae*—The Wellcome Trust, National Medical Slide Bank, London, UK; *Leukoplakia*—Robinson HBG, Miller AS. Colby, Kerr, and Robinson's Color Atlas of Oral Pathology. Philadelphia, JB Lippincott, 1990.)

TABLE 6-22 Findings in the Gums and Teeth

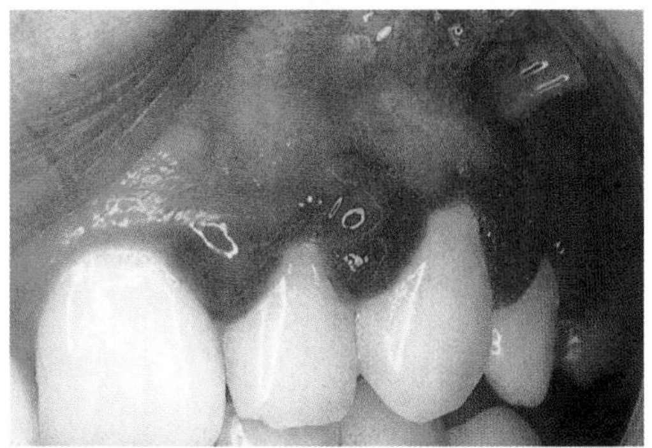

Marginal Gingivitis

Marginal gingivitis is common among teenagers and young adults. The gingival margins are reddened and swollen, and the interdental papillae are blunted, swollen, and red. Brushing the teeth often makes the gums bleed. *Plaque*—the soft white film of salivary salts, protein, and bacteria that covers the teeth and leads to gingivitis—is not readily visible.

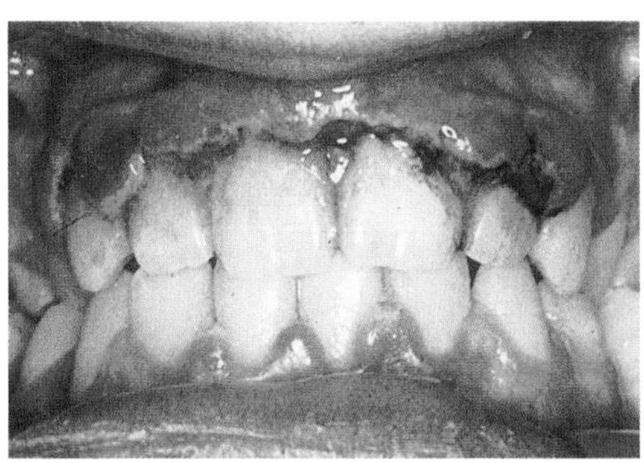

Acute Necrotizing Ulcerative Gingivitis

This uncommon form of gingivitis occurs suddenly in adolescents and young adults and is accompanied by fever, malaise, and enlarged lymph nodes. Ulcers develop in the interdental papillae. Then the destructive (necrotizing) process spreads along the gum margins, where a grayish pseudomembrane develops. The red, painful gums bleed easily; the breath is foul.

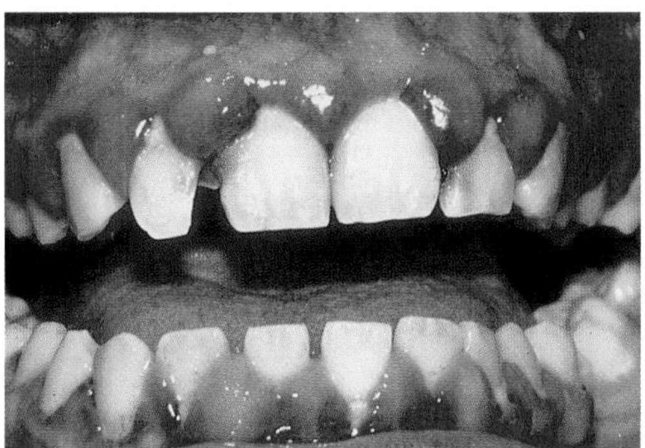

Gingival Hyperplasia

Gums enlarged by hyperplasia are swollen into heaped-up masses that may even cover the teeth. The redness of inflammation may coexist, as in this example. Causes include dilantin therapy (as in this case), puberty, pregnancy, and leukemia.

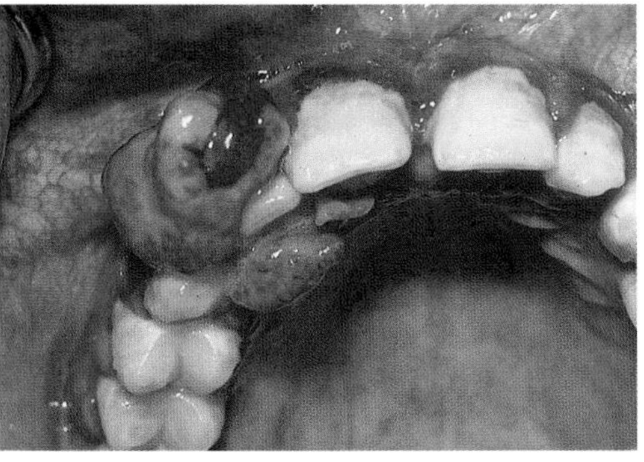

Pregnancy Tumor (Epulis, Pyogenic Granuloma)

Gingival enlargement may be localized, forming a tumorlike mass that usually originates in an interdental papilla. It is red and soft and usually bleeds easily. The estimated incidence of this lesion in pregnancy is about 1%. Note the accompanying gingivitis in this example.

(Sources of photos: *Marginal Gingivitis, Acute Necrotizing Ulcerative Gingivitis*—Tyldesley WR. A Colour Atlas of Orofacial Diseases, 2nd ed. London, Wolfe Medical Publications, 1991; *Gingival Hyperplasia*—Courtesy of Dr. James Cottone; *Pregnancy Tumor*—Langlais RP, Miller CS. Color Atlas of Common Oral Diseases. Philadelphia, Lea & Febiger, 1992. Used with permission.)

(table continues next page)

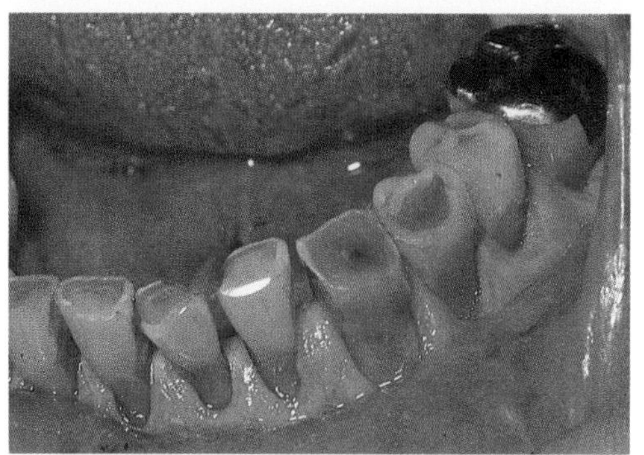

Attrition of Teeth; Recession of Gums

In many elderly people, the chewing surfaces of the teeth have been worn down by repetitive use so that the yellow-brown dentin becomes exposed—a process called *attrition*. Note also the *recession of the gums*, which has exposed the roots of the teeth, giving a "long in the tooth" appearance.

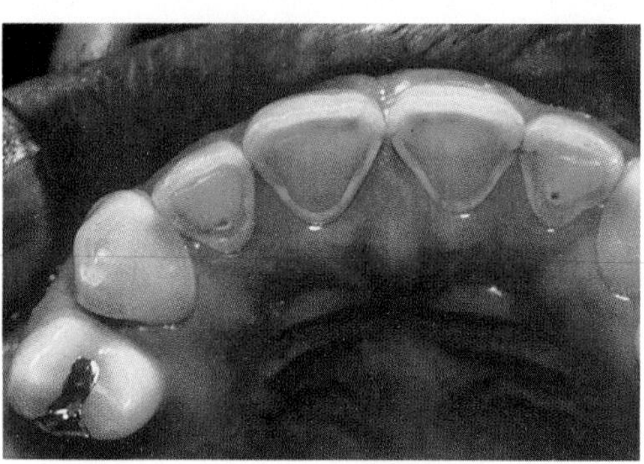

Erosion of Teeth

Teeth may be eroded by chemical action. Note here the erosion of the enamel from the lingual surfaces of the upper incisors, exposing the yellow-brown dentin. This results from recurrent regurgitation of stomach contents, as in bulimia.

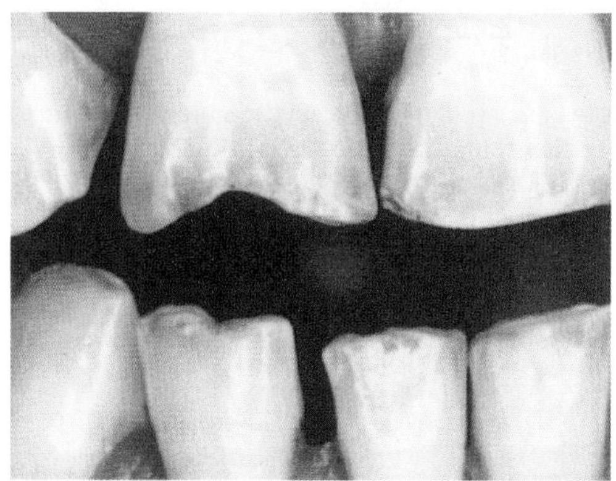

Abrasion of Teeth With Notching

The biting surface of the teeth may become abraded or notched by recurrent trauma, such as holding nails or opening bobby pins between the teeth. Unlike Hutchinson's teeth, the sides of these teeth show normal contours; size and spacing of the teeth are unaffected.

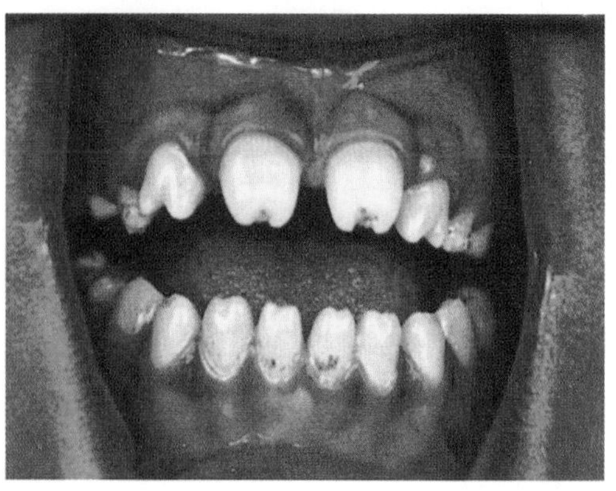

Hutchinson's Teeth

Hutchinson's teeth are smaller and more widely spaced than normal and are notched on their biting surfaces. The sides of the teeth taper toward the biting edges. The upper central incisors of the permanent (not the deciduous) teeth are most often affected. These teeth are a sign of congenital syphilis.

(Sources of photos: *Attrition of Teeth, Erosion of Teeth*—Langlais RP, Miller CS. Color Atlas of Common Oral Diseases. Philadelphia, Lea & Febiger, 1992. Used with permission; *Abrasion of Teeth, Hutchinson's Teeth*—Robinson HBG, Miller AS. Colby, Kerr, and Robinson's Color Atlas of Oral Pathology. Philadelphia, JB Lippincott, 1990.)

TABLE 6-23 Findings in or Under the Tongue

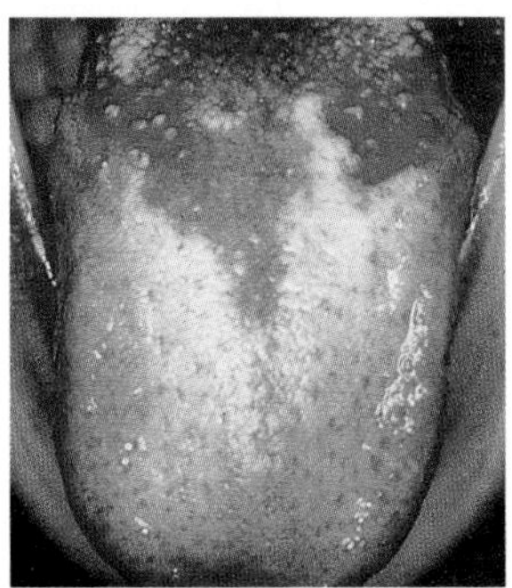

Geographic Tongue. In this benign condition, the dorsum shows scattered smooth red areas denuded of papillae. Together with the normal rough and coated areas, they give a maplike pattern that changes over time.

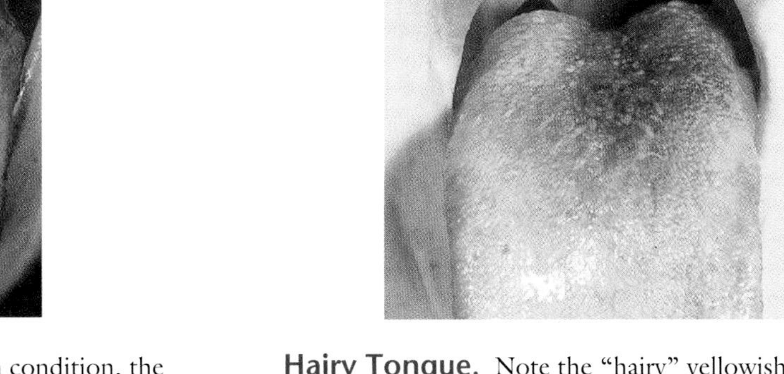

Hairy Tongue. Note the "hairy" yellowish to brown or black elongated papillae on the tongue's dorsum. This benign condition may follow antibiotic therapy; it also may occur spontaneously.

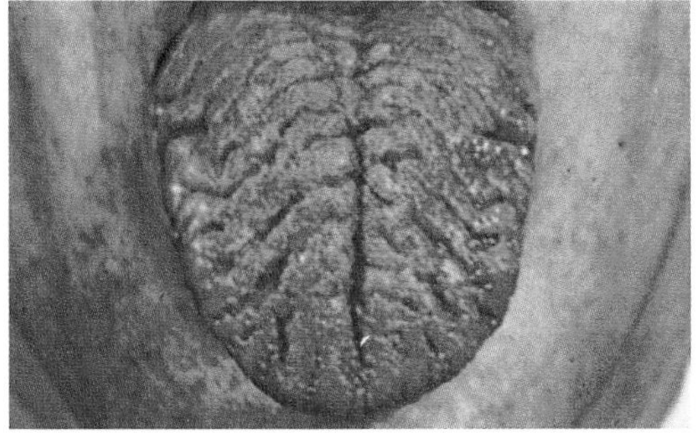

Fissured Tongue. Fissures appear with increasing age, sometimes termed *scrotal tongue*. Food debris may accumulate in the crevices and become irritating, but a fissured tongue is benign.

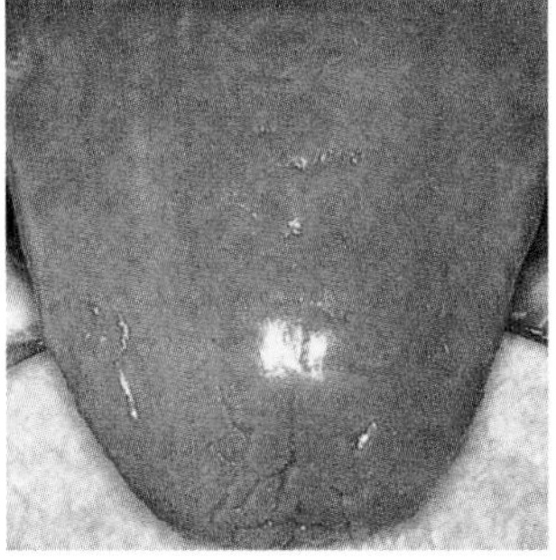

Smooth Tongue (Atrophic Glossitis). A smooth and often sore tongue that has lost its papillae suggests a deficiency in riboflavin, niacin, folic acid, vitamin B_{12}, pyridoxine, or iron, or treatment with chemotherapy.

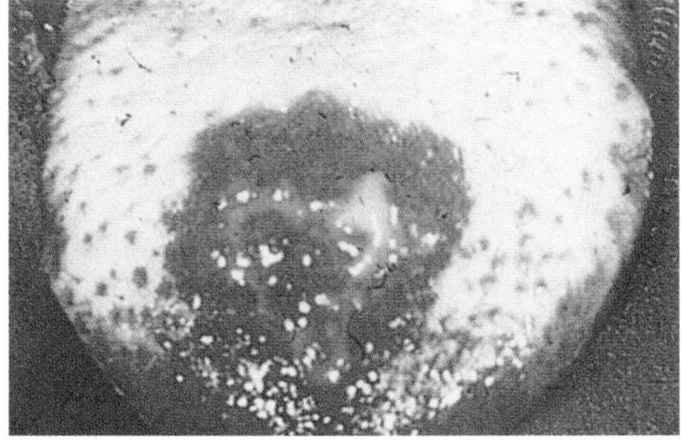

Candidiasis. Note the thick white coating from *Candida* infection. The raw red surface is where the coat was scraped off. Infection may also occur without the white coating. It is seen in immunosuppressed conditions.

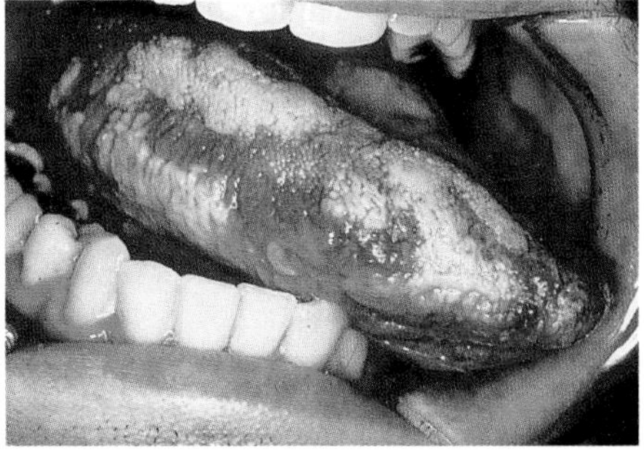

Hairy Leukoplakia. These whitish raised areas with a feathery or corrugated pattern most often affect the sides of the tongue. Unlike candidiasis, these areas cannot be scraped off. They are seen with HIV and AIDS.

(table continues next page)

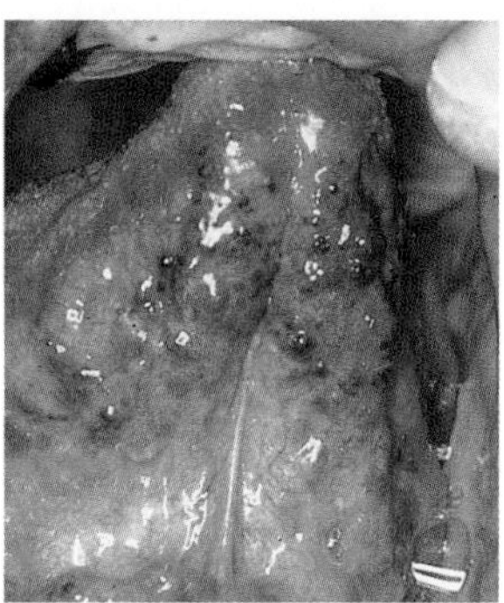

Varicose Veins. Small purplish or blue-black round swellings appear under the tongue with age. These dilatations of the lingual veins have no clinical significance.

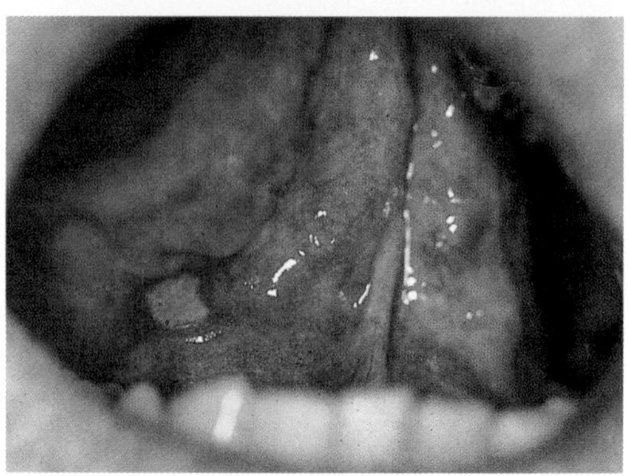

Aphthous Ulcer (Canker Sore). A painful, round or oval ulcer that is white or yellowish gray and surrounded by a halo of reddened mucosa. It may be single or multiple. It heals in 7–10 days, but may recur.

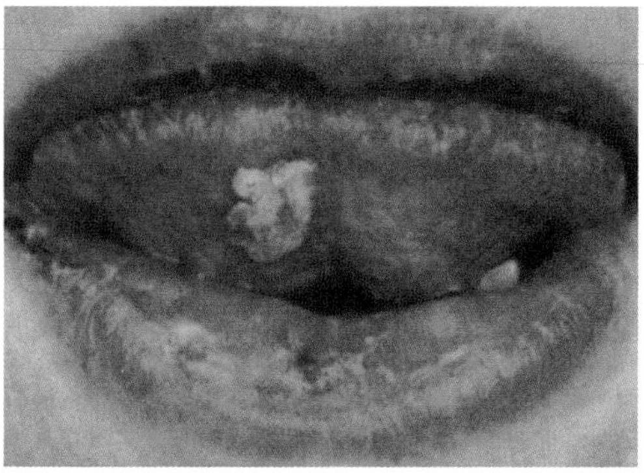

Mucous Patch of Syphilis. This painless lesion in the secondary stage of syphilis is highly infectious. It is slightly raised, oval, and covered by a grayish membrane. It may be multiple and occur elsewhere in the mouth.

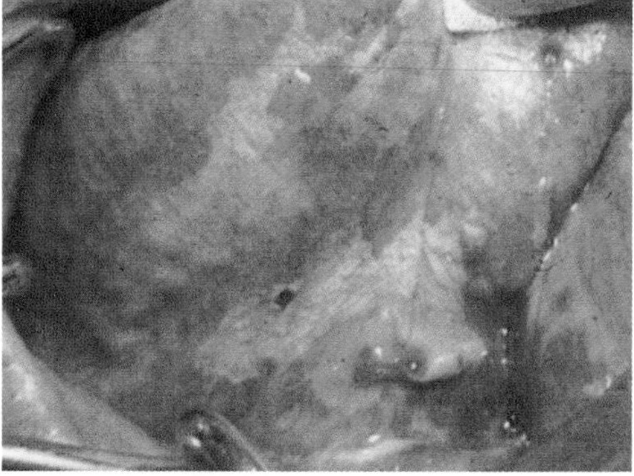

Leukoplakia. With this persisting painless white patch in the oral mucosa, the undersurface of the tongue appears painted white. Patches of any size raise the possibility of malignancy and require a biopsy.

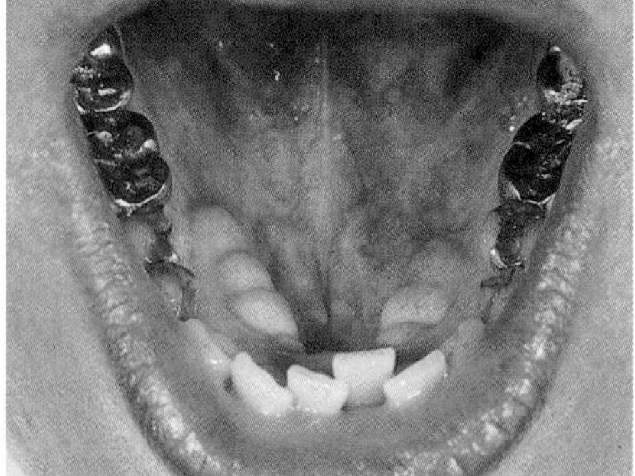

Tori Mandibulares. Rounded bony growths on the inner surfaces of the mandible are typically bilateral, asymptomatic, and harmless.

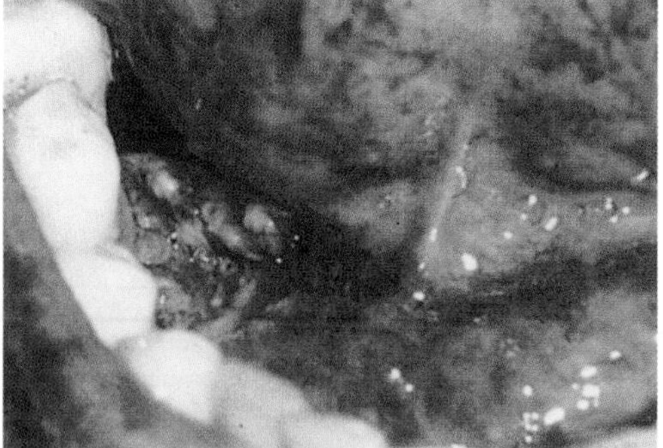

Carcinoma, Floor of the Mouth. This ulcerated lesion is in a common location for carcinoma. Medially, note the reddened area of mucosa, called *erythroplakia,* suggesting possible malignancy.

(Sources of photos: *Fissured Tongue, Candidiasis, Mucous Patch, Leukoplakia, Carcinoma*—Robinson HBG, Miller AS. Colby, Kerr, and Robinson's Color Atlas of Oral Pathology. Philadelphia, JB Lippincott, 1990; *Smooth Tongue*—Courtesy of Dr. R. A. Cawson, from Cawson RA. Oral Pathology, 1st ed. London, UK, Gower Medical Publishing, 1987; *Geographic Tongue*—The Wellcome Trust, National Medical Slide Bank, London, UK; *Hairy Leukoplakia*—Ioachim HL. Textbook and Atlas of Disease Associated With Acquired Immune Deficiency Syndrome. London, UK, Gower Medical Publishing, 1989; *Varicose Veins*—Neville B, et al. Color Atlas of Clinical Oral Pathology. Philadelphia, Lea & Febiger, 1991. Used with permission.)

TABLE 6-24 Thyroid Enlargement and Function

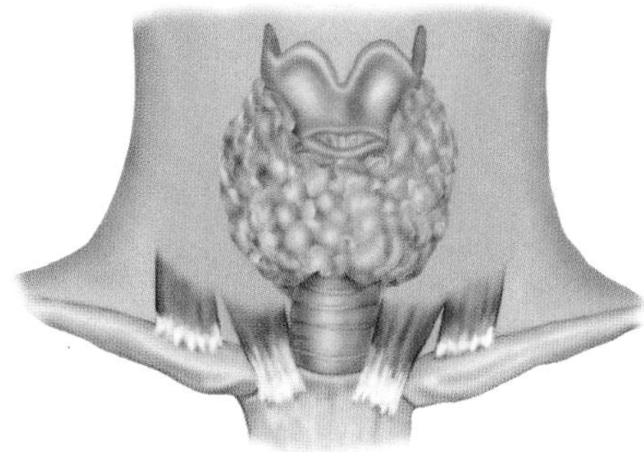

Diffuse Enlargement. Includes the isthmus and lateral lobes; there are no discretely palpable nodules. Causes include Graves' disease, Hashimoto's thyroiditis, and endemic goiter.

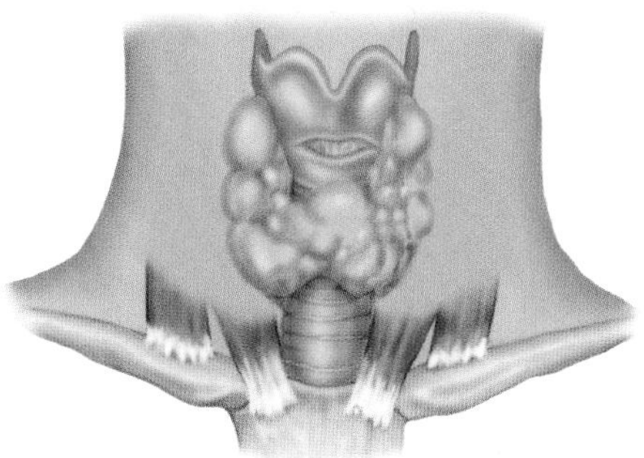

Single Nodule. May be a cyst, a benign tumor, or one nodule within a multinodular gland. It raises the question of malignancy. Risk factors are prior irradiation, hardness, rapid growth, fixation to surrounding tissues, enlarged cervical nodes, and occurrence in males.[17]

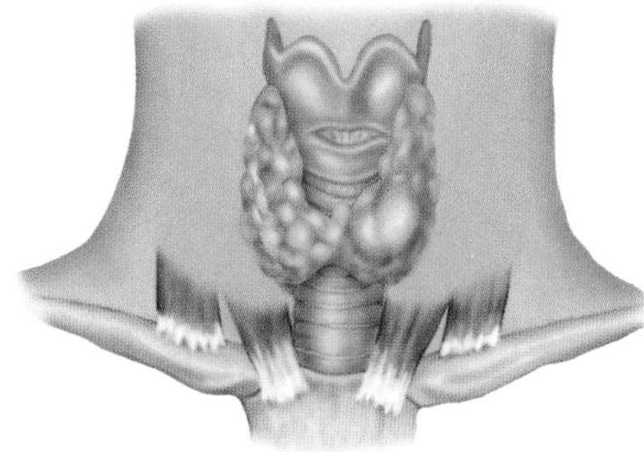

Multinodular Goiter. An enlarged thyroid gland with two or more nodules suggests a metabolic rather than a neoplastic process. Positive family history and continuing nodular enlargement are additional risk factors for malignancy.

TABLE 6-25 Symptoms and Signs of Thyroid Dysfunction[15,16]

	Hyperthyroidism	Hypothyroidism
Symptoms	Nervousness Weight loss despite increased appetite Excessive sweating and heat intolerance Palpitations Frequent bowel movements Muscular weakness of the proximal type and tremor	Fatigue, lethargy Modest weight gain with anorexia Dry, coarse skin and cold intolerance Swelling of face, hands, and legs Constipation Weakness, muscle cramps, arthralgias, paresthesias, impaired memory and hearing
Signs	Warm, smooth, moist skin	Dry, coarse, cool skin, sometimes yellowish from carotene, with nonpitting edema and loss of hair
	With Graves' disease, eye signs such as stare, lid lag, and exophthalmos	Periorbital puffiness
	Increased systolic and decreased diastolic blood pressures	Decreased systolic and increased diastolic blood pressures
	Tachycardia or atrial fibrillation	Bradycardia and, in late stages, hypothermia
	Hyperdynamic cardiac pulsations with an accentuated S_1	Intensity of heart sounds sometimes decreased
	Tremor and proximal muscle weakness	Impaired memory, mixed hearing loss, somnolence, peripheral neuropathy, carpal tunnel syndrome

CHAPTER

7

The Thorax and Lungs

ANATOMY AND PHYSIOLOGY

Study the *anatomy of the chest wall,* identifying the structures illustrated. Note that an interspace between two ribs is numbered by the rib above it.

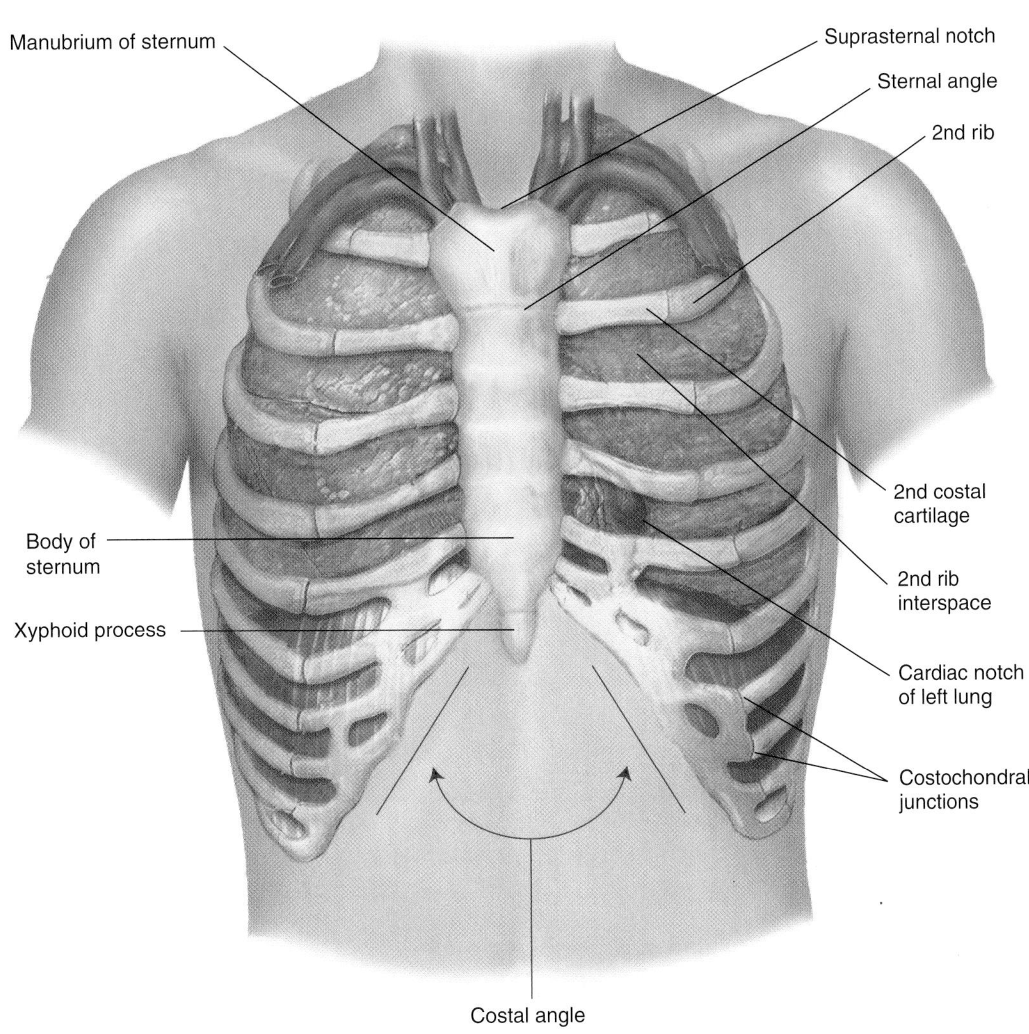

Locating Findings on the Chest. Describe abnormalities of the chest in two dimensions: *along the vertical axis* and *around the circumference of the chest.*

To make *vertical* locations, you must be able to count the ribs and interspaces. The *sternal angle,* also termed the angle of Louis, is the best guide: place your finger in the hollow curve of the suprasternal notch, then move your finger down about 5 cm to the horizontal bony ridge joining the manubrium to the body of the sternum. Then move your finger laterally and find the adjacent 2nd rib and costal cartilage. From here, using two fingers, "walk down the interspaces," one space at a time, on an oblique line illustrated by the red numbers below. Do not try to count interspaces along the lower edge of the sternum; the ribs there are too close together. In a woman, to find the interspaces, either displace the breast laterally or palpate a little more medially than illustrated. Avoid pressing too hard on tender breast tissue.

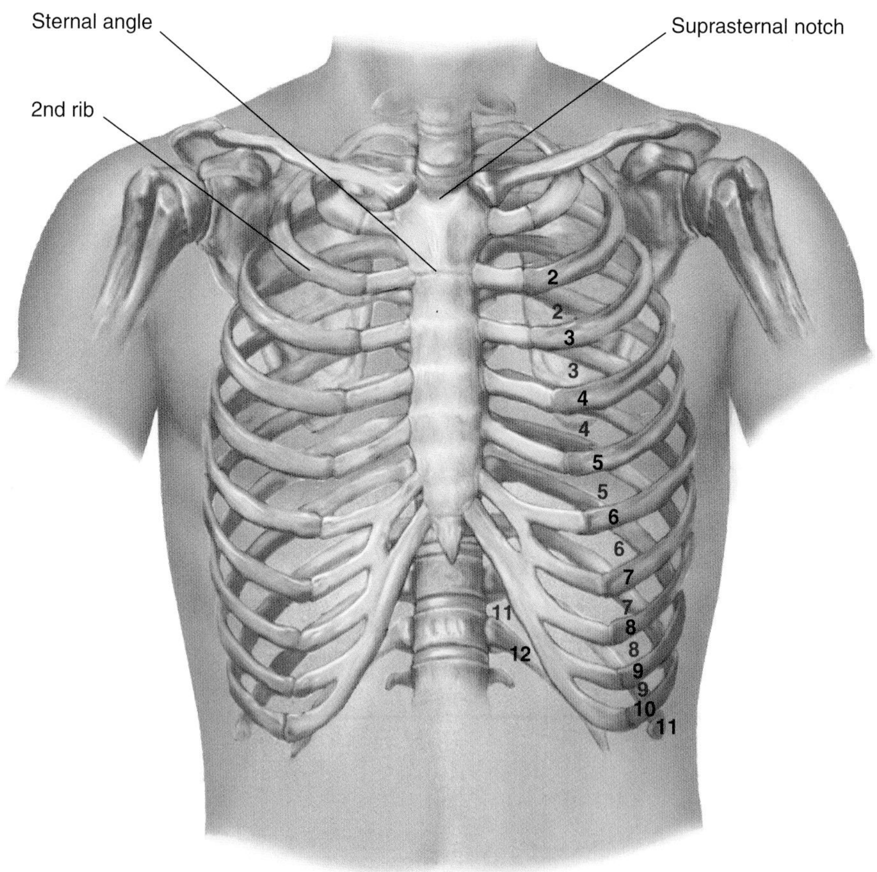

Note that the costal cartilages of the first seven ribs articulate with the sternum; the cartilages of the 8th, 9th, and 10th ribs articulate with the costal cartilages just above them. The 11th and 12th ribs, the "floating ribs," have no anterior attachments. The cartilaginous tip of the 11th rib can usually be felt laterally, and the 12th rib may be felt posteriorly. On palpation, costal cartilages and ribs feel identical.

Posteriorly, the 12th rib is another possible starting point for counting ribs and interspaces: it helps locate findings on the lower posterior chest and provides an option when the anterior approach is unsatisfactory. With the fingers of one hand, press in and up against the lower border of the 12th rib, then "walk up" the interspaces numbered in red below, or follow a more oblique line up and around to the front of the chest.

The inferior tip of the scapula is another useful bony marker—it usually lies at the level of the 7th rib or interspace.

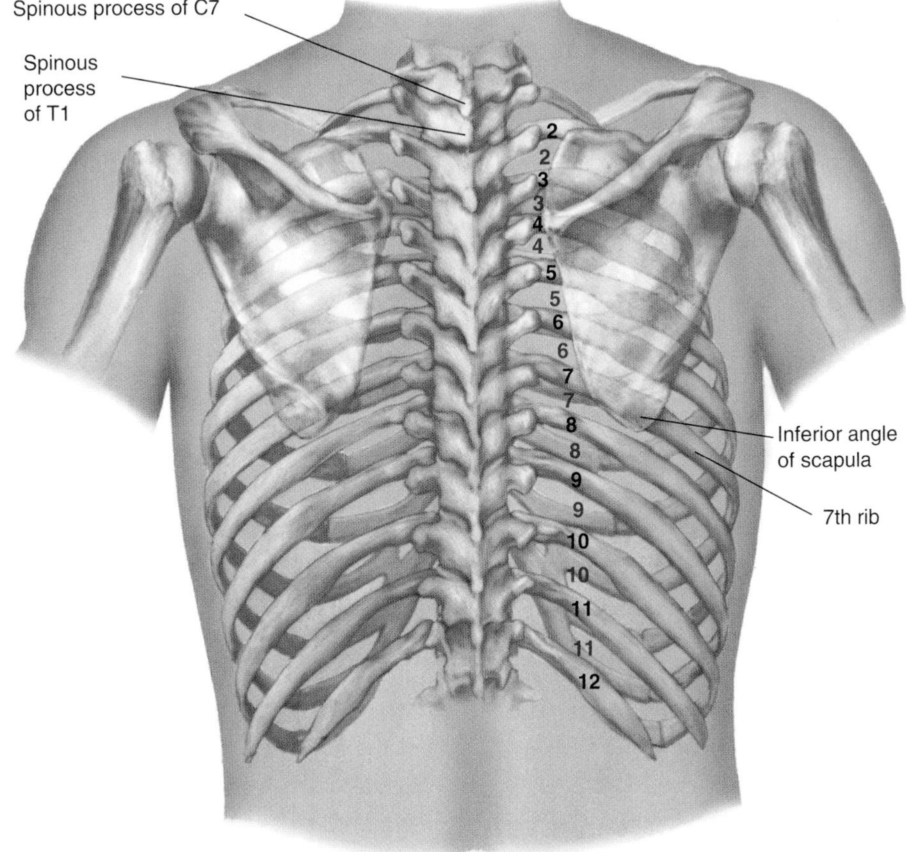

The spinous processes of the vertebrae are also useful anatomical landmarks. When the neck is flexed forward, the most protruding process is usually the vertebra of C7. If two processes are equally prominent, they are C7 and T1. You can often palpate and count the processes below them, especially when the spine is flexed.

To locate findings around the *circumference of the chest,* use a series of vertical lines, shown in the adjacent illustrations. The *midsternal* and *vertebral lines* are precise; the others are estimated. The *midclavicular line* drops vertically from the midpoint of the clavicle. To find it, you must identify both ends of the clavicle accurately (see p. 511).

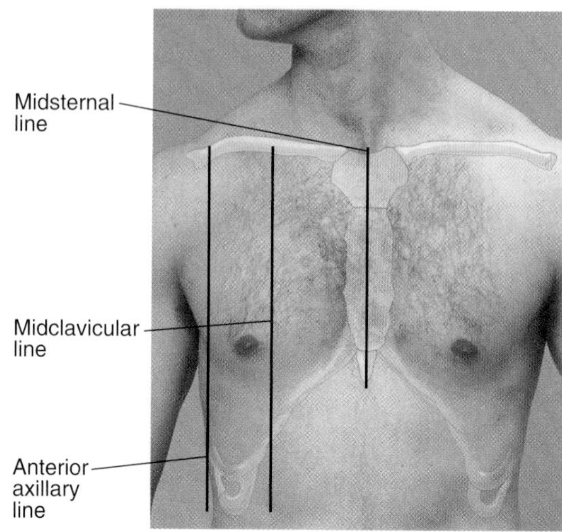

The *anterior* and *posterior axillary lines* drop vertically from the anterior and posterior axillary folds, the muscle masses that border the axilla. The *midaxillary line* drops from the apex of the axilla.

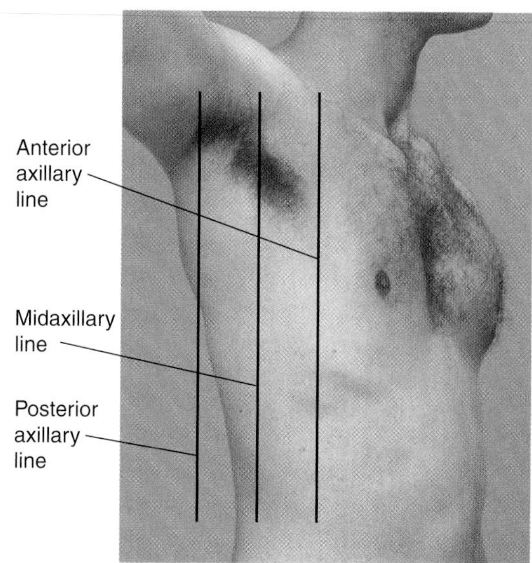

Posteriorly, the *vertebral line* overlies the spinous process of the vertebrae. The scapular line drops from the inferior angle of the scapula.

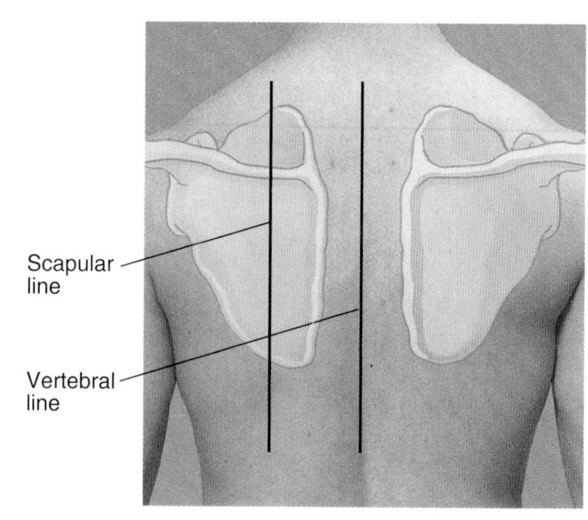

Lungs, Fissures, and Lobes. Picture the lungs and their fissures and lobes on the chest wall. Anteriorly, the apex of each lung rises about 2 cm to 4 cm above the inner third of the clavicle. The lower border of the lung crosses the 6th rib at the midclavicular line and the 8th rib at the midaxillary line. Posteriorly, the lower border of the lung lies at about the level of the T10 spinous process. On inspiration, it descends farther.

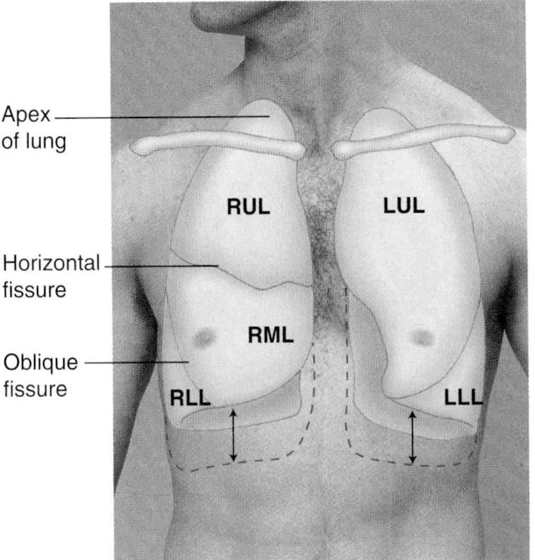

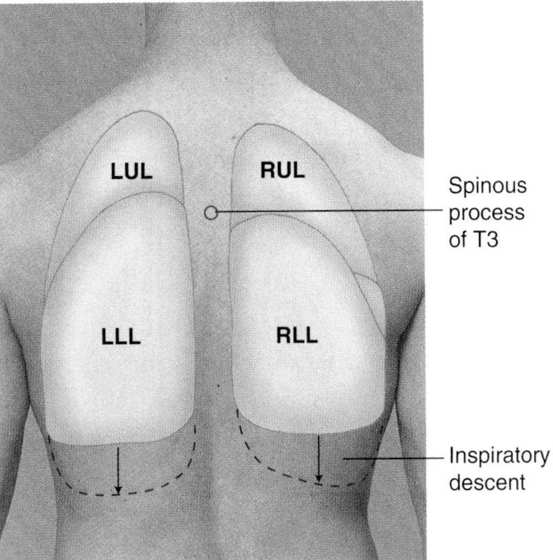

Each lung is divided roughly in half by an *oblique (major) fissure*. This fissure may be approximated by a string that runs from the T3 spinous process obliquely down and around the chest to the 6th rib at the midclavicular line. The right lung is further divided by the *horizontal (minor) fissure*. Anteriorly, this fissure runs close to the 4th rib and meets the oblique fissure in the midaxillary line near the 5th rib. The right lung is thus divided into *upper, middle,* and *lower lobes*. The left lung has only two lobes, upper and lower.

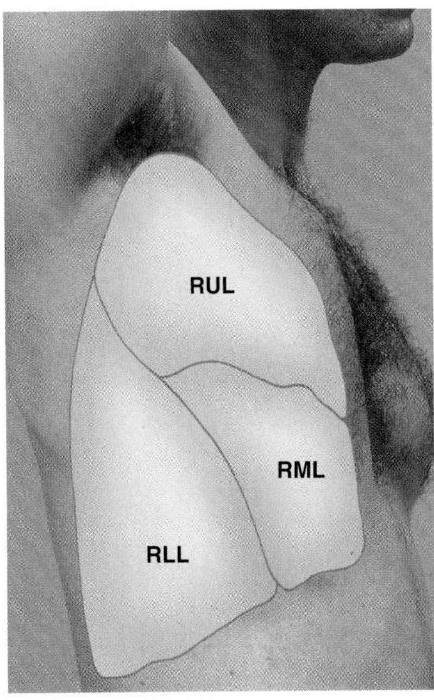

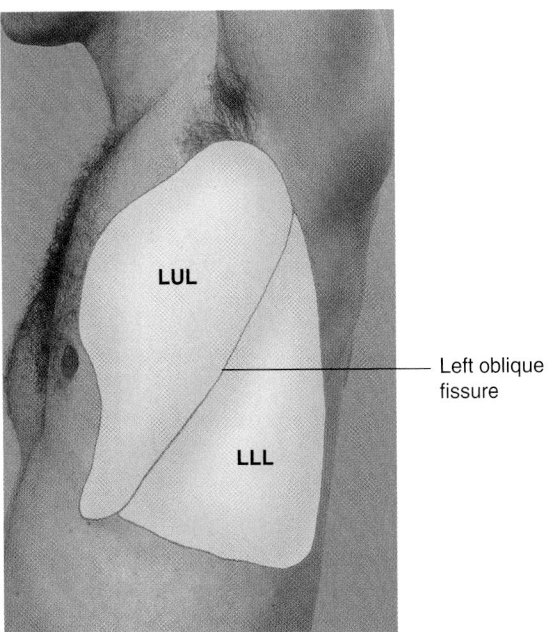

Locations on the Chest. Learn the general anatomic terms used to locate chest findings, such as:

Supraclavicular—above the clavicles
Infraclavicular—below the clavicles
Interscapular—between the scapulae
Infrascapular—below the scapulae
Bases of the lungs—the lowermost portions
Upper, middle, and lower lung fields

You may then infer what parts of the lungs are affected by an abnormal process. Signs in the right upper lung field, for example, almost certainly originate in the right upper lobe. Signs in the right middle lung field laterally, however, could come from any of three different lobes.

The Trachea and Major Bronchi. Breath sounds over the trachea and bronchi have a different quality than breath sounds over the lung parenchyma. Be sure you know the location of these structures. The trachea bifurcates into its mainstem bronchi at the levels of the sternal angle anteriorly and the T4 spinous process posteriorly.

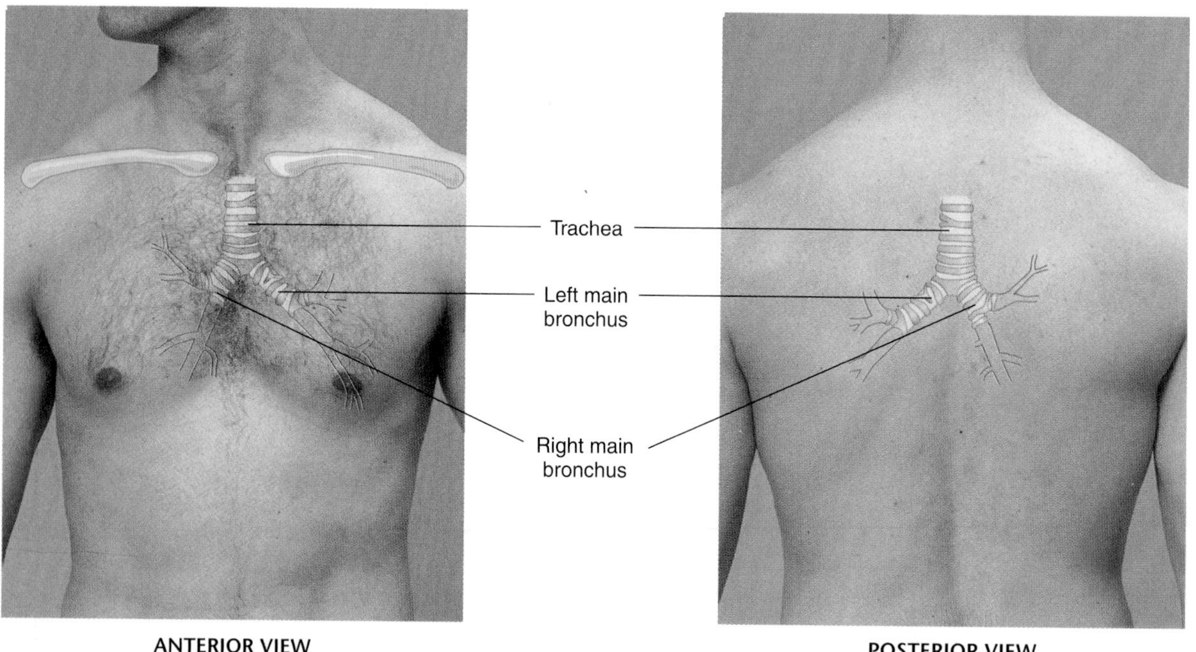

The Pleurae. The pleurae are serous membranes that cover the outer surface of each lung, the *visceral pleura,* and also line the inner rib cage and upper surface of the diaphragm, the *parietal pleura*. Their smooth opposing surfaces, lubricated by pleural fluid, allow the lungs to move easily within the rib cage during inspiration and expiration. The *pleural space* is the potential space between visceral and parietal pleurae.

Breathing. Breathing is largely an automatic act, controlled in the brainstem and mediated by the muscles of respiration. The dome-shaped *diaphragm* is the primary muscle of inspiration. When it contracts, it descends in the chest and enlarges the thoracic cavity. At the same time, it compresses the abdominal contents, pushing the abdominal wall outward. Muscles in the rib cage and neck expand the thorax during inspiration, especially the *parasternals,* which run obliquely from sternum to ribs, and the *scalenes,* which run from the cervical vertebrae to the first two ribs.

During inspiration, as these muscles contract, the thorax expands. Intrathoracic pressure decreases, drawing air through the tracheobronchial tree into the *alveoli,* or distal air sacs, and expanding the lungs. Oxygen diffuses into the blood of adjacent pulmonary capillaries, and carbon dioxide diffuses from the blood into the alveoli.

After inspiratory effort stops, the expiratory phase begins. The chest wall and lungs recoil, the diaphragm relaxes and rises passively, air flows outward, and the chest and abdomen return to their resting positions.

Normal breathing is quiet and easy—barely audible near the open mouth as a faint whish. When a healthy person lies supine, the breathing movements of the thorax are relatively slight. In contrast, the abdominal movements are usually easy to see. In the sitting position, movements of the thorax become more prominent.

During exercise and in certain diseases, extra work is required to breathe, and accessory muscles join the inspiratory effort. The sternomastoids are the most important of these, and the scalenes may become visible. Abdominal muscles assist in expiration.

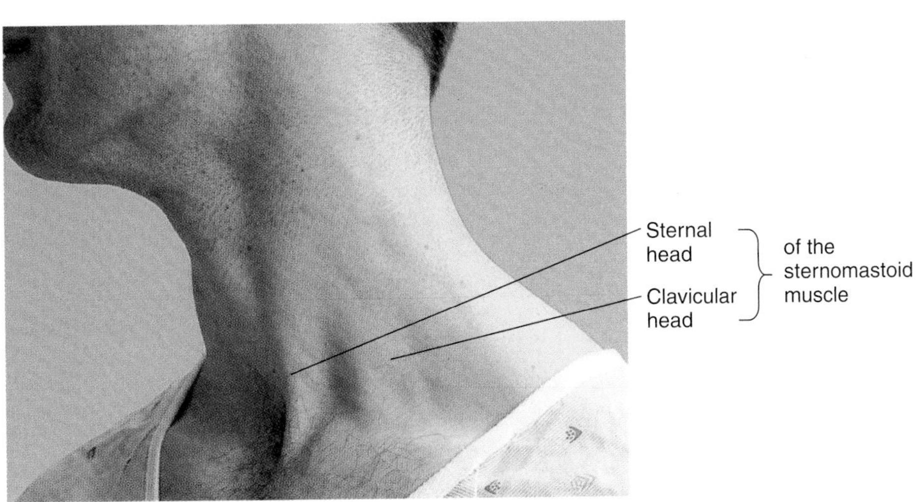

THE HEALTH HISTORY

Common or Concerning Symptoms

- Chest pain
- Dyspnea
- Wheezing
- Cough
- Blood-streaked sputum (hemoptysis)

Complaints of *chest pain* or *chest discomfort* raise the specter of heart disease, but often arise from structures in the thorax and lung as well. To assess this symptom, you must pursue a dual investigation of both thoracic and cardiac causes. Sources of chest pain are listed below. For this important symptom, you must keep all of these in mind.

See Table 7-1. Chest Pain, pp. 268–269.

- The myocardium — Angina pectoris, myocardial infarction
- The pericardium — Pericarditis
- The aorta — Dissecting aortic aneurysm
- The trachea and large bronchi — Bronchitis
- The parietal pleura — Pericarditis, pneumonia
- The chest wall, including the musculoskeletal system and skin — Costochondritis, herpes zoster
- The esophagus — Reflux esophagitis, esophageal spasm
- Extrathoracic structures such as the neck, gallbladder, and stomach. — Cervical arthritis, biliary colic, gastritis

This section focuses on *pulmonary complaints*, including general questions about chest symptoms, dyspnea, wheezing, cough, and hemoptysis. For health history questions about exertional chest pain, palpitations, orthopnea, paroxysmal nocturnal dyspnea, and edema, see Chapter 8, The Cardiovascular System.

Your initial questions should be as broad as possible. "Do you have any discomfort or unpleasant feelings in your chest?" As you proceed to the full history, ask the patient to point to where the pain is in the chest. Watch for any

A clenched fist over the sternum suggests *angina pectoris;* a finger pointing to a tender area on the

gestures as the patient describes the pain. You should elicit all seven attributes of this symptom (see p. 32) to distinguish among the various causes of chest pain.

chest wall suggests musculoskeletal pain; a hand moving from neck to epigastrum suggests heartburn.

Lung tissue itself has no pain fibers. Pain in lung conditions such as pneumonia or pulmonary infarction usually arises from inflammation of the adjacent parietal pleura. Muscle strain from prolonged recurrent coughing may also be responsible. The pericardium also has few pain fibers—the pain of pericarditis stems from inflammation of the adjacent parietal pleura. (Chest pain is commonly associated with anxiety, too, but the mechanism remains obscure.)

Anxiety is the most frequent cause of chest pain in children; costochondritis is also common.

Dyspnea is a nonpainful but uncomfortable awareness of breathing that is inappropriate to the level of exertion. This serious symptom warrants a full explanation and assessment because dyspnea commonly results from cardiac or pulmonary disease.

See Table 7-2, Dyspnea, pp. 270–271.

Ask "Have you had any difficulty breathing?" Find out when the symptom occurs, at rest or with exercise, and how much effort produces onset. Because of variations in age, body weight, and physical fitness, there is no absolute scale for quantifying dyspnea. Instead, make every effort *to determine its severity based on the patient's daily activities.* How many steps or flights of stairs can the patient climb before pausing for breath? What about work such as carrying bags of groceries, mopping the floor, or making the bed? Has dyspnea altered the patient's lifestyle and daily activities? How? Carefully elicit the timing and setting of dyspnea, any associated symptoms, and relieving or aggravating factors.

Most patients with dyspnea relate shortness of breath to their level of activity. Anxious patients present a different picture. They may describe difficulty taking a deep enough breath, or a smothering sensation with inability to get enough air, along with *paresthesias,* or sensations of tingling or "pins and needles" around the lips or in the extremities.

Anxious patients may have episodic dyspnea during both rest and exercise, and *hyperventilation,* or rapid, shallow breathing. At other times, they may have frequent sighs.

Wheezes are musical respiratory sounds that may be audible to the patient and to others.

Wheezing suggests partial airway obstruction from secretions, tissue inflammation, or a foreign body.

Cough is a common symptom that ranges in significance from trivial to ominous. Typically, cough is a reflex response to stimuli that irritate receptors in the larynx, trachea, or large bronchi. These stimuli include mucus, pus, and blood, as well as external agents such as dusts, foreign bodies, or even extremely hot or cold air. Other causes include inflammation of the respiratory mucosa and pressure or tension in the air passages from a tumor or enlarged peribronchial lymph nodes. Although cough typically signals a problem in the respiratory tract, it may also be cardiovascular in origin.

See Table 7-3, Cough and Hemoptysis, p. 272.

Cough can be a symptom of left-sided heart failure.

For complaints of cough, a thorough assessment is in order. Ask whether the cough is dry or produces *sputum*, or phlegm. Ask the patient to describe the volume of any sputum and its color, odor, and consistency.

Dry hacking cough in Mycoplasma pneumonia; productive cough in bronchitis, viral or bacterial pneumonia

Mucoid sputum is translucent, white, or gray; *purulent* sputum is yellowish or greenish.

Foul-smelling sputum in anaerobic lung abscess; tenacious sputum in cystic fibrosis

To help patients quantify volume, a multiple-choice question may be helpful . . . "How much do you think you cough up in 24 hours; a teaspoon, tablespoon, a quarter cup, half cup, cupful?" If possible, ask the patient to cough into a tissue; inspect the phlegm and note its characteristics. The symptoms associated with a cough often lead you to its cause.

Large volumes of purulent sputum in bronchiectasis or lung abscess

Diagnostically helpful symptoms include fever, chest pain, dyspnea, orthopnea, and wheezing.

Hemoptysis is the coughing up of blood from the lungs; it may vary from blood-streaked phlegm to frank blood. For patients reporting hemoptysis, assess the volume of blood produced as well as the other sputum attributes; ask about the related setting and activity and any associated symptoms.

See Table 7-3, Cough and Hemoptysis, p. 272. Hemoptysis is rare in infants, children, and adolescents; it is seen most often in cystic fibrosis.

Before using the term "hemoptysis," try to confirm the source of the bleeding by both history and physical examination. Blood or blood-streaked material may originate in the mouth, pharynx, or gastrointestinal tract and is easily mislabeled. When vomited, it probably originates in the gastrointestinal tract. Occasionally, however, blood from the nasopharynx or the gastrointestinal tract is aspirated and then coughed out.

Blood originating in the stomach is usually darker than blood from the respiratory tract and may be mixed with food particles.

HEALTH PROMOTION AND COUNSELING

Important Topics for Health Promotion and Counseling

- Tobacco cessation

Despite declines in smoking over the past several decades, 22.5% of all adults, or 46 million Americans, still smoke.[1] Eighty percent of smokers have their first cigarette before age 18, and smoking rates are highest among high school students and young adults ages 18 to 24. Smoking wreaks a heavy toll on health, accounting for approximately 440,000 deaths each year, or roughly 20% of annual U.S. mortality. These figures include an estimated

35,000 deaths from exposure to secondhand smoke. Risk for death from lung cancer is 22 times higher among male smokers and approximately 12 times higher among female smokers compared with those who have never smoked. Risk for death from chronic obstructive heart disease increases ten-fold for smokers. Smokers have a 2 to 4 times increased risk for heart disease, double the risk for stroke, and 10 times the risk for peripheral vascular disease. Nonsmokers exposed to smoke also have increased risk for lung cancer, ear and respiratory infection, asthma, low birth weight, and residential fires. Smoking exposes patients not only to carcinogens but also to nicotine, an addictive drug.

Smoking is the leading cause of preventable death in the United States. More than 70% of smokers express interest in quitting, although less than 10% are successful.[1] Clinicians should query smokers on every visit about quitting, especially teenagers and pregnant women, and should adopt the five "As":

- **A**sk about smoking at each visit.
- **A**dvise patients regularly to stop smoking using a clear personalized message.
- **A**ssess patient readiness to quit.
- **A**ssist patients to set stop dates and provide educational materials for self-help.
- **A**rrange for follow-up visits to monitor and support patient progress.

The disease risks of smoking drop significantly within 1 year of smoking cessation. Study the addictive features of nicotine: tolerance over time, physical dependence, and the features of withdrawal ranging from irritability, anger, and insomnia to anxiety and depressed mood. Learn to make effective interventions to promote sustained quit rates, including targeted messages, group counseling, and use of nicotine-replacement therapies.[2] Combining clinician and group counseling with nicotine replacement therapy is especially effective for highly addicted patients.

Relapses are common and should be expected. Nicotine withdrawal, weight gain, stress, social pressure, and use of alcohol are often cited as explanations. Help patients to learn from these experiences: work with the patient to pinpoint the precipitating circumstances and develop strategies for alternative responses and health-promoting behaviors.

TECHNIQUES OF EXAMINATION

It is helpful to examine the posterior thorax and lungs while the patient is sitting, and the anterior thorax and lungs with the patient supine. Proceed in an orderly fashion: inspect, palpate, percuss, and auscultate. Try to visualize the underlying lobes, and compare one side with the other, so that the patient serves as his or her own control. For men, arrange the patient's gown so that you can see the chest fully. For women, cover the anterior chest when you examine the back. For the anterior examination, drape the gown over each half of the chest as you examine the other half.

With the patient sitting, examine the posterior thorax and lungs. The patient's arms should be folded across the chest with hands resting, if possible, on the opposite shoulders. This position moves the scapulae partly out of the way and increases your access to the lung fields. Then ask the patient to lie down.

With the patient supine, examine the anterior thorax and lungs. The supine position makes it easier to examine women because the breasts can be gently displaced. Furthermore, wheezes, if present, are more likely to be heard. (Some authorities, however, prefer to examine both the back and the front of the chest with the patient sitting. This technique is also satisfactory).

For patients unable to sit up without aid, try to get help so that you can examine the posterior chest in the sitting position. If this is impossible, roll the patient to one side and then to the other. Percuss the upper lung, and auscultate both lungs in each position. Because ventilation is relatively greater in the dependent lung, your chances of hearing abnormal wheezes or crackles are greater on the dependent side (see p. 260).

INITIAL SURVEY OF RESPIRATION AND THE THORAX

Even though you may have already recorded the respiratory rate when you took the vital signs, it is wise to again *observe the rate, rhythm, depth, and effort of breathing.* A normal resting adult breathes quietly and regularly about 14 to 20 times a minute. An occasional sigh is to be expected. Note whether expiration lasts longer than usual.

See Table 4-8, Abnormalities in Rate and Rhythm of Breathing, p. 120.

Always inspect the patient for any signs of respiratory difficulty.

- *Assess the patient's color* for cyanosis. Recall any relevant findings from earlier parts of your examination, such as the shape of the fingernails.

Cyanosis signals hypoxia. Clubbing of the nails (see p. 150) in lung abscesses or malignancy, congenital heart disease

- *Listen to the patient's breathing.* Is there any *audible wheezing*? If so, where does it fall in the respiratory cycle?

Audible *stridor,* a high-pitched wheeze, is an ominous sign of airway obstruction in the larynx or trachea.

- *Inspect the neck.* During inspiration, is there contraction of the sternomastoid or other accessory muscles, or supraclavicular retraction? Is the trachea midline?

Inspiratory contraction of the sternomastoids at rest signals severe difficulty breathing. Lateral displacement of the trachea in *pneumothorax, pleural effusion,* or *atelectasis*

Also *observe the shape of the chest.* The anteroposterior (AP) diameter may increase with aging.

The AP diameter also may increase in *chronic obstructive pulmonary disease* (COPD).

EXAMINATION OF THE POSTERIOR CHEST

INSPECTION

From a midline position behind the patient, note the *shape of the chest* and *the way in which it moves,* including:

- Deformities or asymmetry

See Table 7-4, Deformities of the Thorax (p. 273).

- Abnormal retraction of the interspaces during inspiration. Retraction is most apparent in the lower interspaces. Supraclavicular retraction is often present.

Retraction in severe asthma, COPD, or upper airway obstruction

- Impaired respiratory movement on one or both sides or a unilateral lag (or delay) in movement.

Unilateral impairment or lagging of respiratory movement suggests disease of the underlying lung or pleura.

PALPATION

As you palpate the chest, focus on areas of tenderness and abnormalities in the overlying skin, respiratory expansion, and fremitus.

Intercostal tenderness over inflamed pleura

Identify tender areas. Carefully palpate any area where pain has been reported or where lesions or bruises are evident.

Bruises over a fractured rib

Assess any observed abnormalities such as masses or sinus tracts (blind, inflammatory, tubelike structures opening onto the skin).

Although rare, sinus tracts usually indicate infection of the underlying pleura and lung (as in tuberculosis, actinomycosis).

Test chest expansion. Place your thumbs at about the level of the 10th ribs, with your fingers loosely grasping and parallel to the lateral rib cage. As you position your hands, slide them medially just enough to raise a loose fold of skin on each side between your thumb and the spine.

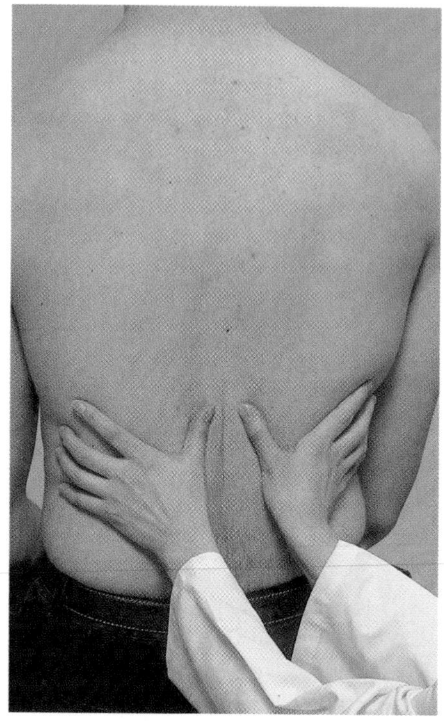

Ask the patient to inhale deeply. Watch the distance between your thumbs as they move apart during inspiration, and feel for the range and symmetry of the rib cage as it expands and contracts.

Causes of unilateral decrease or delay in chest expansion include chronic fibrotic disease of the underlying lung or pleura, pleural effusion, lobar pneumonia, pleural pain with associated splinting, and unilateral bronchial obstruction.

Feel for tactile fremitus. Fremitus refers to the palpable vibrations transmitted through the bronchopulmonary tree to the chest wall when the patient speaks. To detect fremitus, use either the ball (the bony part of the palm at the base of the fingers) or the ulnar surface of your hand to optimize the vibratory sensitivity of the bones in your hand. Ask the patient to repeat the words "ninety-nine" or "one-one-one." If fremitus is faint, ask the patient to speak more loudly or in a deeper voice.

Use one hand until you have learned the feel of fremitus. Some clinicians find using one hand more accurate. The simultaneous use of both hands to compare sides, however, increases your speed and may facilitate detection of differences.

Fremitus is decreased or absent when the voice is soft or when the transmission of vibrations from the larynx to the surface of the chest is impeded. Causes include an obstructed bronchus; COPD; separation of the pleural surfaces by fluid (pleural effusion), fibrosis (pleural thickening), air (pneumothorax), or an infiltrating tumor; and a very thick chest wall.

Palpate and compare symmetric areas of the lungs in the pattern shown in the photograph. Identify and locate any areas of increased, decreased, or absent fremitus. Fremitus is typically more prominent in the interscapular area than in the lower lung fields and is often more prominent on the right side than on the left. It disappears below the diaphragm.

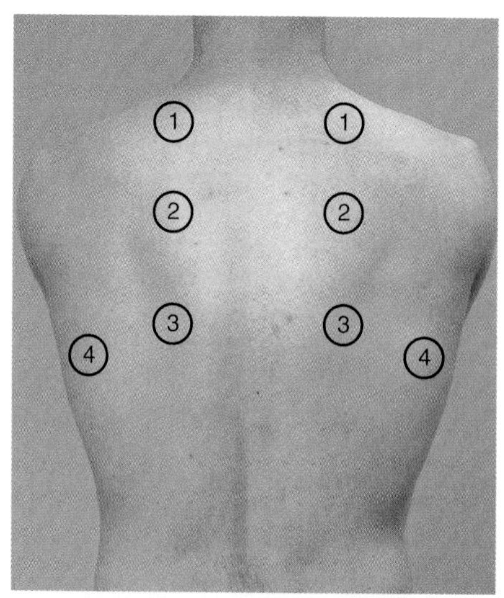

LOCATIONS FOR FEELING FREMITUS

Tactile fremitus is a relatively rough assessment tool, but as a scouting technique, it directs your attention to possible abnormalities. Later in the examination you will check any suggested findings by listening for breath sounds, voice sounds, and whispered voice sounds. All these attributes tend to increase or decrease together.

PERCUSSION

Percussion is one of the most important techniques of physical examination. Percussion of the chest sets the chest wall and underlying tissues into motion, producing audible sound and palpable vibrations. Percussion helps you establish whether the underlying tissues are air-filled, fluid-filled, or solid. It penetrates only about 5 cm to 7 cm into the chest, however, and will not help you to detect deep-seated lesions.

The technique of percussion can be practiced on any surface. As you practice, listen for changes in percussion notes over different types of materials or different parts of the body. The key points for good technique, described for a right-handed person, are as follows:

- Hyperextend the middle finger of your left hand, known as the pleximeter finger. Press its distal interphalangeal joint firmly on the surface to be percussed. Avoid surface contact by any other part of the hand, because this dampens out vibrations. Note that the thumb and 2nd, 4th, and 5th fingers are not touching the chest.

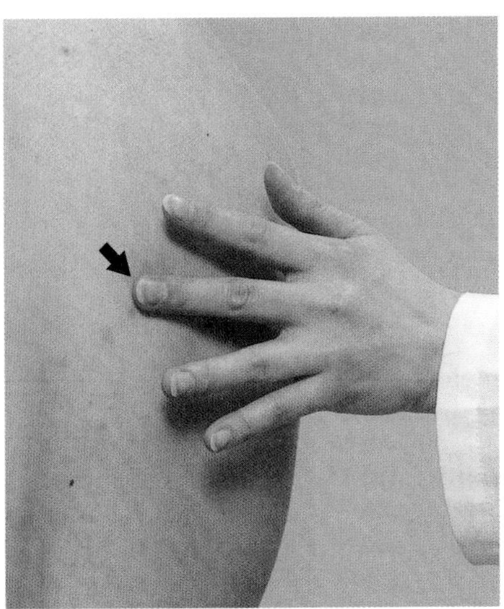

- Position your right forearm quite close to the surface, with the hand cocked upward. The middle finger should be partially flexed, relaxed, and poised to strike.

- With a *quick sharp but relaxed wrist motion*, strike the pleximeter finger with the right middle finger, or plexor finger. Aim at your distal interphalangeal joint. You are trying to transmit vibrations through the bones of this joint to the underlying chest wall.

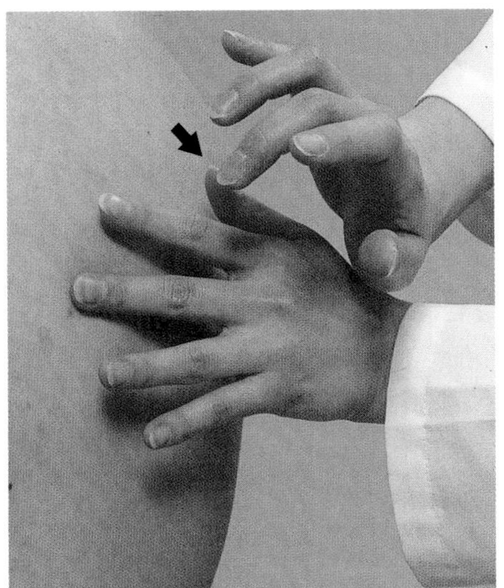

Strike using the *tip of the plexor finger,* not the finger pad. Your finger should be almost at right angles to the pleximeter. A short fingernail is recommended to avoid self-injury.

- Withdraw your striking finger quickly to avoid damping the vibrations you have created.

In summary, the movement is at the wrist. It is directed, brisk yet relaxed, and a bit bouncy.

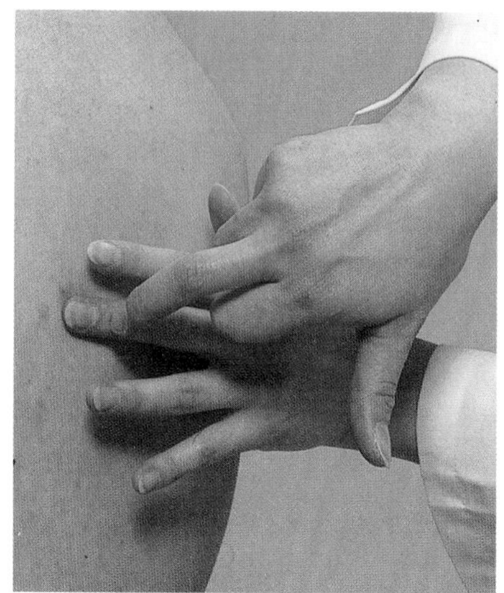

Percussion Notes. With your plexor or tapping finger, use the lightest percussion that produces a clear note. A thick chest wall requires stronger percussion than a thin one. However, if a *louder* note is needed, apply more pressure with the *pleximeter* finger (this is more effective for increasing percussion note volume than tapping harder with the plexor finger).

When percussing the lower posterior chest, stand somewhat to the side rather than directly behind the patient. This allows you to place your pleximeter finger more firmly on the chest and your plexor is more effective, making a better percussion note.

When comparing two areas, use the same percussion technique in both areas. Percuss or strike twice in each location. It is easier to detect differences in percussion notes by comparing one area with another than by striking repetitively in one place.

Learn to identify five percussion notes. You can practice four of them on yourself. These notes differ in their basic qualities of sound: intensity, pitch, and duration. Train your ear to distinguish these differences by concentrating on one quality at a time as you percuss first in one location, then in another. Review the table below. Normal lungs are *resonant.*

■ *Percussion Notes and Their Characteristics*

	Relative Intensity	Relative Pitch	Relative Duration	Example of Location	Pathologic Examples
Flatness	Soft	High	Short	Thigh	Large pleural effusion
Dullness	Medium	Medium	Medium	Liver	Lobar pneumonia
Resonance	Loud	Low	Long	Normal lung	Simple chronic bronchitis
Hyperresonance	Very loud	Lower	Longer	None normally	Emphysema, pneumothorax
Tympany	Loud	High*	*	Gastric air bubble or puffed-out cheek	Large pneumothorax

* Distinguished mainly by its musical timbre.

While the patient keeps both arms crossed in front of the chest, percuss the thorax in symmetric locations from the apices to the lung bases.

Percuss one side of the chest and then the other at each level in a ladder-like pattern, as shown by the numbers below. Omit the areas over the scapulae—the thickness of muscle and bone alters the percussion notes over the lungs. Identify and locate the area and quality of any abnormal percussion note.

Dullness replaces resonance when fluid or solid tissue replaces air-containing lung or occupies the pleural space beneath your percussing fingers. Examples include: lobar pneumonia, in which the alveoli are filled with fluid and blood cells; and pleural accumulations of serous fluid (pleural effusion), blood (hemothorax), pus (empyema), fibrous tissue, or tumor.

Generalized hyperresonance may be heard over the hyperinflated lungs of emphysema or asthma, but it is not a reliable sign. *Unilateral hyperresonance* suggests a large pneumothorax or possibly a large air-filled bulla in the lung.

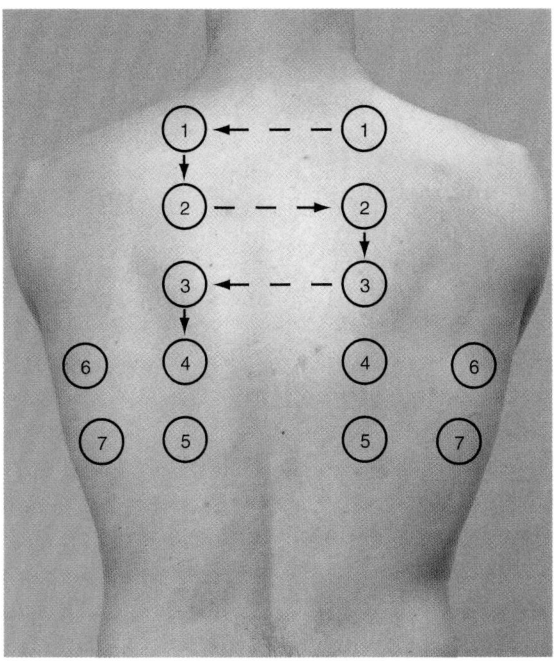

"LADDER" PATTERNS FOR PERCUSSION AND AUSCULTATION

Identify the descent of the diaphragms, or *diaphragmatic excursion.* First, *determine the level of diaphragmatic dullness* during quiet respiration. Holding the pleximeter finger *above and parallel* to the expected level of dullness, percuss downward in progressive steps until dullness clearly replaces resonance. Confirm this level of change by percussion near the middle of the hemothorax and also more laterally.

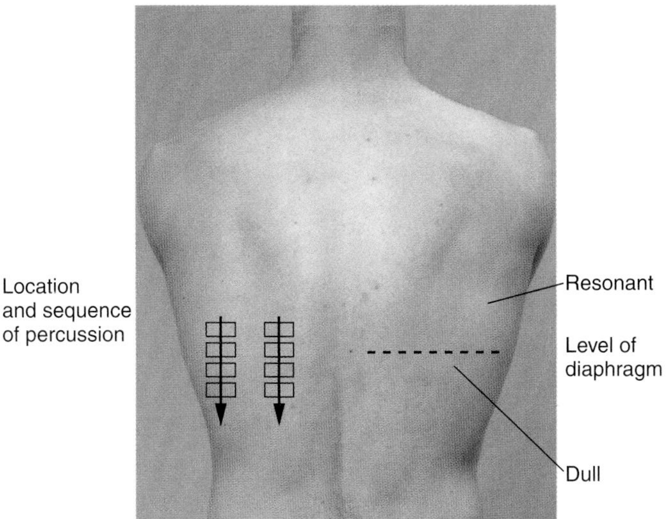

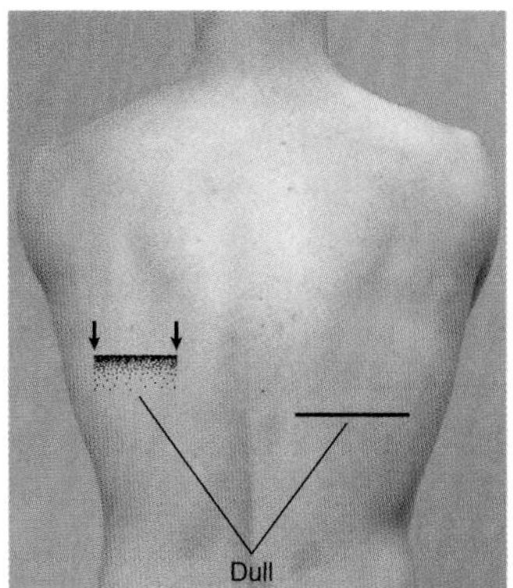

An abnormally high level suggests pleural effusion, or a high diaphragm as in atelectasis or diaphragmatic paralysis.

Note that with this technique, you are identifying the boundary between the resonant lung tissue and the duller structures below the diaphragm. You are not percussing the diaphragm itself. You can infer the probable location of the diaphragm from the level of dullness.

Now, *estimate the extent of diaphragmatic excursion* by determining the distance between the level of dullness on full expiration and the level of dullness on full inspiration, normally about 5 or 6 cm. This estimate does not correlate well, however, with radiologic assessment of diaphragmatic movement.

AUSCULTATION

Auscultation of the lungs is the most important examining technique for assessing air flow through the tracheobronchial tree. Together with percussion, it also helps the clinician to assess the condition of the surrounding lungs and pleural space. Auscultation involves (1) listening to the sounds generated by breathing, (2) listening for any adventitious (added) sounds, and (3) if abnormalities are suspected, listening to the sounds of the patient's spoken or whispered voice as they are transmitted through the chest wall.

Sounds from bedclothes, paper gowns, and the chest itself can generate confusion in auscultation. Hair on the chest may cause crackling sounds. Either press harder or wet the hair. If the patient is cold or tense, you may hear muscle contraction sounds—muffled, low-pitched rumbling or roaring noises. A change in the patient's position may eliminate this noise. You can reproduce this sound on yourself by doing a Valsalva maneuver (straining down) as you listen to your own chest.

Breath Sounds (Lung Sounds). You will learn to identify patterns of breath sounds by their intensity, their pitch, and the relative duration of their inspiratory and expiratory phases. Normal breath sounds are:

- *Vesicular,* or soft and low pitched. They are heard through inspiration, continue without pause through expiration, and then fade away about one third of the way through expiration.
- *Bronchovesicular,* with inspiratory and expiratory sounds about equal in length, at times separated by a silent interval. Detecting differences in pitch and intensity is often easier during expiration.
- *Bronchial,* or louder and higher in pitch, with a short silence between inspiratory and expiratory sounds. Expiratory sounds last longer than inspiratory sounds.

The characteristics of these three kinds of breath sounds are summarized in the table below. Also shown are the *tracheal* breath sounds—very loud, harsh sounds that are heard by listening over the trachea in the neck.

Listen to the breath sounds with the diaphragm of a stethoscope after instructing the patient to breathe deeply through an open mouth. Use the pattern suggested for percussion, moving from one side to the other and comparing symmetric areas of the lungs. If you hear or suspect abnormal sounds, auscultate adjacent areas so that you can fully describe the extent of any abnormality. Listen to at least one full breath in each location. Be alert for patient discomfort due to hyperventilation (e.g., lightheadedness, faintness), and allow the patient to rest as needed.

Note the *intensity* of the breath sounds. Breath sounds are usually louder in the lower posterior lung fields and may also vary from area to area. If the

Breath sounds may be decreased when air flow is decreased (as by

Characteristics of Breath Sounds

	Duration of Sounds	Intensity of Expiratory Sound	Pitch of Expiratory Sound	Locations Where Heard Normally
Vesicular*	Inspiratory sounds last longer than expiratory ones.	Soft	Relatively low	Over most of both lungs
Broncho-vesicular	Inspiratory and expiratory sounds are about equal.	Intermediate	Intermediate	Often in the 1st and 2nd interspaces anteriorly and between the scapulae
Bronchial	Expiratory sounds last longer than inspiratory ones.	Loud	Relatively high	Over the manubrium, if heard at all
Tracheal	Inspiratory and expiratory sounds are about equal.	Very loud	Relatively high	Over the trachea in the neck

* The thickness of the bars indicates intensity; the steeper their incline, the higher the pitch.

If bronchovesicular or bronchial breath sounds are heard in locations distant from those listed, suspect that air-filled lung has been replaced by fluid-filled or solid lung tissue. See Table 7-5, Normal and Altered Breath and Voice Sounds (p. 274).

breath sounds seem faint, ask the patient to breathe more deeply. You may then hear them easily. When patients do not breathe deeply enough or have a thick chest wall, as in obesity, breath sounds may remain diminished.

obstructive lung disease or muscular weakness) or when the transmission of sound is poor (as in pleural effusion, pneumothorax, or emphysema).

Is there a *silent gap* between the inspiratory and expiratory sounds?

A gap suggests bronchial breath sounds.

Listen for the *pitch, intensity, and duration of the expiratory and inspiratory sounds.* Are vesicular breath sounds distributed normally over the chest wall? Or are there bronchovesicular or bronchial breath sounds in unexpected places? If so, where are they?

Adventitious (Added) Sounds. Listen for any added, or adventitious, sounds that are superimposed on the usual breath sounds. Detection of adventitious sounds—*crackles* (sometimes called *rales*), *wheezes,* and *rhonchi*—is an important part of your examination, often leading to diagnosis of cardiac and pulmonary conditions. The most common kinds of these sounds are described on the next page:

For further discussion and other added sounds, see Table 7-6, Adventitious (Added) Lung Sounds: Causes and Qualities (p. 275).

■ *Adventitious or Added Breath Sounds*

Crackles (or Rales)	Wheezes and Rhonchi
▪ **Discontinuous**	▪ **Continuous**
▪ Intermittent, nonmusical, and brief	▪ ≥250 msec, musical, prolonged (but not necessarily persisting throughout the respiratory cycle)
▪ Like dots in time	▪ Like dashes in time
▪ *Fine crackles:* soft, high-pitched, very brief (5–10 msec) · · · · ·	▪ *Wheezes:* relatively high-pitched (≥400 Hz) with hissing or shrill quality
Coarse crackles: somewhat louder, lower in pitch, brief (20–30 msec) • • • • •	▪ *Rhonchi:* relatively low-pitched (≤200 Hz) with snoring quality

Crackles may be due to abnormalities of the lungs (pneumonia, fibrosis, early congestive heart failure) or of the airways (bronchitis, bronchiectasis).

Wheezes suggest narrowed airways, as in asthma, COPD, or bronchitis.

Rhonchi suggest secretions in large airways.

If you hear *crackles,* especially those that do not clear after cough, listen carefully for the following characteristics. These are clues to the underlying condition:

- Loudness, pitch, and duration (summarized as fine or coarse crackles)
- Number (few to many)
- Timing in the respiratory cycle
- Location on the chest wall
- Persistence of their pattern from breath to breath
- Any change after a cough or a change in the patient's position

Fine late inspiratory crackles that persist from breath to breath suggest abnormal lung tissue.

Clearing of crackles, wheezes, or rhonchi after cough or position change suggests inspissated secretions, as in bronchitis or atelectasis.

In some normal people, crackles may be heard at the lung bases anteriorly after maximal expiration. Crackles in dependent portions of the lungs may also occur after prolonged recumbency.

If you hear *wheezes* or *rhonchi,* note their timing and location. Do they change with deep breathing or coughing?

Transmitted Voice Sounds. If you hear abnormally located bronchovesicular or bronchial breath sounds, assess transmitted voice sounds. With a stethoscope, listen in symmetric areas over the chest wall as you:

Increased transmission of voice sounds suggests that air-filled lung has become airless. See Table 7-5, Normal and Altered Breath and Voice Sounds (p. 274).

- Ask the patient to say "ninety-nine." Normally the sounds transmitted through the chest wall are muffled and indistinct.

Louder, clearer voice sounds are called *bronchophony.*

- Ask the patient to say "ee." You will normally hear a muffled long E sound.

When "ee" is heard as "ay," an *E-to-A change (egophony)* is present, as in lobar consolidation from pneumonia. The quality sounds nasal.

- Ask the patient to whisper "ninety-nine" or "one-two-three." The whispered voice is normally heard faintly and indistinctly, if at all.

Louder, clearer whispered sounds are called *whispered pectoriloquy.*

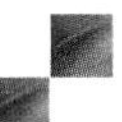

EXAMINATION OF THE ANTERIOR CHEST

When examined in the supine position, the patient should lie comfortably with arms somewhat abducted. A patient who is having difficulty breathing should be examined in the sitting position or with the head of the bed elevated to a comfortable level.

Persons with severe COPD may prefer to sit leaning forward, with lips pursed during exhalation and arms supported on their knees or a table.

INSPECTION

Observe *the shape of the patient's chest* and *the movement of the chest wall.* Note:

- Deformities or asymmetry

See Table 7-4, Deformities of the Thorax (p. 273).

- Abnormal retraction of the lower interspaces during inspiration

Severe asthma, COPD, or upper airway obstruction

- Local lag or impairment in respiratory movement

Underlying disease of lung or pleura

PALPATION

Palpation has four potential uses:

- *Identification of tender areas*

Tender pectoral muscles or costal cartilages tend to corroborate, but do not prove, that chest pain has a musculoskeletal origin.

- *Assessment of observed abnormalities*
- *Further assessment of chest expansion.* Place your thumbs along each costal margin, your hands along the lateral rib cage. As you position your hands, slide them medially a bit to raise loose skin folds between your thumbs. Ask the patient to inhale deeply. Observe how far your thumbs diverge as the thorax expands, and feel for the extent and symmetry of respiratory movement.

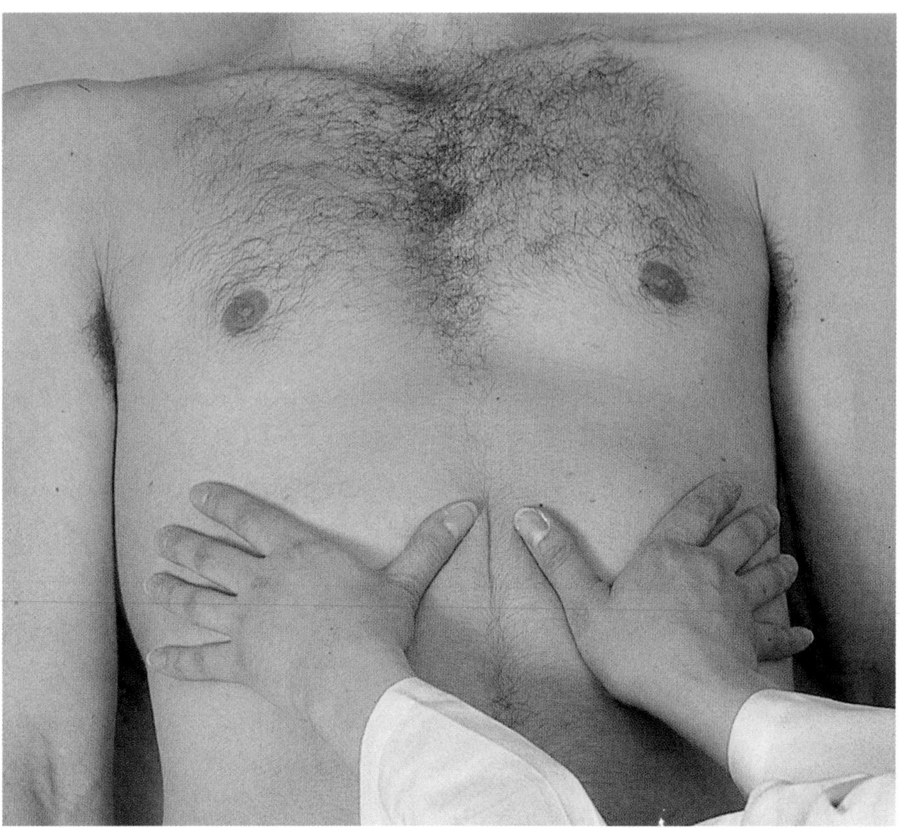

- *Assessment of tactile fremitus.* Compare both sides of the chest, using the ball or ulnar surface of your hand. Fremitus is usually decreased or absent over the precordium. When examining a woman, gently displace the breasts as necessary.

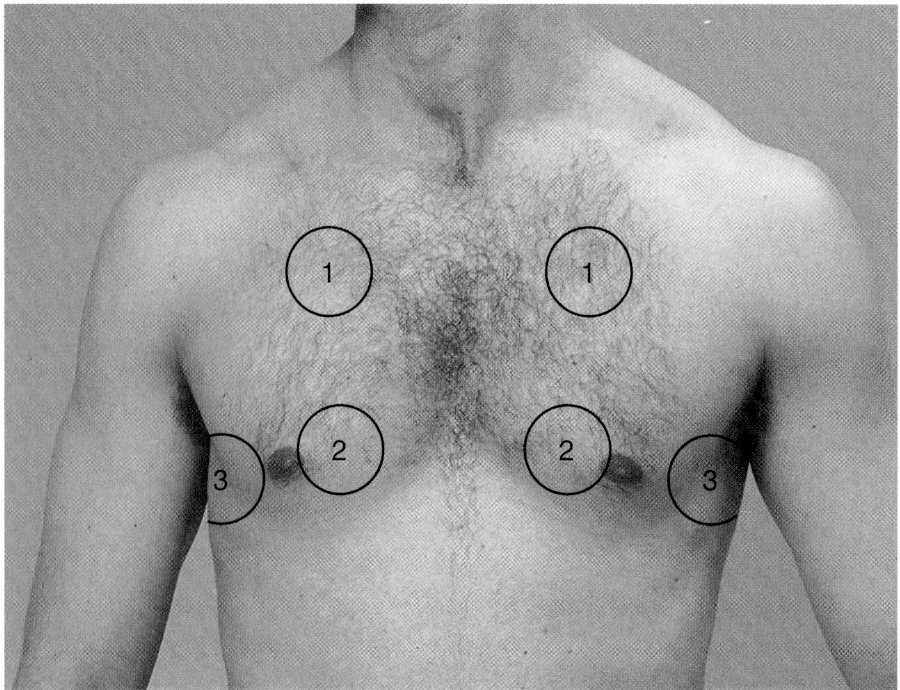

LOCATIONS FOR FEELING FREMITUS

PERCUSSION

Percuss the anterior and lateral chest, again comparing both sides. The heart normally produces an area of dullness to the left of the sternum from the 3rd to the 5th interspaces. Percuss the left lung lateral to it.

Dullness replaces resonance when fluid or solid tissue replaces air-containing lung or occupies the pleural space. Because pleural fluid usually sinks to the lowest part of the pleural space (posteriorly in a supine patient), only a very large effusion can be detected anteriorly.

The hyperresonance of COPD may totally replace cardiac dullness.

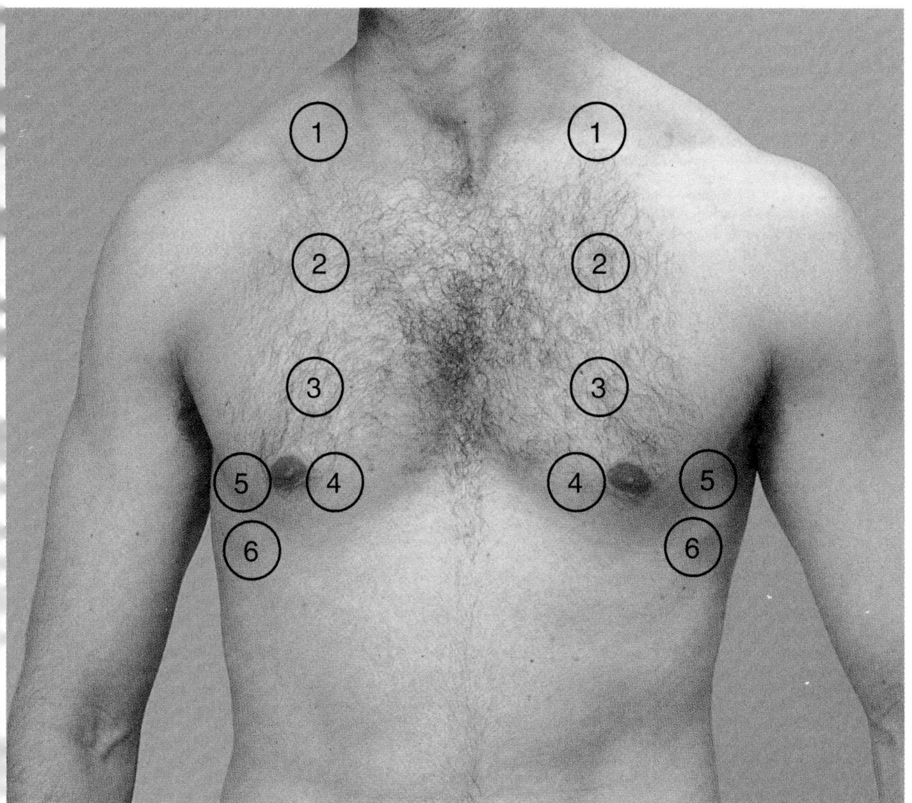

LOCATIONS FOR PERCUSSION AND AUSCULTATION

In a woman, to enhance percussion, gently displace the breast with your left hand while percussing with the right.

The dullness of right middle lobe pneumonia typically occurs behind the right breast. Unless you displace the breast, you may miss the abnormal percussion note.

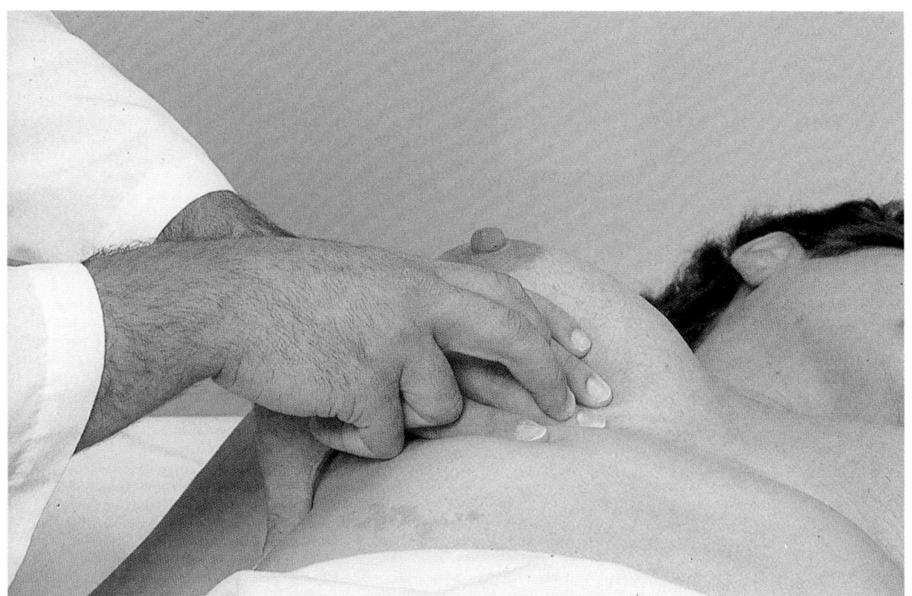

Alternatively, you may ask the patient to move her breast for you.

Identify and locate any area with an abnormal percussion note.

With your pleximeter finger above and parallel to the expected upper border of liver dullness, percuss in progressive steps downward in the right midclavicular line. Identify the upper border of liver dullness. Later, during the abdominal examination, you will use this method to estimate the size of the liver. As you percuss down the chest on the left, the resonance of normal lung usually changes to the tympany of the gastric air bubble.

A lung affected by COPD often displaces the upper border of the liver downward. It also lowers the level of diaphragmatic dullness posteriorly.

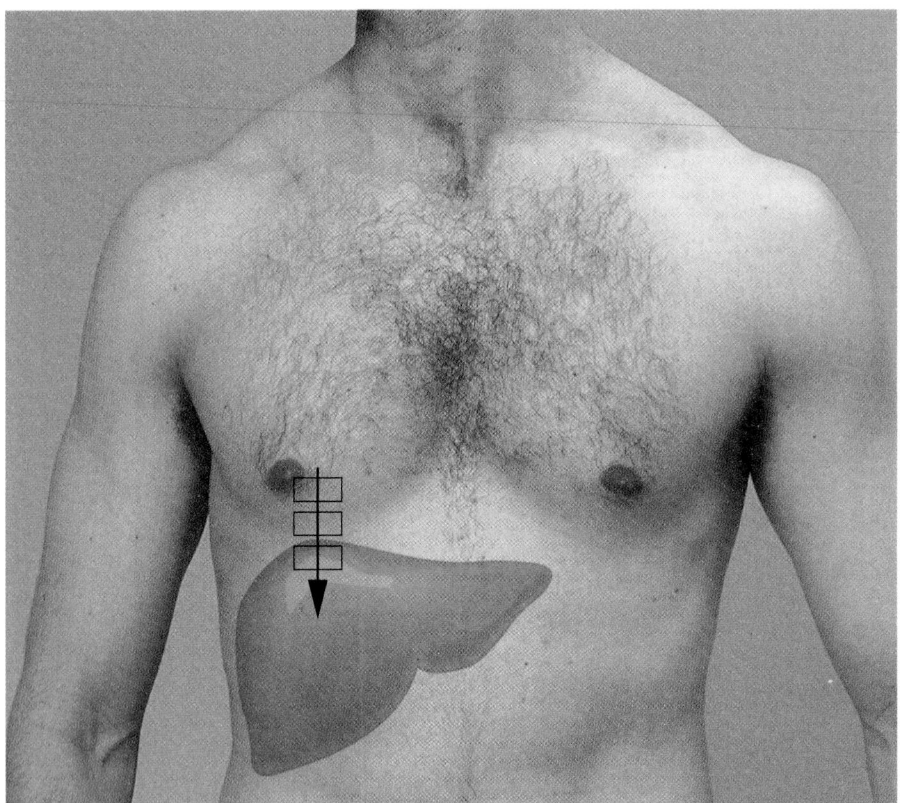

AUSCULTATION

Listen to the chest anteriorly and laterally as the patient breathes with mouth open, somewhat more deeply than normal. Compare symmetric areas of the lungs, using the pattern suggested for percussion and extending it to adjacent areas as indicated.

Listen to the breath sounds, noting their intensity and identifying any variations from normal vesicular breathing. Breath sounds are usually louder in the upper anterior lung fields. Bronchovesicular breath sounds may be heard over the large airways, especially on the right.

Identify any adventitious sounds, time them in the respiratory cycle, and locate them on the chest wall. Do they clear with deep breathing?

If indicated, *listen for transmitted voice sounds.*

See Table 7-6, Adventitious (Added) Lung Sounds: Causes and Qualities (p. 275), and Table 7-7, Physical Findings in Selected Chest Disorders (pp. 276–277).

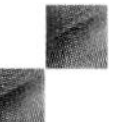

SPECIAL TECHNIQUES

Clinical Assessment of Pulmonary Function. A simple but informative way to assess the complaint of breathlessness in an ambulatory patient is to walk with the patient down the hall or climb one flight of stairs. Observe the rate, effort, and sound of the patient's breathing.

Forced Expiratory Time. This test assesses the expiratory phase of breathing, which is typically slowed in obstructive pulmonary disease. Ask the patient to take a deep breath in and then breathe out as quickly and completely as possible with mouth open. Listen over the trachea with the diaphragm of a stethoscope and time the audible expiration. Try to get three consistent readings, allowing a short rest between efforts if necessary.

If the patient understands and cooperates in performing the test, a forced expiration time of 6 seconds or more suggests obstructive pulmonary disease.

Identification of a Fractured Rib. Local pain and tenderness of one or more ribs raise the question of fracture. By anteroposterior compression of the chest, you can help to distinguish a fracture from soft-tissue injury. With one hand on the sternum and the other on the thoracic spine, squeeze the chest. Is this painful, and where?

An increase in the local pain (distant from your hands) suggests rib fracture rather than just soft-tissue injury.

RECORDING YOUR FINDINGS

Note that initially you may use sentences to describe your findings; later you will use phrases. The style below contains phrases appropriate for most write-ups.

Recording the Physical Examination— The Thorax and Lungs

"Thorax is symmetric with good expansion. Lungs resonant. Breath sounds vesicular; no rales, wheezes, or rhonchi. Diaphragms descend 4 cm bilaterally."

OR

"Thorax symmetric with moderate kyphosis and increased anteroposterior (AP) diameter, decreased expansion. Lungs are hyperresonant. Breath sounds distant with delayed expiratory phase and scattered expiratory wheezes. Fremitus decreased; no bronchophony, egophony, or whispered pectoriloquy. Diaphragms descend 2 cm bilaterally."

Suggests chronic obstructive lung disease

Bibliography

CITATIONS

1. Centers for Disease Control and Prevention (CDC). At a glance. Targeting tobacco use: the nation's leading cause of death, 2004. Available at: http://www.cdc.gov/nccdphp/aag/pdf/aag_osh2004.pdf. Accessed October 29, 2004. [See also Centers for Disease Control Tobacco Information and Prevention Source (TIPS). Available at: http://www.cdc.gov/tobacco/issue.htm. Accessed October 29, 2004.]
2. Rigotti NA. Putting the research into practice. BMJ 327(7428): 1395–1396, 2003.

ADDITIONAL REFERENCES

Examination of the Lungs

Badgett RG, et al. Can moderate obstructive pulmonary disease be diagnosed by historical and physical findings alone? Am J Med 94:188, 1993.

Bettancourt PE, DelBono EA, Speigelman D, et al. Clinical utility of chest auscultation in common pulmonary disease. Am J Resp Crit Care Med 150:1921, 1994.

Cugell DW. Lung sound nomenclature. Am Rev Respir Dis 136: 1016, 1987.

Epler GR, Carrington CB, Gaensler EA. Crackles (rales) in the interstitial pulmonary diseases. Chest 73:333, 1978.

Holleman DR, Simel DL. Does the clinical examination predict airflow limitation? JAMA 273:313, 1995.

Koster MEY, Baughmann RP, Loudon RG. Continuous adventitious lung sounds. J Asthma 27:237, 1990.

Kraman SS. Lung sounds for the clinician. Arch Intern Med 146: 1411, 1986.

Lehrer S. Understanding Lung Sounds, 3rd ed. Philadelphia, WB Saunders, 2002.

Lichtenstein D, Goldstein I, Mourgeon E, et al. Comparative diagnostic performances of auscultation, chest radiography, and lung ultrasonography in acute respiratory distress syndrome. Anesthesiology 100(1):9–15, 2004.

Loudon RG. The lung exam. Clin Chest Med 8:265, 1987.

Metlay JP, Kapoor WN, Fine MJ. Does this patient have community-acquired pneumonia? Diagnosing pneumonia by history and physical examination. JAMA 278(17):1440, 1997.

Nath AR, Carpel LH. Inspiratory crackles—early and late. Thorax 29:223, 1974.

Nath AR, Carpel LH. Lung crackles in bronchiectasis. Thorax 35:694, 1980.

Schapira RM, et al. The value of the forced expiratory time in the physical diagnosis of obstructive airways disease. JAMA 270:731, 1993.

Straus SE, Finaly AM, Sackett DL, et al, for the CARE-COAD1 Group. The accuracy of patient history, wheezing, and laryngeal measurements in diagnosing obstructive airway disease. JAMA 283(14):1853–1857, 2000.

Pulmonary Conditions

American Thoracic Society and Centers for Disease Control and Prevention. Diagnostic standards and classification of tuberculosis in adults and children. Am J Respir Crit Care Med 161(4 Pt 1):1376–1395, 2000.

Baum GL, Crapo JD, et al (eds). Baum's Textbook of Pulmonary Diseases, 7th ed. Philadelphia, Lippincott Williams & Wilkins, 2004.

Chunilal SD, Eikelboom JW, Attia J, et al. Does this patient have pulmonary embolism? JAMA 290(20):2849–2858, 2003.

Fiore MC, Bailey WC, Cohen SJ, et al. Treating Tobacco Use and Dependence. Quick Reference Guide for Clinicians. Rockville, MD, U.S. Department of Health and Human Services, Public Health Service, 2000. Available at: http://www.surgeongeneral.gov/tobacco/tobaqrg.pdf. Accessed May 22, 2005.

Global Initiative for Chronic Obstructive Lung Disease (GOLD), World Health Organization (WHO), National Heart, Lung and Blood Institute (NHLBI). Global Strategy for the Diagnosis, Management, and Prevention of Chronic Obstructive Pulmonary Disease. Bethesda, MD, Global Initiative for Chronic Obstructive Lung Disease, World Health Organization, National Heart, Lung and Blood Institute, 2004. Available at: http://www.guideline.gov. Accessed May 22, 2005.

Irwin RS, Madison JM. The diagnosis and treatment of cough. N Engl J Med 343(23):1715–1721, 2000.

Treatment of tuberculosis. MMWR Recomm Rep 52(RR-11):1–77, 2003.

Weinberger S. Principles of Pulmonary Medicine, 4th ed. Philadelphia, WB Saunders, 2004.

Williams SG, Schmidt DK, Redd SC, Storms W. Key clinical activities for quality asthma care: recommendations of the National Asthma Education and Prevention Program. MMWR Recomm Rep 52(RR-6):1–8, 2003.

Woodruff PG, Fahy JV. Asthma: prevalence, pathogenesis, and prospects for novel therapies. JAMA 286(4):395–398, 2001.

TABLE 7-1 Chest Pain

Problem	Process	Location	Quality	Severity
Cardiovascular				
Angina Pectoris	Temporary myocardial ischemia, usually secondary to coronary atherosclerosis	Retrosternal or across the anterior chest, sometimes radiating to the shoulders, arms, neck, lower jaw, or upper abdomen	Pressing, squeezing, tight, heavy, occasionally burning	Mild to moderate, sometimes perceived as discomfort rather than pain
Myocardial Infarction	Prolonged myocardial ischemia, resulting in irreversible muscle damage or necrosis	Same as in angina	Same as in angina	Often but not always a severe pain
Pericarditis	■ Irritation of parietal pleura adjacent to the pericardium	Precordial, may radiate to the tip of the shoulder and to the neck	Sharp, knifelike	Often severe
	■ Mechanism unclear	Retrosternal	Crushing	Severe
Dissecting Aortic Aneurysm	A splitting within the layers of the aortic wall, allowing passage of blood to dissect a channel	Anterior chest, radiating to the neck, back, or abdomen	Ripping, tearing	Very severe
Pulmonary				
Tracheobronchitis	Inflammation of trachea and large bronchi	Upper sternal or on either side of the sternum	Burning	Mild to moderate
Pleural Pain	Inflammation of the parietal pleura, as in pleurisy, pneumonia, pulmonary infarction, or neoplasm	Chest wall overlying the process	Sharp, knifelike	Often severe
Gastrointestinal and Other				
Reflex Esophagitis	Inflammation of the esophageal mucosa by reflux of gastric acid	Retrosternal, may radiate to the back	Burning, may be squeezing	Mild to severe
Diffuse Esophageal Spasm	Motor dysfunction of the esophageal muscle	Retrosternal, may radiate to the back, arms, and jaw	Usually squeezing	Mild to severe
Chest Wall Pain	Variable, often unclear	Often below the left breast or along the costal cartilages; also elsewhere	Stabbing, sticking, or dull, aching	Variable
Anxiety	Unclear	Precordial, below the left breast, or across the anterior chest	Stabbing, sticking, or dull, aching	Variable

Note: Remember that chest pain may be referred from extrathoracic structures such as the neck (arthritis) and abdomen (biliary colic, acute cholecystitis). Pleural pain may be due to abdominal conditions such as subdiaphragmatic abscess.

Timing	Factors That Aggravate	Factors That Relieve	Associated Symptoms
Usually 1–3 min but up to 10 min. Prolonged episodes up to 20 min	Exertion, especially in the cold; meals; emotional stress. May occur at rest	Rest, nitroglycerin	Sometimes dyspnea, nausea, sweating
20 min to several hours			Nausea, vomiting, sweating, weakness
Persistent	Breathing, changing position, coughing, lying down, sometimes swallowing	Sitting forward may relieve it.	Of the underlying illness
Persistent			Of the underlying illness
Abrupt onset, early peak, persistent for hours or more	Hypertension		Syncope, hemiplegia, paraplegia
Variable	Coughing	Lying on the involved side may relieve it.	Cough
Persistent	Breathing, coughing, movements of the trunk		Of the underlying illness
Variable	Large meal; bending over, lying down	Antacids, sometimes belching	Sometimes regurgitation, dysphagia
Variable	Swallowing of food or cold liquid; emotional stress	Sometimes nitroglycerin	Dysphagia
Fleeting to hours or days	Movement of chest, trunk, arms		Often local tenderness
Fleeting to hours or days	May follow effort, emotional stress		Breathlessness, palpitations, weakness, anxiety

TABLE 7-2 Dyspnea

Problem	Process	Timing
Left-Sided Heart Failure ***(left ventricular failure or mitral stenosis)***	Elevated pressure in pulmonary capillary bed with transudation of fluid into interstitial spaces and alveoli, decreased compliance (increased stiffness) of the lungs, increased work of breathing	Dyspnea may progress slowly, or suddenly as in acute pulmonary edema.
Chronic Bronchitis*	Excessive mucus production in bronchi, followed by chronic obstruction of airways	Chronic productive cough followed by slowly progressive dyspnea
Chronic Obstructive Pulmonary Disease (COPD)*	Overdistention of air spaces distal to terminal bronchioles, with destruction of alveolar septa and chronic obstruction of the airways	Slowly progressive dyspnea; relatively mild cough later
Asthma	Bronchial hyperresponsiveness involving release of inflammatory mediators, increased airway secretions, and bronchoconstriction	Acute episodes, separated by symptom-free periods. Nocturnal episodes common
Diffuse Interstitial Lung Diseases ***(such as sarcoidosis, widespread neoplasms, asbestosis, and idiopathic pulmonary fibrosis)***	Abnormal and widespread infiltration of cells, fluid, and collagen into interstitial spaces between alveoli. Many causes	Progressive dyspnea, which varies in its rate of development with the cause
Pneumonia	Inflammation of lung parenchyma from the respiratory bronchioles to the alveoli	An acute illness, timing varies with the causative agent
Spontaneous Pneumothorax	Leakage of air into pleural space through blebs on visceral pleura, with resulting partial or complete collapse of the lung	Sudden onset of dyspnea
Acute Pulmonary Embolism	Sudden occlusion of all or part of pulmonary arterial tree by a blood clot that usually originates in deep veins of legs or pelvis	Sudden onset of dyspnea
Anxiety With Hyperventilation	Overbreathing, with resultant respiratory alkalosis and fall in the partial pressure of carbon dioxide in the blood	Episodic, often recurrent

*Chronic bronchitis and *chronic obstructive pulmonary disease (COPD)* may coexist.

Factors That Aggravate	Factors That Relieve	Associated Symptoms	Setting
Exertion, lying down	Rest, sitting up, though dyspnea may become persistent	Often cough, orthopnea, paroxysmal nocturnal dyspnea; sometimes wheezing	History of heart disease or its predisposing factors
Exertion, inhaled irritants, respiratory infections	Expectoration; rest, though dyspnea may become persistent	Chronic productive cough, recurrent respiratory infections; wheezing may develop	History of smoking, air pollutants, recurrent respiratory infections
Exertion	Rest, though dyspnea may become persistent	Cough, with scant mucoid sputum	History of smoking, air pollutants, sometimes a familial deficiency in $alpha_1$-antitrypsin
Variable, including allergens, irritants, respiratory infections, exercise, and emotion	Separation from aggravating factors	Wheezing, cough, tightness in chest	Environmental and emotional conditions
Exertion	Rest, though dyspnea may become persistent	Often weakness, fatigue. Cough less common than in other lung diseases	Varied. Exposure to one of many substances may be causative.
		Pleuritic pain, cough, sputum, fever, though not necessarily present	Varied
		Pleuritic pain, cough	Often a previously healthy young adult
		Often none. Retrosternal oppressive pain if the occlusion is massive. Pleuritic pain, cough, and hemoptysis may follow an embolism if pulmonary infarction ensues. Symptoms of anxiety (see below).	Postpartum or postoperative periods; prolonged bed rest; congestive heart failure, chronic lung disease, and fractures of hip or leg; deep venous thrombosis (often not clinically apparent)
More often occurs at rest than after exercise. An upsetting event may not be evident.	Breathing in and out of a paper or plastic bag sometimes helps the associated symptoms.	Sighing, lightheadedness, numbness or tingling of the hands and feet, palpitations, chest pain	Other manifestations of anxiety may be present.

TABLE 7-3 Cough and Hemoptysis*

Problem	Cough and Sputum	Associated Symptoms and Setting
Acute Inflammation		
Laryngitis	Dry cough (without sputum), may become productive of variable amounts of sputum	An acute, fairly minor illness with hoarseness. Often associated with viral nasopharyngitis
Tracheobronchitis	Dry cough, may become productive (as above)	An acute, often viral illness, with burning retrosternal discomfort
Mycoplasma and Viral Pneumonias	Dry hacking cough, often becoming productive of mucoid sputum	An acute febrile illness, often with malaise, headache, and possibly dyspnea
Bacterial Pneumonias	Pneumococcal: sputum mucoid or purulent; may be blood-streaked, diffusely pinkish, or rusty	An acute illness with chills, high fever, dyspnea, and chest pain. Often preceded by acute upper respiratory infection
	Klebsiella: similar; or sticky, red, and jellylike	Typically occurs in older alcoholic men
Chronic Inflammation		
Postnasal Drip	Chronic cough; sputum mucoid or mucopurulent	Repeated attempts to clear the throat. Postnasal discharge may be sensed by patient or seen in posterior pharynx. Associated with chronic rhinitis, with or without sinusitis
Chronic Bronchitis	Chronic cough; sputum mucoid to purulent, may be blood-streaked or even bloody	Often long-standing cigarette smoking. Recurrent superimposed infections. Wheezing and dyspnea may develop.
Bronchiectasis	Chronic cough; sputum purulent, often copious and foul-smelling; may be blood-streaked or bloody	Recurrent bronchopulmonary infections common; sinusitis may coexist.
Pulmonary Tuberculosis	Cough dry or sputum that is mucoid or purulent; may be blood-streaked or bloody	Early, no symptoms. Later, anorexia, weight loss, fatigue, fever, and night sweats
Lung Abscess	Sputum purulent and foul-smelling; may be bloody	A febrile illness. Often poor dental hygiene and a prior episode of impaired consciousness
Asthma	Cough, with thick mucoid sputum, especially near end of an attack	Episodic wheezing and dyspnea, but cough may occur alone. Often a history of allergy
Gastroesophageal Reflux	Chronic cough, especially at night or early in the morning	Wheezing, especially at night (often mistaken for asthma), early morning hoarseness, and repeated attempts to clear the throat. Often a history of heartburn and regurgitation
Neoplasm		
Cancer of the Lung	Cough dry to productive; sputum may be blood-streaked or bloody	Usually a long history of cigarette smoking. Associated manifestations are numerous.
Cardiovascular Disorders		
Left Ventricular Failure or Mitral Stenosis	Often dry, especially on exertion or at night; may progress to the pink frothy sputum of pulmonary edema or to frank hemoptysis	Dyspnea, orthopnea, paroxysmal nocturnal dyspnea
Pulmonary Emboli	Dry to productive; may be dark, bright red, or mixed with blood	Dyspnea, anxiety, chest pain, fever; factors that predispose to deep venous thrombosis
Irritating Particles, Chemicals, or Gases	Variable. There may be a latent period between exposure and symptoms.	Exposure to irritants. Eyes, nose, and throat may be affected.

*Characteristics of hemoptysis are printed in red.

TABLE 7-4 Deformities of the Thorax

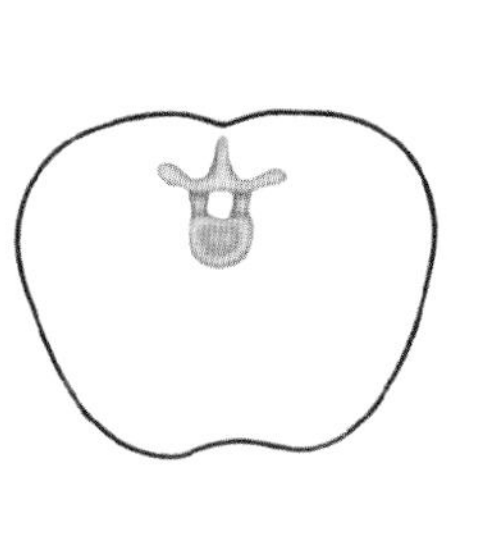
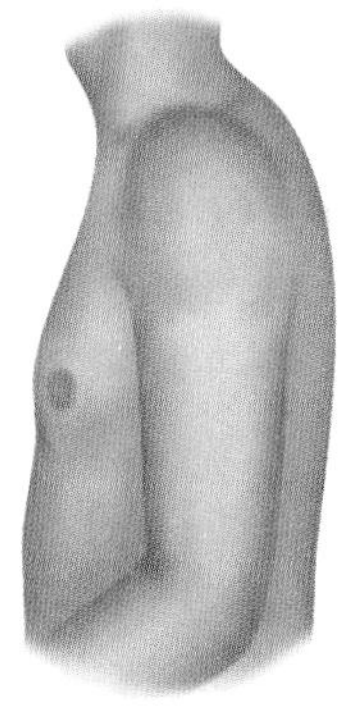

Normal Adult

The thorax in the normal adult is wider than it is deep. Its lateral diameter is larger than its anteroposterior diameter.

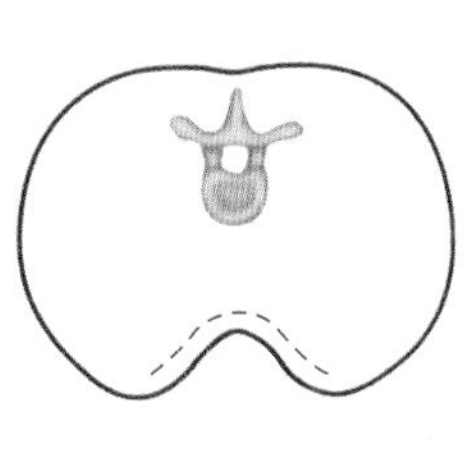
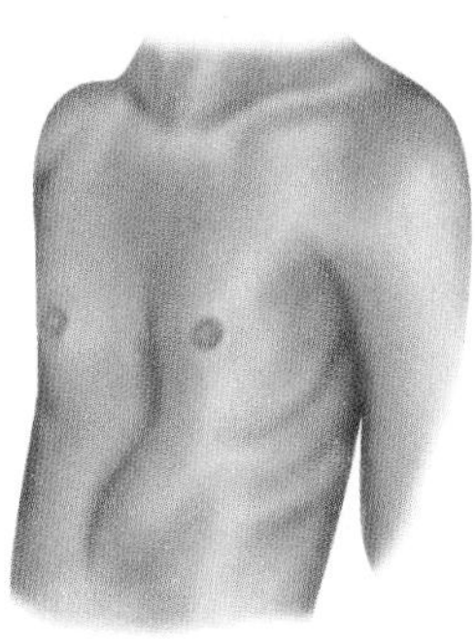

Funnel Chest (*Pectus Excavatum*)

Note depression in the lower portion of the sternum. Compression of the heart and great vessels may cause murmurs.

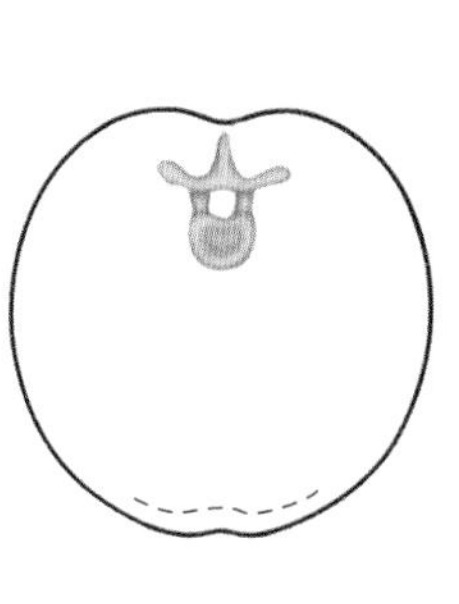
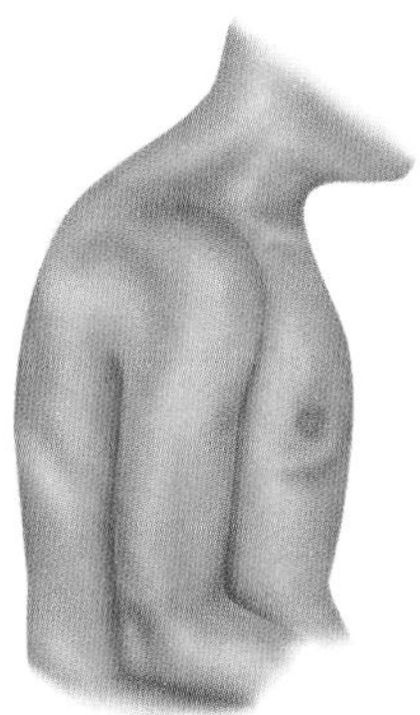

Barrel Chest

There is an increased anteroposterior diameter. This shape is normal during infancy, and often accompanies normal aging and chronic obstructive pulmonary disease.

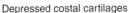

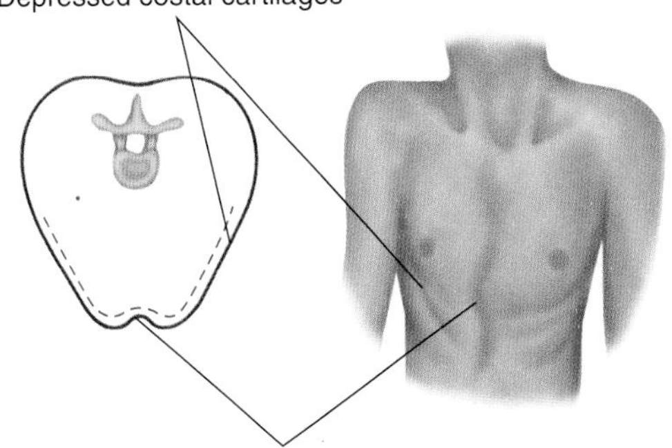

Pigeon Chest (*Pectus Carinatum*)

The sternum is displaced anteriorly, increasing the anteroposterior diameter. The costal cartilages adjacent to the protruding sternum are depressed.

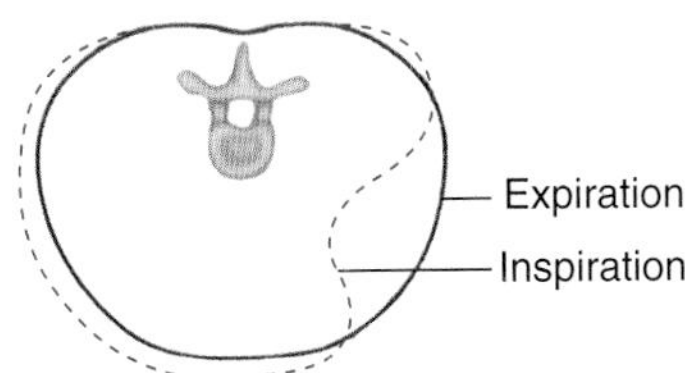

Traumatic Flail Chest

Multiple rib fractures may result in paradoxical movements of the thorax. As descent of the diaphragm decreases intrathoracic pressure, on inspiration the injured area caves inward; on expiration, it moves outward.

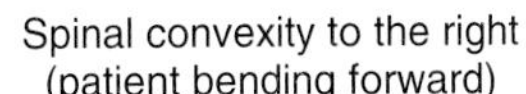

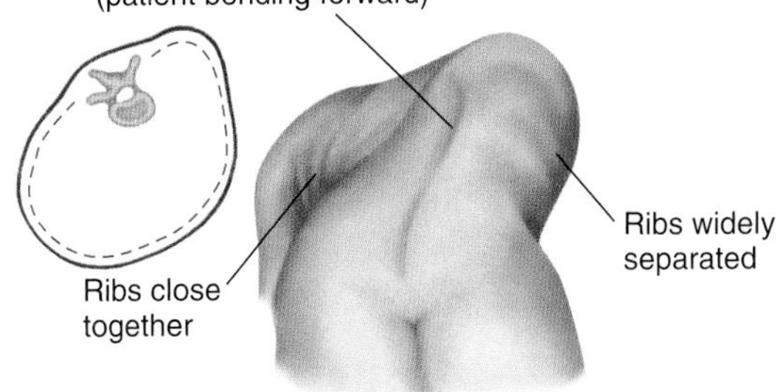

Thoracic Kyphoscoliosis

Abnormal spinal curvatures and vertebral rotation deform the chest. Distortion of the underlying lungs may make interpretation of lung findings very difficult.

TABLE 7-5 Normal and Altered Breath and Voice Sounds

The origins of breath sounds are still unclear. According to leading theories, turbulent air flow in the central airways produces the tracheal and bronchial breath sounds. As these sounds pass through the lungs to the periphery, lung tissue filters out their higher-pitched components, and only the soft and lower-pitched components reach the chest wall, where they are heard as vesicular breath sounds. Normally, tracheal and bronchial sounds may be heard over the trachea and mainstem bronchi; vesicular breath sounds predominate throughout most of the lungs.

When lung tissue loses its air, it transmits high-pitched sounds much better. If the tracheobronchial tree is open, bronchial breath sounds may replace the normal vesicular sounds over airless areas of the lung. This change is seen in lobar pneumonia when the alveoli fill with fluid, red cells, and white cells—a process called *consolidation*. Other causes include pulmonary edema or hemorrhage. Bronchial breath sounds usually correlate with an increase in tactile fremitus and transmitted voice sounds. These findings are summarized below.

	Normal Air-Filled Lung	**Airless Lung, as in Lobar Pneumonia**
	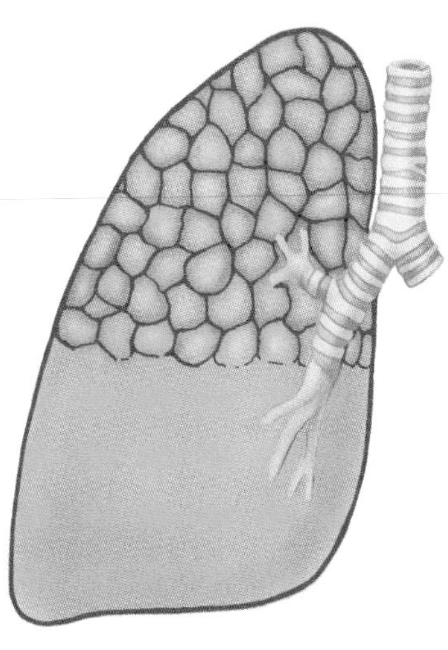	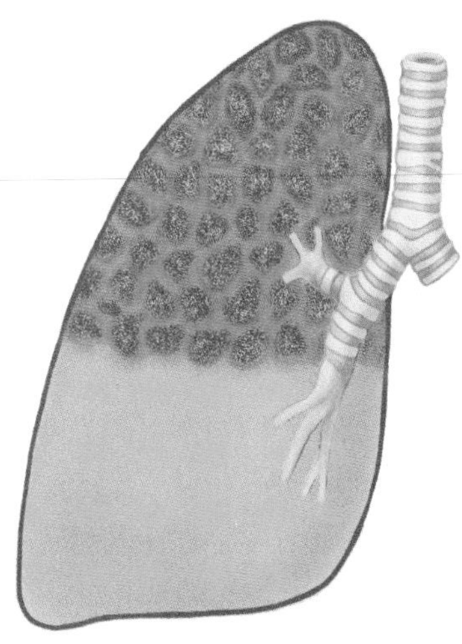
Breath Sounds	Predominantly vesicular	Bronchial or bronchovesicular over the involved area
Transmitted Voice Sounds	Spoken words muffled and indistinct Spoken "ee" heard as "ee" Whispered words faint and indistinct, if heard at all	Spoken words louder, clearer (*bronchophony*) Spoken "ee" heard as "ay" (*egophony*) Whispered words louder, clearer (*whispered pectoriloquy*)
Tactile Fremitus	Normal	Increased

TABLE 7-6 Adventitious (Added) Lung Sounds: Causes and Qualities

Crackles

Crackles have two leading explanations. (1) They result from a series of tiny explosions when small airways, deflated during expiration, pop open during inspiration. This mechanism probably explains the late inspiratory crackles of interstitial lung disease and early congestive heart failure. (2) Crackles result from air bubbles flowing through secretions or lightly closed airways during respiration. This mechanism probably explains at least some coarse crackles.

Inspiration Expiration

Late inspiratory crackles may begin in the first half of inspiration but must continue into late inspiration. They are usually fine and fairly profuse, and persist from breath to breath. These crackles appear first at the bases of the lungs, spread upward as the condition worsens, and shift to dependent regions with changes in posture. Causes include interstitial lung disease (such as fibrosis) and early congestive heart failure.

Early inspiratory crackles appear soon after the start of inspiration and do not continue into late inspiration. They are often but not always coarse and are relatively few in number. Expiratory crackles are sometimes associated. Causes include chronic bronchitis and asthma.

Midinspiratory and expiratory crackles are heard in bronchiectasis but are not specific for this diagnosis. Wheezes and rhonchi may be associated.

Wheezes and Rhonchi

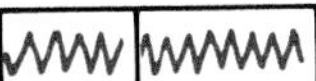

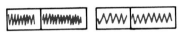

Wheezes occur when air flows rapidly through bronchi that are narrowed nearly to the point of closure. They are often audible at the mouth as well as through the chest wall. Causes of wheezes that are generalized throughout the chest include asthma, chronic bronchitis, COPD, and congestive heart failure (cardiac asthma). In asthma, wheezes may be heard only in expiration or in both phases of the respiratory cycle. Rhonchi suggest secretions in the larger airways. In chronic bronchitis, wheezes and rhonchi often clear with coughing.

Occasionally in severe obstructive pulmonary disease, the patient is no longer able to force enough air through the narrowed bronchi to produce wheezing. The resulting *silent chest* should raise immediate concern and not be mistaken for improvement.

A persistent localized wheeze suggests a partial obstruction of a bronchus, as by a tumor or foreign body. It may be inspiratory, expiratory, or both.

Stridor

A wheeze that is entirely or predominantly inspiratory is called *stridor*. It is often louder in the neck than over the chest wall. It indicates a partial obstruction of the larynx or trachea, and demands immediate attention.

Pleural Rub

Inflamed and roughened pleural surfaces grate against each other as they are momentarily and repeatedly delayed by increased friction. These movements produce creaking sounds known as a *pleural rub* (or pleural friction rub).

Pleural rubs resemble crackles acoustically, although they are produced by different pathologic processes. The sounds may be discrete, but sometimes are so numerous that they merge into a seemingly continuous sound. A rub is usually confined to a relatively small area of the chest wall, and typically is heard in both phases of respiration. When inflamed pleural surfaces are separated by fluid, the rub often disappears.

Mediastinal Crunch (*Hamman's Sign*)

A *mediastinal crunch* is a series of precordial crackles synchronous with the heart beat, not with respiration. Best heard in the left lateral position, it is due to mediastinal emphysema (pneumomediastinum).

TABLE 7-7 Physical Findings in Selected Chest Disorders

The black boxes in this table suggest a framework for clinical assessment. Start with the three boxes under Percussion Note: resonant, dull, and hyperresonant. Then move from each of these to other boxes that emphasize some of the key differences among various conditions. The changes described vary with the extent and severity of the disorder. Abnormalities deep in the chest usually produce fewer signs than superficial ones, and may cause no signs at all. Use the table for the direction of typical changes, not for absolute distinctions.

Condition	Percussion Note	Trachea	Breath Sounds	Adventitious Sounds	Tactile Fremitus and Transmitted Voice Sounds
Normal The tracheobronchial tree and alveoli are clear; pleurae are thin and close together; mobility of the chest wall is unimpaired.	**Resonant**	Midline	Vesicular, except perhaps bronchovesicular and bronchial sounds over the large bronchi and trachea, respectively	None, except perhaps a few transient inspiratory crackles at the bases of the lungs	Normal
Chronic Bronchitis The bronchi are chronically inflamed and a productive cough is present. Airway obstruction may develop.	**Resonant**	Midline	Vesicular (normal)	None; or scattered coarse *crackles* in early inspiration and perhaps expiration; or *wheezes* or *rhonchi*	Normal
Left-Sided Heart Failure (*Early*) Increased pressure in the pulmonary veins causes congestion and interstitial edema (around the alveoli); bronchial mucosa may become edematous.	**Resonant**	Midline	Vesicular	*Late inspiratory crackles* in the dependent portions of the lungs; possibly *wheezes*	Normal
Consolidation Alveoli fill with fluid or blood cells, as in pneumonia, pulmonary edema, or pulmonary hemorrhage.	**Dull** over the airless area	Midline	*Bronchial* over the involved area	*Late inspiratory crackles* over the involved area	*Increased* over the involved area, with *bronchophony, egophony,* and *whispered pectoriloquy*
Atelectasis (*Lobar Obstruction*) When a plug in a mainstem bronchus (as from mucus or a foreign object) obstructs air flow, affected lung tissue collapses into an airless state.	**Dull** over the airless area	May be *shifted toward involved side*	*Usually absent* when bronchial plug persists. Exceptions include right upper lobe atelectasis, where adjacent tracheal sounds may be transmitted.	None	*Usually absent* when the bronchial plug persists. In exceptions (e.g., right upper lobe atelectasis) may be increased

(table continues next page)

TABLE 7-7 Physical Findings in Selected Chest Disorders *(Continued)*

Condition	Percussion Note	Trachea	Breath Sounds	Adventitious Sounds	Tactile Fremitus and Transmitted Voice Sounds
Pleural Effusion Fluid accumulates in the pleural space, separates air-filled lung from the chest wall, blocking the transmission of sound.	**Dull** to flat over the fluid	*Shifted toward opposite side* in a large effusion	*Decreased to absent,* but bronchial breath sounds may be heard near top of large effusion.	None, except a *possible pleural* rub	*Decreased to absent, but may be increased* toward the top of a large effusion
Pneumothorax When air leaks into the pleural space, usually unilaterally, the lung recoils from the chest wall. Pleural air blocks transmission of sound.	**Hyperresonant** or tympanitic over the pleural air	*Shifted toward opposite side* if much air	*Decreased to absent* over the pleural air	None, except a *possible pleural* rub	*Decreased to absent* over the pleural air
Chronic Obstructive Pulmonary Disease (COPD) Slowly progressive disorder in which the distal air spaces enlarge and lungs become hyperinflated. Chronic bronchitis is often associated.	Diffusely **hyperresonant**	Midline	*Decreased to absent*	None, or the crackles, wheezes, and rhonchi of associated chronic bronchitis	*Decreased*
Asthma Widespread narrowing of the tracheobronchial tree diminishes air flow to a fluctuating degree. During attacks, air flow decreases further, and lungs hyperinflate.	**Resonant** to diffusely **hyperresonant**	Midline	*Often obscured by wheezes*	*Wheezes, possibly crackles*	*Decreased*

CHAPTER

8

The Cardiovascular System

ANATOMY AND PHYSIOLOGY

SURFACE PROJECTIONS OF THE HEART AND GREAT VESSELS

Understanding cardiac anatomy and physiology is particularly important in the examination of the cardiovascular system. Learn to visualize the underlying structures of the heart as you examine the anterior chest.

Note that the *right ventricle* occupies most of the anterior cardiac surface. This chamber and the pulmonary artery form a wedgelike structure behind and to the left of the sternum, outlined in red.

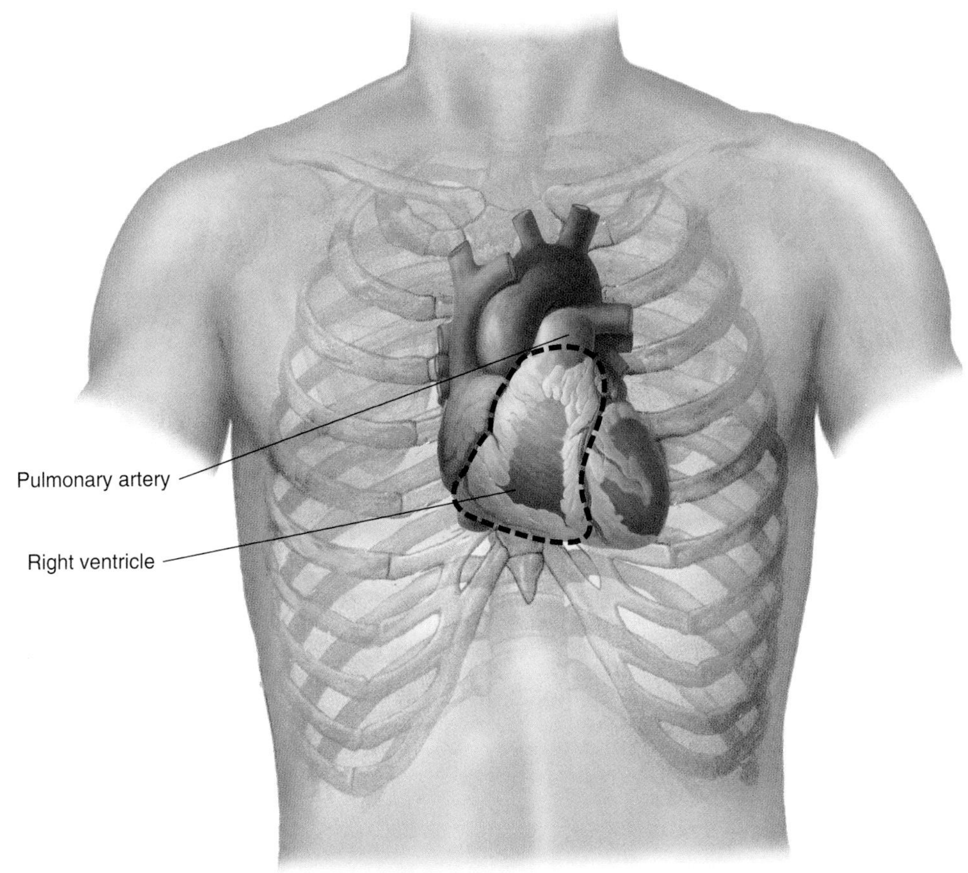

The inferior border of the right ventricle lies below the junction of the sternum and the xiphoid process. The right ventricle narrows superiorly and meets the pulmonary artery at the level of the sternum or "base of the heart"—a clinical term that refers to the proximal surface of the heart at the right and left 2nd interspaces close to the sternum.

The *left ventricle,* behind the right ventricle and to the left, as outlined, forms the left lateral margin of the heart. Its tapered inferior tip is often termed the cardiac "apex." It is clinically important because it produces the *apical impulse,* sometimes called the *point of maximal impulse,* or *PMI.* This impulse locates the left border of the heart and is usually found in the 5th interspace 7 cm to 9 cm lateral to the midsternal line. It is approximately the size of a quarter, roughly 1 to 2.5 cm in diameter. Because the most prominent cardiac impulse may not be apical, some authorities discourage use of the term PMI.

The right heart border is formed by the *right atrium,* a chamber not usually identifiable on physical examination. The *left atrium* is mostly posterior and cannot be examined directly, although its small atrial appendage may make up a segment of the left heart border between the pulmonary artery and the left ventricle.

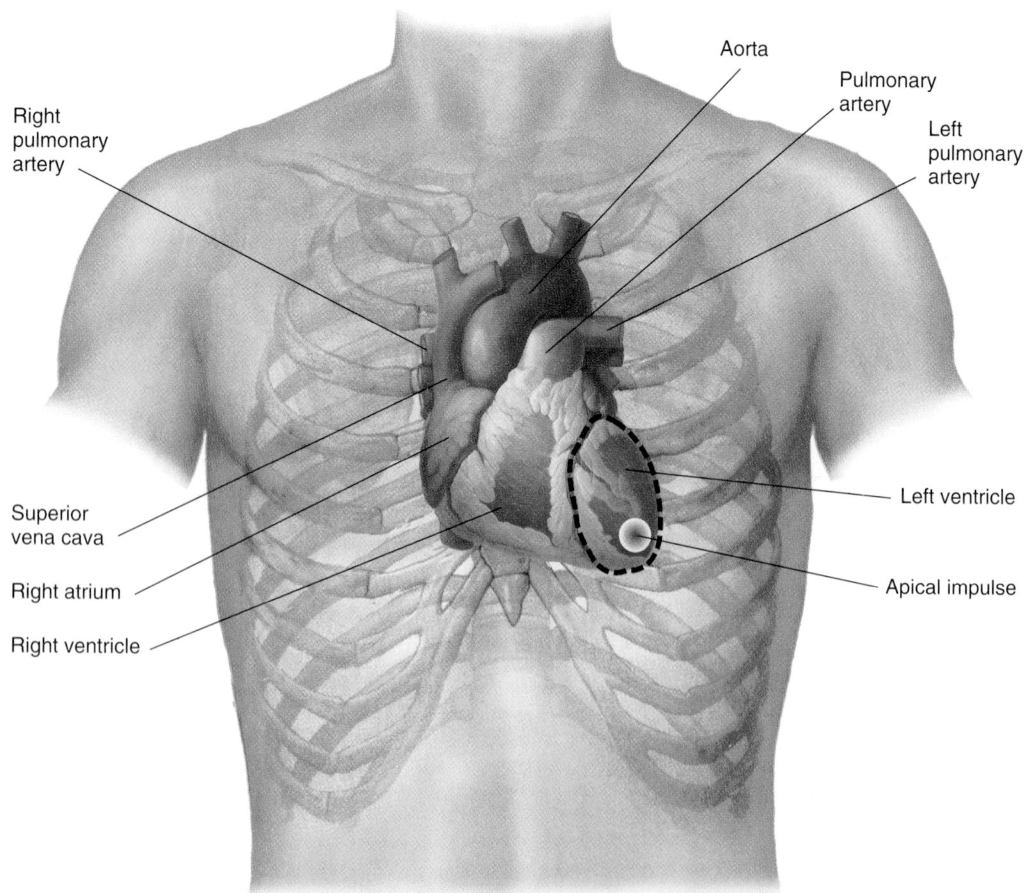

Above the heart lie the great vessels. The *pulmonary artery,* already mentioned, bifurcates quickly into its left and right branches. The *aorta* curves upward from the left ventricle to the level of the sternal angle, where it arches backward to the left and then down. On the right, the superior vena cava empties into the right atrium.

Although not illustrated, the inferior vena cava also empties into the right atrium. The *superior* and *inferior venae cavae* carry venous blood to the heart from the upper and lower portions of the body.

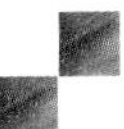

CARDIAC CHAMBERS, VALVES, AND CIRCULATION

Circulation through the heart is shown in the diagram below, which identifies the cardiac chambers, valves, and direction of blood flow. Because of their positions, the *tricuspid* and *mitral valves* are often called *atrioventricular valves.* The *aortic* and *pulmonic valves* are called *semilunar valves* because each of their leaflets is shaped like a half moon. Although this diagram shows all valves in an open position, they do not open simultaneously in the living heart.

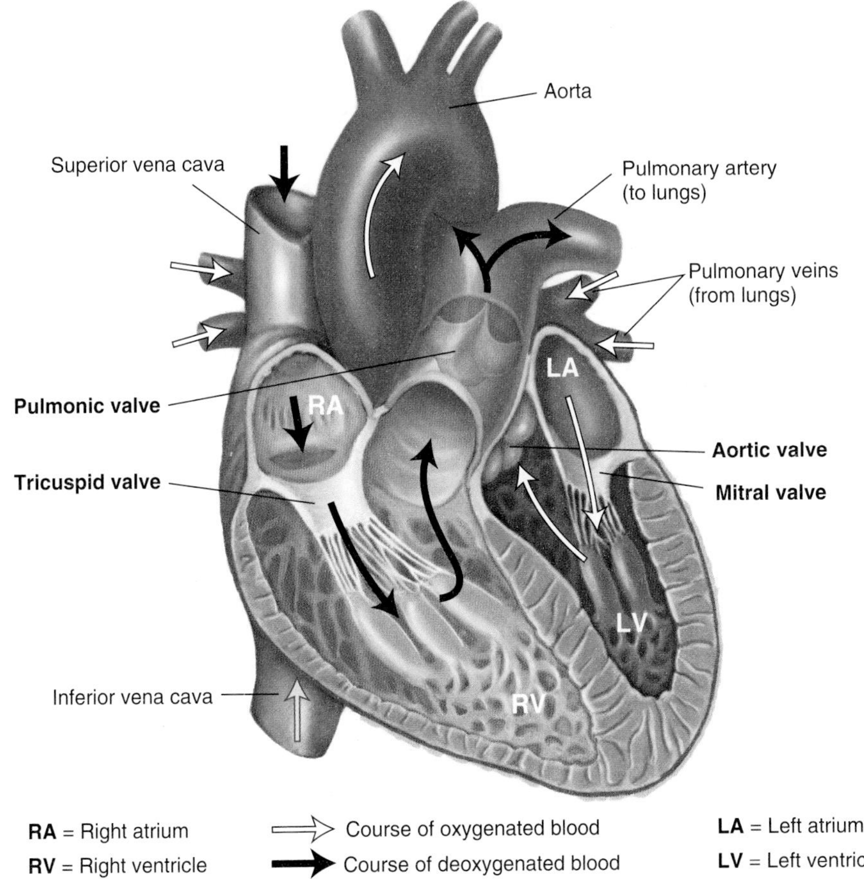

As the heart valves close, the heart sounds arise from vibrations emanating from the leaflets, the adjacent cardiac structures, and the flow of blood. It is essential to understand the positions and movements of the valves in relation to events in the cardiac cycle.

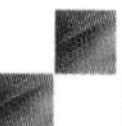

EVENTS IN THE CARDIAC CYCLE

The heart serves as a pump that generates varying pressures as its chambers contract and relax. *Systole is the period of ventricular contraction.* In the diagram below, pressure in the left ventricle rises from less than 5 mm Hg in its resting state to a normal peak of 120 mm Hg. After the ventricle ejects much of its blood into the aorta, the pressure levels off and starts to fall. *Diastole is the period of ventricular relaxation.* Ventricular pressure falls further to below 5 mm Hg, and blood flows from atrium to ventricle. Late in diastole, ventricular pressure rises slightly during inflow of blood from atrial contraction.

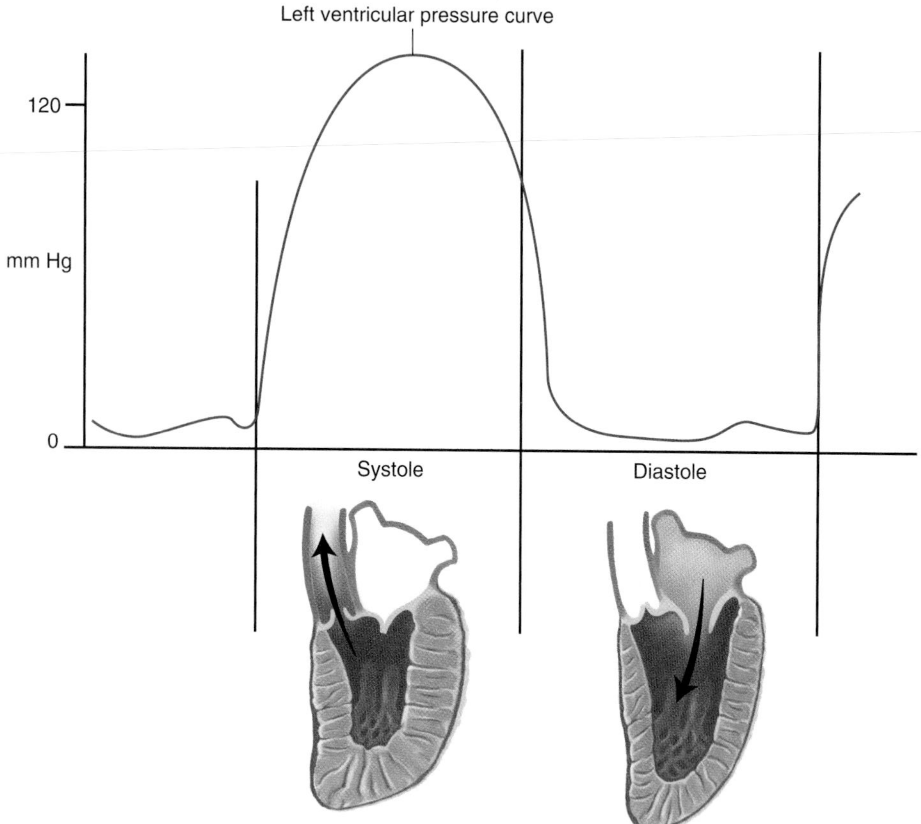

Note that during *systole* the aortic valve is open, allowing ejection of blood from the left ventricle into the aorta. The mitral valve is closed, preventing blood from regurgitating back into the left atrium. In contrast, during *diastole* the aortic valve is closed, preventing regurgitation of blood from the aorta back into the left ventricle. The mitral valve is open, allowing blood to flow from the left atrium into the relaxed left ventricle.

Understanding the interrelationships of the *pressure gradients* in these three chambers—left atrium, left ventricle, and aorta—together with the position and movement of the valves is fundamental to understanding heart sounds. Trace these changing pressures and sounds through one cardiac cycle. Note that during auscultation the first and second heart sounds define the duration of *systole* and *diastole.* An extensive literature deals with the exact causes of heart sounds. Possible explanations include actual closure of valve leaflets, tensing of related structures, leaflet positions and pressure gradients at the time of atrial and ventricular systole, and the effects of columns of blood. The explanations given here are oversimplified but retain clinical usefulness.

During *diastole,* pressure in the blood-filled left atrium slightly exceeds that in the relaxed left ventricle, and blood flows from left atrium to left ventricle across the open mitral valve. Just before the onset of ventricular systole, atrial contraction produces a slight pressure rise in both chambers.

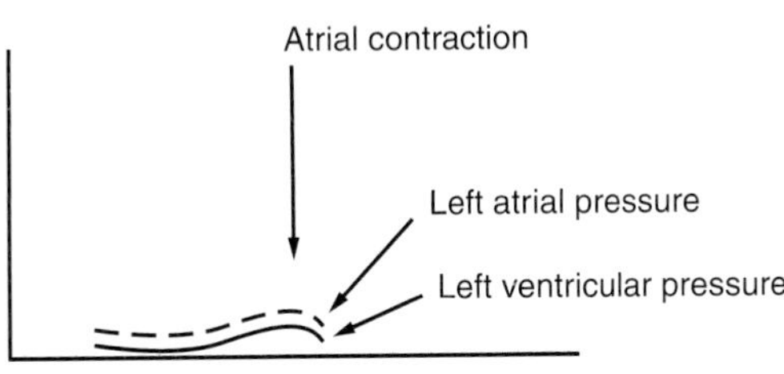

During *systole,* the left ventricle starts to contract and ventricular pressure rapidly exceeds left atrial pressure, thus shutting the mitral valve. *Closure of the mitral valve produces the first heart sound,* S_1.

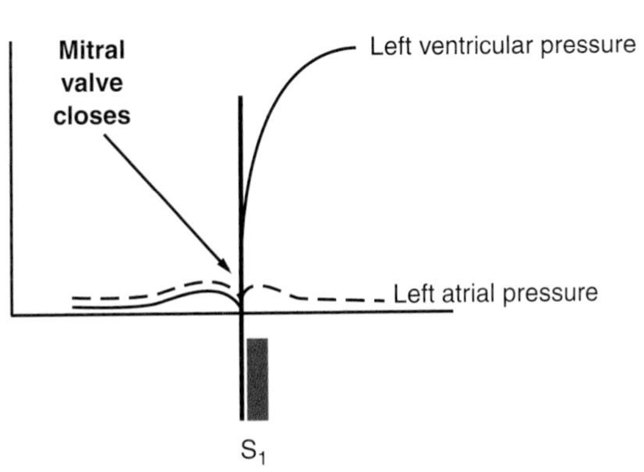

As left ventricular pressure continues to rise, it quickly exceeds the pressure in the aorta and forces the aortic valve open. In some pathologic conditions, opening of the aortic valve is accompanied by an early systolic ejection sound (Ej). *Normally, maximal left ventricular pressure corresponds to systolic blood pressure.*

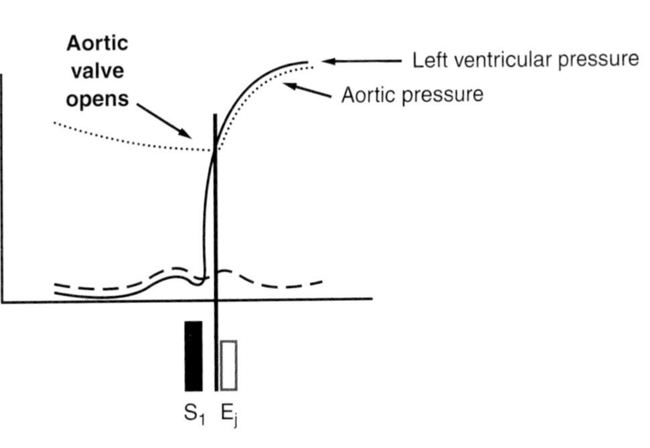

As the left ventricle ejects most of its blood, ventricular pressure begins to fall. When left ventricular pressure drops below aortic pressure, the aortic valve shuts. *Aortic valve closure produces the second heart sound,* S_2, and another diastole begins.

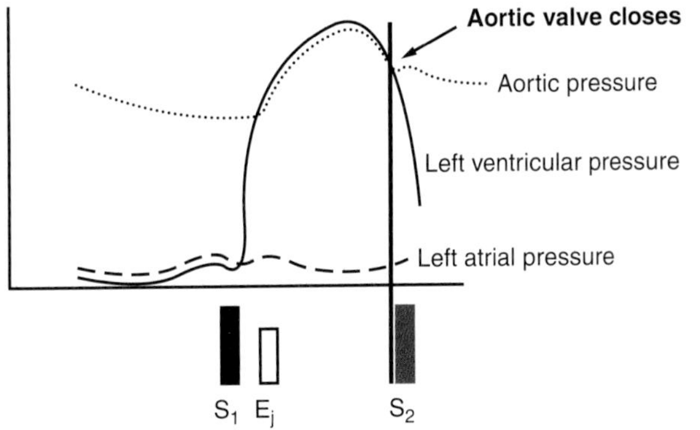

In *diastole,* left ventricular pressure continues to drop and falls below left atrial pressure. The mitral valve opens. This is usually a silent event, but may be audible as a pathologic opening snap (OS) if valve leaflet motion is restricted, as in mitral stenosis.

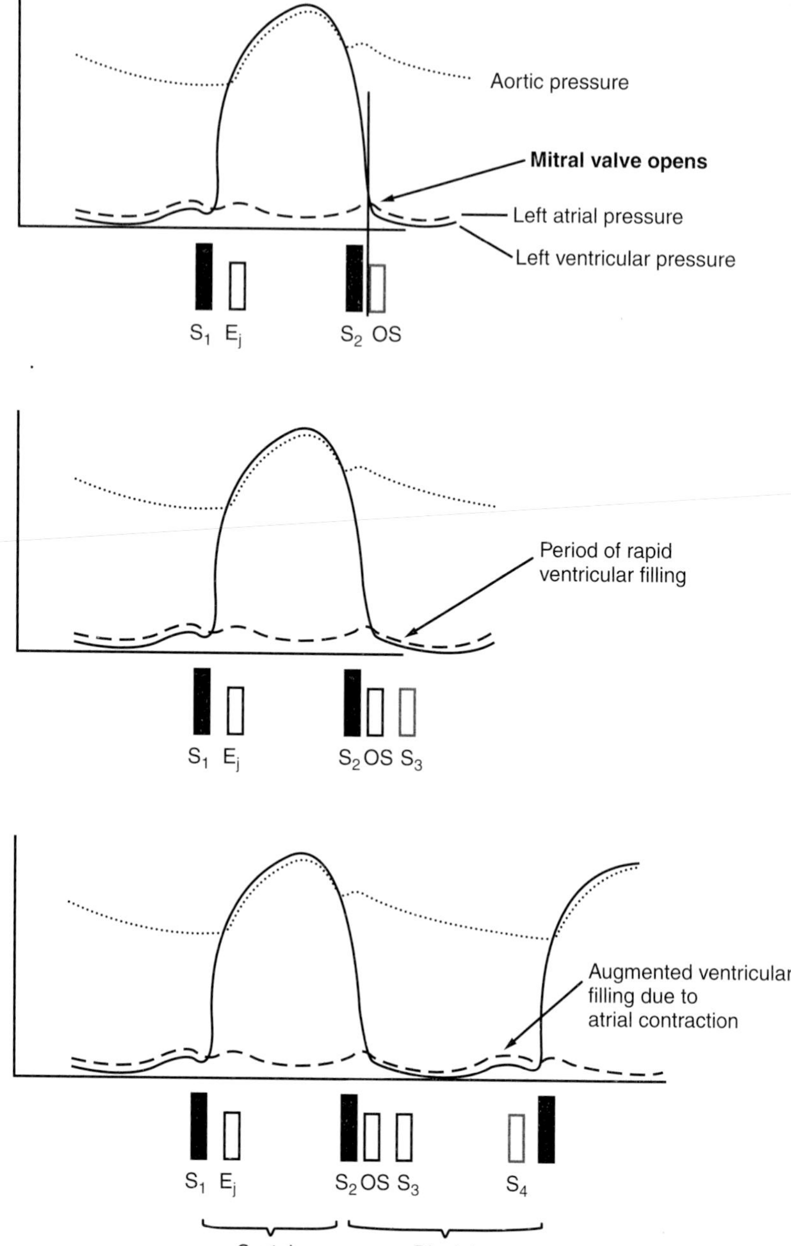

After the mitral valve opens, there is a period of rapid ventricular filling as blood flows early in diastole from left atrium to left ventricle. In children and young adults, a third heart sound, S_3, may arise from rapid deceleration of the column of blood against the ventricular wall. In older adults, an S_3, sometimes termed "an S_3 gallop," usually indicates a pathologic change in ventricular compliance.

Finally, although not often heard in normal adults, a fourth heart sound, S_4, marks atrial contraction. It immediately precedes S_1 of the next beat, and also reflects a pathologic change in ventricular compliance.

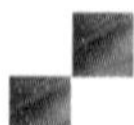

THE SPLITTING OF HEART SOUNDS

While these events are occurring on the left side of the heart, similar changes are occurring on the right, involving the right atrium, right ventricle, tricuspid valve, pulmonic valve, and pulmonary artery. Right ventricular and pulmonary arterial pressures are significantly lower than corresponding pressures on the left side. Furthermore, right-sided events usually occur slightly later than those on the left. Instead of a single heart sound, you may hear two discernible components, the first from left-sided aortic valve closure, or A_2, and the second from right-sided closure of the pulmonic valve, or P_2.

Consider the second heart sound and its two components, A_2 and P_2, which come from closure of the aortic and pulmonic valves, respectively. During inspiration A_2 and P_2 separate slightly, and may split S_2 into its two audible components. During expiration, these two components are fused into a single sound, S_2.

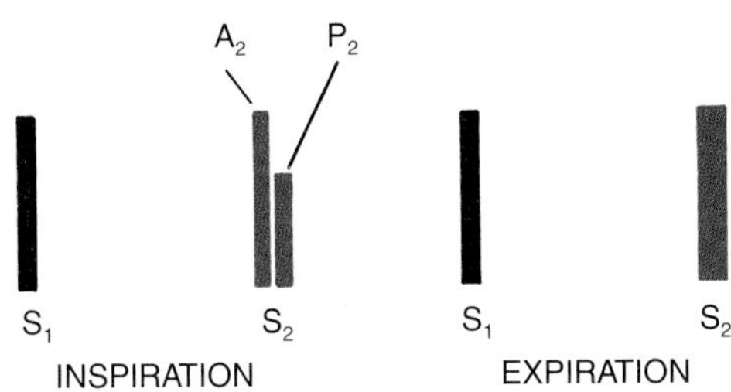

Current explanations of inspiratory splitting cite increased capacitance in the pulmonary vascular bed during inspiration, which prolongs ejection of blood from the right ventricle, delaying closure of the pulmonic valve, or P_2. Ejection of blood from the left ventricle is comparatively shorter, so A_2 occurs slightly earlier.

Of the two components of the second heart sound, A_2 is normally louder, reflecting the high pressure in the aorta. It is heard throughout the precordium. P_2, in contrast, is relatively soft, reflecting the lower pressure in the pulmonary artery. It is heard best in its own area—the 2nd and 3rd left interspaces close to the sternum. It is here that you should search for splitting of the second heart sound.

S_1 also has two components, an earlier mitral and a later tricuspid sound. The mitral sound, its principal component, is much louder, again reflecting the high pressures on the left side of the heart. It can be heard throughout the precordium and is loudest at the cardiac apex. The softer tricuspid component is heard best at the lower left sternal border, and it is here that you may hear a split S_1. The earlier louder mitral component may mask the tricuspid sound, however, and splitting is not always detectable. Splitting of S_1 does not vary with respiration.

HEART MURMURS

Heart murmurs are distinguishable from heart sounds by their longer duration. They are attributed to turbulent blood flow and may be "innocent," as with flow murmurs of young adults, or diagnostic of valvular heart disease. A *stenotic valve* has an abnormally narrowed valvular orifice that obstructs blood flow, as in *aortic stenosis,* and causes a characteristic murmur. So does a valve that fails to fully close, as in *aortic regurgitation* or *insufficiency.* Such a valve allows blood to leak backward in a retrograde direction and produces a *regurgitant* murmur.

To identify murmurs accurately, you must learn to assess the chest wall location where they are best heard, their timing in systole or diastole, and their qualities. In the section on Techniques of Examination, you will learn to integrate several characteristics, including murmur intensity, pitch, duration, and direction of radiation (see pp. 316–319).

RELATION OF AUSCULTATORY FINDINGS TO THE CHEST WALL

The locations on the chest wall where you hear heart sounds and murmurs help to identify the valve or chamber where they originate. Sounds and murmurs arising from the mitral valve are usually heard best at and around the cardiac apex. Those originating in the tricuspid valve are heard best at or near the lower left sternal border. Murmurs arising from the pulmonic valve are usually heard best in the 2nd and 3rd left interspaces close to the sternum, but at times may also be heard at higher or lower levels, and those originating in the aortic valve may be heard anywhere from the right 2nd interspace to the apex. These areas overlap, as illustrated below, and you will need to correlate auscultatory findings with other portions of the cardiac examination to identify sounds and murmurs accurately.

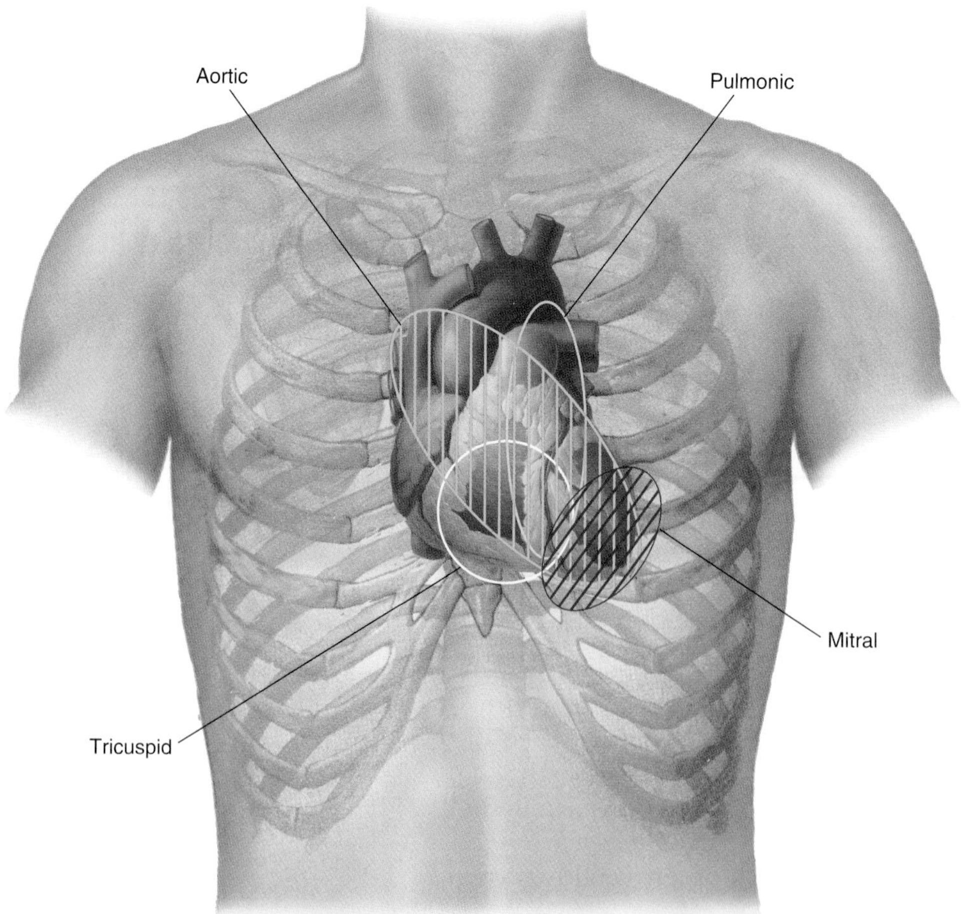

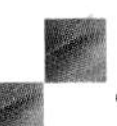

THE CONDUCTION SYSTEM

An electrical conduction system stimulates and coordinates the contraction of cardiac muscle.

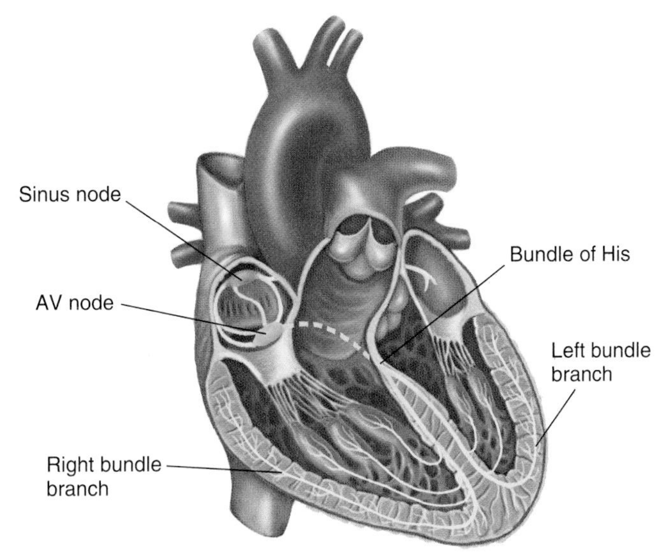

Each normal electrical impulse is initiated in the *sinus node*, a group of specialized cardiac cells located in the right atrium near the junction of the vena cava. The sinus node acts as the cardiac pacemaker and automatically discharges an impulse about 60 to 100 times a minute. This impulse travels through both atria to the *atrioventricular node*, a specialized group of cells located low in the atrial septum. Here the impulse is delayed before passing down the bundle of His and its branches to the ventricular myocardium. Muscular contraction follows: first the atria, then the ventricles. The normal conduction pathway is diagrammed in simplified form above.

The electrocardiogram, or ECG, records these events. Contraction of cardiac smooth muscle produces electrical activity, resulting in a series of waves on the ECG. The components of the *normal ECG* and their duration are briefly summarized here, but you will need further instruction and practice to interpret recordings from actual patients. Note:

- The small *P wave* of atrial depolarization (duration up to 80 milliseconds; *PR interval* 120 to 200 milliseconds)

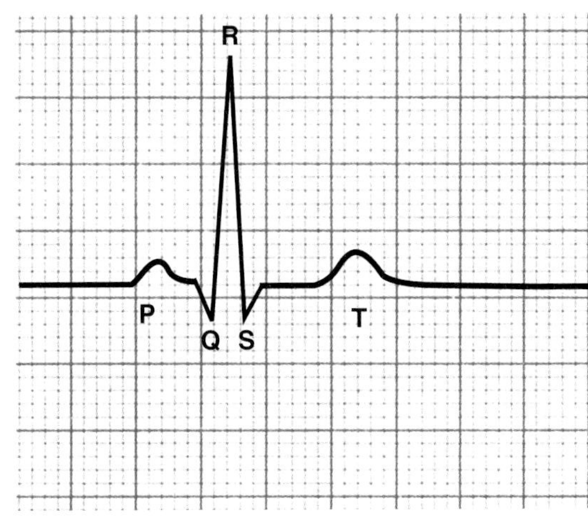

- The larger *QRS complex* of ventricular depolarization (up to 100 milliseconds), consisting of one or more of the following:

  –the *Q wave*, a downward deflection from septal depolarization
  –the *R wave*, an upward deflection from ventricular depolarization
  –the *S wave*, a downward deflection following an R wave

- A *T wave* of ventricular repolarization, or recovery (duration relates to QRS).

The electrical impulse slightly precedes the myocardial contraction that it stimulates. The relation of electrocardiographic waves to the cardiac cycle is shown below.

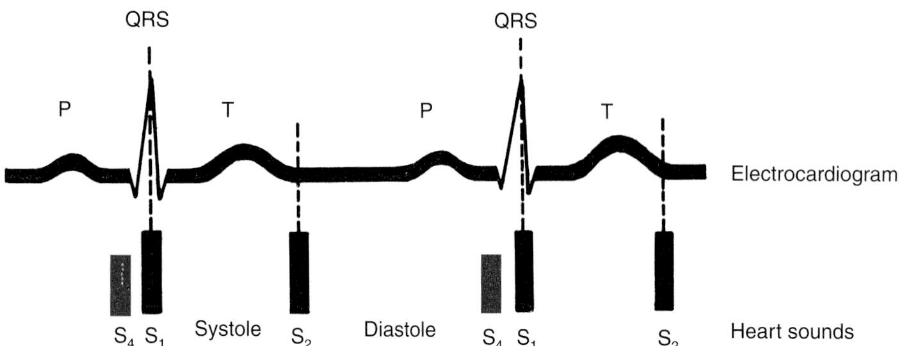

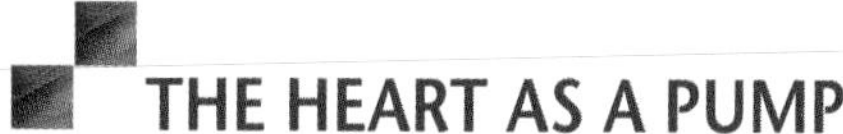

THE HEART AS A PUMP

The left and right ventricles pump blood into the systemic and pulmonary arterial trees, respectively. *Cardiac output,* the volume of blood ejected from each ventricle during 1 minute, is the product of *heart rate* and *stroke volume.* Stroke volume (the volume of blood ejected with each heartbeat) depends in turn on preload, myocardial contractility, and afterload.

Preload refers to the load that stretches the cardiac muscle before contraction. The volume of blood in the right ventricle at the end of diastole, then, constitutes its preload for the next beat. Right ventricular preload is increased by increasing venous return to the right heart. Physiologic causes include inspiration and the increased volume of blood flow from exercising muscles. The increased blood volume in a dilated right ventricle of congestive heart failure also increases preload. Causes of decreased right ventricular preload include exhalation, decreased left ventricular output, and pooling of blood in the capillary bed or the venous system.

Myocardial contractility refers to the ability of the cardiac muscle, when given a load, to shorten. Contractility increases when stimulated by action of the sympathetic nervous system, and decreases when blood flow or oxygen delivery to the myocardium is impaired.

Afterload refers to the degree of vascular resistance to ventricular contraction. Sources of resistance to left ventricular contraction include the tone in the walls of the aorta, the large arteries, and the peripheral vascular tree (primarily the small arteries and arterioles), as well as the volume of blood already in the aorta.

Pathologic increases in preload and afterload, called *volume overload* and *pressure overload,* respectively, produce changes in ventricular function that may be clinically detectable. These changes include alterations in ventricular impulses, detectable by palpation, and in normal heart sounds. Pathologic heart sounds and murmurs may also develop.

ARTERIAL PULSES AND BLOOD PRESSURE

With each contraction, the left ventricle ejects a volume of blood into the aorta and on into the arterial tree. The ensuing pressure wave moves rapidly through the arterial system, where it is felt as the *arterial pulse*. Although the pressure wave travels quickly—many times faster than the blood itself—a palpable delay between ventricular contraction and peripheral pulses makes the pulses in the arms and legs unsuitable for timing events in the cardiac cycle.

Blood pressure in the arterial system varies during the cardiac cycle, peaking in systole and falling to its lowest trough in diastole. These are the levels that are measured with the blood pressure cuff, or sphygmomanometer. The difference between systolic and diastolic pressures is known as the *pulse pressure*.

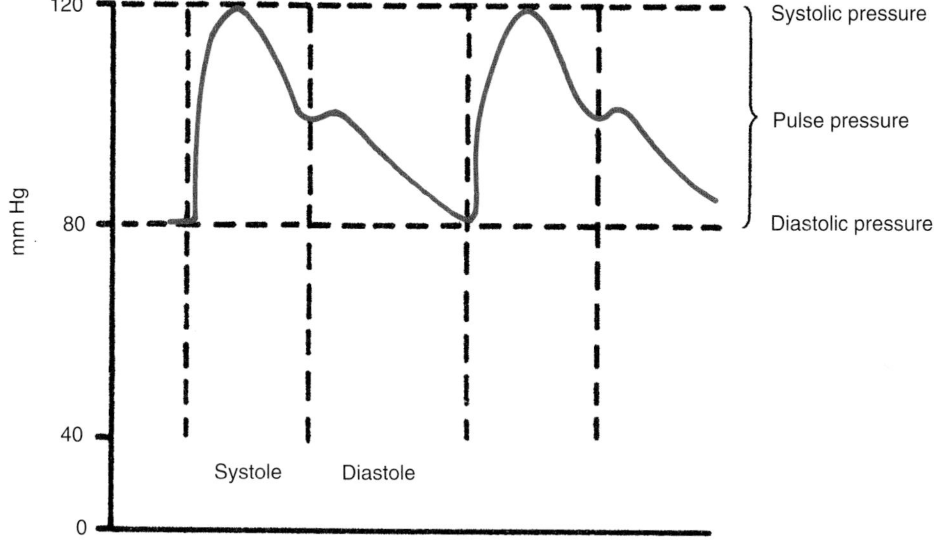

The principal factors influencing arterial pressure are:

- Left ventricular stroke volume
- Distensibility of the aorta and the large arteries
- Peripheral vascular resistance, particularly at the arteriolar level
- Volume of blood in the arterial system.

Changes in any of these four factors alter systolic pressure, diastolic pressure, or both. Blood pressure levels fluctuate strikingly through any 24-hour period, varying with physical activity; emotional state; pain; noise; environmental temperature; the use of coffee, tobacco, and other drugs; and even the time of day.

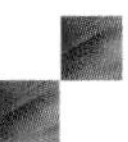

JUGULAR VENOUS PRESSURE (JVP)

Systemic venous pressure is much lower than arterial pressure. Although venous pressure ultimately depends on left ventricular contraction, much of this force is dissipated as blood flows through the arterial tree and the capillary bed. Walls of veins contain less smooth muscle than walls of arteries. This reduces venous tone and makes veins more distensible. Other important determinants of venous pressure include blood volume and the capacity of the right heart to eject blood into the pulmonary arterial system. Cardiac disease may alter these variables, producing abnormalities in central venous pressure. For example, venous pressure falls when left ventricular output or blood volume is significantly reduced; it rises when the right heart fails or when increased pressure in the pericardial sac impedes the return of blood to the right atrium. These venous pressure changes are reflected in the height of the venous column of blood in the internal jugular veins, termed the *jugular venous pressure* or *JVP.*

Pressure in the jugular veins reflects right atrial pressure, giving clinicians an important clinical indicator of cardiac function and right heart hemodynamics. Assessing the JVP is an essential, though challenging, clinical skill. The JVP is best estimated from the internal jugular vein, usually on the *right side,* because the right internal jugular vein has a more direct anatomic channel into the right atrium.[1]

The internal jugular veins lie deep to the sternomastoid muscles in the neck and are not directly visible, so the clinician must learn to identify the *pulsations* of the internal jugular vein that are transmitted to the surface of the neck, making sure to carefully distinguish these venous pulsations from pulsations of the carotid artery. If pulsations from the internal jugular vein cannot be identified, those of the external jugular vein can be used, but they are less reliable.

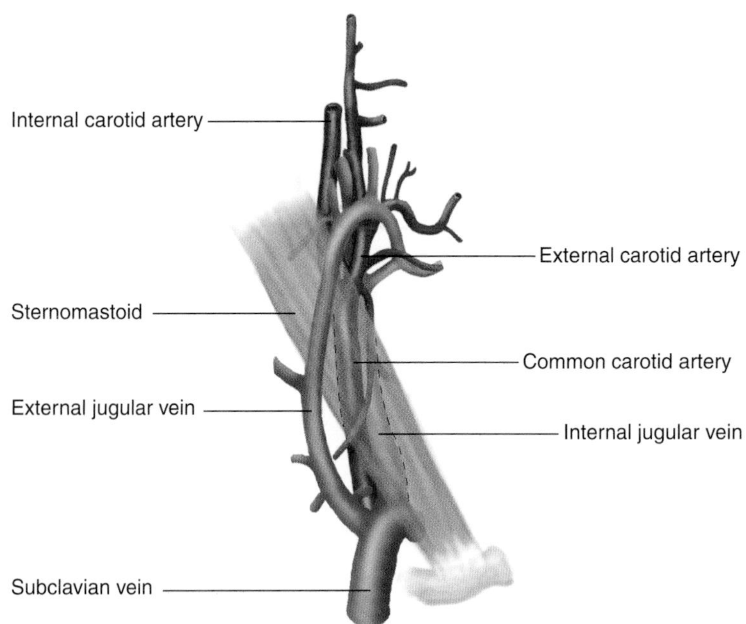

To estimate the level of the JVP, you will learn to find the *highest point of oscillation in the internal jugular vein* or, if necessary, the point above which the external jugular vein appears collapsed. The JVP is usually measured in vertical distance above the *sternal angle*, the bony ridge adjacent to the second rib where the manubrium joins the body of the sternum.

Study carefully the illustrations below. Note that regardless of the patient's position, the sternal angle remains roughly 5 cm above the right atrium. In this patient, however, the pressure in the internal jugular vein is somewhat elevated.

- In *Position A*, the head of the bed is raised to the usual level, about 30°, but the JVP cannot be measured because the meniscus, or level of oscillation, is above the jaw and therefore not visible.
- In *Position B*, the head of the bed is raised to 60°. The "top" of the internal jugular vein is now easily visible, so the vertical distance from the sternal angle or right atrium can now be measured.
- In *Position C*, the patient is upright and the veins are barely discernible above the clavicle, making measurement untenable.

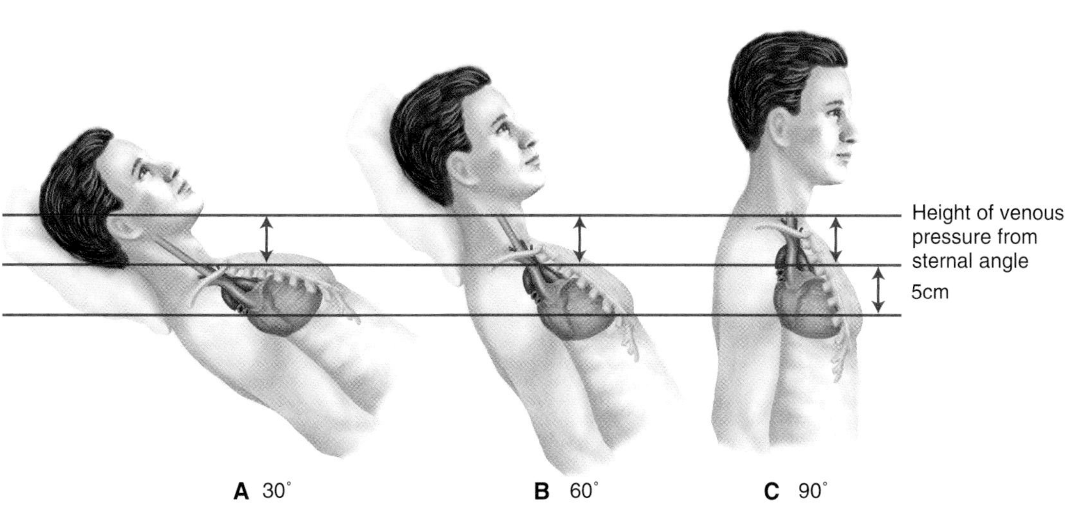

Note that the height of the venous pressure as measured from the sternal angle is the *same* in all three positions, but your ability to *measure* the height of the column of venous blood, or JVP, differs according to how you position the patient. Jugular venous pressure measured at more than 4 cm above the sternal angle, or more than 9 cm above the right atrium, is considered elevated or abnormal. The techniques for measuring the JVP are fully described in Techniques of Examination on pp. 302–304.

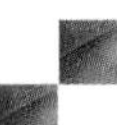

JUGULAR VENOUS PULSATIONS

The oscillations that you see in the internal jugular veins, and often in the externals, reflect changing pressures within the right atrium. The right internal jugular vein empties more directly into the right atrium and reflects these pressure changes best.

Careful observation reveals that the undulating pulsations of the internal jugular veins, and sometimes the externals, are composed of two quick peaks and two troughs.

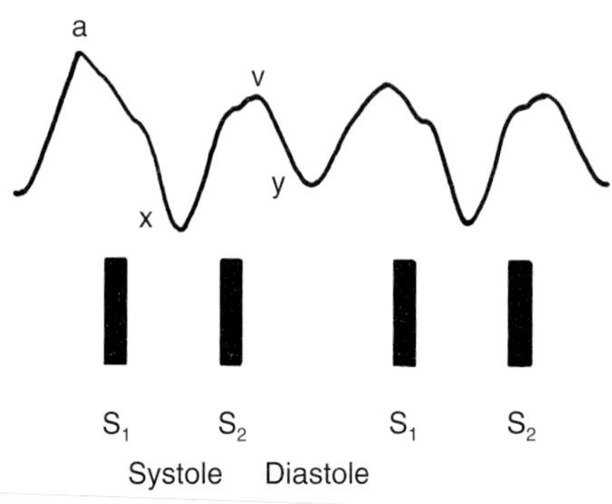

The first elevation, the *a wave,* reflects the slight rise in atrial pressure that accompanies atrial contraction. It occurs just before the first heart sound and before the carotid pulse. The following trough, the *x descent,* starts with atrial relaxation. It continues as the right ventricle, contracting during systole, pulling the floor of the atrium downward. During ventricular systole, blood continues to flow into the right atrium from the venae cavae. The tricuspid valve is closed, the chamber begins to fill, and right atrial pressure begins to rise again, creating the second elevation, the *v wave.* When the tricuspid valve opens early in diastole, blood in the right atrium flows passively into the right ventricle, and right atrial pressure falls again, creating the second trough or *y descent.* To remember these four oscillations in an oversimplified way, think of the following sequence: atrial contraction, atrial relaxation, atrial filling, and atrial emptying. (You can think of the *a* wave as atrial contraction and the *v* wave as venous filling.)

To the naked eye, the two descents are the most obvious events in the normal jugular pulse. Of the two, the sudden collapse of the *x* descent late in systole is more prominent, occurring just before the second heart sound. The *y* descent follows the second heart sound early in diastole.

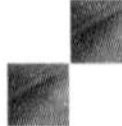

CHANGES OVER THE LIFE SPAN

Aging may affect the location of the apical impulse, the pitch of heart sounds and murmurs, the stiffness of the arteries, and blood pressure. For example, the *apical impulse* is usually felt easily in children and young adults; as the chest deepens in its anteroposterior diameter, the impulse gets harder to find. For the same reason, *splitting of the second heart sound* may be harder to hear in older people as its pulmonic component becomes less audible. Further, at some time over the life span, almost everyone has a *heart murmur.* Most murmurs occur without other evidence of cardiovascular abnormality and may therefore be considered innocent normal variants. These common murmurs vary with age, and familiarity with their patterns helps you to distinguish normal from abnormal. Turn to pp. 671–815, Chapter 18, Assessing Children:

Infancy Through Adolescence, and to pp. 817–838, Chapter 19, The Pregnant Woman, for information on how to distinguish these innocent murmurs.

Murmurs may originate in large blood vessels as well as in the heart. The *jugular venous hum,* which is very common in children, may still be heard through young adulthood (see p. 762). A second, more important example is the *cervical systolic murmur* or *bruit,* which may be innocent in children but suspicious for arterial obstruction in adults.

THE HEALTH HISTORY

Common or Concerning Symptoms

- Chest pain
- Palpitations
- Shortness of breath: dyspnea, orthopnea, or paroxysmal nocturnal dyspnea
- Swelling or edema

Chest pain or discomfort is one of the most important symptoms you will assess as a clinician. As you listen to the patient's story, you must always keep serious adverse events in mind, such as *angina pectoris, myocardial infarction,* or even a *dissecting aortic aneurysm.*[2–4] This section approaches chest symptoms from the *cardiac standpoint,* including chest pain, palpitations, orthopnea, paroxysmal nocturnal dyspnea (PND), and edema. For this complaint, however, it is wise to think through the range of possible cardiac, pulmonary, and extrathoracic etiologies. You should review the Health History section of Chapter 7, The Thorax and Lungs, which enumerates the various possible sources of chest pain: the myocardium, the pericardium, the aorta, the trachea and large bronchi, the parietal pleura, the esophagus, the chest wall, and extrathoracic structures such as the neck, gallbladder, and stomach. This review is important, because symptoms such as dyspnea, wheezing, cough, and even hemoptysis (see pp. 248–250) can be cardiac as well as pulmonary in origin.

See Table 7-1, Chest Pain, pp. 268–269.

Your initial questions should be broad . . . "Do you have any pain or discomfort in your chest?" Ask the patient to point to the pain and to describe all seven of its attributes. After listening closely to the patient's description, move on to more specific questions such as "Is the pain related to exertion?" and "What kinds of activities bring on the pain?" Also "How intense is the pain, on a scale of 1 to 10?" . . . "Does it radiate into the neck, shoulder, back, or down your arm?" . . . "Are there any associated symptoms like shortness of breath, sweating, palpitations, or nausea?" . . . "Does it ever wake you up at night?" . . . "What do you do to make it better?"

Exertional chest pain with radiation to the left side of the neck and down the left arm in *angina pectoris;* sharp pain radiating into the back or into the neck in *aortic dissection.*

Palpitations are an unpleasant awareness of the heartbeat. When reporting these sensations, patients use various terms such as skipping, racing, fluttering, pounding, or stopping of the heart. Palpitations may result from an irregular heartbeat, from rapid acceleration or slowing of the heart, or from increased forcefulness of cardiac contraction. Such perceptions, however, also depend on how patients respond to their own body sensations. Palpitations do not necessarily mean heart disease. In contrast, the most serious dysrhythmias, such as ventricular tachycardia, often do not produce palpitations.

See Tables 8-1 and 8-2 for selected heart rates and rhythms (pp. 324–325)

Symptoms or signs of irregular heart action warrant an electrocardiogram. Only *atrial fibrillation,* which is "irregularly irregular," can be reliably identified at the bedside.

You may ask directly about palpitations, but if the patient does not understand your question, reword it. "Are you ever aware of your heartbeat? What is it like?" Ask the patient to tap out the rhythm with a hand or finger. Was it fast or slow? Regular or irregular? How long did it last? If there was an episode of rapid heartbeats, did they start and stop suddenly or gradually? (For this group of symptoms, an electrocardiogram is indicated.)

It is helpful to teach selected patients how to make serial measurements of their pulse rates in case they have further episodes.

Clues in the history include transient skips and flipflops (possible premature contractions); rapid regular beating of sudden onset and offset (possible paroxysmal supraventricular tachycardia); a rapid regular rate of less than 120 beats per minute, especially if starting and stopping more gradually (possible sinus tachycardia).

Shortness of breath is a common patient concern and may represent dyspnea, orthopnea, or paroxysmal nocturnal dyspnea. *Dyspnea* is an uncomfortable awareness of breathing that is inappropriate to a given level of exertion. This complaint is often made by patients with cardiac or pulmonary problems, as discussed in Chapter 7, The Thorax and Lungs, p. 249.

Orthopnea is dyspnea that occurs when the patient is lying down and improves when the patient sits up. Classically, it is quantified according to the number of pillows the patient uses for sleeping, or by the fact that the patient needs to sleep sitting up. Make sure, however, that the reason the patient uses extra pillows or sleeps upright is shortness of breath when supine and not other causes.

Orthopnea suggests *left ventricular heart failure* or *mitral stenosis;* it may also accompany *obstructive lung disease.*

Paroxysmal nocturnal dyspnea, or *PND,* describes episodes of sudden dyspnea and orthopnea that awaken the patient from sleep, usually 1 or 2 hours after going to bed, prompting the patient to sit up, stand up, or go to a window for air. There may be associated wheezing and coughing. The episode usually subsides but may recur at about the same time on subsequent nights.

PND suggests *left ventricular heart failure* or *mitral stenosis* and may be mimicked by *nocturnal asthma* attacks.

Edema refers to the accumulation of excessive fluid in the interstitial tissue spaces and appears as swelling. Questions about edema are typically included in the cardiac history, but edema has many other causes, both local and general. Focus your questions on the location, timing, and setting of the swelling, and on associated symptoms. "Have you had any swelling anywhere? Where? . . . Anywhere else? When does it occur? Is it worse in the morning or at night? Do your shoes get tight?"

Dependent edema appears in the lowest body parts: the feet and lower legs when sitting, or the sacrum when bedridden. Causes may be cardiac (*congestive heart failure*), nutritional (*hypoalbuminemia*), or positional.

Continue with "Are the rings tight on your fingers? Are your eyelids puffy or swollen in the morning? Have you had to let out your belt?" Also, "Have your clothes gotten too tight around the middle?" It is useful to ask patients

Edema occurs in renal and liver disease: periorbital puffiness, tight rings in *nephrotic syndrome;*

who retain fluid to record daily morning weights, because edema may not be obvious until several liters of extra fluid have accumulated.

enlarged waistline from *ascites* and *liver failure.*

HEALTH PROMOTION AND COUNSELING

Important Topics for Health Promotion and Counseling

- Preventing hypertension
- Preventing cardiovascular disease and stroke
- Lowering cholesterol and low-density lipoprotein (LDL)
- Lifestyle modification and risk intervention, including healthy eating and counseling about weight and exercise

Despite improvements in risk factor modification, cardiovascular disease remains the leading cause of death for both men and women, accounting for approximately one third of all U.S. deaths. Both *primary prevention,* in those without evidence of cardiovascular disease, and *secondary prevention,* in those with known cardiovascular events such as angina or myocardial infarction, remain important priorities for the office, the hospital, and the nation's public health. Education and counseling will guide your patients to maintain optimal levels of blood pressure, cholesterol, weight, and exercise and reduce risk factors for cardiovascular disease and stroke.

Preventing Hypertension. According to the U.S. Preventive Services Task Force, hypertension accounts for "35% of all myocardial infarctions and strokes, 49% of all episodes of heart failure, and 24% of all premature deaths."[5] The Task Force strongly recommends *screening of adults 18 years and older for high blood pressure.* Recent long-term population-based studies have fueled a dramatic shift in national strategies to prevent and reduce blood pressure (BP). "The Seventh Report of the Joint National Committee on Prevention, Detection, Evaluation, and Treatment of High Blood Pressure," known as JNC 7, the National High Blood Pressure Education Program, and clinical investigators have issued several key messages (see box on next page)[6,7]: These findings underlie the tougher and simpler blood pressure classification of JNC 7 (see table on p. 109)[10]:

- The former six categories of blood pressure have been collapsed to four, with normal blood pressure defined as <120/80 mm Hg.
- Systolic blood pressures of 120 to 139 mm Hg and diastolic blood pressures of 80 to 89 mm Hg are no longer "high normal"; they are "prehypertension."

- Drug therapy should begin with stage 1 hypertension, namely systolic blood pressure of 140 to 159 mm Hg or diastolic blood pressure of 90 to 99 mm Hg.
- Adoption of healthy lifestyles by all people is now considered "indispensable."

KEY MESSAGES ABOUT HYPERTENSION

- "Individuals who are normotensive at 55 years have a 90% lifetime risk for developing hypertension."[6]
- "More than 1 of every 2 adults older than 60 years of age has hypertension,"[7] and only 34% of those with hypertension have achieved blood pressure goals.[6]
- "The relationship between pressure and risk of cardiovascular disease (CVD) events is continuous, consistent, and independent of other risk factors. . . . For individuals aged 40 to 70 years, each increment of 20 mm Hg in systolic BP or 10 mm Hg in diastolic BP doubles the risk of CVD across the entire BP range from 115/75 to 185/115 mm Hg."[6,8]
- Recent large population studies of cardiovascular risk factors reveal two striking findings[9]:
  1. Only approximately 4.8% to 9.9% of the young and middle-aged population is at low risk.
  2. The benefits of low-risk status are enormous: a 72% to 85% reduction in CVD mortality and a 40% to 58% reduction in mortality from all causes, leading to a gain of 5.8 to 9.5 years in life expectancy. This gain "holds for both African Americans and whites, and for those of lower and higher socioeconomic status."[9]
- Hence, identifying and treating people with risk factors are not enough. *A population-wide strategy is critical to prevent and reduce the magnitude of all the major risk factors* so that people develop favorable behaviors in childhood and *remain* at *low risk for life.*[9]

Risk factors for hypertension include physical inactivity, microalbuminuria or estimated GFR less than 60 mL/min, family history of premature CVD (<55 years for men and <65 years for women), excess intake of dietary sodium, insufficient intake of potassium, and excess consumption of alcohol.[6]

Preventing Cardiovascular Disease and Stroke. The American Heart Association (AHA) in its 2002 update placed the challenge for implementing risk factor reduction squarely on clinicians: "The challenge for health care professionals is to engage greater numbers of patients, at an earlier stage of their disease, in comprehensive cardiovascular risk reduction" to expand the benefits of primary prevention. "The continuing message is that adoption of healthy life habits remains the cornerstone of primary prevention." "The imperative is to prevent the first episode of coronary disease or stroke or the development of aortic aneurysm and peripheral vascular disease because of the still-high rate of first events that are fatal or disabling."[11]

As a first step, clinicians need to identify not only elevated blood pressure but also other well-studied risk factors for coronary heart disease (CHD). In its "Guidelines for Primary Prevention of Cardiovascular Disease and Stroke," the AHA recommends *risk factor screening* for adults beginning at age 20, and *global absolute CHD risk estimation* for all adults 40 years and

RISK FACTORS AND SCREENING FREQUENCY FOR ADULTS BEGINNING AT AGE 20

Risk Factor	*Frequency*
Family history of coronary heart disease (CHD)	Update regularly
Smoking status Diet Alcohol intake Physical activity	At each routine visit
Blood pressure Body mass index Waist circumference Pulse (to detect atrial fibrillation)	At each routine visit (at least every 2 years)
Fasting lipoprotein profile Fasting glucose	At least every 5 years If risk factors for hyperlipidemia or diabetes present, every 2 years

Source: Pearson TA, Blair SN, Daniels SR, et al. AHA guidelines for primary prevention of cardiovascular disease and stroke: 2000 update. Circulation 106:388–391, 2002.

GLOBAL RISK ESTIMATION FOR 10-YEAR RISK FOR CHD FOR ADULTS ≥ AGE 40

Establish multiple risk score for CHD based on:

- Age
- Sex
- Smoking status
- Systolic (and sometimes diastolic) blood pressure
- Total (and sometimes LDL) cholesterol
- HDL cholesterol
- Diabetes

For calculation of global CHD risk, use the risk calculators found at either of the Web sites below (or other equations):

http://www.americanheart.org/presenter.jhtml?identifier=3003499
http://hin.nhlbi.nih.gov/atpiii/calculator.asp?usertype=prof

Source: Pearson TA, Blair SN, Daniels SR, et al. AHA guidelines for primary prevention of cardiovascular disease and stroke: 2000 update. Circulation 106:388–391, 2002.

older.[11] The goal of global risk estimation is to help patients keep their risk as low as possible. Note that diabetes, or 10-year risk of more than 20%, is considered equivalent to established CHD risk equivalents.

Lowering Cholesterol and LDL. In 2001 the National Heart, Lung, and Blood Institute of the National Institutes of Health published the "Third Report of the National Cholesterol Education Program Expert Panel," known as ATP III.[12] Publication of the full NCEP report followed in 2002.[13] These reports provide evidence-based recommendations on the management of high cholesterol and related lipid disorders, and document that "epidemiological surveys have shown that serum cholesterol levels are continuously correlated with CHD risk over a broad range of cholesterol values," in many of the world's populations.[14] Key features of ATP III are as follows:

- Identifying LDL as the primary target of cholesterol-lowering therapy
- Classifying three risk categories:
    - *High risk (10-year risk > 20%):* established CHD and CHD risk equivalents
    - *Moderately high risk (10-year risk 10%–20%):* multiple, or 2+, risk factors
    - *Low risk (10-year risk < 10%):* zero to 1 risk factor

    Risk factors include cigarette smoking, BP >140/90 mm Hg or use of antihypertensive medication, HDL <40 mg/dL, family history of CHD in male first-degree relative <age 55 or female first-degree relative <age 65, and age ≥45 for men or ≥55 for women.

    CHD includes history of myocardial infarction, stable or unstable angina, coronary artery procedures such as angioplasty or bypass surgery, or evidence of significant myocardial ischemia.

    CHD risk equivalents include *noncoronary atherosclerotic disease,* such as peripheral arterial disease, abdominal aortic aneurysm, and carotid artery disease (transient ischemic attacks or stroke of carotid origin or > 50% obstruction of the carotid artery); *diabetes;* and *2+ risk factors with 10-year risk for CHD of> 20%.*

- Defining *high risk* as "all persons with CHD or CHD risk equivalents," with an *LDL goal for high-risk people of ≤ 100 mg/dL*

In July 2004, NCEP updated these reports based on the findings in five major clinical trials.[14] For *high-risk people,* NCEP now recommends an LDL goal of less than 70 mg/dL and intensive lipid therapy as a *therapeutic option.*[15] The NCEP cites data showing that high-risk patients benefit from a further 30% to 40% drop in LDL even when LDL is less than 100 mg/dL.

The U.S. Preventive Services Task Force recommends routine screening of LDL for men 35 years or older and for women 45 years or older.[16] Screening should begin at 20 years for those with risk factors for CHD.[17,18]

Counsel your patients to obtain a *fasting lipid profile* to determine levels of total and LDL cholesterol. Use the risk calculators on p. 297, or consult ATP III, to *establish your patient's 10-year risk category*. Use the 2004 guidelines below, which now have four risk groups, to plan your interventions regarding lifestyle change and lipid-lowering medications.

■ *Updated ATP III Guidelines*

10-year Risk Category	LDL Goal	Consider Drug Therapy if LDL:
High risk (>20%)	<100 mg/dL *Optional goal:* <70 mg/dL	≥100 mg/dL (<100 mg/dL: consider drug options, including further 30%–40% reduction in LDL)
Moderately high risk (10%–20%)	<130 mg/dL *Optional goal:* <100 mg/dL	≥130 mg/dL (100–129 mg/dL: consider drug options to achieve goal of <100 mg/dL)
Moderate risk (<10%)	<130 mg/dL	≥160 mg/dL
Lower risk (0–1 risk factor)	<160 mg/dL	≥190 mg/dL (160–189 mg/dL: drug therapy *optional*)

(Source: Adapted from Grundy SM, Cleeman JI, Merz NB, et al, for the Coordinating Committee of the National Cholesterol Education Program. Implications of recent clinical trials for the National Cholesterol Education Adult Treatment Panel III guidelines. Circulation 110(2):227–239, 2004.)

Lifestyle Modification and Risk Intervention. JNC VII, the National High Blood Pressure Education Program, and the AHA encourage a series of well-studied effective lifestyle modifications and risk interventions

LIFESTYLE MODIFICATIONS TO PREVENT OR MANAGE HYPERTENSION

- Optimal weight, or BMI of 18.5–24.9 kg/m^2
- Salt intake of less than 6 grams of sodium chloride or 2.4 grams of sodium per day
- Regular aerobic exercise such as brisk walking for at least 30 minutes per day, most days of the week
- Moderate alcohol consumption per day of 2 drinks or fewer for men and 1 drink or fewer for women (2 drinks = 1 oz ethanol, 24 oz beer, 10 oz wine, or 2–3 oz whiskey)
- Dietary intake of more than 3,500 mg of potassium
- Diet rich in fruits, vegetables, and low-fat dairy products with reduced content of saturated and total fat

Source: Whelton PK, He J, Appel LJ, et al. Primary prevention of hypertension. Clinical and Public Health Advisory from the National High Blood Pressure Education Program. JAMA 288(15):1882–1888, 2002.

to prevent hypertension, CVD, and stroke. Lifestyle modifications for hypertension can lower systolic blood pressure from 2 to 20 mm Hg.[6] Lifestyle modifications to reduce hypertension overlap with those recommended for reducing risk for CVD and stroke, as seen below.

RISK INTERVENTIONS TO PREVENT CARDIOVASCULAR DISEASE AND STROKE

- Complete cessation of smoking
- Optimal blood pressure control—see table for JNC VII guidelines on p. 109
- Healthy eating—see diet recommendations on previous page
- Lipid management—see table on p. 299
- Regular aerobic exercise—see previous page
- Optimal weight—see previous page
- Diabetes management so that fasting glucose level is below 110 mg/dL and HgA1C is less than 7%
- Conversion of atrial fibrillation to normal sinus rhythm or, if chronic, anticoagulation

Source: Pearson TA, Blair SN, Daniels SR, et al. AHA guidelines for primary prevention of cardiovascular disease and stroke: 2002 update. Circulation 106:388–391, 2002.

Healthy Eating. Begin with a dietary history (see pp. 92–93), then target low intake of cholesterol and total fat, especially less saturated and *trans* fat. Foods with monounsaturated fats, polyunsaturated fats, and omega-3 fatty acids in fish oils help to lower blood cholesterol. Review the food sources of these healthy and unhealthy fats.[19]

Sources of Unhealthy Fats

- *Foods high in cholesterol:* dairy products, egg yolks, liver and organ meats, high-fat meat and poultry
- *Foods high in saturated fat:* high-fat dairy products—cream, cheese, ice cream, whole and 2% milk, and sour cream; bacon, butter; chocolate; coconut oil; lard and gravy from meat drippings; high-fat meats like ground beef, bologna, hot dogs, and sausage
- *Foods high in* trans *fat:* snacks and baked goods with hydrogenated or partially hydrogenated oil, stick margarines, shortening, french fries

Sources of Healthy Fats

- *Foods high in monounsaturated fat:* nuts, such as almonds, pecans, and peanuts; sesame seeds; avocados; canola oil; olive and peanut oil; peanut butter
- *Foods high in polyunsaturated fat:* corn, safflower, cottonseed, and soy-

bean oil; walnuts; pumpkin or sunflower seeds; soft (tub) margarine; mayonnaise; salad dressings

- *Foods high in omega-3 fatty acids:* albacore tuna, herring, mackerel, rainbow trout, salmon, sardines

Counseling About Weight and Exercise. The January 2004 "Progress Review—Nutrition and Overweight" in Healthy People 2010 reports that "Dietary factors are associated with 4 of the 10 leading causes of death—coronary heart disease, some types of cancer, stroke, and type 2 diabetes—as well as with high blood pressure and osteoporosis. Overall, the data on the three Healthy People 2010 objectives for the weight status of adults and children reflect a trend for the worse."[20] More than 60% of all Americans are now obese or overweight, with a BMI greater than or equal to 25.

Counseling about weight has become a clinician imperative. Assess body mass index (BMI) as described in Chapter 4, pp. 90–92. Discuss the principles of healthy eating—patients with high fat intake are more likely to accumulate body fat than patients with high intake of protein and carbohydrate. Review the patient's eating habits and weight patterns in the family. Set realistic goals that will help the patient maintain healthy eating habits *for life.*

Regular exercise is the number one health indicator for Healthy People 2010. In its April 2004 "Progress Review—Physical Activity and Fitness," Healthy People 2010 states that "in 2000, poor diet coupled with lack of exercise was the second leading actual cause of death. The gap between this risk factor and tobacco use, the leading cause, has narrowed substantially over the past decade."[21] To reduce risk for CHD, counsel patients to pursue aerobic exercise, or exercise that increases muscle oxygen uptake, for at least 30 minutes on most days of the week. Spur motivation by emphasizing the immediate benefits to health and well-being. Deep breathing, sweating in cool temperatures, and pulse rates exceeding 60% of the maximum normal age-adjusted heart rate, or 220 minus the person's age, are markers that help patients recognize onset of aerobic metabolism. Be sure to evaluate any cardiovascular, pulmonary, or musculoskeletal conditions that present risks before selecting an exercise regimen.

TECHNIQUES OF EXAMINATION

As you begin the cardiovascular examination, review the blood pressure and heart rate recorded during the General Survey and Vital Signs at the start of the physical examination. If you need to repeat these measurements, or if they have not already been done, take the time to measure the blood pressure and heart rate using optimal technique (see Chapter 4, Beginning the Physical Examination: General Survey and Vital Signs, especially pp. 106–112).[22–26]

In brief, for *blood pressure,* after letting the patient rest for at least 5 minutes in a quiet setting, choose a correctly sized cuff and position the patient's arm at heart level, either resting on a table if seated or supported at midchest level if standing. Make sure the bladder of the cuff is centered over the brachial artery. Inflate the cuff about 30 mm Hg above the pressure at which the brachial or radial pulse disappears. As you deflate the cuff, listen first for the sounds of at least two consecutive heartbeats—these mark the *systolic* pressure. Then listen for the disappearance point of the heartbeats, which marks the *diastolic* pressure. For *heart rate,* measure the radial pulse using the pads of your index and middle fingers, or assess the apical pulse using your stethoscope (see p. 111).

Now you are ready to systematically assess the components of the cardiovascular system:

- The jugular venous pressure and pulsations
- The carotid upstrokes and presence or absence of bruits
- The point of maximal impulse (PMI) and any heaves, lifts, or thrills
- The first and second heart sounds, S_1 and S_2
- Presence or absence of extra heart sounds such as S_3 or S_4
- Presence or absence of any cardiac murmurs.

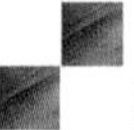

JUGULAR VENOUS PRESSURE AND PULSATIONS

Jugular Venous Pressure (JVP). Estimating the JVP is one of the most important and frequently used skills of physical examination. At first it will seem difficult, but with practice and supervision you will find that the JVP provides valuable information about the patient's volume status and cardiac function. As you have learned, the JVP reflects pressure in the right atrium, or central venous pressure, and is best assessed from pulsations in the right internal jugular vein. Note, however, that the jugular veins and pulsations are difficult to see in children younger than 12 years of age, so they are not useful for evaluating the cardiovascular system in this age group.

To assist you in learning this portion of the cardiac examination, steps for assessing the JVP are outlined on the next page. As you begin your assessment, take a moment to reflect on the patient's volume status and consider how you may need to alter the elevation of the head of the bed or examining table. The usual starting point for assessing the JVP is to elevate the head of the bed to 30°. Identify the external jugular vein on each side, then find the internal jugular venous pulsations transmitted from deep in the neck to the overlying soft tissues. The JVP is the elevation at which the highest oscillation point, or meniscus, of the jugular venous pulsations is usually evident in euvolemic patients. In patients who are *hypovolemic,* you may anticipate that *the JVP will be low,* causing you to subsequently *lower the head of the bed,* sometimes even to 0°, to see the point of oscillation best. Likewise, in volume-overloaded or *hypervolemic* patients, you may anticipate that *the JVP will be high,* causing you to subsequently *raise the head of the bed.*

A hypovolemic patient may have to lie flat before you see the neck veins. In contrast, when jugular venous pressure is increased, an elevation up to 60° or even 90° may be required. In all these positions, the sternal angle usually remains about 5 cm above the right atrium, as diagrammed on p. 291.

STEPS FOR ASSESSING THE JUGULAR VENOUS PRESSURE (JVP)

- Make the patient comfortable. *Raise the head slightly on a pillow* to relax the sternomastoid muscles.
- *Raise the head of the bed or examining table to about 30°. Turn the patient's head slightly away from the side you are inspecting.*
- Use *tangential lighting* and examine both sides of the neck. Identify the external jugular vein on each side, then find the internal jugular venous pulsations.
- *If necessary, raise or lower the head of the bed* until you can see the oscillation point or meniscus of the internal jugular venous pulsations in the lower half of the neck.
- Focus on the *right internal jugular vein.* Look for pulsations in the suprasternal notch, between the attachments of the sternomastoid muscle on the sternum and clavicle, or just posterior to the sternomastoid. The table below helps you distinguish internal jugular pulsations from those of the carotid artery.
- *Identify the highest point of pulsation in the right internal jugular vein.* Extend a long rectangular object or card horizontally from this point and a centimeter ruler vertically from the sternal angle, making an exact right angle. Measure the vertical distance in centimeters above the sternal angle where the horizontal object crosses the ruler. *This distance, measured in centimeters above the sternal angle or the right atrium, is the JVP.*

The following features help to distinguish jugular from carotid artery pulsations:[1]

■ *Distinguishing Internal Jugular and Carotid Pulsations*

Internal Jugular Pulsations	Carotid Pulsations
Rarely palpable	Palpable
Soft, rapid, undulating quality, usually with two elevations and two troughs per heart beat	A more vigorous thrust with a single outward component
Pulsations eliminated by light pressure on the vein(s) just above the sternal end of the clavicle	Pulsations not eliminated by this pressure
Level of the pulsations changes with position, dropping as the patient becomes more upright.	Level of the pulsations unchanged by position
Level of the pulsations usually descends with inspiration.	Level of the pulsations not affected by inspiration

Establishing the true vertical and horizontal lines to measure the JVP is difficult, much like the problem of hanging a picture straight when you are close to it. Place your ruler on the sternal angle and line it up with something in the room that you know to be vertical. Then place a card or rectangular object at an exact right angle to the ruler. This constitutes your horizontal line. Move it up or down—still horizontal—so that the lower edge rests at the top of the jugular pulsations, and read the vertical distance on the ruler. Round your measurement off to the nearest centimeter.

Increased pressure suggests *right-sided congestive heart failure* or, less commonly, *constrictive pericarditis, tricuspid stenosis,* or *superior vena cava obstruction.*[27–33]

In patients with obstructive lung disease, venous pressure may appear elevated on expiration only; the veins collapse on inspiration. This finding does not indicate congestive heart failure.

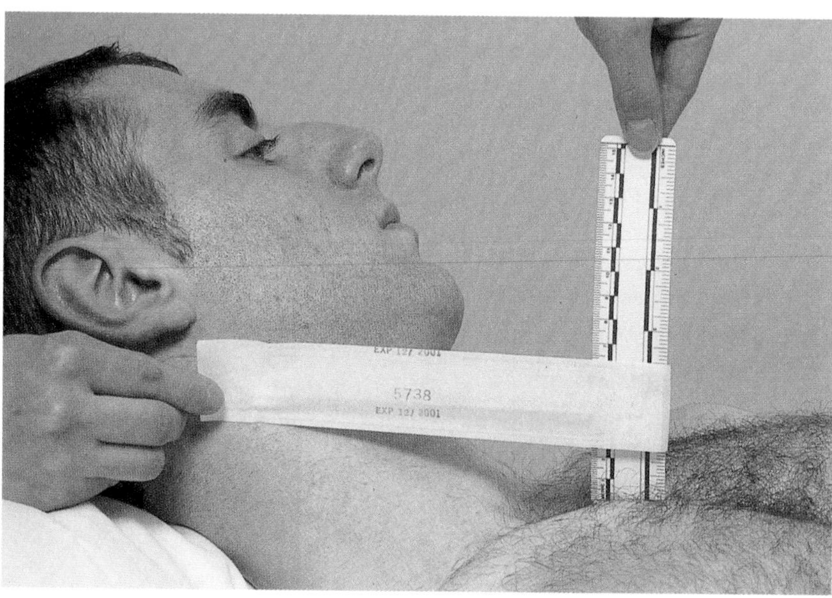

Venous pressure measured at greater than 3 cm or possibly 4 cm above the sternal angle, or more than 8 cm or 9 cm in total distance above the right atrium, is considered elevated *above normal.*

If you are unable to see pulsations in the internal jugular vein, look for them in the external jugular vein. If you see no pulsation, use *the point above which the external jugular veins appear to collapse.* Make this observation on each side of the neck. Measure the vertical distance of this point from the sternal angle.

Unilateral distention of the external jugular vein is usually caused by local kinking or obstruction. Occasionally, even bilateral distention has a local cause.

The highest point of venous pulsations may lie below the level of the sternal angle. Under these circumstances, venous pressure is not elevated and seldom needs to be measured.

Even though students may not see clinicians making these measurements very frequently in clinical settings, practicing exact techniques for measuring the JVP is important. Eventually, with experience, clinicians and cardiologists come to identify the JVP and estimate its height visually.

Jugular Venous Pulsations. *Observe the amplitude and timing of the jugular venous pulsations.* In order to time these pulsations, feel the left carotid artery with your right thumb or listen to the heart simultaneously. The *a* wave just precedes S_1 and the carotid pulse, the *x* descent can be seen

Prominent *a* waves indicate increased resistance to right atrial contraction, as in *tricuspid stenosis,* or, more commonly, the decreased

as a systolic collapse, the *v* wave almost coincides with S_2, and the *y* descent follows early in diastole. Look for absent or unusually prominent waves.

compliance of a hypertrophied right ventricle. The *a* waves disappear in atrial fibrillation. Larger *v* waves characterize tricuspid regurgitation.

Jugular venous pulsations

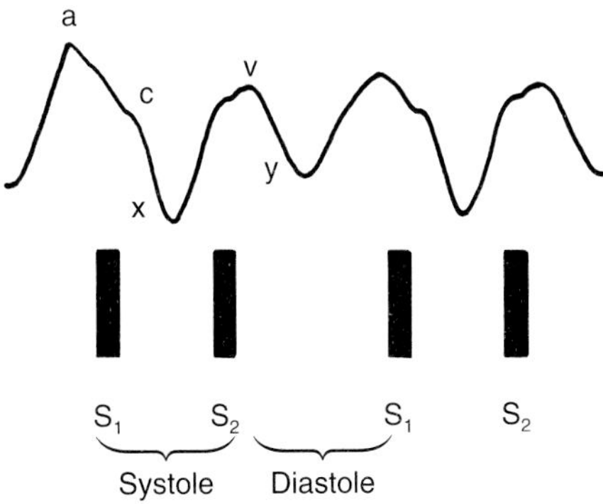

Jugular venous pressure curves

a = atrial contraction
c = carotid transmission not visible clinically
x = descent in right atrium following *a*
v = passive venous filling of atria from the vena cavae
y = descent during atrial resting phase before contraction

Considerable practice and experience are required to master jugular venous pulsations. A beginner is well-advised to concentrate primarily on jugular venous pressure.

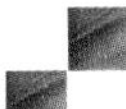

THE CAROTID PULSE

After you measure the JVP, move on to assessment of the *carotid pulse.* The carotid pulse provides valuable information about cardiac function and is especially useful for detecting stenosis or insufficiency of the aortic valve. Take the time to assess the quality of the carotid upstroke, its amplitude and contour, and presence or absence of any overlying *thrills* or *bruits.*

For irregular rhythms, see Table 8-1, Selected Heart Rates and Rhythms (p. 324), and Table 8-2, Selected Irregular Rhythms (p. 325).

To assess *amplitude and contour,* the patient should be lying down with the head of the bed still elevated to about 30°. When feeling for the carotid artery, first inspect the neck for carotid pulsations. These may be visible just medial to the sternomastoid muscles. Then place your left index and middle fingers (or left thumb) on the right carotid artery in the lower third of the neck, press posteriorly, and feel for pulsations.

A tortuous and kinked carotid artery may produce a unilateral pulsatile bulge.

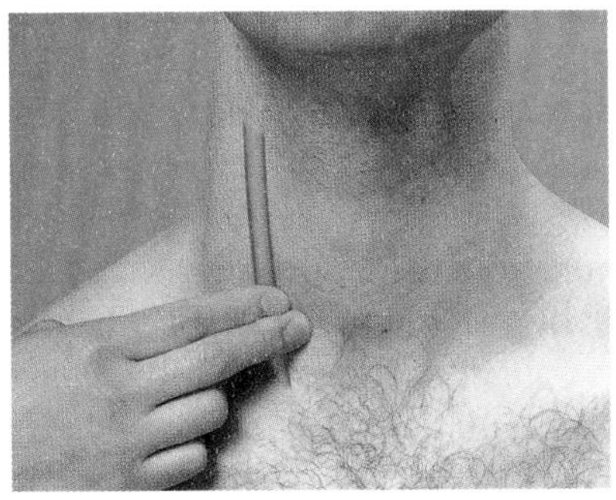

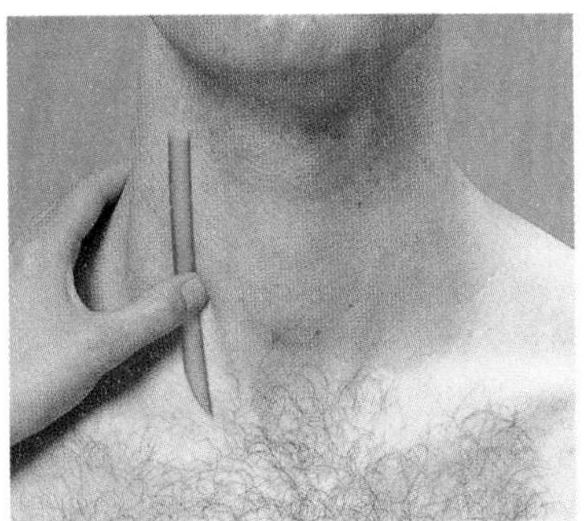

Decreased pulsations may be caused by decreased stroke volume, but may also result from local factors in the artery such as atherosclerotic narrowing or occlusion.

- Identify the *timing of impulses or sounds* in relation to the cardiac cycle. Timing of sounds is often possible through auscultation alone. In most people with normal or slow heart rates, it is easy to identify the paired heart sounds by listening through a stethoscope. S_1 is the first of these sounds, S_2 is the second, and the relatively long diastolic interval separates one pair from the next.

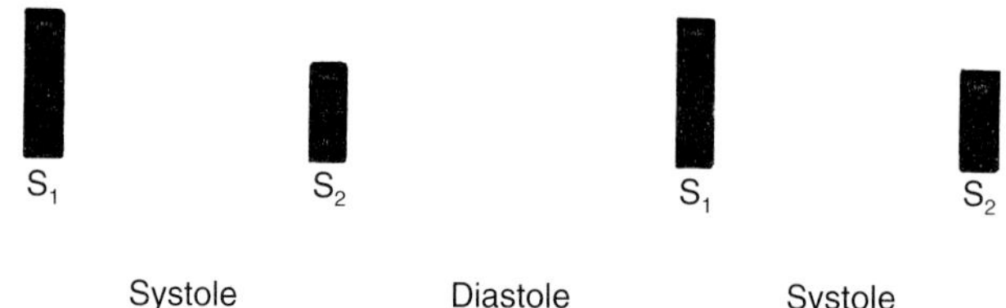

The relative intensity of these sounds may also be helpful. S_1 is usually louder than S_2 at the apex; more reliably, S_2 is usually louder than S_1 at the base.

Even experienced clinicians are sometimes uncertain about the timing of heart sounds, especially extra sounds and murmurs. "Inching" can then be helpful. Return to a place on the chest—most often the base—where it is easy to identify S_1 and S_2. Get their rhythm clearly in mind. Then inch your stethoscope down the chest in steps until you hear the new sound.

Auscultation alone, however, can be misleading. The intensities of S_1 and S_2, for example, may be abnormal. At rapid heart rates, moreover, diastole shortens, and at about a rate of 120, the durations of systole and diastole become indistinguishable. *Use palpation of the carotid pulse or of the apical impulse to help determine whether the sound or murmur is systolic or diastolic.* Because both the carotid upstroke and the apical impulse occur in systole, right after S_1, sounds or murmurs coinciding with them are systolic; sounds or murmurs occurring after the carotid upstroke or apical impulse are diastolic.

For example, S_1 is decreased in *first-degree heart block*, and S_2 is decreased in *aortic stenosis*.

INSPECTION AND PALPATION

Overview. Careful *inspection* of the anterior chest may reveal the location of the *apical impulse* or *point of maximal impulse (PMI)*, or less commonly, the ventricular movements of a left-sided S_3 or S_4. Tangential light is best for making these observations. Use *palpation* to confirm the characteristics of the apical impulse. Palpation is also valuable for detecting thrills and the ventricular movements of an S_3 or S_4.

Begin with general palpation of the chest wall. First palpate for heaves, lifts, or thrills using your *fingerpads.* Hold them flat or obliquely on the body surface, using light pressure for an S_3 or S_4, and firmer pressure for S_1 and S_2. Ventricular impulses may heave or lift your fingers. Then check for *thrills* by pressing the *ball of your hand* firmly on the chest. If subsequent auscultation reveals a loud murmur, go back and check for thrills over that area again. Be sure to assess the right ventricle by palpating the right ventricular area at the lower left sternal border and in the subxiphoid area, the pulmonary artery in the left 2nd interspace, and the aortic area in the right 2nd interspace. Review the diagram on the next page. *Note that the "areas" designated for the left and right ventricle, the pulmonary artery, and the aorta pertain to the majority of patients whose hearts are situated in the left chest, with normal anatomy of the great vessels.*

Thrills may accompany loud, harsh, or rumbling murmurs as in *aortic stenosis, patent ductus arteriosus, ventricular septal defect,* and, less commonly, *mitral stenosis.* They are palpated more easily in patient positions that accentuate the murmur.

On rare occasions, a patient has *dextrocardia*—a heart situated on the right side. The apical impulse

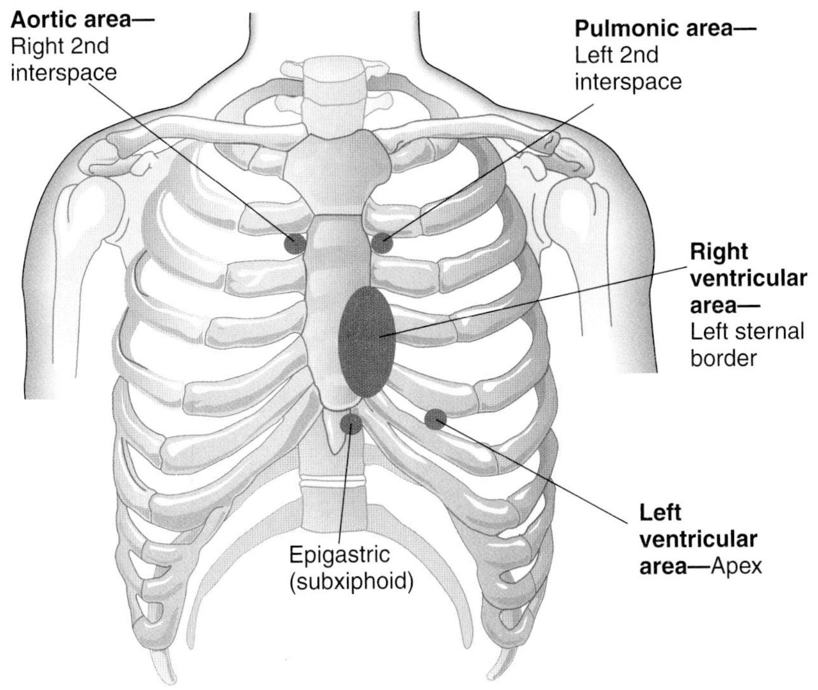

Left Ventricular Area—The Apical Impulse or Point of Maximal Impulse (PMI). The apical impulse represents the brief early pulsation of the left ventricle as it moves anteriorly during contraction and touches the chest wall. Note that in most examinations the apical impulse is the point of maximal impulse, or PMI; however, some pathologic conditions may produce a pulsation that is more prominent than the apex beat, such as an enlarged right ventricle, a dilated pulmonary artery, or an aneurysm of the aorta.

If you cannot identify the apical impulse with the patient supine, ask the patient to roll partly onto the left side—this is the *left lateral decubitus* position. Palpate again using the palmar surfaces of several fingers. If you cannot find

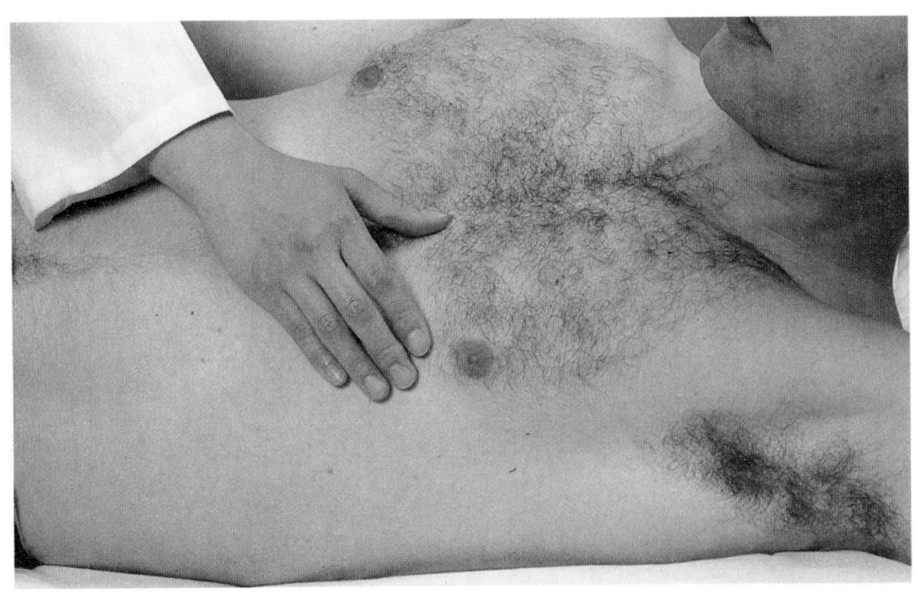

will then be found on the right. If you cannot find an apical impulse, percuss for the dullness of heart and liver and for the tympany of the stomach. In *situs inversus,* all three of these structures are on opposite sides from normal. A right-sided heart with a normally placed liver and stomach is usually associated with congenital heart disease.

the apical impulse, ask the patient to exhale fully and stop breathing for a few seconds. When examining a woman, it may be helpful to displace the left breast upward or laterally as necessary; alternatively, ask her to do this for you.

Once you have found the apical impulse, make finer assessments with your fingertips, and then with one finger.

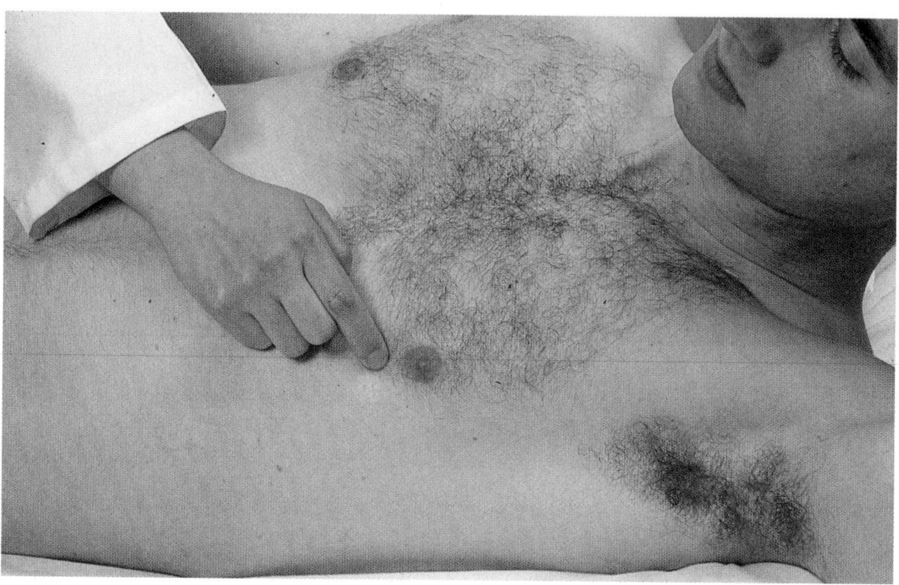

With experience, you will learn to feel the apical impulse in a high percentage of patients. Obesity, a very muscular chest wall, or an increased anteroposterior diameter of the chest, however, may make it undetectable. Some apical impulses hide behind the rib cage, despite positioning.

Now assess the location, diameter, amplitude, and duration of the apical impulse. You may wish to have the patient breathe out and briefly stop breathing to check your findings.

See Table 8-3, Variations and Abnormalities of the Ventricular Impulses (p. 326).

- *Location.* Try to assess location with the patient *supine* because the left lateral decubitus position displaces the apical impulse to the left. Locate two points: the interspaces, usually the 5th or possibly the 4th, which give the vertical location; and the distance in centimeters from the midsternal line, which gives the horizontal location. Note that even though the apical impulse normally falls roughly at the midclavicular line, measurements from this line are less reproducible because clinicians vary in their estimates of the midpoint of the clavicle.

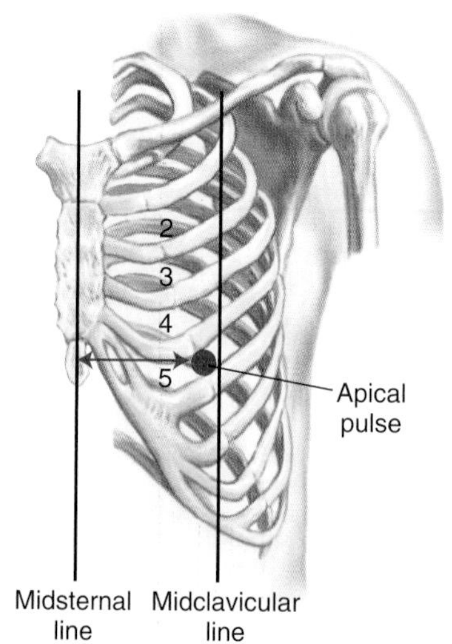

The apical impulse may be displaced upward and to the left by pregnancy or a high left diaphragm.

Lateral displacement from cardiac enlargement in *congestive heart failure, cardiomyopathy, ischemic heart disease.* Displacement in deformities of the thorax and mediastinal shift.

- *Diameter*. Palpate the diameter of the apical impulse. In the supine patient, it usually measures less than 2.5 cm and occupies only one interspace. It may feel larger in the left lateral decubitus position.

In the left lateral decubitus position, a diameter greater than 3 cm indicates left ventricular enlargement.

- *Amplitude*. Estimate the amplitude of the impulse. It is usually small and feels *brisk* and *tapping*. Some young people have an increased amplitude, or hyperkinetic impulse, especially when excited or after exercise; its duration, however, is normal.

Increased amplitude may also reflect *hyperthyroidism, severe anemia,* pressure overload of the left ventricle (e.g., *aortic stenosis*), or volume overload of the left ventricle (e.g., *mitral regurgitation*).

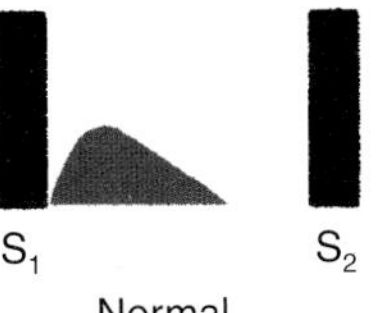

Normal

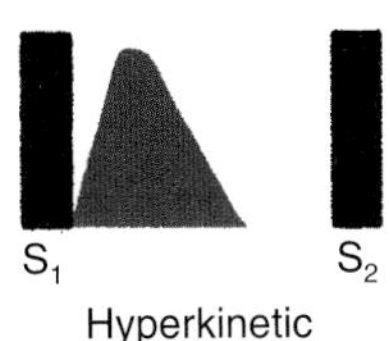

Hyperkinetic

- *Duration*. Duration is the most useful characteristic of the apical impulse for identifying hypertrophy of the left ventricle. To assess duration, listen to the heart sounds as you feel the apical impulse, or watch the movement of your stethoscope as you listen at the apex. Estimate the proportion of systole occupied by the apical impulse. Normally it lasts through the first two thirds of systole, and often less, but does not continue to the second heart sound.

A sustained, high-amplitude impulse that is normally located suggests left ventricular hypertrophy from pressure overload (as in hypertension). If such an impulse is displaced laterally, consider volume overload.

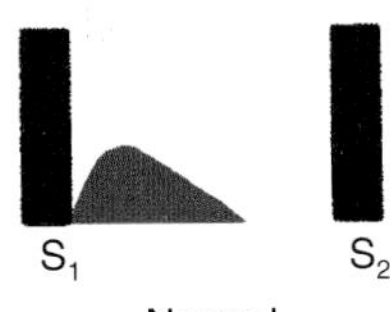

Normal

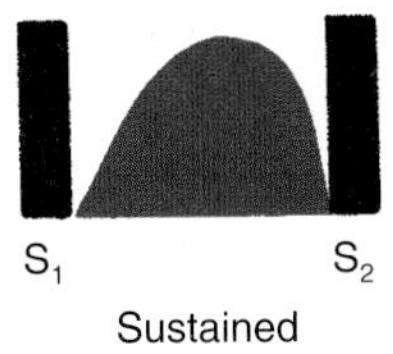

Sustained

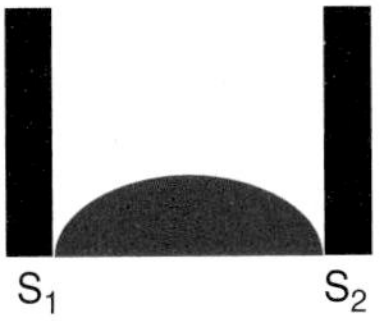

A sustained low-amplitude (hypokinetic) impulse may result from dilated cardiomyopathy.

S_3 and S_4. By inspection and palpation, you may detect ventricular movements that are synchronous with pathologic third and fourth heart sounds. For the left ventricular impulses, feel the apical beat gently with one finger. The patient should lie partly on the left side, breathe out, and briefly stop breathing. By inking an X on the apex, you may be able to see these movements.

A brief middiastolic impulse indicates an S_3; an impulse just before the systolic apical beat itself indicates an S_4.

Right Ventricular Area—The Left Sternal Border in the 3rd, 4th, and 5th Interspaces. The patient should rest supine at 30°. Place the tips of your curved fingers in the 3rd, 4th, and 5th interspaces and try to feel the systolic impulse of the right ventricle. Again, asking the patient to breathe out and then briefly stop breathing improves your observation.

If an impulse is palpable, assess its location, amplitude, and duration. A brief systolic tap of low or slightly increased amplitude is sometimes felt in thin or shallow-chested people, especially when stroke volume is increased, as by anxiety.

A marked increase in amplitude with little or no change in duration occurs in chronic volume overload of the right ventricle, as from an *atrial septal defect.*

An impulse with increased amplitude and duration occurs with pressure overload of the right ventricle, as in *pulmonic stenosis* or *pulmonary hypertension.*

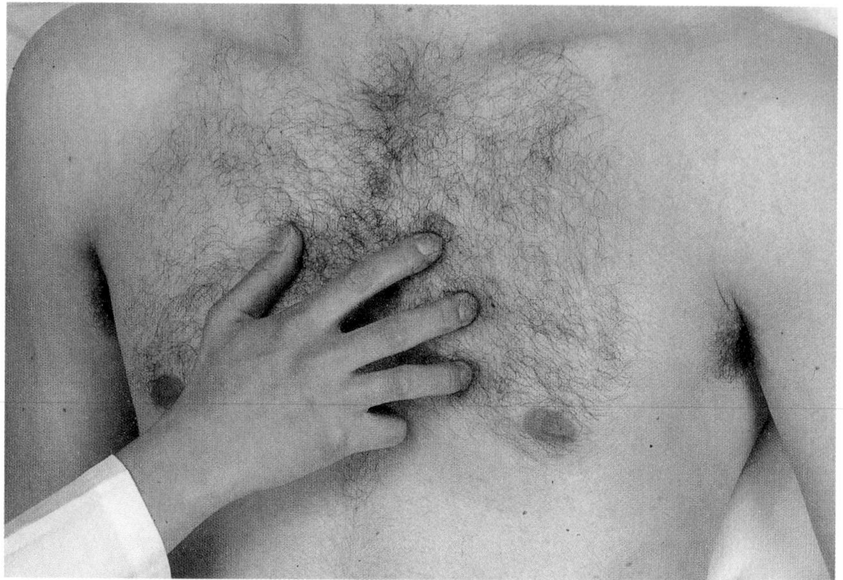

The diastolic movements of *right-sided third and fourth heart sounds* may be felt occasionally. Feel for them in the 4th and 5th left interspaces. Time them by auscultation or carotid palpation.

In patients with an increased anteroposterior (AP) diameter, palpation of the *right ventricle* in the *epigastric* or *subxiphoid area* is also useful. With your hand flattened, press your index finger just under the rib cage and up toward the left shoulder and try to feel right ventricular pulsations.

In obstructive pulmonary disease, hyperinflated lung may prevent palpation of an enlarged right ventricle in the left parasternal area. The impulse is felt easily, however, high in the epigastrium where heart sounds are also often heard best.

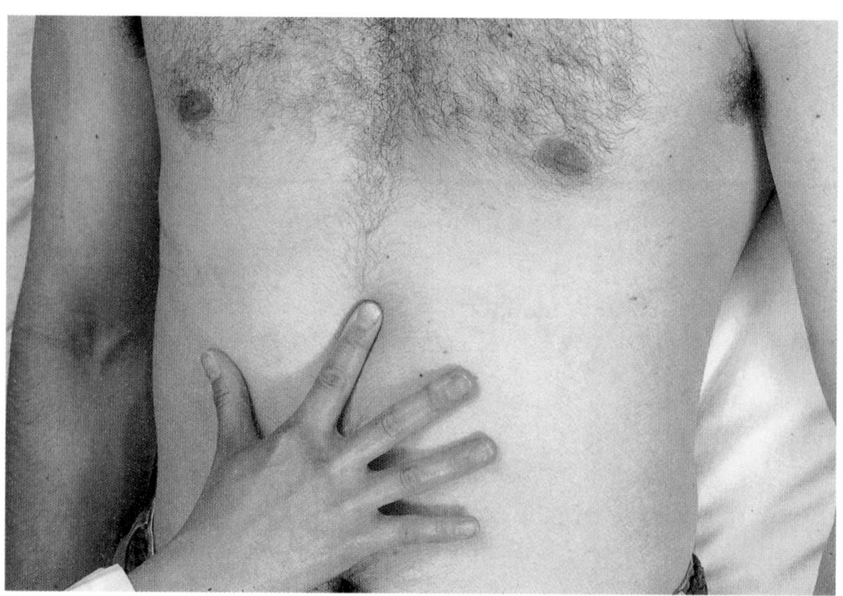

Asking the patient to inhale and briefly stop breathing is helpful. The inspiratory position moves your hand well away from the pulsations of the abdominal aorta, which might otherwise be confusing. The diastolic movements of S_3 and S_4, if present, may also be felt here.

Pulmonic Area—The Left 2nd Interspace. This interspace overlies the *pulmonary artery*. As the patient holds expiration, look and feel for an impulse and feel for possible heart sounds. In thin or shallow-chested patients, the pulsation of a pulmonary artery may sometimes be felt here, especially after exercise or with excitement.

A prominent pulsation here often accompanies dilatation or increased flow in the pulmonary artery. A palpable S_2 suggests increased pressure in the pulmonary artery (*pulmonary hypertension*).

Aortic Area—The Right 2nd Interspace. This interspace overlies the aortic outflow tract. Search for pulsations and palpable heart sounds.

A palpable S_2 suggests systemic *hypertension.* A pulsation here suggests a dilated or aneurysmal aorta.

PERCUSSION

In most cases, palpation has replaced percussion in the estimation of cardiac size. When you cannot feel the apical impulse, however, percussion may suggest where to search for it. Occasionally, percussion may be your only tool. Under these circumstances, cardiac dullness often occupies a large area. Starting well to the left on the chest, percuss from resonance toward cardiac dullness in the 3rd, 4th, 5th, and possibly 6th interspaces.

A markedly dilated failing heart may have a hypokinetic apical impulse that is displaced far to the left. A large pericardial effusion may make the impulse undetectable.

AUSCULTATION

Overview. Auscultation of heart sounds and murmurs is a rewarding and important skill of physical examination that leads directly to several clinical diagnoses. In this section, you will learn the techniques for identifying S_1 and S_2, extra sounds in systole and diastole, and systolic and diastolic murmurs. Review the auscultatory areas on the next page with the following caveats: (1) some authorities discourage use of these names because murmurs of more than one origin may occur in a given area; and (2) these areas may not apply to patients with dextrocardia or anomalies of the great vessels. Also, if the heart is enlarged or displaced, your pattern of auscultation should be altered accordingly.

In a quiet room, listen to the heart with your stethoscope *in the right 2nd interspace* close to the sternum, *along the left sternal border* in each interspace from the 2nd through the 5th, and *at the apex*. Recall that the upper margins of the heart are sometimes termed the "base" of the heart. Some clinicians begin auscultation at the apex, others at the base. Either pattern is satisfactory. You should also listen in any area where you detect an abnormality and in areas adjacent to murmurs to determine where they are loudest and where they radiate.

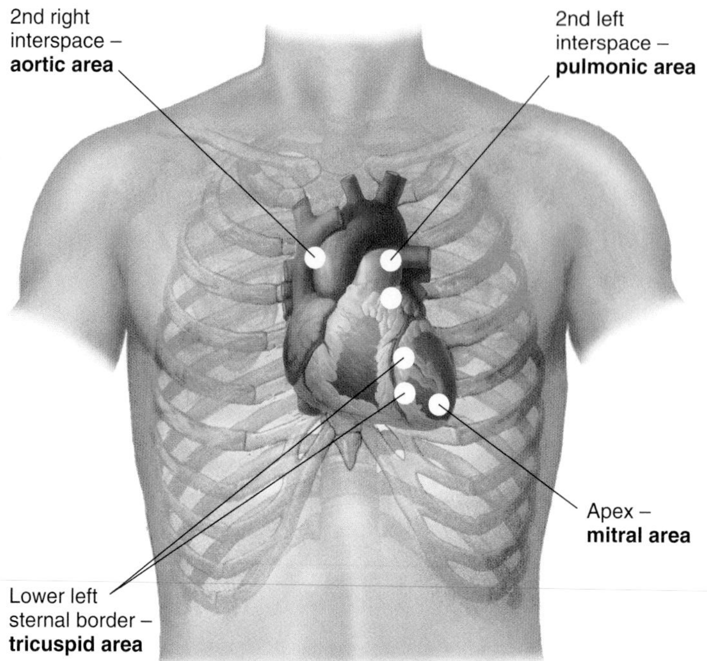

Heart sounds and murmurs that originate in the four valves are illustrated in the diagram below. Pulmonic sounds are usually heard best in the 2nd and 3rd left interspaces, but may extend further.

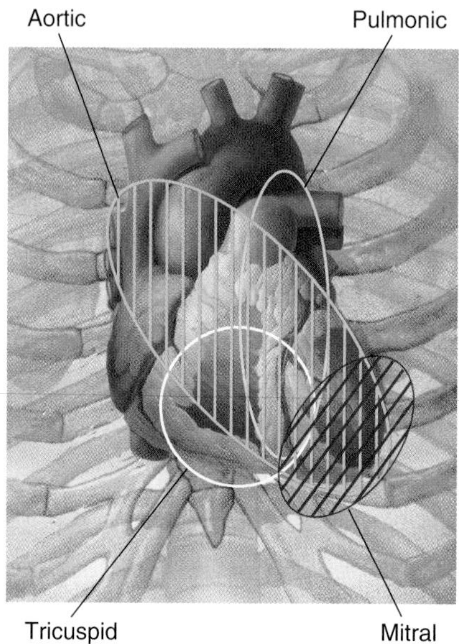

(Redrawn from Leatham A: Introduction to the Examination of the Cardiovascular System, 2nd ed. Oxford, Oxford University Press, 1979)

Know your stethoscope! It is important to understand the uses of both the diaphragm and the bell.

- *The diaphragm.* The diaphragm is better for picking up the relatively high-pitched sounds of S_1 and S_2, the murmurs of aortic and mitral regurgitation, and pericardial friction rubs. *Listen throughout the precordium* with the diaphragm, pressing it firmly against the chest.

- *The bell.* The bell is more sensitive to the low-pitched sounds of S_3 and S_4 and the murmur of mitral stenosis. Apply the bell lightly, with just enough pressure to produce an air seal with its full rim. *Use the bell at the apex, then move medially along the lower sternal border.* Resting the heel of your hand on the chest like a fulcrum may help you to maintain light pressure.

  Pressing the bell firmly on the chest makes it function more like the diaphragm by stretching the underlying skin. Low-pitched sounds such as S_3 and S_4 may disappear with this technique—an observation that may help to identify them. In contrast, high-pitched sounds such as a midsystolic click, an ejection sound, or an opening snap, will persist or get louder.

  Listen to the entire precordium with the patient supine. For new patients and patients needing a complete cardiac examination, use two other important positions to listen for mitral stenosis and aortic regurgitation.

- Ask the patient to *roll partly onto the left side into the left lateral decubitus position,* bringing the left ventricle close to the chest wall. Place the bell of your stethoscope lightly on the apical impulse.

This position accentuates or brings out a left-sided S_3 and S_4 and mitral murmurs, especially *mitral stenosis.* You may otherwise miss these important findings.

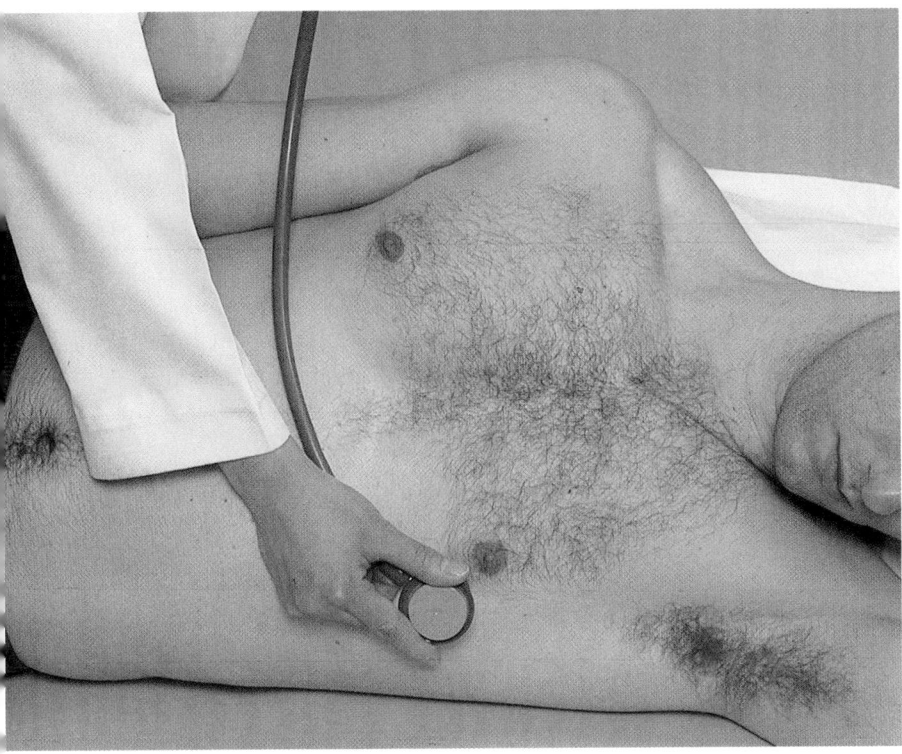

- Ask the patient to *sit up, lean forward, exhale completely, and stop breathing in expiration*. Pressing the diaphragm of your stethoscope on the chest, listen along the left sternal border and at the apex, pausing periodically so the patient may breathe.

This position accentuates or brings out aortic murmurs. You may easily miss the soft diastolic murmur of *aortic regurgitation* unless you listen at this position.

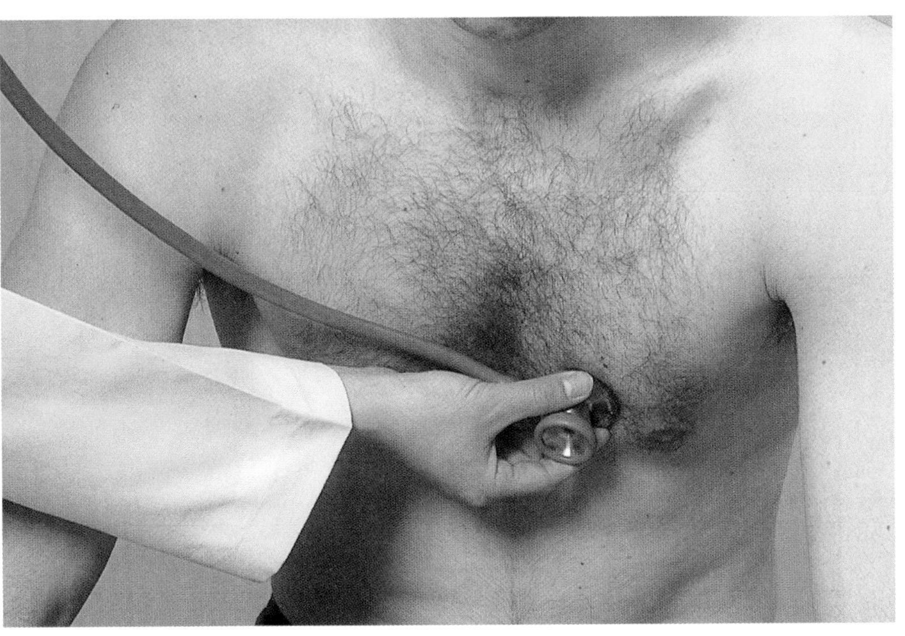

Listening for Heart Sounds. Throughout your examination, take your time at each auscultatory area. Concentrate on each of the events in the cardiac cycle listed on the next page and sounds you may hear in systole and diastole.

■ Auscultatory Sounds

Heart Sounds	Guides to Auscultation	Examples of Abnormalities
S_1	Note its intensity and any apparent splitting. Normal splitting is detectable along the lower left sternal border.	See Table 8-4, Variations in the First Heart Sound—S_1 (p. 327).
S_2	Note its intensity.	
Split S_2	Listen for splitting of this sound in the 2nd and 3rd left interspaces. Ask the patient to breathe quietly, and then slightly more deeply than normal. Does S_2 split into its two components, as it normally does? If not, ask the patient to (1) breathe a little more deeply, or (2) sit up. Listen again. A thick chest wall may make the pulmonic component of S_1 inaudible.	See Table 8-5, Variations in the Second Heart Sound—S_2 (p. 328). When either A_2 or P_2 is absent, as in disease of the respective valves, S_2 is persistently single.
	Width of split. How wide is the split? It is normally quite narrow.	
	Timing of split. When in the respiratory cycle do you hear the split? It is normally heard late in inspiration.	Expiratory splitting suggests an abnormality (p. 328).
	Does the split disappear as it should, during exhalation? If not, listen again with the patient sitting up.	Persistent splitting results from delayed closure of the pulmonic valve or early closure of the aortic valve.
	Intensity of A_2 and P_2. Compare the intensity of the two components, A_2 and P_2. A_2 is usually louder.	A loud P_2 suggests pulmonary hypertension.
Extra Sounds in Systole	Such as ejection sounds or systolic clicks Note their location, timing, intensity, and pitch, and the effects of respiration on the sounds.	The systolic click of mitral valve prolapse is the most common of these sounds. See Table 8-6, Extra Heart Sounds in Systole (p. 329).
Extra Sounds in Diastole	Such as S_3, S_4, or an opening snap Note the location, timing, intensity, and pitch, and the effects of respiration on the sounds. (An S_3 or S_4 in athletes is a normal finding.)	See Table 8-7, Extra Heart Sounds in Diastole (p. 330).
Systolic and Diastolic Murmurs	Murmurs are differentiated from heart sounds by their longer duration.	See Table 8-8, Pansystolic (Holosystolic) Murmurs (p. 331), Table 8-9, Midsystolic Murmurs (pp. 332–333), and Table 8-10, Diastolic Murmurs (p. 334).

Attributes of Heart Murmurs. If you detect a heart murmur, you must learn to identify and describe its *timing, shape, location of maximal intensity, radiation* or transmission from this location, *intensity, pitch,* and *quality.*

- *Timing.* First decide if you are hearing a *systolic murmur,* falling between S_1 and S_2, or a *diastolic murmur,* falling between S_2 and S_1. Palpating the carotid pulse as you listen can help you with timing. *Murmurs that coincide with the carotid upstroke are systolic.*

  Systolic murmurs are usually *midsystolic* or *pansystolic.* Late systolic murmurs may also be heard.

Diastolic murmurs usually indicate valvular heart disease. Systolic murmurs may indicate valvular disease, but often occur when the heart valves are entirely normal.

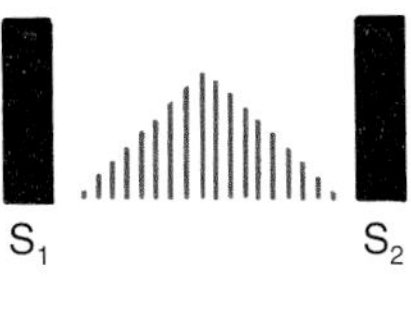

S_1

A *midsystolic murmur* begins after S_1 and stops before S_2. Brief gaps are audible between the murmur and the heart sounds. Listen carefully for the gap just before S_2. It is heard more easily and, if present, usually confirms the murmur as midsystolic, not pansystolic.

Midsystolic murmurs most often are related to blood flow across the semilunar (aortic and pulmonic) valves. See Table 8-9, Midsystolic Murmurs (p. 331).

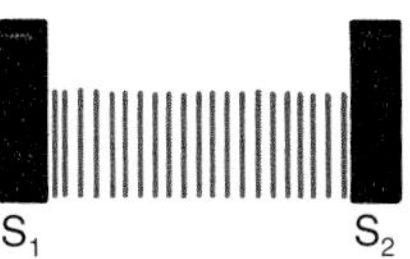

S_1

A *pansystolic (holosystolic) murmur* starts with S_1 and stops at S_2, without a gap between murmur and heart sounds.

Pansystolic murmurs often occur with regurgitant (backward) flow across the atrioventricular valves. See Table 8-8, Pansystolic (Holosystolic) Murmurs (pp. 332–333).

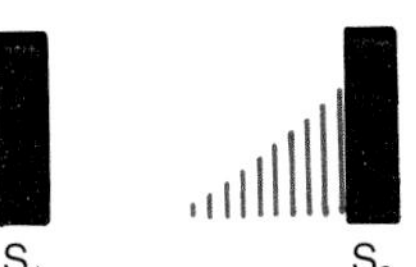

S_1

A *late systolic murmur* usually starts in mid- or late systole and persists up to S_2.

This is the murmur of mitral valve prolapse and is often, but not always, preceded by a systolic click (see p. 329).

Diastolic murmurs may be *early diastolic, middiastolic*, or *late diastolic.*

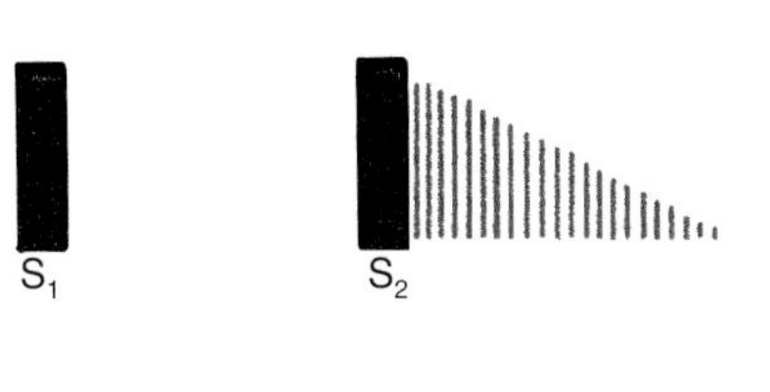

S_1

An *early diastolic murmur* starts right after S_2, without a discernible gap, and then usually fades into silence before the next S_1.

Early diastolic murmurs typically accompany regurgitant flow across incompetent semilunar valves.

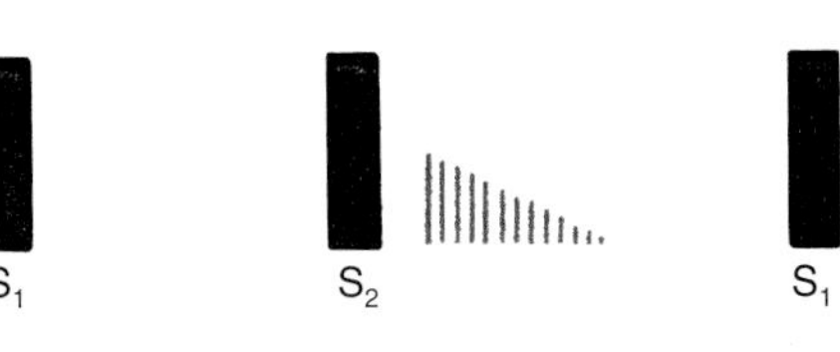

S_1

A *middiastolic murmur* starts a short time after S_2. It may fade away, as illustrated, or merge into a late diastolic murmur.

Middiastolic and presystolic murmurs reflect turbulent flow across the atrioventricular valves. See Table 8-10, Diastolic Murmurs (p. 334).

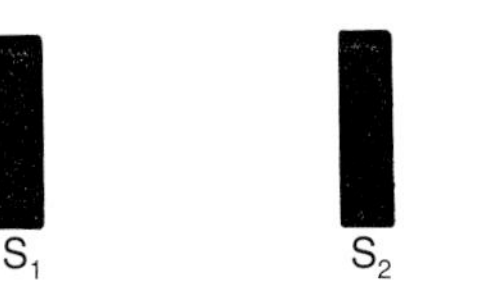

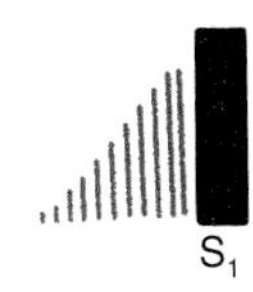

S_1

A *late diastolic (presystolic) murmur* starts late in diastole and typically continues up to S_1.

An occasional murmur, such as the murmur of a patent ductus arteriosus, starts in systole and continues without pause through S_2 into but not necessarily throughout diastole. It is then called a *continuous murmur.* Other cardiovascular sounds, such as pericardial friction rubs or venous hums, have *both systolic and diastolic components.* Observe and describe these sounds according to the characteristics used for systolic and diastolic murmurs.

See Table 8-11, Cardiovascular Sounds With Both Systolic and Diastolic Components (p. 335).

- *Shape.* The shape or configuration of a murmur is determined by its intensity over time.

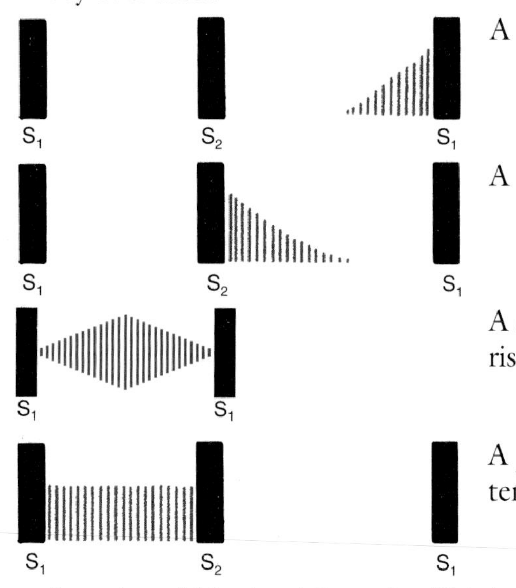

A *crescendo murmur* grows louder.

The presystolic murmur of *mitral stenosis* in normal sinus rhythm

A *decrescendo murmur* grows softer.

The early diastolic murmur of *aortic regurgitation*

A *crescendo–decrescendo murmur* first rises in intensity, then falls.

The midsystolic murmur of *aortic stenosis* and *innocent flow murmurs*

A *plateau murmur* has the same intensity throughout.

The pansystolic murmur of *mitral regurgitation*

- *Location of Maximal Intensity.* This is determined by the site where the murmur originates. Find the location by exploring the area where you hear the murmur. Describe where you hear it best in terms of the interspace and its relation to the sternum, the apex, or the midsternal, the midclavicular, or one of the axillary lines.

For example, a murmur best heard in the 2nd right interspace (the aortic area) usually originates at or near the aortic valve.

- *Radiation or Transmission From the Point of Maximal Intensity.* This reflects not only the site of origin but also the intensity of the murmur and the direction of blood flow. Explore the area around a murmur and determine where else you can hear it.

A loud murmur of *aortic stenosis* often radiates into the neck (in the direction of arterial flow).

- *Intensity.* This is usually graded on a 6-point scale and expressed as a fraction. The numerator describes the intensity of the murmur wherever it is loudest, and the denominator indicates the scale you are using. Intensity is influenced by the thickness of the chest wall and the presence of intervening tissue.

An identical degree of turbulence would cause a louder murmur in a thin person than in a very muscular or obese person. Emphysematous lungs may diminish the intensity of murmurs.

Learn to grade murmurs using the 6-point scale below. Note that grades 4 through 6 require the added presence of a palpable thrill.

Gradations of Murmurs

Grade	Description
Grade 1	Very faint, heard only after listener has "tuned in"; may not be heard in all positions
Grade 2	Quiet, but heard immediately after placing the stethoscope on the chest
Grade 3	Moderately loud
Grade 4	Loud, with palpable thrill
Grade 5	Very loud, with thrill. May be heard when the stethoscope is partly off the chest
Grade 6	Very loud, with thrill. May be heard with stethoscope entirely off the chest

- *Pitch.* This is categorized as high, medium, or low.
- *Quality.* This is described in terms such as blowing, harsh, rumbling, and musical.

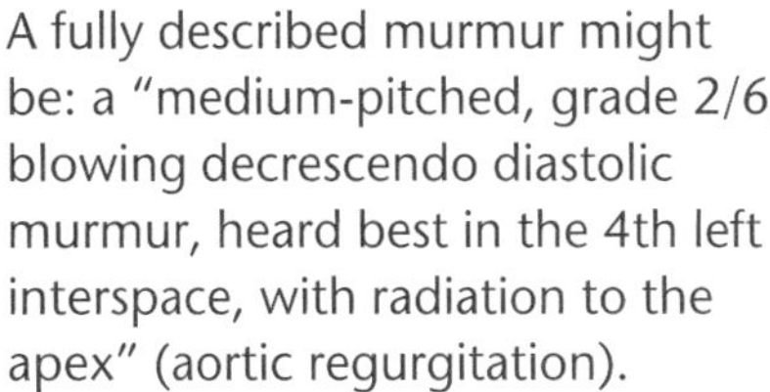

A fully described murmur might be: a "medium-pitched, grade 2/6, blowing decrescendo diastolic murmur, heard best in the 4th left interspace, with radiation to the apex" (aortic regurgitation).

Other useful characteristics of murmurs—and heart sounds too—include variation with respiration, with the position of the patient, or with other special maneuvers.

Murmurs originating in the right side of the heart tend to change more with respiration than left-sided murmurs.

INTEGRATING CARDIOVASCULAR ASSESSMENT

A good cardiovascular examination requires more than observation. You need to think about the possible meanings of your individual observations, fit them together in a logical pattern, and correlate your cardiac findings with the patient's blood pressure, arterial pulses, venous pulsations, jugular venous pressure, the remainder of your physical examination, and the patient's history.

Evaluating the common systolic murmur illustrates this point. In examining an asymptomatic teenager, for example, you might hear a grade 2/6 midsystolic murmur in the 2nd and 3rd left interspaces. Because this suggests a murmur of pulmonic origin, you should assess the size of the right ventricle by carefully palpating the left parasternal area. Because pulmonic stenosis and atrial septal defects can occasionally cause such murmurs, listen carefully to the splitting of the second heart sound and try to hear any ejection sounds. Listen to the murmur after the patient sits up. Look for evidence of anemia, hyperthyroidism, or pregnancy that could produce such a murmur by increasing the flow across the aortic or the pulmonic valve. If all your findings are normal, your patient probably has an *innocent murmur*—one with no pathologic significance.

In a 60-year-old person with angina, you might hear a harsh 3/6 midsystolic crescendo–decrescendo murmur in the right 2nd interspace radiating to the neck. These findings suggest *aortic stenosis,* but could arise from *aortic sclerosis* (leaflets sclerotic but not stenotic), a dilated aorta, or increased flow across a normal valve. Assess any delay in the carotid upstroke and the blood pressure for evidence of *aortic stenosis.* Check the apical impulse for left ventricular hypertrophy. Listen for *aortic regurgitation* as the patient leans forward and exhales.

Put all this information together to make a hypothesis about the origin of the murmur.

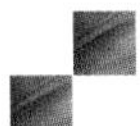

SPECIAL TECHNIQUES

Aids to Identify Systolic Murmurs. Elsewhere in this chapter you have learned how to improve your auscultation of heart sounds and murmurs by placing the patient in different positions. Two additional techniques help you distinguish the murmurs of mitral valve prolapse and hypertrophic cardiomyopathy from aortic stenosis.

(1) Standing and Squatting. When a person stands, venous return to the heart decreases, as does peripheral vascular resistance. Arterial blood pressure, stroke volume, and the volume of blood in the left ventricle all decline. When squatting, changes occur in the opposite direction. These changes help (1) to identify a prolapsed mitral valve, and (2) to distinguish hypertrophic cardiomyopathy from aortic stenosis.

Secure the patient's gown so that it will not interfere with your examination, and ready yourself for prompt auscultation. Instruct the patient to squat next to the examining table and hold on to it for balance. Listen to the heart with the patient in the squatting position and again in the standing position.

(2) Valsalva Maneuver. When a person strains down against a closed glottis, venous return to the right heart is decreased, and after a few seconds, left ventricular volume and arterial blood pressure both fall. Release of the effort has the opposite effects. These changes help to distinguish prolapse of the mitral valve and hypertrophic cardiomyopathy from aortic stenosis.

The patient should be lying down. Ask the patient to "bear down," or place one hand on the midabdomen and instruct the patient to strain against it. By adjusting the pressure of your hand you can alter the patient's effort to the desired level. Use your other hand to place your stethoscope on the patient's chest.

■ *Maneuvers to Identify Systolic Murmurs*

		Effect on Systolic Sounds and Murmurs		
Maneuver	**Cardiovascular Effect**	*Mitral Valve Prolapse*	*Hypertrophic Cardiomyopathy*	*Aortic Stenosis*
Standing; Strain Phase of Valsalva	**Decreased left ventricular volume** from ↓ venous return to heart	↑ prolapse of mitral valve	↑ outflow obstruction	↓ blood volume ejected into aorta
	Decreased vascular tone: ↓ arterial blood pressure	*Click moves earlier in systole* and *murmur lengthens*	**↑ intensity of murmur**	**↓ intensity of murmur**
Squatting; Release of Valsalva	**Increased left ventricular volume** from ↑ venous return to heart	↓ prolapse of mitral valve	↓ outflow obstruction	↑ blood volume ejected into aorta
	Increased vascular tone: ↑ arterial blood pressure; ↑ peripheral vascular resistance	*Delay of click* and *murmur shortens*	**↓ intensity of murmur**	**↑ intensity of murmur**

Pulsus Alternans. In *pulsus alternans,* the rhythm of the pulse remains regular, but the *force* of the arterial pulse alternates because of alternating strong and weak ventricular contractions. *Pulsus alternans* almost always indicates severe left-sided heart failure and is usually best felt by applying light pressure on the radial or femoral arteries.[35] Use a blood pressure cuff to confirm your finding. After raising the cuff pressure, lower it slowly to the systolic level—the initial Korotkoff sounds are the strong beats. As you lower the cuff, you will hear the softer sounds of the alternating weak beats.

Alternately loud and soft Korotkoff sounds or a sudden doubling of the apparent heart rate as the cuff pressure declines indicates a *pulsus alternans* (see p. 119).

The upright position may accentuate the alternation.

Paradoxical Pulse. If you have noted that the pulse varies in amplitude with respiration or if you suspect pericardial tamponade (because of increased jugular venous pressure, a rapid and diminished pulse, and dyspnea, for example), use a blood-pressure cuff to check for a *paradoxical pulse.* This is a greater than normal drop in systolic pressure during inspiration. As the

The level identified by first hearing Korotkoff sounds is the highest systolic pressure during the respiratory cycle. The level identified by hearing sounds throughout the cycle is the

patient breathes, quietly if possible, lower the cuff pressure slowly to the systolic level. Note the pressure level at which the first sounds can be heard. Then drop the pressure very slowly until sounds can be heard throughout the respiratory cycle. Again note the pressure level. The difference between these two levels is normally no greater than 3 or 4 mm Hg.

lowest systolic pressure. A difference between these levels of more than 10 mm Hg indicates a paradoxical pulse and suggests *pericardial tamponade,* possible *constrictive pericarditis,* but most commonly *obstructive airway disease* (see p. 119).

RECORDING YOUR FINDINGS

Note that initially you may use sentences to describe your findings; later you will use phrases. The style below contains phrases appropriate for most write-ups.

Recording the Physical Examination— The Cardiovascular Examination

"The jugular venous pulse (JVP) is 3 cm above the sternal angle with the head of bed elevated to 30°. Carotid upstrokes are brisk, without bruits. The point of maximal impulse (PMI) is tapping, 7 cm lateral to the midsternal line in the 5th intercostal space. Good S_1 and S_2. No murmurs or extra sounds."

OR

"The JVP is 5 cm above the sternal angle with the head of bed elevated to 50°. Carotid upstrokes are brisk; a bruit is heard over the left carotid artery. The PMI is diffuse, 3 cm in diameter, palpated at the anterior axillary line in the 5th and 6th intercostal spaces. S_1 and S_2 are soft. S_3 present. Harsh 2/6 holosystolic murmur best heard at the apex, radiating to the lower left sternal border (LLSB). No S_4 or diastolic murmurs."

Suggests *congestive heart failure* with possible *left carotid occlusion* and *mitral regurgitation.*[36–38]

Bibliography

CITATIONS

1. Cook DJ, Simel DL. Does this patient have abnormal central venous pressure? JAMA 275(8):630–634, 1996.
2. Lee TH, Goldman L. Evaluation of the patient with acute chest pain. N Engl J Med 342(16):1187–1195, 2000.
3. Goldman L, Kirtane AJ. Triage of patient with acute chest syndrome and possible cardiac ischemia: the elusive search for diagnostic perfection. Ann Intern Med 139(12):987–995, 2003.
4. Snow V, Barry P, Fihn SD, et al. Evaluation of primary care patients with chronic stable angina: guidelines from the American College of Physicians. Ann Intern Med 141(1):57–64, 2004.
5. U.S. Preventive Services Task Force. Screening for high blood pressure: recommendations and rationale. Rockville, MD, Agency for Healthcare Research and Quality, July 2003. Available at: http://www.ahrq.gov/clinic/3rduspstf/hibloodrr.htm. Accessed March 6, 2005.
6. Chobanion AV, Bakris GL, Black HR, et al. The seventh report of the Joint National Committee on Preventions, Detection, Evaluation, and Treatment of High Blood Pressure—the JNC 7 report. JAMA 289(19):2560–2572, 2003. Available at: www.nhlbi.nih.gov/guidelines/hypertension/jncintro.htm.
7. Whelton PK, He J, Appel LJ, et al. Primary prevention of hypertension. Clinical and Public Health Advisory from the National High Blood Pressure Education Program. JAMA 288(15):1882–1888, 2002.
8. Vasan RS, Larson MG, Leip EP, et al. Impact of high-normal blood pressure on the risk of cardiovascular disease. N Engl J Med 345(18):1291–1297, 2001.
9. Stamler J, Stamler R, Neaton JD, et al. Low risk-factor profile and long-term cardiovascular and noncardiovascular mortality and life expectancy—findings for 5 large cohorts of young adult and middle-aged men and women. JAMA 282(21):2012–2018, 1999.
10. Vidt DG, Borazanian RA. Treat high blood pressure sooner: tougher, simpler JNC 7 guidelines. Cleve Clin J Med 70(8): 721–728, 2003.
11. Pearson TA, Blair SN, Daniels SR, et al. AHA guidelines for primary prevention of cardiovascular disease and stroke: 2002 update. Circulation 106:388–391, 2002.

12. Third Report of the National Cholesterol Education Program (NCEP) Expert Panel. Detection, evaluation, and treatment of high blood cholesterol in adults—executive summary. National Cholesterol Education Program, National Heart, Lung, and Blood Institute, National Institutes of Health. NIH Publication No. 01-3670. May 2001. Available at: www.nhlbi.nih.gov/guidelines/cholesterol/index.htm. Accessed August 31, 2004.
13. National Cholesterol Education Panel. Third report of the National Cholesterol Education Program (NCEP) Expert Panel on detection, evaluation, and treatment of high blood cholesterol in adults (Adult Treatment Panel III) final report. Circulation 106:3143–3421, 2002.
14. Grundy SM, Cleeman JI, Merz NB, et al, for the Coordinating Committee of the National Cholesterol Education Program. Implications of recent clinical trials for the National Cholesterol Education Program Adult Treatment Panel III guidelines. Circulation 110:227–239, 2004.
15. Heart Protection Study Collaborative Group. MRC/BHF Heart Protection Study of cholesterol lowering with simvastatin in 20,356 high risk individuals: a randomized placebo-controlled trial. Lancet 360(9326):7–22, 2002.
16. Screening for lipid disorders: recommendations and rationale. Am J Prev Med 20(3S):73–76, 2001. Agency for Healthcare Research and Quality, Rockville, MD. Available at: http://www.ahrq.gov/clinic/ajpmsuppl/lipidrr.htm. Accessed January 15, 2005.
17. Pignone MP, Phillips CJ, Atkins D, et al. Summary of the evidence. Screening and treating adults for lipid disorders. Agency for Healthcare Research and Quality, Rockville, MD. Available at: http://www.ahrq.gov/clinic/ajpmsuppl/pignone1.htm. Accessed January 15, 2005.
18. Walsh JME, Pignone M. Drug treatment of hyperlipidemia in women. JAMA 291(18):2243–2252, 2004.
19. American Diabetes Association. Toolkit No. 7—protect your heart: choose fats wisely. March 2004. Available at: http://www.diabetes.org/type-1-diabetes/well-being/Choose-Fats.jsp. Accessed March 17, 2005.
20. Healthy People 2010. Progress review—nutrition and overweight. U.S. Department of Health and Human Services—Public Health Service. January 21, 2004. Available at: http://www.healthypeople.gov/data/2010prog/focus19/default.htm. Accessed March 17, 2005.
21. Healthy People 2010. Progress review—physical activity and fitness. U.S. Department of Health and Human Services—Public Health Service. April 14, 2004. Available at: http://www.healthypeople.gov/data/2010prog/focus22/. Accessed March 17, 2005.
22. Beevers G, Lip GY, O'Brien E. ABC of hypertension. Blood pressure measurement. Part I. Sphygmomanometry: factors common in all techniques. BMJ 322:981–985, 2001.
23. Beevers G, Lip GY, O'Brien E. ABC of hypertension. Blood pressure measurement. Part II. Conventional sphygmomanometry: technique of auscultatory blood pressure measurement. BMJ 322:1043–1047, 2001.
24. McAlister FA, Straus SE. Evidence-based treatment of hypertension. measurement of blood pressure: an evidence based review. BMJ 322:098–911, 2001.
25. Tholl U, Forstner K, Anlauf M. Measuring blood pressure: pitfalls and recommendations. Nephrol Dial Transplant 19:766, 2004.
26. Edmonds ZV, Mower WR, Lovato LM, et al. The reliability of vital sign measurements. Ann Emerg Med 39(3):233–237, 2002.
27. Lange RA, Hillis LD. Acute pericarditis. N Engl J Med 351(21):2195–2202, 2004.
28. Spodick D. Acute pericarditis: current concepts and practice. JAMA 289(9): 1150–1153, 2003.
29. Drazner MH, Rame E, Stevenson LW, et al. Prognostic importance of elevated jugular venous pressure and a third heart sound in patients with heart failure. N Engl J Med 345(8):574–581, 2001.
30. Khot UN. Prognostic importance of physical examination for heart failure in non-ST elevation acute coronary syndromes. The enduring value of Killip classification. JAMA 290(16): 2174–2181, 2003.
31. Jessup M, Brozena S. Medical progress: heart failure. N Engl J Med 348(20):2007–2017, 2003.
32. Aurigemma GP, Gaasch WH. Diastolic heart failure. N Engl J Med 351(11):1097–1104, 2004.
33. Badgett RG, Lucey CR, Muirow CD. Can the clinical examination diagnose left-sided heart failure in adults? JAMA 277(21):1712–1719, 1997.
34. Sauve JS, Laupacis A, Ostbye T, et al. Does this patient have a clinically important carotid bruit? JAMA 270(23): 2843–2845, 1993.
35. Cha K, Falk RH. Images in clinical medicine: pulsus alternans. N Engl J Med 334(13):834, 1996.
36. Halder AW, Larson MG, Franklin SS, et al. Systolic blood pressure, diastolic blood pressure, and pulse pressure as predictors of risk for congestive heart failure in the Framingham Heart Study. Ann Intern Med 138(1):10–16, 2003.
37. Thomas JT, Kelly RF, Thomas SJ, et al. Utility of history, physical examination, electrocardiogram, and chest radiograph for differentiating normal from decreased systolic function in patients with heart failure. Am J Med 112(6): 437–445, 2002.
38. Fonarow GC, Adams KF, Abraham WT, et al. Risk stratification for in-hospital mortality in acutely decompensated heart failure. Classification and regression tree analysis. JAMA 293(5):572–580, 2005.
39. Etchells E, Bell C, Robb K. Does this patient have an abnormal systolic murmur? JAMA 277(7):564–571, 1997.
40. Lembo NJ, Dell'Italia LJ, Crawford MH, et al. Bedside diagnosis of systolic murmurs. N Engl J Med 318:1572–1578, 1988.
41. Etchells E, Glenns, Shadowitz S, et al. A bedside clinical prediction rule for detecting moderate or severe aortic stenosis. J Gen Intern Med 13:699–704, 1998.
42. Pierard LA, Lancellotti P. The role of ischemic mitral regurgitation in the pathogenesis of acute pulmonary edema. N Engl J Med 351(16):1627–1634, 2004.
43. Enriquez-Serano M, Tajik AJ. Aortic regurgitation. N Engl J Med 351(15):1539–1546, 2004.
44. Babu AN, Kymes SM, Fryer SMC. Eponyms and the diagnosis of aortic regurgitation: what says the evidence? Ann Intern Med 138(9):736–742, 2003.

ADDITIONAL REFERENCES

Beckman JA, Creager MA, Libby P. Diabetes and atherosclerosis: epidemiology, pathophysiology, and management. JAMA 287(19):2570–2581, 2002.

Cohn JN, Hoke L, Whitwam W, et al. Screening for early detection of cardiovascular disease in asymptomatic individuals. Am Heart J 146(4):679–685, 2003.

Dosh SA. The diagnosis of essential and secondary hypertension in adults. J Fam Pract 50(8):707–712, 2001.

Drezner JA. Sudden cardiac death in young athletes: causes, athlete's heart, and screening guidelines. Postgrad Med 108(5):37–44, 47–50, 2000.

Fletcher GF, Balady GJ, Amsterdam EA, et al. Exercise standards for testing and training: a statement for healthcare professionals from the American Heart Association. Circulation 104(14): 1694–1740, 2001.

Fuster V, Alexander RW, O'Rourke RA, et al. Hurst's the Heart, 11th ed. New York, McGraw-Hill, Medical Pub Division, 2004.

Hansson GK. Inflammation, atherosclerosis, and coronary artery disease. N Engl J Med 352(16):1685–1695, 2005.

Kuperstein R, Feinberg MS, Eldar M, Schwammenthal E. Physical determinants of systolic murmur intensity in aortic stenosis. Am J Cardiol 95(6):774–776, 2005.

Lee AJ, Price JF, Russell MJ, et al. Improved prediction of fatal myocardial infarction using the ankle brachial index in addition to conventional risk factors: the Edinburgh Artery Study. Circulation 110(19):3075–3080, 2004.

Oparil S, Saman MA, Calhoun DA. Pathogenesis of hypertension. Ann Intern Med 139(9):761–776, 2003.

Perloff, JK. Physical Examination of the Heart and Circulation, 3rd ed. Philadelphia, WB Saunders, 2000.

Pryor DB, Shaw L, McCants CB. Value of the history and physical in identifying patients at increased risk for coronary artery disease. Ann Intern Med 118(2):81–90, 1993.

Selvanayagam J, De Pasquale C, Arnolda L. Usefulness of clinical assessment of the carotid pulse in the diagnosis of aortic stenosis. Am J Cardiol 93(4):493–495, 2004.

Selvin E, Erlinger TP. Prevalence of and risk factors for peripheral arterial disease in the United States: results from the National Health and Nutrition Examination Survey. Circulation 110(6):738–743, 2004.

Smulyan H, Safar ME. The diastolic blood pressure in systolic hypertension. Ann Intern Med 132(3):233–237, 2000.

Stein RA, Zusman R. Management of sexual dysfunction in patients with cardiovascular disease: recommendations of the Princeton Consensus Panel. Am J Cardiol 86(2A):62F–68F, 2000.

Taylor HA Jr. Sexual activity and the cardiovascular patient: guidelines. Am J Cardiol 84(5B):6N–10N, 1999.

Thomas JT, Kelly RF, Thomas SJ, et al. Utility of history, physical examination, electrocardiogram, and chest radiograph for differentiating normal from decreased systolic function in patients with heart failure. Am J Med 112(6):437–445, 2002.

Zipes DP, Braunwald E (eds). Braunwald's Heart Disease: A Textbook of Cardiovascular Medicine, 7th ed. Philadelphia, Elsevier Saunders, 2005.

TABLE 8-1 Selected Heart Rates and Rhythms

Cardiac rhythms may be classified as *regular* or *irregular*. When rhythms are irregular or rates are fast or slow, obtain an ECG to identify the origin of the beats (sinus node, AV node, atrium, or ventricle) and the pattern of conduction. Note that with AV (atrioventricular) block, arrhythmias may have a fast, normal, or slow ventricular rate.

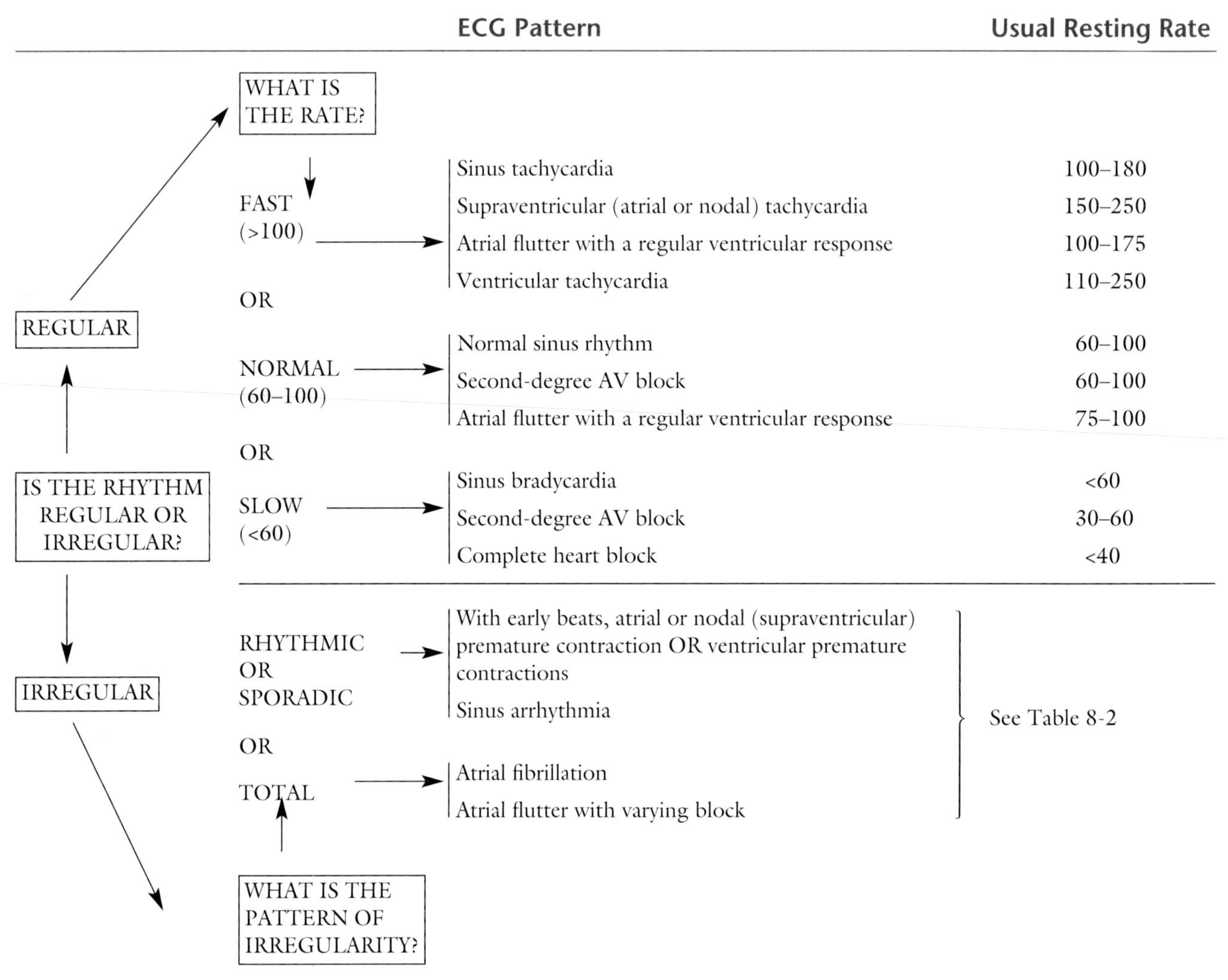
IS THE RHYTHM REGULAR OR IRREGULAR?
REGULAR
WHAT IS THE RATE?
IRREGULAR
WHAT IS THE PATTERN OF IRREGULARITY?

		ECG Pattern	Usual Resting Rate
REGULAR	FAST (>100)	Sinus tachycardia	100–180
		Supraventricular (atrial or nodal) tachycardia	150–250
		Atrial flutter with a regular ventricular response	100–175
		Ventricular tachycardia	110–250
	OR NORMAL (60–100)	Normal sinus rhythm	60–100
		Second-degree AV block	60–100
		Atrial flutter with a regular ventricular response	75–100
	OR SLOW (<60)	Sinus bradycardia	<60
		Second-degree AV block	30–60
		Complete heart block	<40
IRREGULAR	RHYTHMIC OR SPORADIC	With early beats, atrial or nodal (supraventricular) premature contraction OR ventricular premature contractions	See Table 8-2
		Sinus arrhythmia	
	OR TOTAL	Atrial fibrillation	
		Atrial flutter with varying block	

TABLE 8-2 Selected Irregular Rhythms

Type of Rhythm	ECG Waves and Heart Sounds	
Atrial or Nodal Premature Contractions (*Supraventricular*)	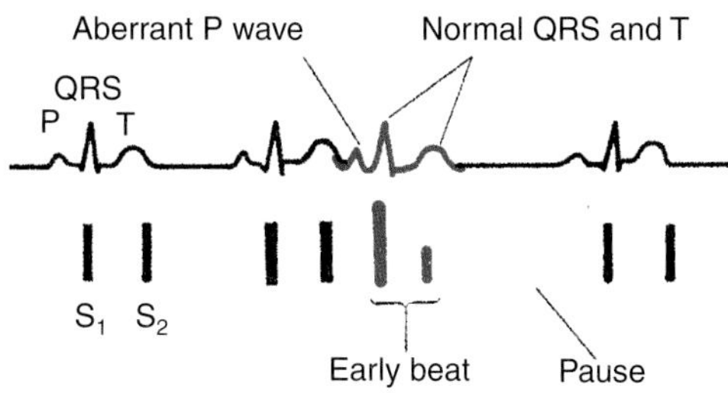	**Rhythm.** A beat of atrial or nodal origin comes earlier than the next expected normal beat. A pause follows, and then the rhythm resumes. **Heart Sounds.** S_1 may differ in intensity from the S_1 of normal beats, and S_2 may be decreased. Both sounds are otherwise similar to those of normal beats.
Ventricular Premature Contractions	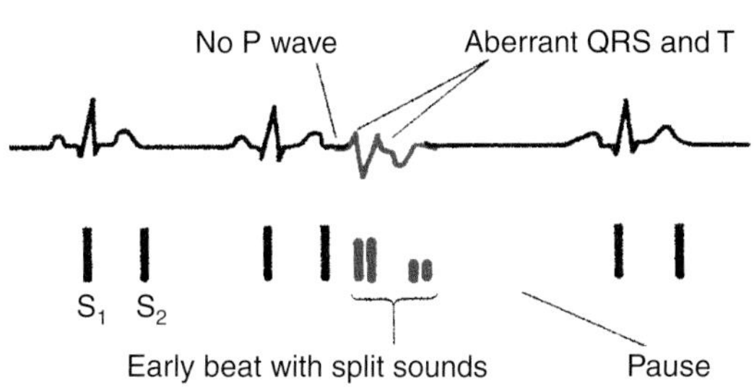	**Rhythm.** A beat of ventricular origin comes earlier than the next expected normal beat. A pause follows, and the rhythm resumes. **Heart Sounds.** S_1 may differ in intensity from the S_1 of the normal beats, and S_2 may be decreased. Both sounds are likely to be split.
Sinus Arrhythmia	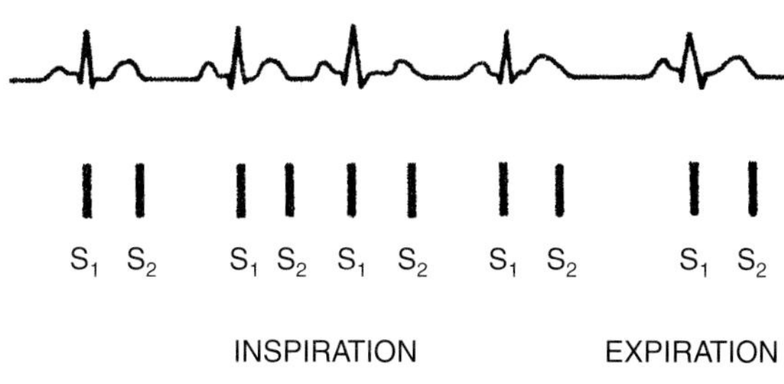	**Rhythm.** The heart varies cyclically, usually speeding up with inspiration and slowing down with expiration. **Heart Sounds.** Normal, although S_1 may vary with the heart rate.
Atrial Fibrillation and Atrial Flutter With Varying AV Block	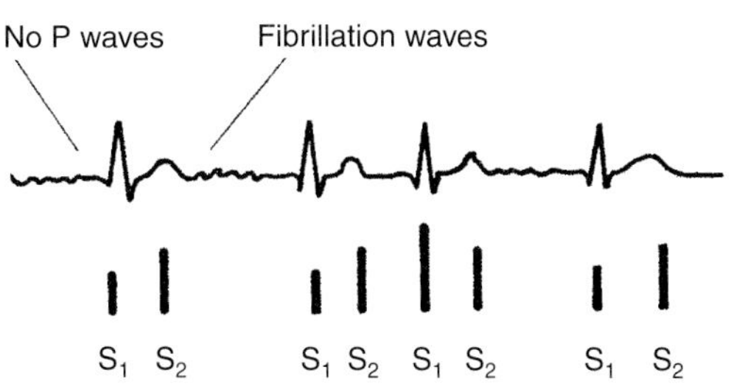	**Rhythm.** The ventricular rhythm is totally irregular, although short runs of the irregular ventricular rhythm may seem regular. **Heart Sounds.** S_1 varies in intensity.

TABLE 8-3 Variations and Abnormalities of the Ventricular Impulses

In the healthy heart, the *left ventricular impulse* is usually the *point of maximal impulse*, or *PMI*. This brief impulse is generated by the movement of the ventricular apex against the chest wall during contraction. The *right ventricular impulse* is normally not palpable beyond infancy, and its characteristics are indeterminate. In contrast, learn the classical descriptors of the left ventricular PMI:

- *Location:* in the 4th or 5th interspace, ~7–10 cm lateral to the midsternal line, depending on the diameter of the chest
- *Diameter: discrete,* or ≤2 cm
- *Amplitude: brisk* and *tapping*
- *Duration:* ≤2/3 of systole

Careful examination of the ventricular impulse gives you important clues about underlying cardiovascular hemodynamics. The quality of the ventricular impulse changes as the left and right ventricles adapt to high-output states (anxiety, hyperthyroidism, and severe anemia) and to the more pathologic conditions of chronic pressure or volume overload. Note below the distinguishing features of three types of ventricular impulses: the *hyperkinetic ventricular impulse* from transiently increased stroke volume—this change does not necessarily indicate heart disease; the *sustained* ventricular impulse of ventricular hypertrophy from chronic pressure load, known as *increased afterload* (see p. 311); and the *diffuse* ventricular impulse of ventricular dilation from chronic volume overload, or *increased preload.*

	Left Ventricular Impulse			Right Ventricular Impulse		
	Hyperkinetic	*Pressure Overload*	*Volume Overload*	*Hyperkinetic*	*Pressure Overload*	*Volume Overload*
Examples of Causes	Anxiety, hyperthyroidism, severe anemia	Aortic stenosis, hypertension	Aortic or mitral regurgitation	Anxiety, hyperthyroidism, severe anemia	Pulmonic stenosis, pulmonary hypertension	Atrial septal defect
Location	Normal	Normal	Displaced to the left and possibly downward	3rd, 4th, or 5th left interspaces	3rd, 4th, or 5th left interspaces, also subxiphoid	Left sternal border, extending toward the left cardiac border, also subxiphoid
Diameter	~2 cm, though increased amplitude may make it seem larger	>2 cm	>2 cm	Not useful	Not useful	Not useful
Amplitude	More forceful tapping	More forceful tapping	*Diffuse*	Slightly more forceful	More forceful	Slightly to markedly more forceful
Duration	<2/3 systole	*Sustained* (up to S_2)	Often slightly sustained	Normal	Sustained	Normal to slightly sustained

TABLE 8-4 Variations in the First Heart Sound—S_1

Normal Variations	S_1 S_2	S_1 is softer than S_2 at the *base* (right and left 2nd interspaces).
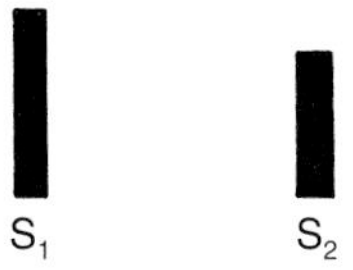	S_1 S_2	S_1 is often but not always louder than S_2 at the *apex*.
Accentuated S_1	S_1 S_2	S_1 is accentuated in (1) tachycardia, rhythms with a short PR interval, and high cardiac output states (e.g., exercise, anemia, hyperthyroidism), and (2) mitral stenosis. In these conditions, the mitral valve is still open wide at the onset of ventricular systole, and then closes quickly.
Diminished S_1	S_1 S_2	S_1 is diminished in first-degree heart block (delayed conduction from atria to ventricles). Here the mitral valve has had time after atrial contraction to float back into an almost closed position before ventricular contraction shuts it. It closes less loudly. S_1 is also diminished (1) when the mitral valve is calcified and relatively immobile, as in mitral regurgitation, and (2) when left ventricular contractility is markedly reduced, as in congestive heart failure or coronary heart disease.
Varying S_1	S_1 S_2 S_1 S_2	S_1 varies in intensity (1) in complete heart block, when atria and ventricles are beating independently of each other, and (2) in any totally irregular rhythm (e.g., atrial fibrillation). In these situations, the mitral valve is in varying positions before being shut by ventricular contraction. Its closure sound, therefore, varies in loudness.
Split S_1	S_1 S_2	S_1 may be split normally along the lower left sternal border where the tricuspid component, often too faint to be heard, becomes audible. This split may sometimes be heard at the apex, but consider also an S_4, an aortic ejection sound, and an early systolic click. Abnormal splitting of both heart sounds may be heard in right bundle branch block and in premature ventricular contractions.

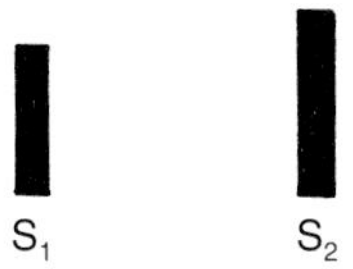

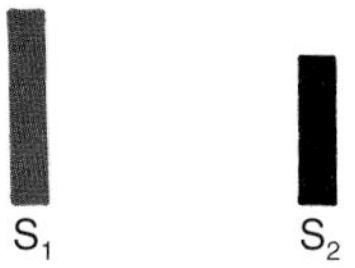

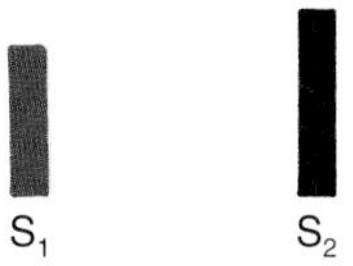

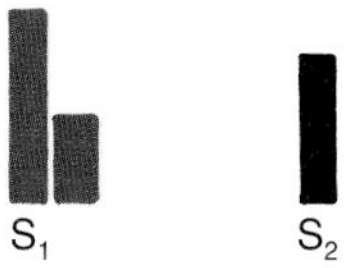

TABLE 8-5 Variations in the Second Heart Sound—S_2

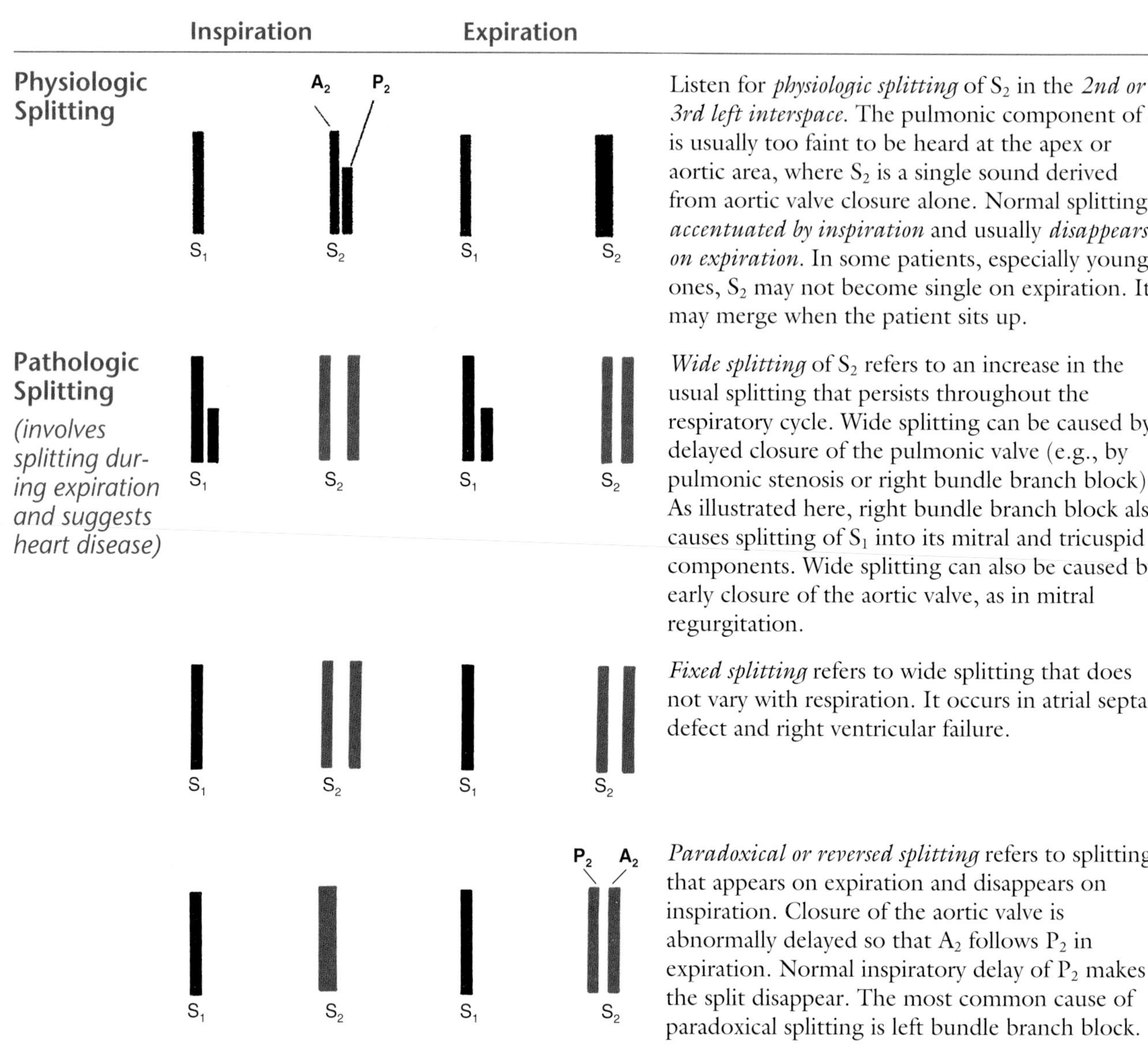

Listen for *physiologic splitting* of S_2 in the *2nd or 3rd left interspace*. The pulmonic component of S_2 is usually too faint to be heard at the apex or aortic area, where S_2 is a single sound derived from aortic valve closure alone. Normal splitting is *accentuated by inspiration* and usually *disappears on expiration*. In some patients, especially younger ones, S_2 may not become single on expiration. It may merge when the patient sits up.

Wide splitting of S_2 refers to an increase in the usual splitting that persists throughout the respiratory cycle. Wide splitting can be caused by delayed closure of the pulmonic valve (e.g., by pulmonic stenosis or right bundle branch block). As illustrated here, right bundle branch block also causes splitting of S_1 into its mitral and tricuspid components. Wide splitting can also be caused by early closure of the aortic valve, as in mitral regurgitation.

Fixed splitting refers to wide splitting that does not vary with respiration. It occurs in atrial septal defect and right ventricular failure.

Paradoxical or reversed splitting refers to splitting that appears on expiration and disappears on inspiration. Closure of the aortic valve is abnormally delayed so that A_2 follows P_2 in expiration. Normal inspiratory delay of P_2 makes the split disappear. The most common cause of paradoxical splitting is left bundle branch block.

Increased Intensity of A_2 in the Right Second Interspace (where only A_2 can usually be heard) occurs in systemic hypertension because of the increased pressure load. It also occurs when the aortic root is dilated, probably because the aortic valve is then closer to the chest wall.

Decreased or Absent A_2 in the Right Second Interspace is noted in calcific aortic stenosis because of valve immobility. If A_2 is inaudible, no splitting is heard.

Increased Intensity of P_2. When P_2 is equal to or louder than A_2, suspect pulmonary hypertension. Other causes include a dilated pulmonary artery and an atrial septal defect. When a split S_2 is heard widely, even at the apex and the right base, P_2 is accentuated.

Decreased or Absent P_2 is usually due to the increased anteroposterior diameter of the chest associated with aging. It can also result from pulmonic stenosis. If P_2 is inaudible, no splitting is heard.

TABLE 8-6 Extra Heart Sounds in Systole

There are two kinds of extra heart sounds in systole: (1) early ejection sounds, and (2) clicks, commonly heard in mid- and late systole.

Early Systolic Ejection Sounds

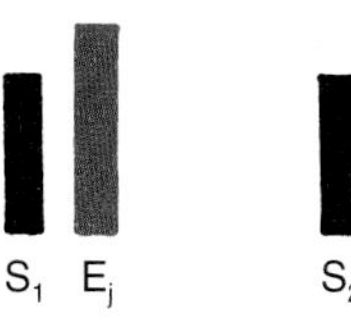

Early systolic ejection sounds occur shortly after S_1, coincident with opening of the aortic and pulmonic valves. They are relatively high in pitch, have a sharp, clicking quality, and are heard better with the diaphragm of the stethoscope. An ejection sound indicates cardiovascular disease.

Listen for an *aortic ejection sound* at both the base and apex. It may be louder at the apex and usually does not vary with respiration. An aortic ejection sound may accompany a dilated aorta, or aortic valve disease from congenital stenosis or a bicuspid valve.

A *pulmonic ejection sound* is heard best in the 2nd and 3rd left interspaces. When S_1, usually relatively soft in this area, appears to be loud, you may be hearing a pulmonic ejection sound. Its intensity often *decreases with inspiration.* Causes include dilatation of the pulmonary artery, pulmonary hypertension, and pulmonic stenosis.

Systolic Clicks

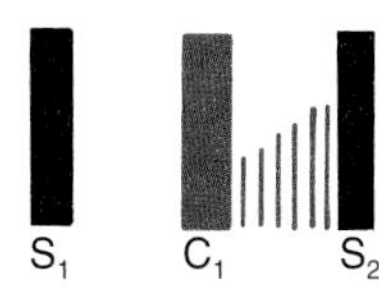

Systolic clicks are usually due to *mitral valve prolapse*—an abnormal systolic ballooning of part of the mitral valve into the left atrium. The clicks are usually mid- or late systolic. Prolapse of the mitral valve is a common cardiac condition, affecting about 5% of the general population. There is equal prevalence in men and women.

The click is usually single, but you may hear more than one, usually *at or medial to the apex,* but also *at the lower left sternal border.* It is high-pitched, so listen with the diaphragm. The click is often followed by a late systolic murmur from mitral regurgitation—a flow of blood from left ventricle to left atrium. The murmur usually crescendos up to S_2. Auscultatory findings are notably variable. Most patients have only a click, some have only a murmur, and some have both. Systolic clicks may also be of extracardial or mediastinal origin.

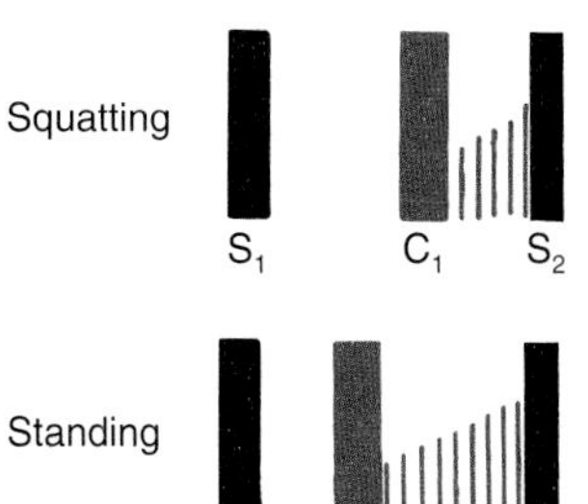

Findings vary from time to time and often change with body position. Several positions are recommended to identify the syndrome: supine, seated, squatting, and standing. *Squatting delays the click and murmur; standing moves them closer to S_1.*

TABLE 8-7 Extra Heart Sounds in Diastole

Opening Snap

S_1 S_2 OS S_1

The *opening snap* is a very early diastolic sound usually produced by the opening of a *stenotic mitral valve.* It is heard best just medial to the apex and along the lower left sternal border. When it is loud, an opening snap radiates to the apex and to the pulmonic area, where it may be mistaken for the pulmonic component of a split S_2. Its high pitch and snapping quality help to distinguish it from an S_2. It is heard better with the diaphragm.

S_3

S_1 S_2 S_3 S_1

You will detect *physiologic* S_3 frequently in children and in young adults to the age of 35 or 40. It is common during the last trimester of pregnancy. Occurring early in diastole during rapid ventricular filling, it is later than an opening snap, dull and low in pitch, and heard best at the apex in the left lateral decubitus position. Use the bell of the stethoscope should be used with very light pressure.

A *pathologic S_3* or *ventricular gallop* sounds just like a physiologic S_3. An S_3 in a person over age 40 (possibly a little older in women) is almost certainly pathologic. Causes include decreased myocardial contractility, congestive heart failure, and volume overloading of a ventricle, as in mitral or tricuspid regurgitation. A *left-sided S_3* is heard typically at the apex in the left lateral decubitus position. A *right-sided S_3* is usually heard along the lower left sternal border or below the xiphoid with the patient supine, and is louder on inspiration. The term *gallop* comes from the cadence of three heart sounds, especially at rapid heart rates, and sounds like "Kentucky."

S_4

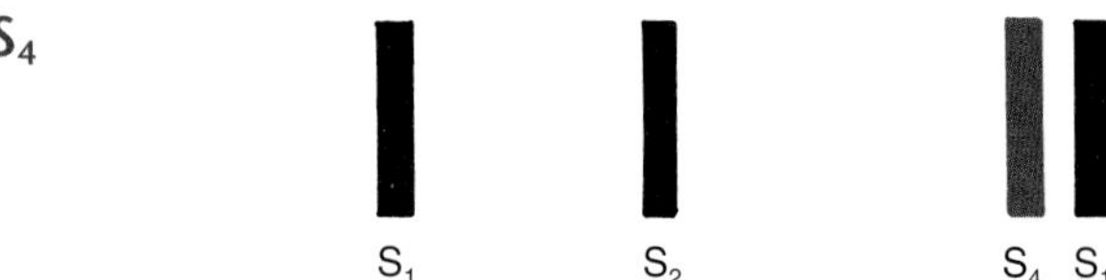

An S_4 (*atrial sound* or *atrial gallop*) occurs just before S_1. It is dull, low in pitch, and heard better with the bell. An S_4 is heard occasionally in an apparently normal person, especially in trained athletes and older age groups. More commonly, it is due to increased resistance to ventricular filling following atrial contraction. This increased resistance is related to decreased compliance (increased stiffness) of the ventricular myocardium.

Causes of a left-sided S_4 include hypertensive heart disease, coronary artery disease, aortic stenosis, and cardiomyopathy. A *left-sided S_4* is heard best at the apex in the left lateral position; it may sound like "Tennessee." The less common *right-sided S_4* is heard along the lower left sternal border or below the xiphoid. It often gets louder with inspiration. Causes of a right-sided S_4 include pulmonary hypertension and pulmonic stenosis.

An S_4 may also be associated with delayed conduction between atria and ventricles. This delay separates the normally faint atrial sound from the louder S_1 and makes it audible. An S_4 is never heard in the absence of atrial contraction, which occurs with atrial fibrillation.

Occasionally, a patient has both an S_3 and an S_4, producing a *quadruple rhythm* of four heart sounds. At rapid heart rates, the S_3 and S_4 may merge into one loud extra heart sound, called a *summation gallop.*

TABLE 8-8 Pansystolic (Holosystolic) Murmurs

Pansystolic (holosystolic) murmurs are pathologic, arising from blood flow from a chamber with high pressure to one of lower pressure, through a valve or other structure that should be closed. The murmur begins immediately with S_1 and continues up to S_2.

	Mitral Regurgitation	Tricuspid Regurgitation	Ventricular Septal Defect
	Decreased S_1 S_2 S_3	S_1 S_2 S_3	S_1 S_2
Murmur	*Location.* Apex *Radiation.* To the left axilla, less often to the left sternal border *Intensity.* Soft to loud; if loud, associated with an apical thrill *Pitch.* Medium to high *Quality.* Harsh, holosystolic *Aids.* Unlike tricuspid regurgitation, it does not become louder in inspiration.	*Location.* Lower left sternal border *Radiation.* To the right of the sternum, to the xiphoid area, and perhaps to the left midclavicular line, but not into the axilla *Intensity.* Variable *Pitch.* Medium *Quality.* Blowing, holosystolic *Aids.* Unlike mitral regurgitation, the intensity may increase slightly with inspiration.	*Location.* 3rd, 4th, and 5th left interspaces *Radiation.* Often wide *Intensity.* Often very loud, with a thrill *Pitch.* High, holosystolic *Quality.* Often harsh
Associated Findings	S_1 is often decreased. An apical S_3 reflects volume overload on the left ventricle. The apical impulse is increased in amplitude and may be *sustained.*	The right ventricular impulse is increased in amplitude and may be *sustained.* An S_3 may be audible along the lower left sternal border. The jugular venous pressure is often elevated, and large *v* waves may be seen in the jugular veins.	A_2 may be obscured by the loud murmur. Findings vary with the severity of the defect and with associated lesions.
Mechanism	When the *mitral valve fails to close fully in systole,* blood regurgitates from left ventricle to left atrium, causing a murmur. This leakage creates volume overload on the left ventricle, with subsequent dilatation and hypertrophy. Several structural abnormalities cause this condition, and findings may vary accordingly.	When the *tricuspid valve fails to close fully in systole,* blood regurgitates from right ventricle to right atrium, producing a murmur. The most common cause is right ventricular failure and dilatation, with resulting enlargement of the tricuspid orifice. Either pulmonary hypertension or left ventricular failure is the usual initiating cause.	A ventricular septal defect is a congenital abnormality in which *blood flows from the relatively high-pressure left ventricle into the low-pressure right ventricle through a hole.* The defect may be accompanied by other abnormalities, but an uncomplicated lesion is described here.

TABLE 8-9 Midsystolic Murmurs

Midsystolic ejection murmurs are the most common kind of heart murmur. They may be (1) *innocent*—without any detectable physiologic or structural abnormality; (2) *physiologic*—from physiologic changes in body metabolism; or (3) *pathologic*—arising from a structural abnormality in the heart or great vessels.[39,40] Midsystolic murmurs tend to peak near midsystole and usually stop before S_2. The crescendo–decrescendo or "diamond" shape is not always audible, but the gap between the murmur and S_2 helps to distinguish midsystolic from pansystolic murmurs.

	Innocent Murmurs	Physiologic Murmurs
	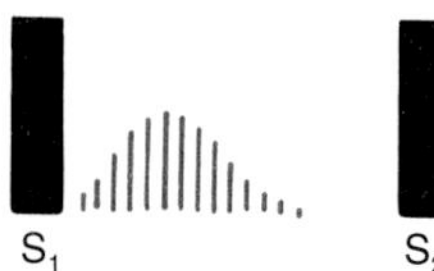	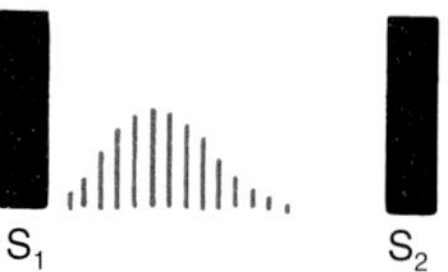
Murmur	*Location.* 2nd to 4th left interspaces between the left sternal border and the apex *Radiation.* Little *Intensity.* Grade 1 to 2, possibly 3 *Pitch.* Soft to medium *Quality.* Variable *Aids.* Usually decreases or disappears on sitting	Similar to innocent murmurs
Associated Findings	None: normal splitting, no ejection sounds, no diastolic murmurs, and no palpable evidence of ventricular enlargement. Occasionally, both an innocent murmur and another kind of murmur are present.	Possible signs of a likely cause
Mechanism	Innocent murmurs result from turbulent blood flow, probably generated by ventricular ejection of blood into the aorta from the left and occasionally the right ventricle. Very common in children and young adults—may also be heard in older people. There is no underlying cardiovascular disease.	Turbulence due to a temporary increase in blood flow in predisposing conditions such as anemia, pregnancy, fever, and hyperthyroidism.

Pathologic Murmurs

Aortic Stenosis[41]	*Hypertrophic Cardiomyopathy*	*Pulmonic Stenosis*
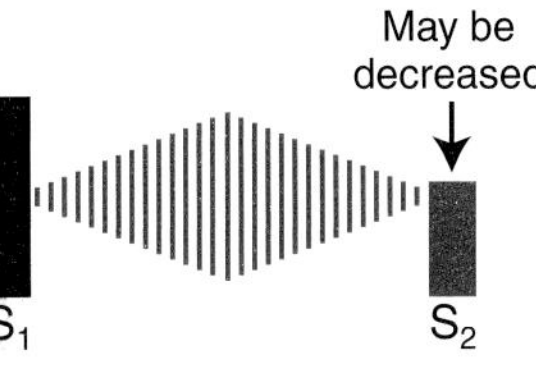	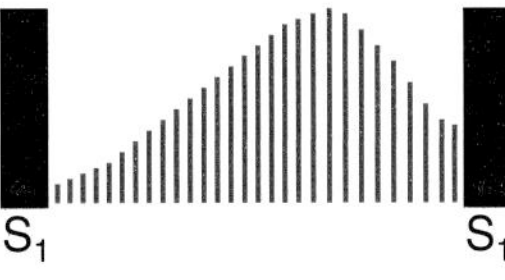	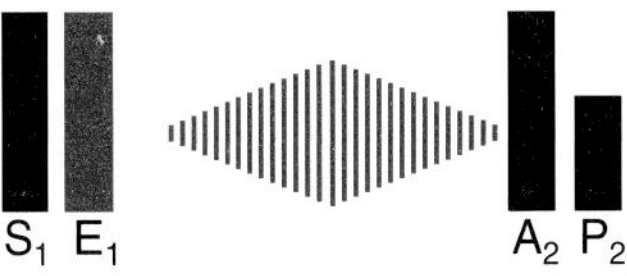
Location. Right 2nd interspace	*Location.* 3rd and 4th left interspaces	*Location.* 2nd and 3rd left interspaces
Radiation. Often to the carotids, down the left sternal border, even to the apex	*Radiation.* Down the left sternal border to the apex, possibly to the base, but not to the neck	*Radiation.* If loud, toward the left shoulder and neck
Intensity. Sometimes soft but often loud, with a thrill	*Intensity.* Variable	*Intensity.* Soft to loud; if loud, associated with a thrill
Pitch. Medium, harsh; crescendo–decrescendo may be higher at the apex	*Pitch.* Medium	*Pitch.* Medium; crescendo–decrescendo
Quality. Often harsh; may be more musical at the apex	*Quality.* Harsh	*Quality.* Often harsh
Aids. Heard best with the patient sitting and leaning forward	*Aids.* Decreases with squatting, increases with straining down from Valsalva	
A_2 decreases as aortic stenosis worsens. A_2 may be delayed and merge with $P_2 \rightarrow$ single S_2 on expiration or paradoxical S_2 split. Carotid upstroke may be ***delayed*** with slow rise and small amplitude. Hypertrophied left ventricle may $\rightarrow$ ***sustained*** apical impulse and an S_4 from decreased compliance.	An S_3 may be present. An S_4 is often present at the apex (unlike mitral regurgitation). The apical impulse may be ***sustained*** and have two palpable components. The carotid pulse rises ***quickly,*** unlike the pulse in aortic stenosis.	In severe stenosis, S_2 is widely split, and P_2 is diminished or inaudible. An early pulmonic ejection sound is common. May hear a right-sided S_4. Right ventricular impulse often increased in amplitude and ***sustained.***
Significant aortic valve stenosis impairs blood flow across the valve, causing turbulence, and increases left ventricular afterload. Causes are congenital, rheumatic, and degenerative; findings may differ with each cause. Other conditions mimic aortic stenosis without obstructing flow: *aortic sclerosis,* a stiffening of aortic valve leaflets associated with aging; a ***bicuspid aortic valve,*** a congenital condition that may not be recognized until adulthood; ***a dilated aorta,*** as in arteriosclerosis, syphilis, or Marfan's syndrome; ***pathologically increased flow across the aortic valve*** during systole, as in aortic regurgitation.	Massive ventricular hypertrophy is associated with unusually rapid ejection of blood from the left ventricle during systole. Outflow tract obstruction to flow may coexist. Accompanying distortion of the mitral valve may cause mitral regurgitation.	Pulmonic valve stenosis impairs flow across the valve, increasing right ventricular afterload. Congenital and usually found in children. In an ***atrial septal defect,*** the systolic murmur from pathologically increased flow across the pulmonic valve may mimic pulmonic stenosis.

TABLE 8-10 Diastolic Murmurs

Diastolic murmurs almost always indicate heart disease. There are two basic types. *Early decrescendo diastolic murmurs* signify regurgitant flow through an incompetent semilunar valve, more commonly the aortic. *Rumbling diastolic murmurs in mid- or late diastole* suggest stenosis of an atrioventricular valve, usually the mitral.

	Aortic Regurgitation[43,44]	Mitral Stenosis
	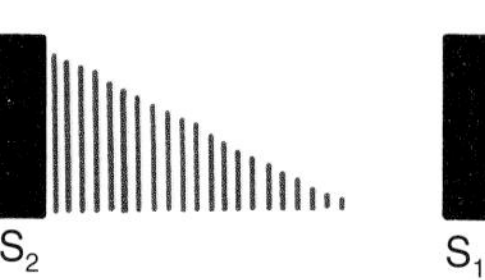	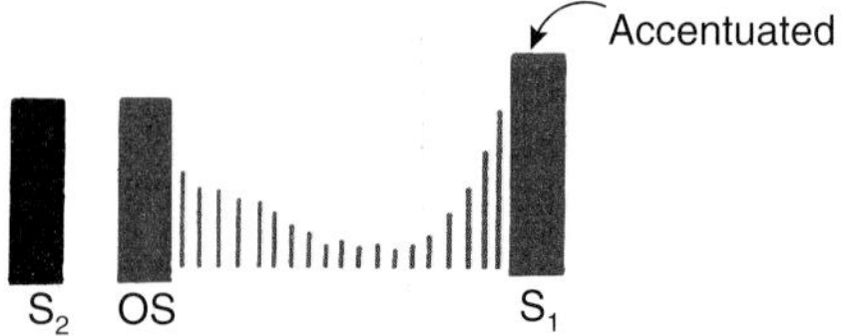
Murmur	*Location.* 2nd to 4th left interspaces *Radiation.* If loud, to the apex, perhaps to the right sternal border *Intensity.* Grade 1 to 3 *Pitch.* High. *Use the diaphragm.* *Quality.* Blowing decrescendo; may be mistaken for breath sounds *Aids.* The murmur is heard best with the *patient sitting, leaning forward,* with breath held after exhalation.	*Location.* Usually limited to the apex *Radiation.* Little or none *Intensity.* Grade 1 to 4 *Pitch.* Decrescendo low-pitched rumble. *Use the bell.* *Aids.* Placing the bell exactly on the apical impulse, turning the patient into a *left lateral position,* and mild exercise all help to make the murmur audible. It is heard better in exhalation.
Associated Findings	An ejection sound may be present. An S_3 or S_4, if present, suggests severe regurgitation. Progressive changes in the apical impulse include increased amplitude, displacement laterally and downward, widened diameter, and increased duration. The pulse pressure increases, and *arterial pulses are often large and bounding.* A midsystolic flow murmur or an Austin Flint murmur suggests large regurgitant flow.	S_1 is accentuated and may be palpable at the apex. An opening snap (OS) often follows S_2 and initiates the murmur. If pulmonary hypertension develops, P_2 is accentuated, and the right ventricular impulse becomes palpable. Mitral regurgitation and aortic valve disease may be associated with mitral stenosis.
Mechanism	The leaflets of the aortic valve fail to close completely during diastole, and blood regurgitates from the aorta back into the left ventricle. Volume overload on the left ventricle results. Two other murmurs may be associated: (1) a midsystolic murmur from the resulting increased forward flow across the aortic valve, and (2) a mitral diastolic (*Austin Flint*) murmur, attributed to diastolic impingement of the regurgitant flow on the anterior leaflet of the mitral valve.	When the leaflets of the mitral valve thicken, stiffen, and become distorted from the effects of rheumatic fever, the *mitral valve fails to open sufficiently in diastole.* The resulting murmur has two components: (1) middiastolic (during rapid ventricular filling), and (2) presystolic (during atrial contraction). The latter disappears if atrial fibrillation develops, leaving only a middiastolic rumble.

TABLE 8-11 Cardiovascular Sounds With Both Systolic and Diastolic Components

Some cardiovascular sounds extend beyond one phase of the cardiac cycle. Three examples, further described below, are: (1) a *venous hum,* a benign sound produced by turbulence of blood in the jugular veins—common in children; (2) a *pericardial friction rub,* produced by inflammation of the pericardial sac; and (3) *patent ductus arteriosus,* a congenital abnormality in which an open channel persists between aorta and pulmonary artery. *Continuous murmurs* begin in systole and extend through S_2 into all or part of diastole, as in *patent ductus arteriosus.*

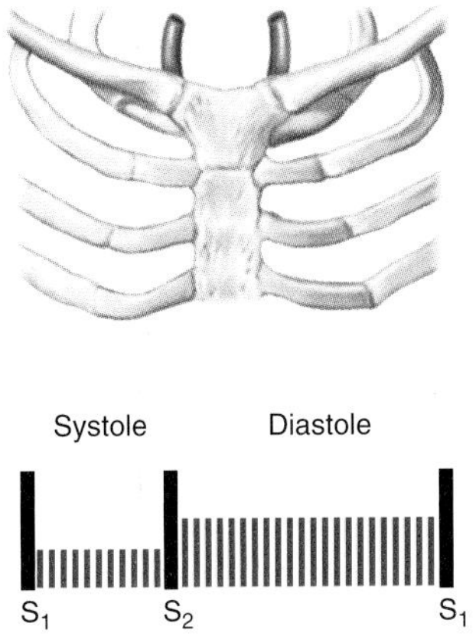

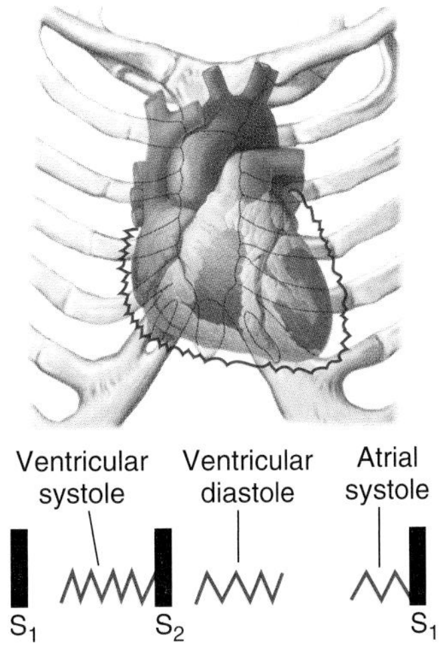

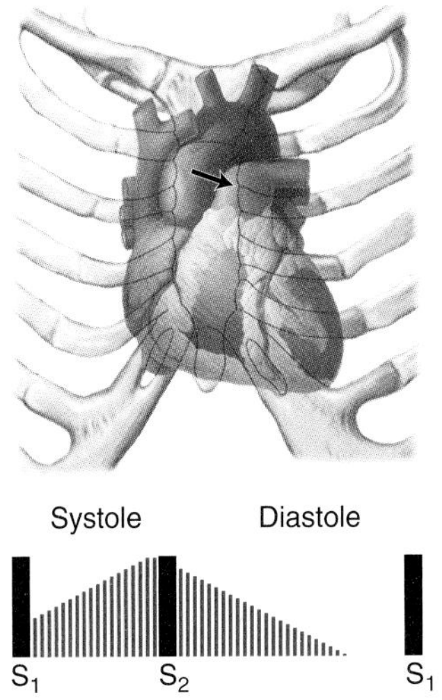

	Venous Hum	Pericardial Friction Rub	Patent Ductus Arteriosus
	Systole, Diastole; S_1 S_2 S_1	Ventricular systole, Ventricular diastole, Atrial systole; S_1 S_2 S_1	Systole, Diastole; S_1 S_2 S_1
Timing	Continuous murmur without a silent interval. Loudest in diastole	May have three short components, each associated with friction from cardiac movement in the pericardial sac: (1) atrial systole, (2) ventricular systole, and (3) ventricular diastole. Usually the first two components are present; all three make diagnosis easy; only one (usually the systolic) invites confusion with a murmur.	Continuous murmur in both systole and diastole, often with a silent interval late in diastole. Loudest in late systole, obscures S_2, and fades in diastole
Location	Above the medial third of the clavicles, especially on the right	Variable, but usually heard best in the 3rd interspace to the left of the sternum	Left 2nd interspace
Radiation	1st and 2nd interspaces	Little	Toward the left clavicle
Intensity	Soft to moderate. Can be obliterated by pressure on the jugular veins	Variable. May increase when the patient leans forward, exhales, and holds breath (in contrast to pleural rub)	Usually loud, sometimes associated with a thrill
Quality	Humming, roaring	Scratchy, scraping	Harsh, machinery-like
Pitch	Low (heard better with a bell)	High (heard better with a diaphragm)	Medium

CHAPTER 9

The Breasts and Axillae

ANATOMY AND PHYSIOLOGY

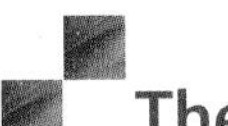

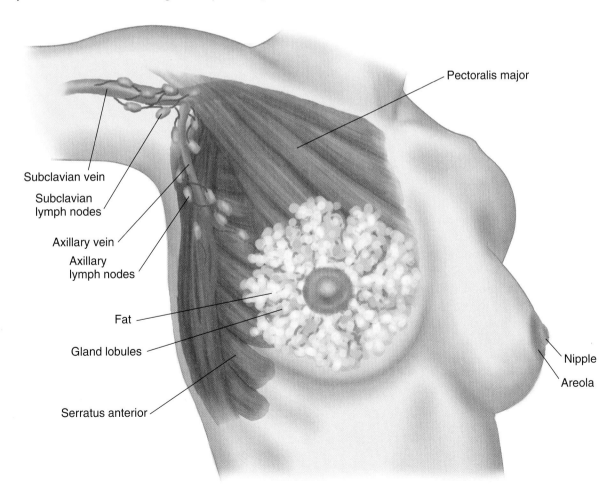

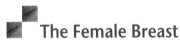

The Female Breast

The female breast lies against the anterior thoracic wall, extending from the clavicle and 2nd rib down to the 6th rib, and from the sternum across to the midaxillary line. Its surface area is generally rectangular rather than round.

The breast overlies the pectoralis major and at its inferior margin, the serratus anterior.

To describe clinical findings, the breast is often divided into four quadrants based on horizontal and vertical lines crossing at the nipple. An axillary tail of breast tissue extends toward the anterior axillary fold. Alternatively, findings can be localized as the time on the face of a clock (e.g., 3 o'clock) and the distance in centimeters from the nipple.

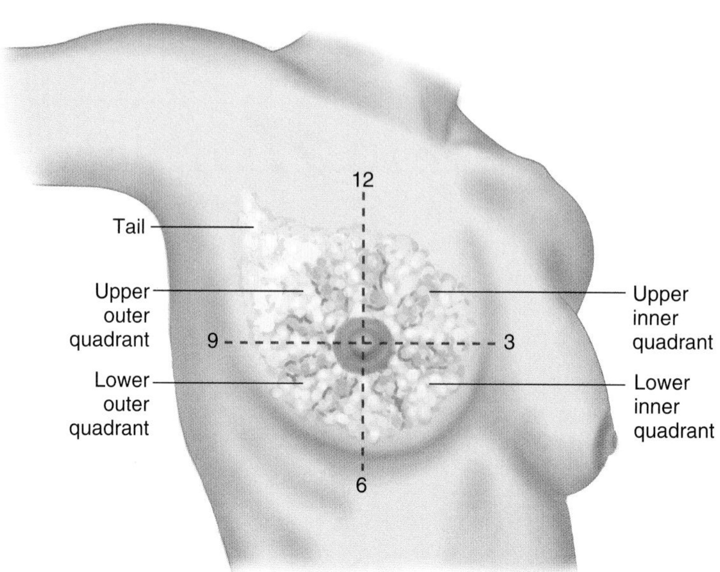

The breast is hormonally sensitive tissue, responsive to the changes of monthly cycling and aging. *Glandular tissue,* namely secretory tubuloalveolar glands and ducts, forms 15 to 20 septated *lobes* radiating around the nipple. Within each lobe are many smaller *lobules.* These drain into milk-producing ducts and sinuses that open onto the surface of the *areola,* or nipple. *Fibrous connective tissue* provides structural support in the form of fibrous bands or suspensory ligaments connected to both the skin and the underlying fascia. *Adipose tissue,* or fat, surrounds the breast, predominantly in the superficial and peripheral areas. The proportions of these components vary with age, the general state of nutrition, pregnancy, exogenous hormone use, and other factors.

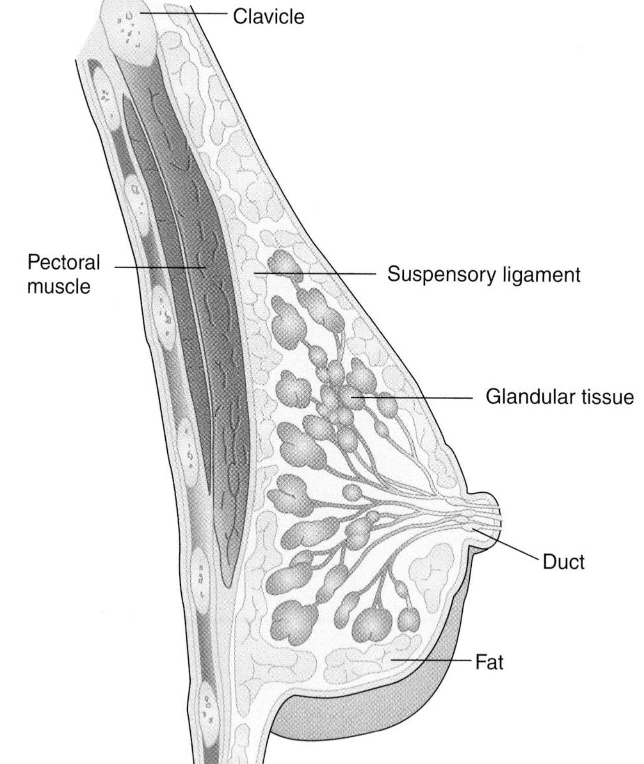

The surface of the areola has small, rounded elevations formed by sebaceous glands, sweat glands, and accessory areolar glands. A few hairs are often seen on the areola.

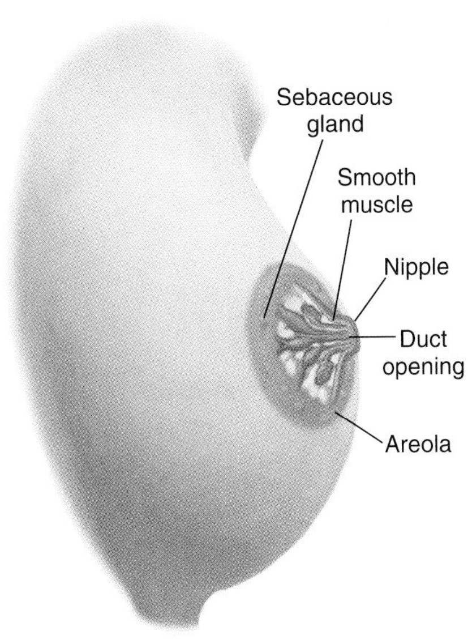

Both the nipple and the areola are well supplied with smooth muscle that contracts to express milk from the ductal system during breast-feeding. Rich sensory innervation, especially in the nipple, triggers "milk letdown" following neurohormonal stimulation from infant sucking. Tactile stimulation of the area, including the breast examination, makes the nipple smaller, firmer, and more erect, whereas the areola puckers and wrinkles. These smooth muscle reflexes are normal and should not be mistaken for signs of breast disease.

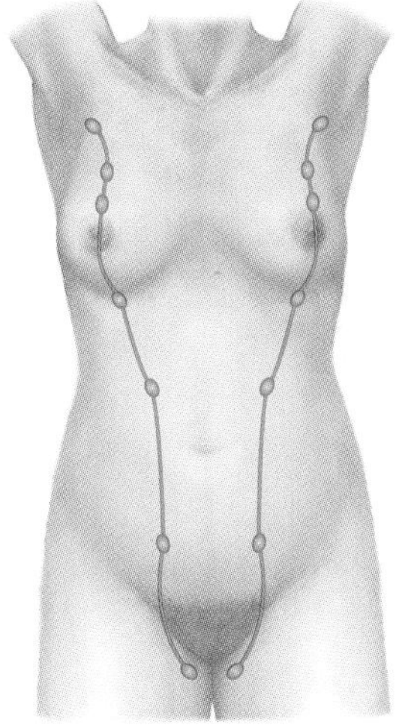

The adult breast may be soft, but it often feels granular, nodular, or lumpy. This uneven texture is normal and may be termed *physiologic nodularity.* It is often bilateral. It may be evident throughout the breast or only in parts of it. The nodularity may increase before menses—a time when breasts often enlarge and become tender or even painful. For breast changes during adolescence and pregnancy, see pp. 778–779 and p. 818.

Occasionally, one or more extra or supernumerary nipples are located along the "milk line," illustrated on the right. Only a small nipple and areola are usually present, often mistaken for a common mole. There may be underlying glandular tissue. An extra nipple has no pathologic significance.

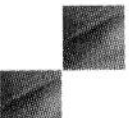

THE MALE BREAST

The *male breast* consists chiefly of a small nipple and areola. These overlie a thin disc of undeveloped breast tissue that may not be distinguishable clinically from the surrounding tissues. A firm button of breast tissue 2 cm or more in diameter has been described in roughly one of three adult men. The limits of normal have not yet been clearly established.

LYMPHATICS

Lymphatics from most of the breast drain toward the axilla. Of the axillary lymph nodes, the *central nodes* are palpable most frequently. They lie along the chest wall, usually high in the axilla and midway between the anterior and posterior axillary folds. Into them drain channels from three other groups of lymph nodes, which are seldom palpable:

- *Pectoral nodes—anterior,* located along the lower border of the pectoralis major inside the anterior axillary fold. These nodes drain the anterior chest wall and much of the breast.
- *Subscapular nodes—posterior,* located along the lateral border of the scapula; palpated deep in the posterior axillary fold. They drain the posterior chest wall and a portion of the arm.
- *Lateral nodes*—located *along the upper humerus.* They drain most of the arm.

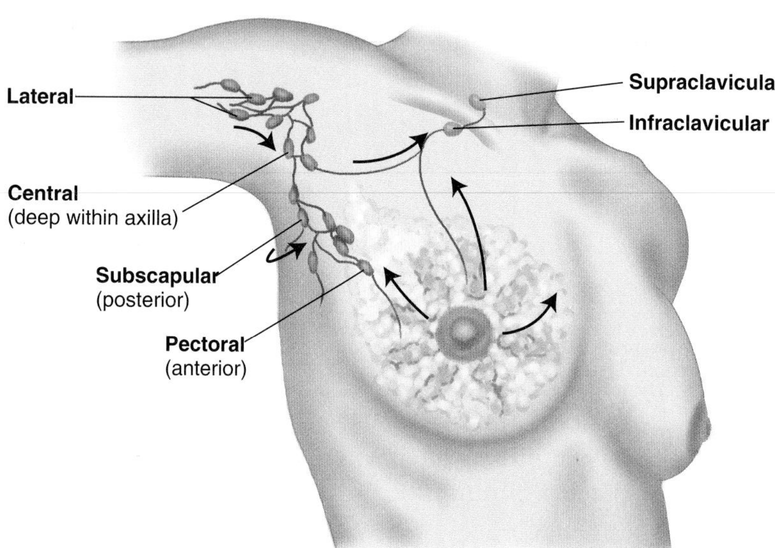

ARROWS INDICATE DIRECTION OF LYMPH FLOW

Lymph drains from the central axillary nodes to the *infraclavicular* and *supraclavicular* nodes.

Not all the lymphatics of the breast drain into the axilla. Malignant cells from a breast cancer may spread directly to the infraclavicular nodes or into deep channels within the chest.

THE HEALTH HISTORY

Common or Concerning Symptoms

- Breast lump or mass
- Breast pain or discomfort
- Nipple discharge

Questions about a woman's breasts may be included in the history or deferred to the physical examination. Ask "Do you examine your breasts?" . . . "How often?" In a menstruating woman, ask when she examines the breast during the monthly cycle: self-examination is best done when estrogen stimulation is lowest, approximately 5 to 7 days after onset of menses. Ask whether she has any *discomfort, pain,* or *lumps* in her breasts. About 50% of women have palpable lumps or nodularity, and premenstrual enlargement and tenderness are common. If your patient reports a lump or mass, ask about the precise location, how long it has been present, and any change in size or variation with the menstrual cycle.

Lumps may be physiologic or pathologic, ranging from cysts and fibroadenomas to breast cancer. See Table 9-1, Visible Signs of Breast Cancer (p. 356), and Table 9-2, Common Breast Masses, (p. 357).

Also ask about any *discharge from the nipples* and when it occurs. If it appears only after squeezing the nipple, it is considered physiologic. If the discharge is spontaneous and seen on the underwear or nightclothes without local stimulation, ask about its color, consistency, and quantity. Is it unilateral or bilateral?

A milky bilateral discharge, or *galactorrhea,* may reflect pregnancy or prolactin or other hormonal imbalance.

Spontaneous persistent nonlactational discharge that is bloody or unilateral suggests local breast disease from *papilloma* or, rarely, possible *breast cancer.*

HEALTH PROMOTION AND COUNSELING

Important Topics for Health Promotion and Counseling

- Risk factors for breast cancer
- Breast cancer screening
- Breast self-examination (BSE)

Women may experience a wide range of changes in breast tissue and sensation, from cyclic swelling and nodularity to a distinct lump or mass. The examination of the breast provides a meaningful opportunity for the clinician and the female patient to explore concerns important to women's health—what to do if a lump or mass is detected, risk factors for breast cancer, and screening measures such as breast self-examination, the clinical breast examination (CBE) by a skilled clinician, and mammography.

Breast masses show marked variation in etiology, from fibroadenomas and cysts seen in younger women, to abscess or mastitis, to primary breast cancer. All breast masses warrant careful evaluation. On initial assessment, the woman's age and physical characteristics of the mass provide clues to its origin, but definitive diagnostic measures should be pursued.

■ *Palpable Masses of the Breast*

Age	Common Lesion	Characteristics
15–25	Fibroadenoma	Usually fine, round, mobile, nontender
25–50	Cysts	Usually soft to firm, round, mobile; often tender
	Fibrocystic changes	Nodular, ropelike
	Cancer	Irregular, stellate, firm, not clearly delineated from surrounding tissue
Over 50	Cancer until proven otherwise	As above
Pregnancy/lactation	Lactating adenomas, cysts, mastitis, and cancer	As above

Adapted from Schultz MZ, Ward BA, Reiss M. Breast diseases. In Noble J, Greene HL, Levinson W, et al. (eds). Primary Care Medicine, 2nd ed. St. Louis, Mosby, 1996. See also Venet L, Strax P, Venet W, et al. Adequacies and inadequacies of breast examinations by physicians in mass screenings. Cancer 28(6):1546–1551, 1971.

Risk Factors for Breast Cancer. Breast cancer is the most common cause of cancer in women worldwide, accounting for more than 10% of all female malignancies. In the United States, a woman born now has a 13% lifetime risk for developing breast cancer. The probability of diagnosis increases by decade: from age 30 to 40, ≤0.5%; from age 40 to 50, 1.49%; from age 50 to 60, 2.79%; and from age 60 to 70, 3.38%.[1] Breast cancer is the second leading cause of cancer death in women, with highest mortality rates in women younger than 35 and older than 75. Mortality rates have declined for white women younger than 55, probably as a result of more widespread use of mammography and more aggressive treatment regimens, but have increased for African American women.[2]

Women with *breast symptoms* merit active investigation. Breast cancer may occur in up to 4% of women with breast complaints and in up to 11% of women complaining specifically of a breast lump or mass.[3] Also pursue complaints of nipple discharge. Although most nipple discharge is benign, approximately 5% of women may have associated breast cancer, especially in older age groups.[4]

Rarely, men report concerns about a breast mass. Breast cancer in men is ≤1% of all breast cancers and is usually diagnosed between the ages of 60 and 70. Risk factors include estrogen exposure, including excess estrogen stimulation in Klinefelter's syndrome or cirrhosis; radiation exposure; and positive family history in female relatives.

For *screening of asymptomatic women,* target risk factors, including family history. Risk factors for breast cancer are present in up to 55% of cases, and a positive family history is present in an additional 10%.[2] The clinician and individual patient should review age and demographic data, family history, reproductive history, and any prior history of proliferative breast disease, especially if a biopsy has shown atypical hyperplasia or lobular carcinoma in situ. Several models help establish the woman patient's risk of breast cancer. The Breast Cancer Risk Assessment Tool of the National Cancer Institute (http://bcra.nci.nih.gov/brc/) and the Gail model are among the most widely used.[5,6]

■ *Summary of Breast Cancer Risk Factors*

Factor	Relative Risk (%)
Family History	
First-degree relative with breast cancer	1.2–3.0
Premenopausal	3.1
Premenopausal and bilateral	8.5–9.0
Postmenopausal	1.5
Postmenopausal and bilateral	4.0–5.4
BRCA1/BRCA2 genes	3.0–7.0
Menstrual History	
Age at menarche <12	1.3
Age at menopause >55	1.5–2.0
Pregnancy	
First live birth from ages 25–29	1.5
First live birth after age 30	1.9
First live birth after age 35	2.0–3.0
Nulliparous	3.0
Breast Conditions and Diseases	
Nonproliferative disease	1.0
Proliferative disease	1.9
Proliferative with atypical hyperplasia	4.4
Lobular carcinoma in situ	6.9–12.0
Breast density on mammography	1.8–6.0

Adapted from Bilmoria MM, Morrow M. The woman at increased risk for breast cancer: evaluation and management strategies. CA Cancer J Clin 45(5):263, 1995, and from Clemons M, Goss P. Estrogen and the risk of breast cancer. N Engl J Med 344(4):276–285, 2001.

Demographic Factors—Age, Education and Income, Location, Ethnicity.[2] Currently, the cumulative lifetime risk for breast cancer is approximately one in seven, and approximately one in nine for invasive breast cancer, reflecting earlier diagnosis of in situ cancers on mammography. More than three fourths of breast cancer cases occur in women older than age 50, and more than half in women older than age 65. Higher education and income levels appear to double the risk for breast cancer, possibly because of differences in age at first birth and parity. Risk is highest in urban areas and varies by region (highest in Hawaii and lowest in Utah) and ethnicity. Rates are highest among Caucasian women, then fall successively for African Americans, Latinas, and Asian Americans.

Family History. The relative risk for breast cancer, or risk relative to an individual without a given risk factor, associated with menarche and menopause, age of first pregnancy, and breast conditions and diseases is summarized in the table above. Risk for familial breast cancer falls into two patterns: family history of breast cancer and genetic predisposition. First-degree relatives, namely a mother or sister with breast cancer, establish a "positive family history." Within this group, menopausal status and extent of disease play key roles. Having a first-degree relative with breast cancer who is premenopausal confers highest risk. Even when a mother or sister has bilateral breast cancer, however, the probability of breast cancer is only 25%.[7]

Inherited disease in women carrying the breast cancer susceptibility genes *BRCA1* and *BRCA2* accounts for 5% to 10% of breast cancers.[8] These genes are autosomal dominant, and, when present, risk for cancer is 50% in women younger than age 50 and 80% in women older than age 65. Red flags for these mutations include multiple relatives with breast cancer, ovarian cancer, or both; a woman with more than one primary cancer (e.g., bilateral disease or combined breast and ovarian); and vertical transmission through two or more generations.

Menstrual History and Pregnancy. Early menarche, delayed menopause, and first live birth after age 35 each raise the risk for breast cancer twofold to threefold. These factors, especially when combined, relate to duration of breast tissue exposure to stimulation from unopposed estrogen.[9]

Breast Conditions and Diseases. Benign breast disease with biopsy findings of atypical hyperplasia or lobular carcinoma in situ carries significantly increased relative risks—4.4 and 6.9 to 12.0, respectively.

Breast Cancer Screening. Although not validated as a method for detecting breast cancer, recent guidelines support *breast self-examination* (BSE) as a means of promoting health awareness. Women choosing to do BSE should be instructed about technique and encouraged to report any new breast symptoms. For women at average risk for breast cancer, the American Cancer Society recommends *clinical breast examination* (CBE) by a health professional every 3 years for women between ages 20 and 39 then annually after age 40 and annual *mammography* beginning at age 40.[10, 11] Intervals for mammography between ages 40 and 50, however, are still subject to controversy. Mammography is less accurate in breasts that are glandular and dense, especially when stimulated by higher estrogen levels before menopause, contributing to varying estimates of benefit. For women at increased risk, many clinicians advise initiating screening mammograms between ages 30 and 40, then every 2 to 3 years until age 50. For women between the ages of 50 and 69, annual CBE and mammography are widely recommended.[7]

After age 70, the benefits of mammography are less well defined. The American Geriatrics Society recommends mammography every 1 to 3 years after age 75 for women with a life expectancy of 4 years or more, particularly in the presence of risk factors or long-term exposure to hormone replacement therapy. If comorbid conditions limit life expectancy, including dementia, clinicians should discuss the decision of mammography with the patient and her family because the benefit of screening will be reduced.[12]

TECHNIQUES OF EXAMINATION

THE FEMALE BREAST

The clinical breast examination is an important component of women's health care: it enhances detection of breast cancers that mammography may miss and provides an opportunity to demonstrate techniques for self-examination to the patient. Clinical investigation has shown, however, that variations in examiner experience and technique affect the value of the clinical breast examination. Clinicians are advised to adopt a more standardized approach, especially for palpation, and to use a systemic and thorough search pattern, varying palpation pressure, and a circular motion with the fingerpads.[13] These techniques will be discussed in more detail in the following pages. Inspection is routinely recommended, but its value in breast cancer detection is less well studied.

Risk factors for breast cancer include previous breast cancer, an affected mother or sister, biopsy showing atypical hyperplasia, increasing age, early menarche, late menopause, late or no pregnancies, and previous radiation to the chest wall.

As you begin the examination of the breasts, be aware that women and girls may feel apprehensive. Be reassuring and adopt a courteous and gentle approach. Before you begin, let the patient know that you are about to examine her breasts. This may be a good time to ask if she has noticed any lumps or other problems and if she performs a monthly breast self-examination. If she does not, teach her good technique and watch as she repeats the steps of examination after you, giving helpful correction as needed.

See Patient Instructions for the Breast Self-Examination, p. 353.

An adequate inspection requires full exposure of the chest, but later in the examination, cover one breast while you are palpating the other. Because breasts tend to swell and become more nodular before menses as a result of increasing estrogen stimulation, the best time for examination is 5 to 7 days *after* the onset of menstruation. Nodules appearing during the premenstrual phase should be reevaluated at this later time.

INSPECTION

Inspect the breasts and nipples with the patient in the sitting position and disrobed to the waist. A thorough examination of the breast includes careful inspection for skin changes, symmetry, contours, and retraction in four views—arms at sides, arms over head, arms pressed against hips, and leaning forward. When examining an adolescent girl, assess her breast development according to Tanner's sex maturity ratings described on page 779.

Arms at Sides. Note the clinical features listed below.

- The *appearance of the skin*, including

  Color

  Redness may be from local infection or inflammatory carcinoma.

  Thickening of the skin and unusually prominent pores, which may accompany lymphatic obstruction

  Thickening and prominent pores suggest breast cancer.

- The *size and symmetry of the breasts.* Some difference in the size of the breasts, including the areolae, is common and is usually normal, as shown in the photograph below.

- The *contour of the breasts.* Look for changes such as masses, dimpling, or flattening. Compare one side with the other.

Flattening of the normally convex breast suggests cancer. See Table 9-1, Visible Signs of Breast Cancer (p. 356).

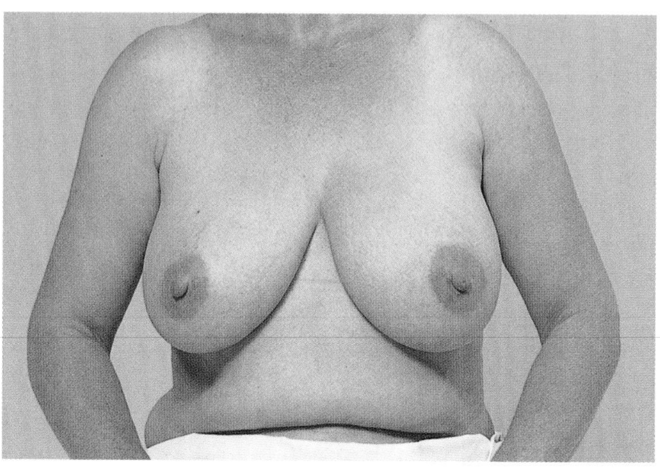

ARMS AT SIDES

- The *characteristics of the nipples,* including *size and shape, direction* in which they point, any *rashes* or *ulceration,* or any *discharge.*

Asymmetry of directions in which nipples point suggests an underlying cancer. Rash or ulceration in Paget's disease of the breast (see p. 356).

Occasionally, the shape of the nipple is *inverted,* or depressed below the areolar surface. It may be enveloped by folds of areolar skin, as illustrated. Long-standing inversion is usually a normal variant of no clinical consequence, except for possible difficulty when breast-feeding.

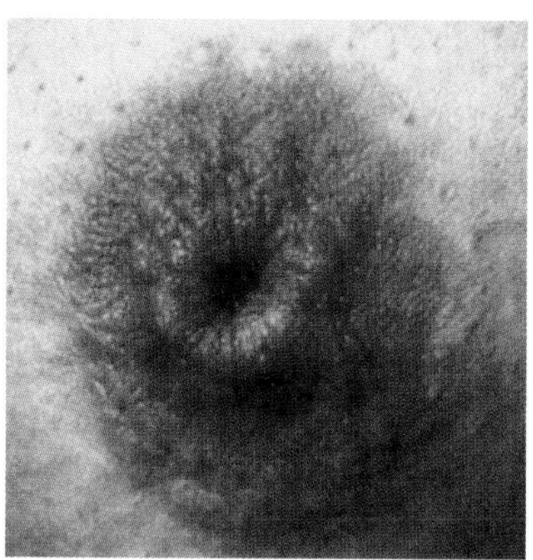

Recent or fixed flattening or depression of the nipple suggests nipple retraction. A retracted nipple may also be broadened and thickened, suggesting an underlying cancer.

Arms Over Head; Hands Pressed Against Hips; Leaning Forward. To bring out dimpling or retraction that may otherwise be invisible, ask the patient to raise her arms over her head, then press her hands against her hips to contract the pectoral muscles. Inspect the breast contours carefully in each position. If the breasts are large or pendulous, it may be useful to have the patient stand and lean forward, supported by the back of the chair or the examiner's hands.

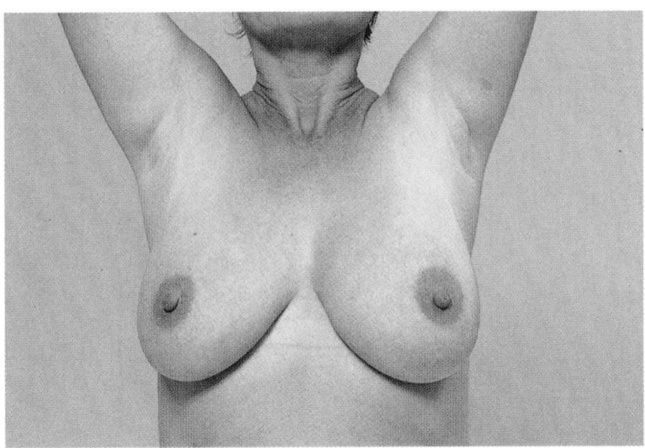

ARMS OVER HEAD

Dimpling or retraction of the breasts in these positions suggests an underlying cancer. When a cancer or its associated fibrous strands are attached to both the skin and the fascia overlying the pectoral muscles, pectoral contraction can draw the skin inward, causing dimpling.

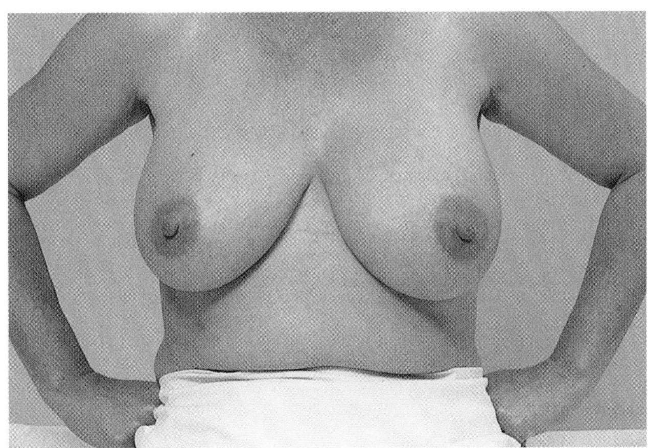

HANDS PRESSED AGAINST HIPS

Occasionally, these signs may be associated with benign lesions such as posttraumatic fat necrosis or mammary duct ectasia, but they must always be further evaluated.

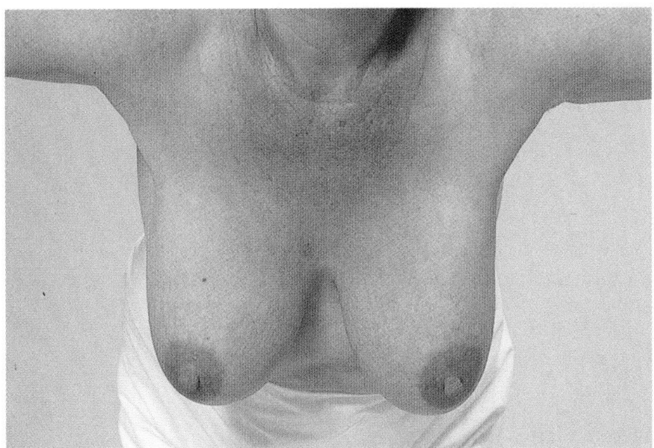

LEANING FORWARD

This position may reveal an asymmetry of the breast or nipple not otherwise visible. Retraction of the nipple and areola suggests an underlying cancer. See Table 9-1, Visible Signs of Breast Cancer (p. 356).

PALPATION

The Breast. Palpation is best performed when the breast tissue is flattened. The patient should be supine. Plan to palpate a rectangular area extending from the clavicle to the inframammary fold or bra line, and from the midsternal line to the posterior axillary line and well into the axilla for the tail of the breast.

A thorough examination will take 3 minutes for each breast. Use the *fingerpads* of the 2nd, 3rd, and 4th fingers, keeping the fingers slightly flexed. It is important to be *systematic*. Although a circular or wedge pattern can be used, the *vertical strip pattern* is currently the best validated technique for detecting breast masses. Palpate in *small, concentric circles* at each examining point, if possible applying light, medium, and deep pressure. You will need to press more firmly to reach the deeper tissues of a large breast. Your examination should cover the entire breast, including the periphery, tail, and axilla.

When pressing deeply on the breast, you may mistake a normal rib for a hard breast mass.

- To examine *the lateral portion of the breast,* ask the patient to roll onto the opposite hip, placing her hand on her forehead but keeping the shoulders pressed against the bed or examining table. This flattens the lateral breast tissue. Begin palpation in the axilla, moving in a straight line down to the bra line, then move the fingers medially and palpate in a vertical strip up the chest to the clavicle. Continue in vertical overlapping strips until you reach the nipple, then reposition the patient to flatten the medial portion of the breast.

Nodules in the tail of the breast are sometimes mistaken for enlarged axillary lymph nodes (and vice versa).

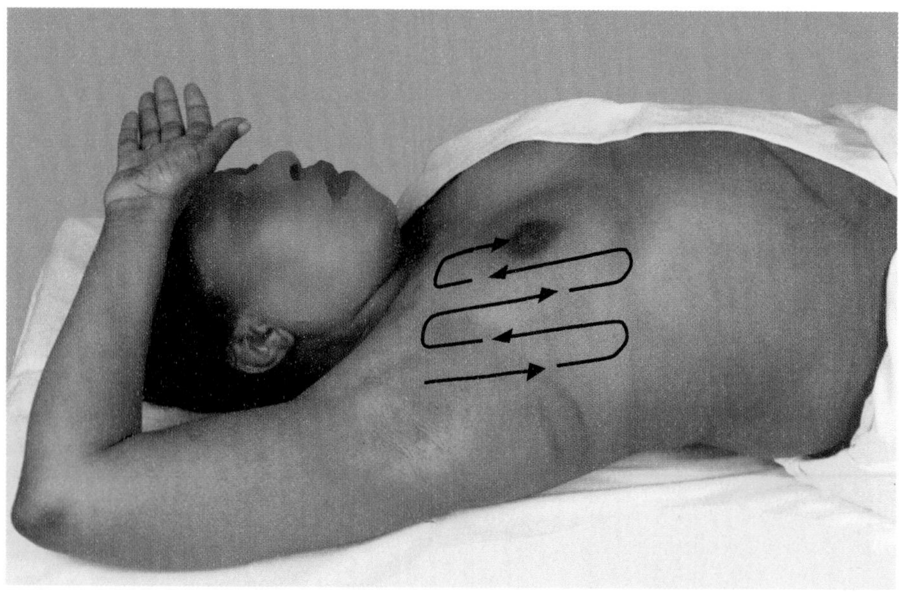

- To examine *the medial portion of the breast,* ask the patient to lie with her shoulders flat against the bed or examining table, placing her hand at her neck and lifting up her elbow until it is even with her shoulder. Palpate in a straight line down from the nipple to the bra line, then back to the clavicle, continuing in vertical overlapping strips to the midsternum.

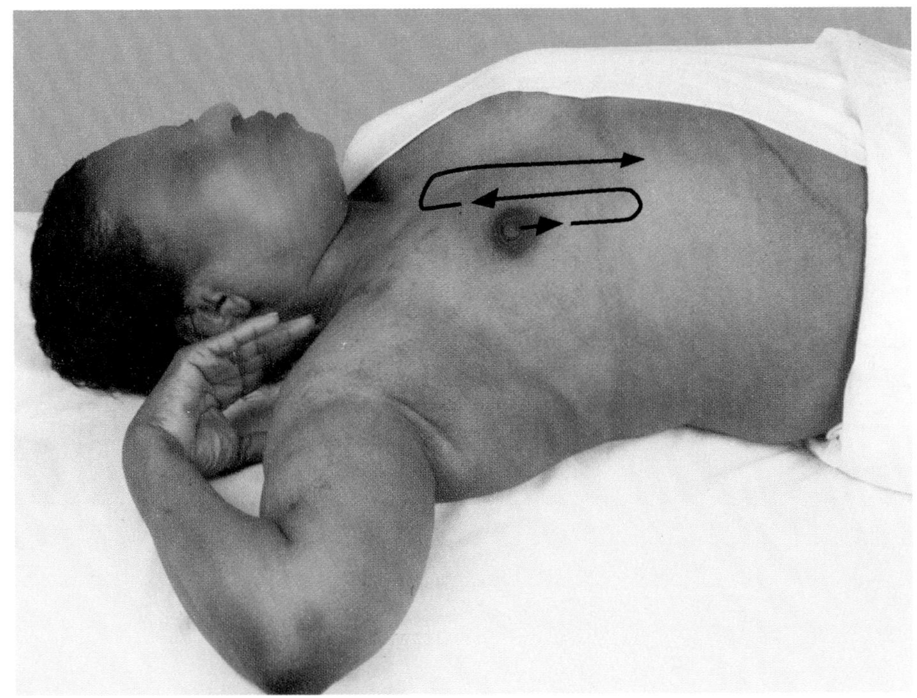

Examine the breast tissue carefully for:

- *Consistency* of the tissues. Normal consistency varies widely, depending in part on the relative proportions of firmer glandular tissue and soft fat. Physiologic nodularity may be present, increasing before menses. There may be a firm transverse ridge of compressed tissue along the lower margin of the breast, especially in large breasts. This is the normal inframammary ridge, not a tumor.

Tender cords suggest *mammary duct ectasia,* a benign but sometimes painful condition of dilated ducts with surrounding inflammation, sometimes with associated masses.

- *Tenderness,* as in premenstrual fullness
- *Nodules.* Palpate carefully for any lump or mass that is qualitatively different from or larger than the rest of the breast tissue. This is sometimes called a dominant mass and may reflect a pathologic change that requires evaluation by mammogram, aspiration, or biopsy. Assess and describe the characteristics of any nodule:

See Table 9-2, Common Breast Masses (p. 357).

Location—by quadrant or clock, with centimeters from the nipple

Size—in centimeters

Shape—round or cystic, disclike, or irregular in contour

Consistency—soft, firm, or hard

Delimitation—well circumscribed or not

Hard, irregular, poorly circumscribed nodules, fixed to the skin or underlying tissues, strongly suggest cancer.

Tenderness

Cysts, inflamed areas; some cancers may be tender.

Mobility—in relation to the skin, pectoral fascia, and chest wall. Gently move the breast near the mass and watch for dimpling.

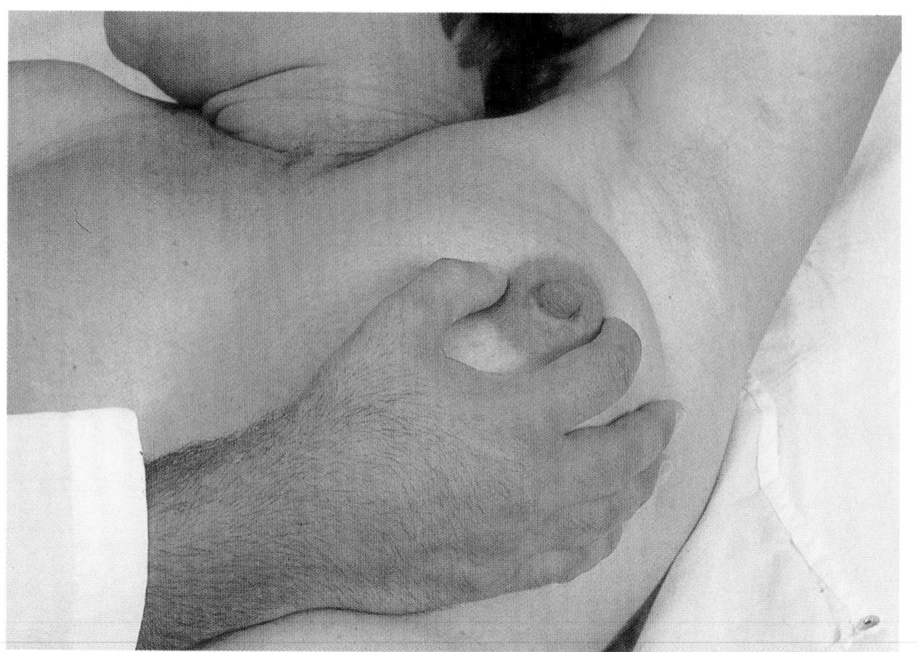

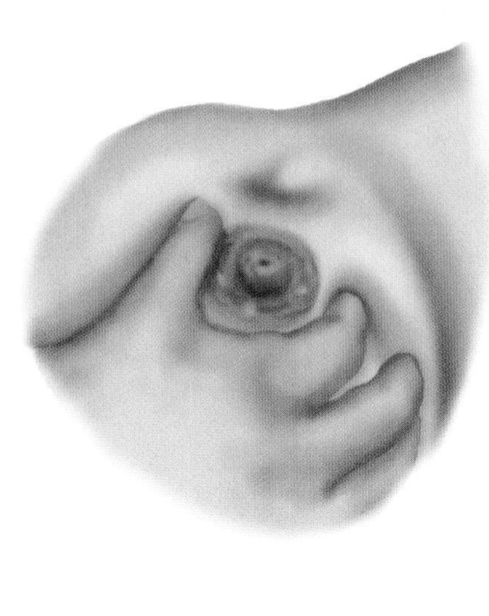

Next, try to move the mass itself while the patient relaxes her arm and then while she presses her hand against her hip.

A mobile mass that becomes fixed when the arm relaxes is attached to the ribs and intercostal muscles; if fixed when the hand is pressed against the hip, it is attached to the pectoral fascia.

The Nipple. Palpate each nipple, noting its elasticity.

Thickening of the nipple and loss of elasticity suggest an underlying cancer.

THE MALE BREAST

Examination of the male breast may be brief but is important. *Inspect the nipple and areola* for nodules, swelling, or ulceration. *Palpate the areola and breast tissue* for nodules. If the breast appears enlarged, distinguish between the soft fatty enlargement of obesity and the firm disc of glandular enlargement, called *gynecomastia*.

Gynecomastia is attributed to an imbalance of estrogens and androgens, sometimes drug related. A hard, irregular, eccentric, or ulcerating nodule is not gynecomastia and suggests breast cancer.

THE AXILLAE

Although the axillae may be examined with the patient lying down, a sitting position is preferable.

INSPECTION

Inspect the skin of each axilla, noting evidence of:

- Rash

Deodorant and other rashes

- Infection

Sweat gland infection (*hidradenitis suppurativa*)

- Unusual pigmentation

Deeply pigmented, velvety axillary skin suggests *acanthosis nigricans*—one form is associated with internal malignancy.

PALPATION

To examine the left axilla, ask the patient to relax with the left arm down. Help by supporting the left wrist or hand with your left hand. Cup together the fingers of your right hand and reach as high as you can toward the apex of the axilla. Warn the patient that this may feel uncomfortable. Your fingers should lie directly behind the pectoral muscles, pointing toward the midclavicle. Now press your fingers in toward the chest wall and slide them downward, trying to feel the central nodes against the chest wall. Of the axillary nodes, these are the most often palpable. One or more soft, small (<1 cm), nontender nodes are frequently felt.

Enlarged axillary nodes from infection of the hand or arm, recent immunizations or skin tests in the arm, or part of a generalized lymphadenopathy. Check the epitrochlear nodes and other groups of lymph nodes.

Nodes that are large (≥1 cm) and firm or hard, matted together, or fixed to the skin or to underlying tissues suggest malignant involvement.

Use your left hand to examine the right axilla.

If the central nodes feel large, hard, or tender, or if there is a suspicious lesion in the drainage areas for the axillary nodes, feel for the other groups of axillary lymph nodes:

- *Pectoral nodes*—grasp the anterior axillary fold between your thumb and fingers, and with your fingers, palpate inside the border of the pectoral muscle.
- *Lateral nodes*—from high in the axilla, feel along the upper humerus.
- *Subscapular nodes*—step behind the patient and, with your fingers, feel inside the muscle of the posterior axillary fold.

Also, feel for infraclavicular nodes and reexamine the supraclavicular nodes.

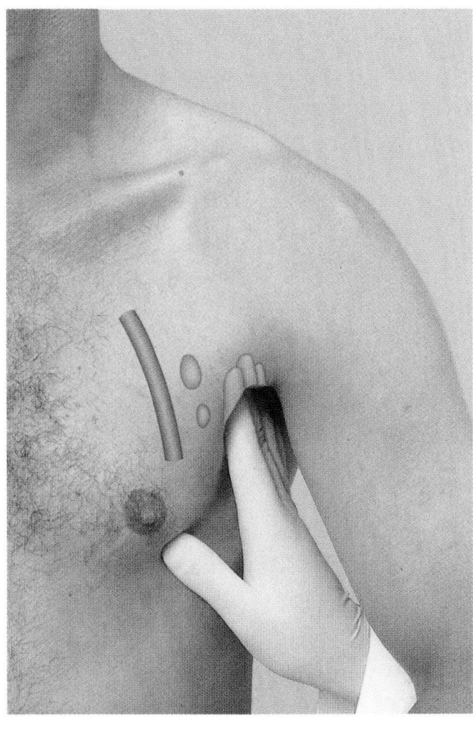

SPECIAL TECHNIQUES

Assessment of Spontaneous Nipple Discharge. If there is a history of spontaneous nipple discharge, try to determine its origin by compressing the areola with your index finger, placed in radial positions around the nipple. Watch for discharge appearing through one of the duct openings on the nipple's surface. Note the color, consistency, and quantity of any discharge and the exact location where it appears.

Milky discharge unrelated to a prior pregnancy and lactation is called *nonpuerperal galactorrhea.* Leading causes are hormonal and pharmacologic.

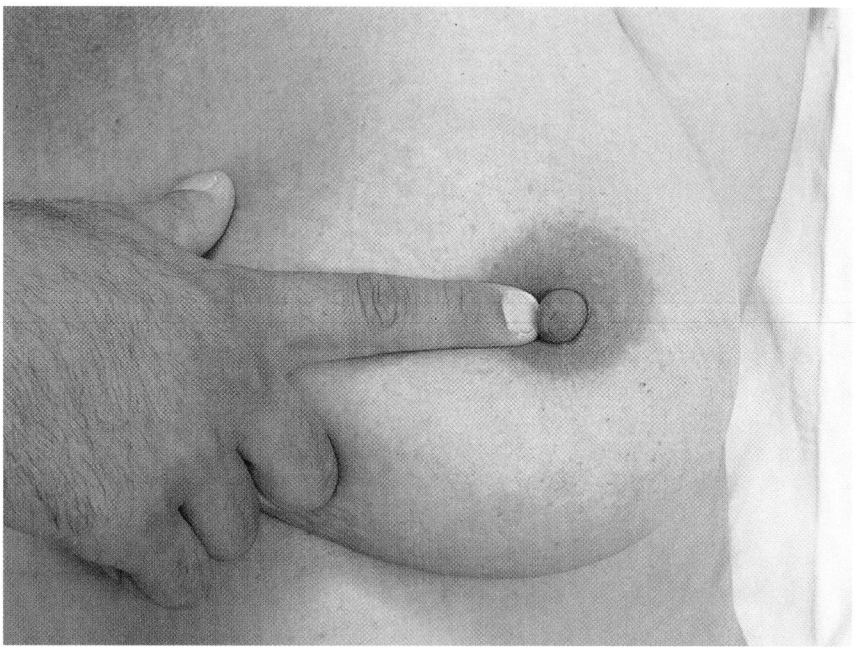

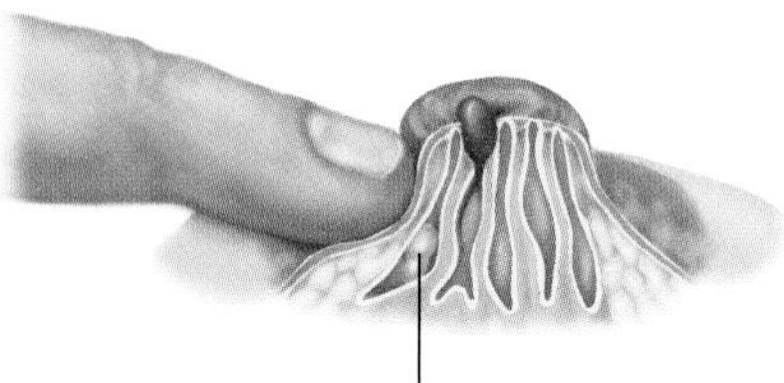

A nonmilky unilateral discharge suggests local breast disease. The causative lesion is usually benign, but may be malignant, especially in elderly women. A benign intraductal papilloma is shown above in its usual subareolar location. Note the drop of blood exuding from a duct opening.

Examination of the Mastectomy Patient. The woman with a mastectomy warrants special care on examination. Inspect the mastectomy scar and axilla carefully for any masses or unusual nodularity. Note any change in color or signs of inflammation. Lymphedema may be present in the axilla and upper arm from impaired lymph drainage after surgery. Palpate gently along the scar—these tissues may be unusually sensitive. Use a circular motion with two or three fingers. Pay special attention to the upper outer quadrant and axilla. Note any enlargement of the lymph nodes or signs of inflammation or infection.

Masses, nodularity, and change in color or inflammation, especially in the incision line, suggest recurrence of breast cancer.

It is especially important to carefully palpate the breast tissue and incision lines of women with breast augmentation or reconstruction.

Instructions for the Breast Self-Examination. The office or hospital visit is an important time to teach the patient how to perform the breast self-examination (BSE). A high proportion of breast masses are detected by women examining their own breasts. Although BSE has not been shown to reduce breast cancer mortality, monthly BSE is inexpensive and may promote stronger health awareness and more active self-care. For early detection of breast cancer, the BSE is most useful when coupled with regular breast examination by an experienced clinician and mammography. The BSE is best timed just after menses, when hormonal stimulation of breast tissue is low.

PATIENT INSTRUCTIONS FOR THE BREAST SELF-EXAMINATION (BSE)

Lying Supine

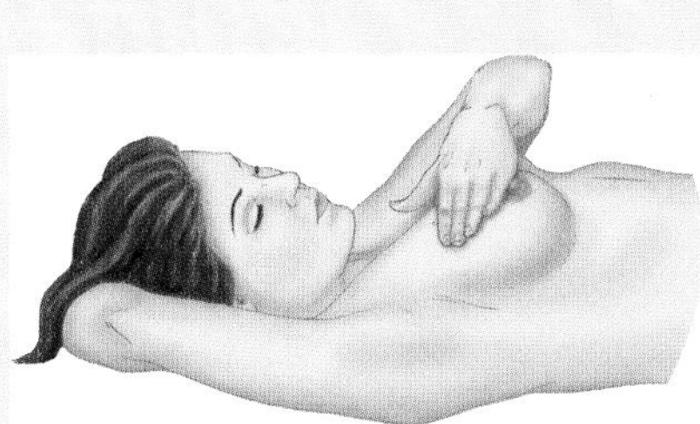

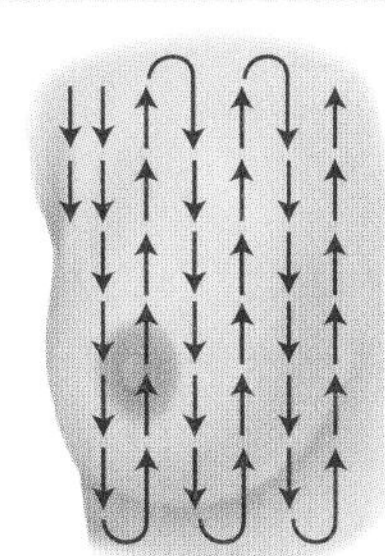

1. Lie down with a pillow under your right shoulder. Place your right arm behind your head.
2. Use the finger pads of the three middle fingers on your left hand to feel for lumps in the right breast. The finger pads are the top third of each finger.
3. Press firmly enough to know how your breast feels. A firm ridge in the lower curve of each breast is normal. If you're not sure how hard to press, talk with your health care provider, or try to copy the way the doctor or nurse does it.
4. Press firmly on the breast in an up-and-down or "strip" pattern. You can also use a circular or wedge pattern, but be sure to use the same pattern every time. Check the entire breast area, and remember how your breast feels from month to month.
5. Repeat the examination on your left breast, using the finger pads of the right hand.
6. If you find any masses, lumps, or skin changes, see your doctor right away.

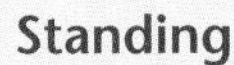

Standing

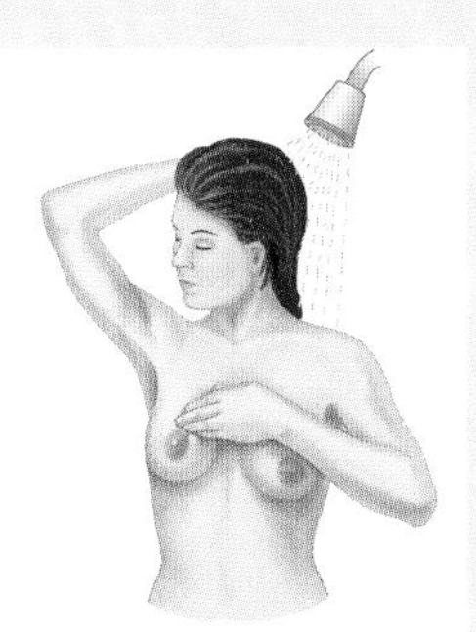

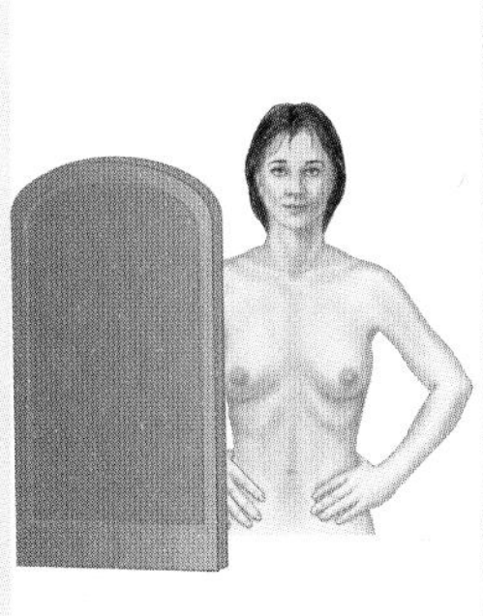

1. Repeat the examination of both breasts while standing, with one arm behind your head. The upright position makes it easier to check the upper outer part of the breasts (toward your armpit). This is where about half of breast cancers are found. You may want to do the upright part of the BSE while you are in the shower. Your soapy hands will make it easy to check how your breasts feel as they glide over the wet skin.
2. For added safety, you might want to check your breasts by standing in front of a mirror right after your BSE each month. See if there are any changes in the way your breasts look, such as dimpling of the skin, changes in the nipple, redness, or swelling.
3. If you find any masses, lumps, or skin changes, see your doctor right away.

Adapted from the American Cancer Society. Available at: www.cancer.org. Accessed November 17, 2004.

RECORDING YOUR FINDINGS

Note that initially you may use sentences to describe your findings; later you will use phrases. The style below contains phrases appropriate for most write-ups.

Recording the Physical Examination—Breasts and Axillae

"Breasts symmetric and without masses. Nipples without discharge." (Axillary adenopathy usually included after Neck in section on Lymph Nodes, see p. 203.)

OR

"Breasts pendulous with diffuse fibrocystic changes. Single firm 1 × 1 cm mass, mobile and nontender, with overlying peau d'orange appearance in right breast, upper outer quadrant at 11 o'clock."

Suggests possible breast cancer

Bibliography

CITATIONS

1. National Cancer Institute. Cancer Facts. Available at: http://cis.nci.nih.gov/fact/5_6.htm. Accessed November 4, 2004.
2. Costanza ME. Epidemiology and risk factors for breast cancer. Available at: www.utdol.com. Accessed November 4, 2004.
3. Barton MB, Elmore JG, Fletcher SW. Breast symptoms among women enrolled in a health maintenance organization: frequency, evaluation, and outcome. Ann Intern Med 130(8): 651–657, 1999.
4. Murad TM, Contesso G, Mouriesse H. Nipple discharge from the breast. Ann Surg 195(3):259–264, 1982.
5. Gail MH, Brinton LA, Byar DP, et al. Projecting individualized probabilities of developing breast cancer for white females who are being examined annually. J Natl Cancer Inst 81: 1879–1886, 1989.
6. Gail MH, Benichou J. Validation studies on a model for breast cancer risk (editorial). J Natl Cancer Inst 86:573–575, 1994.
7. U.S. Preventive Services Task Force. Screening for breast cancer. In: Guide to Clinical Preventive Services, 2nd ed. Baltimore, Williams & Wilkins, 73–87, 1996.
8. Peshkin BN, Isaacs C. Risk assessment in women with an inherited predisposition to cancer. Available at: http://www.utdol.com. Accessed November 4, 2004.
9. Clemons M, Goss P. Estrogen and the risk of breast cancer. N Engl J Med 344(4):276–285, 2001.
10. Smith RA, Saslow D, Sawyer KA, et al. American Cancer Society guidelines for breast cancer screening: update 2003. CA Cancer J Clin 53(3):141–169, 2003.
11. American Cancer Society. How to perform a breast self exam. Available at: www.cancer.org. Accessed November 4, 2004.
12. American Geriatrics Society Clinical Practice Committee. Position statement: breast cancer screening in older women. Available at: http://www.americangeriatrics.org. Accessed November 4, 2004.
13. Barton MB, Harris R, Fletcher S. Does this patient have breast cancer? The screening clinical breast examination: should it be done? How? JAMA 282(13):1270–1280, 1999.

ADDITIONAL REFERENCES

American Geriatrics Society Clinical Practice Committee. Position Statement: Breast Cancer Screening in Older Women. Available at: http://www.americangeriatrics.org. Accessed November 4, 2004.

Bland KI, Vezerdis MP, Copeland EM. Breast (Chapter 16). In Brunicardi FC, Schwartz SI (eds). Schwartz's Principles of Surgery, 8th ed. New York: McGraw-Hill Medical, 2005.

Armstrong K, Eisen A, Weber B. Assessing the risk of breast cancer. N Engl J Med 342(8):564–571, 2000.

Chlebowski RT, Hentrix SL, Langer RD, et al. Influence of estrogen plus progestin on breast cancer and mammography in healthy postmenopausal women: The Women's Health Initiative Randomized Trial. JAMA 289(24):3243–3253, 2003.

Chlebowski RT. Reducing the risk of breast cancer. N Engl J Med 343(3):191–198, 2000.

Fletcher SW, Barton MD. Evaluation of breast lumps. Available at: http://www.utdol.com. Accessed November 4, 2004.

Giordano SH, Cohen DS, Buzdar AU. Breast carcinoma in men: a population-based study. Cancer 101(1):51–57, 2004.

Harris JR, Morrow M, Bonadonna G. Cancer of the breast. In DeVita VT, Hellman S, Rosenberg (eds). Cancer: Principles & Practice of Oncology, 7th ed. Philadelphia, Lippincott Williams & Wilkins, 2004.

BIBLIOGRAPHY

Hollerman DR, Simel DL. Does the clinical examination predict airflow limitation? JAMA 273(4):313–319, 1995.

Kudva YC, Reynolds C, O'Brien TO, et al. "Diabetic mastopathy," or sclerosing lymphocytic lobulitis, is strongly associated with type 1 diabetes. Diabetes Care 25(1):121–126, 2002.

Lannin DR, Mathews HF, Mitchell J, et al. Impacting cultural attitudes in African-American women to decrease breast cancer mortality. Am J Surg 184(5):418–423, 2002.

Mandalblatt J, Saha S, Teusch S, et al. The cost-effectiveness of screening mammography beyond age 65 years: a systematic review for the U.S. Preventive Services Task Force. Ann Intern Med 139(10):835–842, 2003.

U.S. Preventive Services Task Force. Screening for breast cancer: recommendations and rationale. Ann Intern Med 137(5, Part 1): 344–346, 2002.

TABLE 9-1 Visible Signs of Breast Cancer

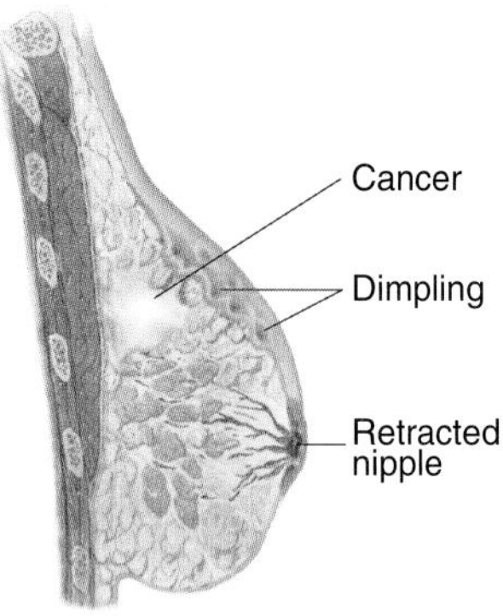

Retraction Signs

As breast cancer advances, it causes fibrosis (scar tissue). Shortening of this tissue produces dimpling, changes in contour, and retraction or deviation of the nipple. Other causes of retraction include fat necrosis and mammary duct ectasia.

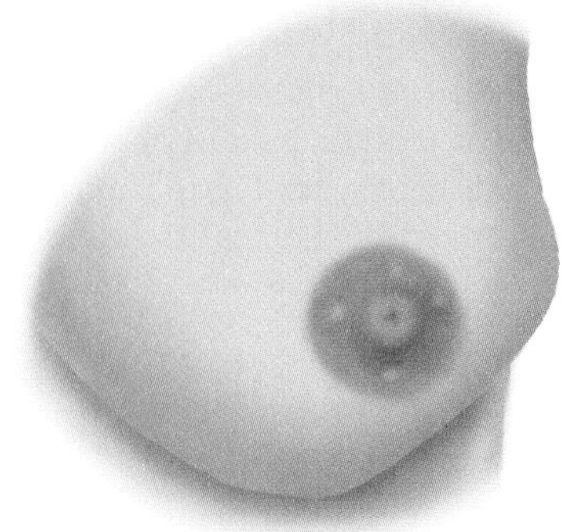

Abnormal Contours

Look for any variation in the normal convexity of each breast, and compare one side with the other. Special positioning may again be useful. Shown here is marked flattening of the lower outer quadrant of the left breast.

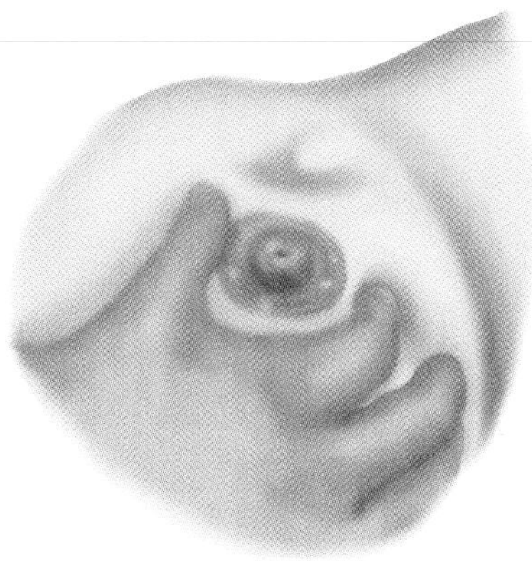

Skin Dimpling

Look for this sign with the patient's arm at rest, during special positioning, and on moving or compressing the breast, as illustrated here.

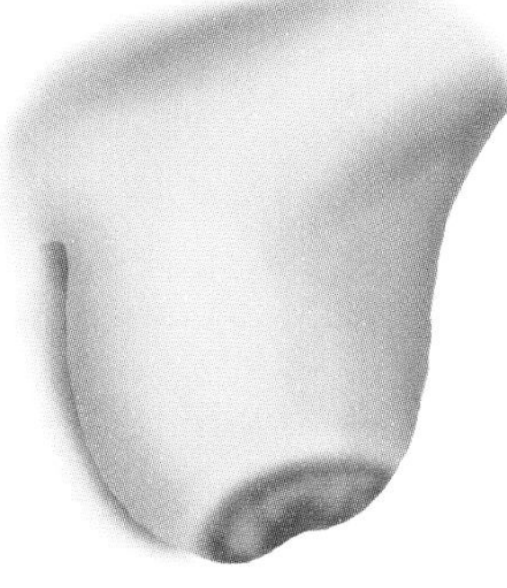

Nipple Retraction and Deviation

A retracted nipple is flattened or pulled inward, as illustrated here. It may also be broadened, and feels thickened. When involvement is radially asymmetric, the nipple may deviate or point in a different direction from its normal counterpart, typically toward the underlying cancer.

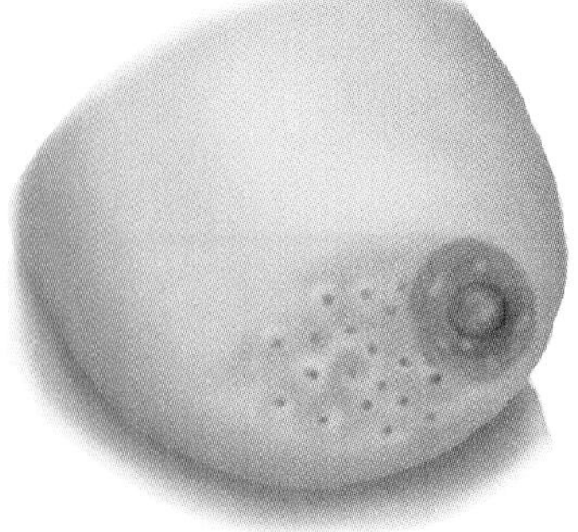

Edema of the Skin

Edema of the skin is produced by lymphatic blockade. It appears as thickened skin with enlarged pores—the so-called *peau d'orange* (orange peel) *sign*. It is often seen first in the lower portion of the breast or areola.

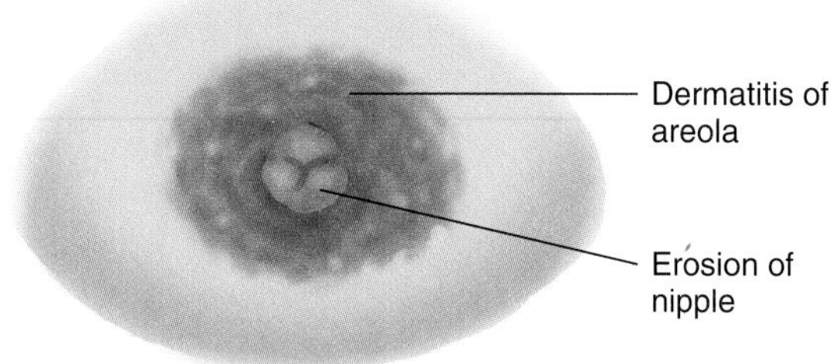

Paget's Disease of the Nipple

This is an uncommon form of breast cancer that usually starts as a scaly, eczemalike lesion. The skin may also weep, crust, or erode. A breast mass may be present. Suspect Paget's disease in any persisting dermatitis of the nipple and areola.

TABLE 9-2 Common Breast Masses

The three most common kinds of breast masses are *fibroadenoma* (a benign tumor), *cysts,* and *breast cancer.* The clinical characteristics of these masses are listed below. However, any breast mass should be carefully evaluated and usually warrants further investigation by ultrasound, aspiration, mammography, or biopsy. The masses depicted below are rather large, for purposes of illustration. Ideally, breast cancer should be identified early, when the mass is small. *Fibrocystic changes,* not illustrated, are also commonly palpable as nodular, ropelike densities in women ages 25–50. They may be tender or painful. They are considered benign and are not viewed as a risk factor for breast cancer.

	Fibroadenoma	Cysts	Cancer
Usual Age	15–25, usually puberty and young adulthood, but up to age 55	30–50, regress after menopause except with estrogen therapy	30–90, most common over 50 in middle-aged and elderly women
Number	Usually single, may be multiple	Single or multiple	Usually single, although may coexist with other nodules
Shape	Round, disclike, or lobular	Round	Irregular or stellate
Consistency	May be soft, usually firm	Soft to firm, usually elastic	Firm or hard
Delimitation	Well delineated	Well delineated	Not clearly delineated from surrounding tissues
Mobility	Very mobile	Mobile	May be fixed to skin or underlying tissues
Tenderness	Usually nontender	Often tender	Usually nontender
Retraction Signs	Absent	Absent	May be present

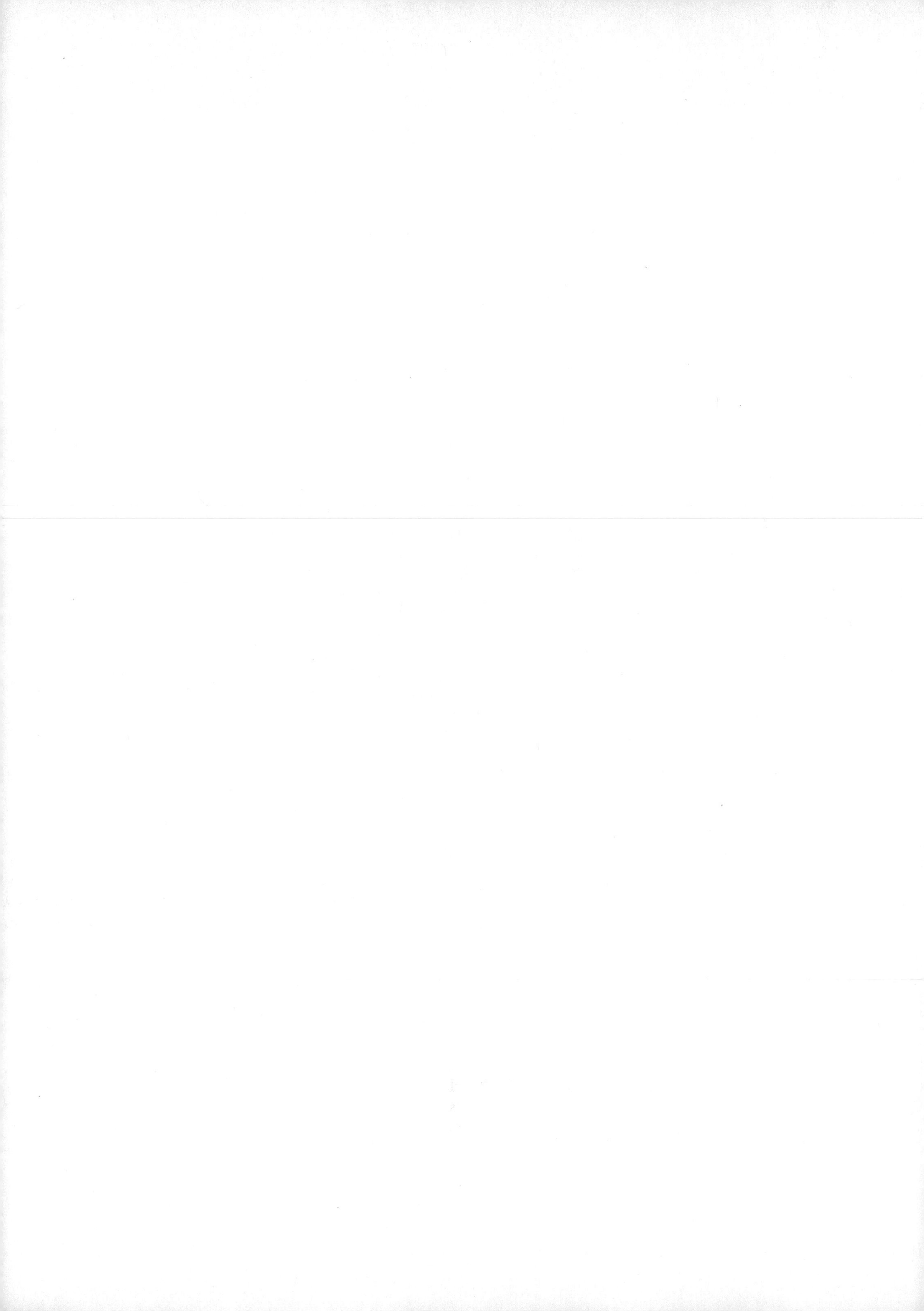

CHAPTER

10

The Abdomen

ANATOMY AND PHYSIOLOGY

Visualize or palpate the landmarks of the abdominal wall and pelvis, as illustrated. The rectus abdominis muscles become more prominent when the patient raises the head and shoulders from the supine position.

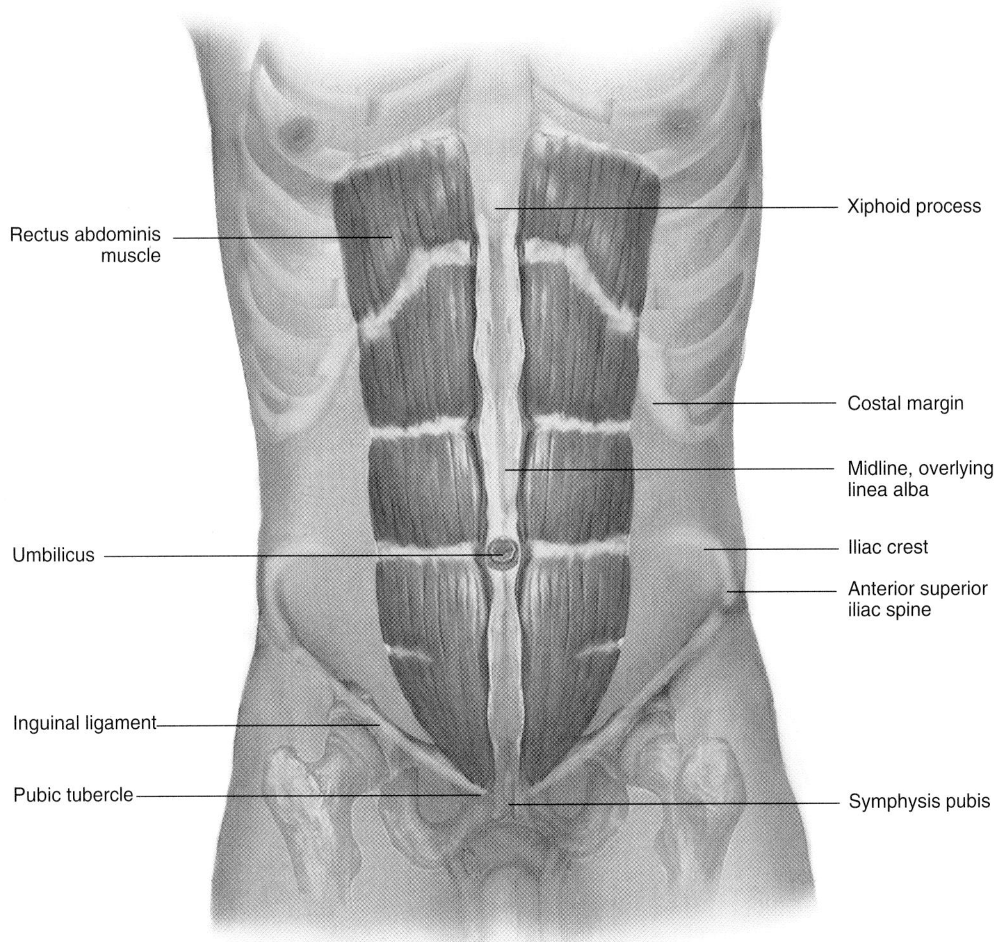

For descriptive purposes, the abdomen is often divided by imaginary lines crossing at the umbilicus, forming the right upper, right lower, left upper, and left lower quadrants. Another system divides the abdomen into nine sections. Terms for three of them are commonly used: epigastric, umbilical, and hypogastric, or suprapubic.

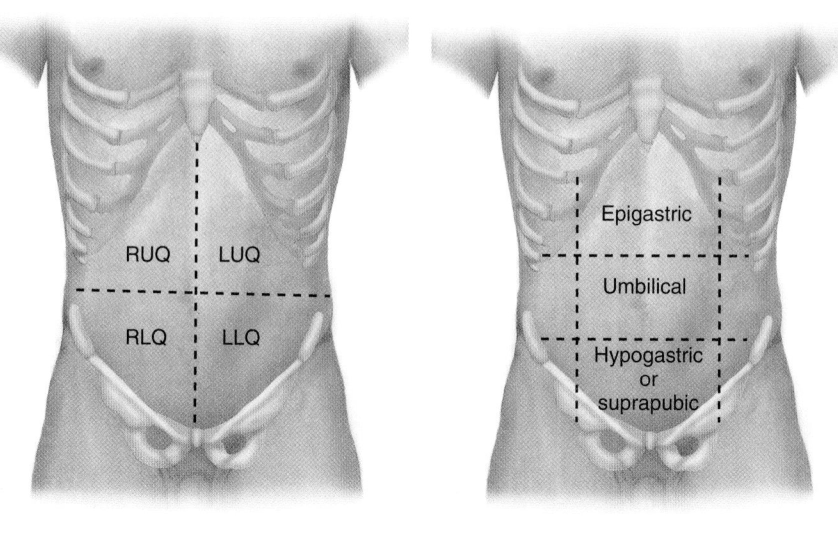

When examining the abdomen, you may be able to feel several normal structures. The sigmoid *colon* is frequently palpable as a firm, narrow tube in the left lower quadrant, whereas the cecum and part of the ascending colon form a softer, wider tube in the right lower quadrant. Portions of the transverse and descending colon may also be palpable. None of these structures should be mistaken for a tumor. Although the normal *liver* often extends down just below the right costal margin, its soft consistency makes it difficult to feel through the abdominal wall. The lower margin of the liver, the liver edge, is often palpable. Also in the right upper quadrant, but usually at a deeper level, lies the lower pole of the right kidney. It is occasionally palpable, especially in thin people with relaxed abdominal muscles. Pulsations of the *abdominal aorta* are frequently visible and usually palpable in the upper abdomen, whereas the pulsations of the *iliac arteries* may sometimes be felt in the lower quadrants.

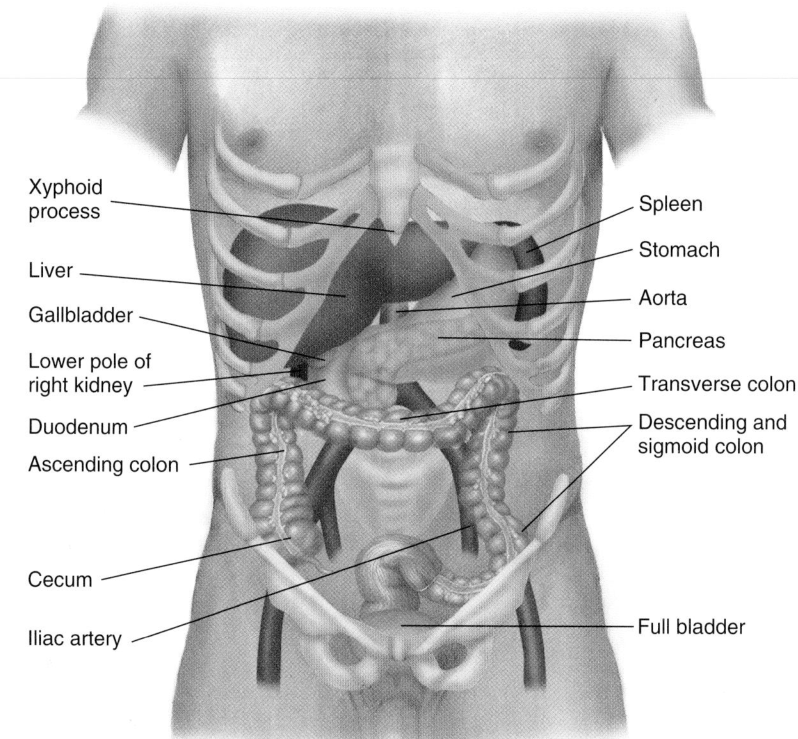

The abdominal cavity extends up under the rib cage to the dome of the diaphragm. In this protected location, beyond the reach of the palpating hand, are much of the liver and *stomach* and all of the usual normal spleen. The *spleen* lies against the diaphragm at the level of the 9th, 10th, and 11th ribs, mostly posterior to the left midaxillary line. It is lateral to and behind the stomach, and just above the left kidney. The tip of a normal spleen is palpable below the left costal margin in a small percentage of adults.

Most of the normal *gallbladder* lies deep to the liver and cannot be distinguished from it clinically. The *duodenum* and *pancreas* lie deep in the upper abdomen, where they are not normally palpable.

A distended *bladder* may be palpable above the symphysis pubis. The bladder accommodates roughly 300 ml of urine filtered by the kidneys into the renal pelvis and the ureters. Bladder expansion stimulates contraction of bladder smooth muscle, the *detrusor muscle,* at relatively low pressures. Rising pressure in the bladder triggers the conscious urge to void.

Increased intraurethral pressure can overcome rising pressures in the bladder and prevent incontinence. Intraurethral pressure is related to such factors as smooth muscle tone in the internal urethral sphincter, the thickness of the urethral mucosa, and in women, sufficient support to the bladder and proximal urethra from pelvic muscles and ligaments to maintain proper anatomical relationships. Striated muscle around the urethra can also contract voluntarily to interrupt voiding.

Neuroregulatory control of the bladder functions at several levels. In infants, the bladder empties by reflex mechanisms in the sacral spinal cord. Voluntary control of the bladder depends on higher centers in the brain and on motor and sensory pathways between the brain and the reflex arcs of the sacral spinal cord. When voiding is inconvenient, higher centers in the brain can inhibit detrusor contractions until the capacity of the bladder, approximately 400 to 500 ml, is exceeded. The integrity of the sacral nerves that innervate the bladder can be tested by assessing perirectal and perineal sensation in the S2, S3, and S4 dermatomes (see p. 606).

Other structures sometimes palpable in the lower abdomen include the *uterus* enlarged by pregnancy or fibroids, which may also rise above the symphysis pubis, and the *sacral promontory,* the anterior edge of the first sacral vertebra. Until you are familiar with this normal structure, you may mistake its stony hard outlines for a tumor. Another stony hard lump that can sometimes mislead you, and may occasionally alarm a patient, is a normal *xiphoid process.*

The *kidneys* are posterior organs. The ribs protect their upper portionss. The *costovertebral angle*—the angle formed by the lower border of the 12th rib and the transverse processes of the upper lumbar vertebrae—defines the region to assess for kidney tenderness.

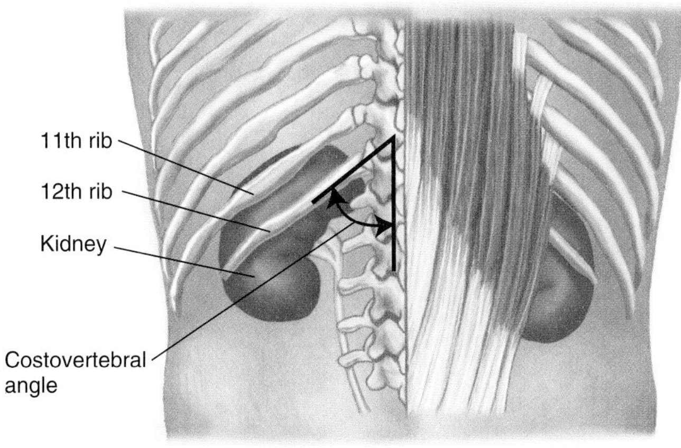

POSTERIOR VIEW

THE HEALTH HISTORY

Common or Concerning Symptoms

Gastrointestinal Disorders
- Indigestion or anorexia
- Nausea, vomiting, or hematemesis
- Abdominal pain
- Dysphagia and/or odynophagia
- Change in bowel function
- Constipation or diarrhea
- Jaundice

Urinary and Renal Disorders
- Suprapubic pain
- Dysuria, urgency, or frequency
- Hesitancy, decreased stream in males
- Polyuria or nocturia
- Urinary incontinence
- Hematuria
- Kidney or flank pain
- Ureteral colic

You will encounter a wide variety of gastrointestinal and urinary complaints in clinical practice. Careful interviewing will often lead you to the underlying disorder. This section addresses such gastrointestinal concerns as *indigestion, anorexia, nausea* or *vomiting, hematemesis, abdominal pain, dysphagia* or *odynophagia, change in bowel function, constipation* and *diarrhea*, and *jaundice*. There is also health history information on disorders of the urinary tract, including complaints of *suprapubic pain, dysuria, urgency, frequency, hesitancy* or *decreased stream* in males, *polyuria, nocturia, incontinence, hematuria, kidney pain,* and *ureteral colic.*

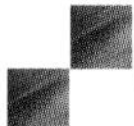

THE GASTROINTESTINAL TRACT

Indigestion, Anorexia, Nausea, Vomiting, Hematemesis. "How is your *appetite*?" is a good starting question and may lead into other important areas such as *indigestion, nausea, vomiting,* and *anorexia*. Patients often complain of *indigestion,* a common complaint that refers to distress associated with eating, but patients use the term for many different symptoms. Find out just what your patient means.

Anorexia, nausea, vomiting in many gastrointestinal disorders; also in pregnancy, diabetic ketoacidosis, adrenal insufficiency, hypercalcemia, uremia, liver disease, emotional states, adverse drug reactions, and other conditions. Induced but without nausea in anorexia/bulimia.

Possible causes include the following:

- *Heartburn*, or a sense of burning or warmth that is retrosternal and may radiate from the epigastrium to the neck. It usually originates in the esophagus. If persistent, especially in the epigastric area, it may raise the question of heart disease. Some patients with coronary artery disease describe their pain as burning, "like indigestion." Pay special attention to what brings on

Heartburn suggests gastric acid reflux into the esophagus; often precipitated by a heavy meal, lying down, or bending forward, also by ingesting alcohol, citrus juices, or

and relieves the discomfort. Is it precipitated by exertion and relieved by rest, suggesting angina, or is it related to meals and made worse during or after eating, suggesting gastroesophageal reflux?

aspirin. If chronic, consider reflux esophagitis. See Table 7-1, Chest Pain, pp. 268–269.

- *Excessive gas*, especially with frequent belching, abdominal bloating or distention, or *flatus*, the passage of gas by rectum, normally about 600 ml per day. Find out if these symptoms are associated with eating specific foods. Ask if symptoms are related to ingestion of milk or milk products.

Belching, but not bloating or excess flatus, is normally seen in *aerophagia*, or swallowing air. Also consider legumes and other gas-producing foods, intestinal lactase deficiency, and irritable bowel syndrome.

- Unpleasant *abdominal fullness* after meals of normal size, or *early satiety*, the inability to eat a full meal.

Consider diabetic gastroparesis, anticholinergic drugs, gastric outlet obstruction, gastric cancer; early satiety in hepatitis.

- *Nausea and vomiting*
- *Abdominal pain*

Anorexia is a loss or lack of appetite. Find out if it arises from intolerance to certain foods or reluctance to eat because of anticipated discomfort. *Nausea*, often described as "feeling sick to my stomach," may progress to retching or vomiting. *Retching* describes the spasmodic movements of the chest and diaphragm that precede and culminate in *vomiting*, the forceful expulsion of gastric contents out through the mouth.

Anorexia, nausea, vomiting in many gastrointestinal disorders; also in pregnancy, diabetic ketoacidosis, adrenal insufficiency, hypercalcemia, uremia, liver disease, emotional states, adverse drug reactions. Induced but without nausea in anorexia/bulimia nervosa.

Some patients may not actually vomit but raise esophageal or gastric contents without nausea or retching, called *regurgitation*.

Regurgitation in esophageal narrowing from stricture or cancer; also in incompetent gastroesophageal sphincter

Ask about any vomitus or regurgitated material and inspect it yourself if possible. What color is it? What does the vomitus smell like? How much has there been? Ask specifically if it contains any blood and try to determine how much. You may have to help the patient with the amount . . . a teaspoon? Two teaspoons? A cupful?

Fecal odor in small bowel obstruction or gastrocolic fistula

Gastric juice is clear or mucoid. Small amounts of yellowish or greenish bile are common and have no special significance. Brownish or blackish vomitus with a "coffee-grounds" appearance suggests blood altered by gastric acid. Coffee-grounds emesis or red blood is termed *hematemesis.*

Hematemesis in duodenal or peptic ulcer, esophageal or gastric varices, gastritis

Do the patient's symptoms suggest any complications of vomiting such as *aspiration* into the lungs, seen in elderly, debilitated, or obtunded patients? Is there dehydration or electrolyte imbalance from prolonged vomiting, or significant loss of blood?

Symptoms of blood loss such as lightheadedness or syncope depend on the rate and volume of bleeding and rarely appear until blood loss exceeds 500 ml.

Abdominal Pain. *Abdominal pain* has several possible mechanisms and clinical patterns and warrants careful clinical assessment. Be familiar with three broad categories of abdominal pain:

See Table 10-1, Abdominal Pain (pp. 394–395).

- *Visceral pain* occurs when hollow abdominal organs such as the intestine or biliary tree contract unusually forcefully or are distended or stretched. Solid organs such as the liver can also become painful when their capsules are stretched. Visceral pain may be difficult to localize. It is typically palpable near the midline at levels that vary according to the structure involved, as illustrated on the next page.

Visceral pain in the right upper quadrant from liver distention against its capsule in alcoholic hepatitis

Visceral pain varies in quality and may be gnawing, burning, cramping, or aching. When it becomes severe, it may be associated with sweating, pallor, nausea, vomiting, and restlessness.

Visceral periumbilical pain in early acute appendicitis from distention of inflamed appendix, gradually changing to parietal pain in the right lower quadrant from inflammation of the adjacent parietal peritoneum

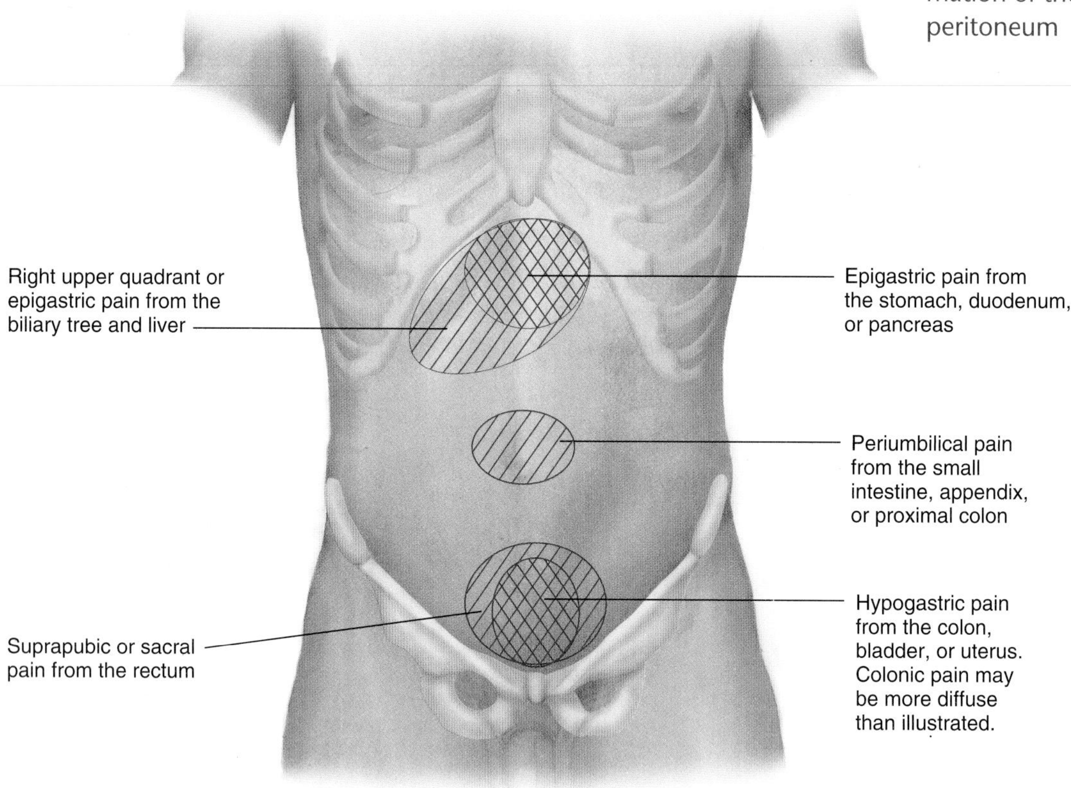

TYPES OF VISCERAL PAIN

- *Parietal pain* originates in the parietal peritoneum and is caused by inflammation. It is a steady aching pain that is usually more severe than visceral pain and more precisely localized over the involved structure. It is typically aggravated by movement or coughing. Patients with this type of pain usually prefer to lie still.

- *Referred pain* is felt in more distant sites, which are innervated at approximately the same spinal levels as the disordered structure. Referred pain often develops as the initial pain becomes more intense and thus

Pain of duodenal or pancreatic origin may be referred to the back; pain from the biliary tree, to the

seems to radiate or travel from the initial site. It may be felt superficially or deeply but is usually well localized.

right shoulder or the right posterior chest.

Pain may also be referred to the abdomen from the chest, spine, or pelvis, thus complicating the assessment of abdominal pain.

Pain from *pleurisy* or *acute myocardial infarction* may be referred to the upper abdomen.

Ask patients to *describe the abdominal pain in their own words,* then ask them to *point to the pain.* If clothes interfere, repeat the question during the physical examination. You may need to pursue important details: "Where does the pain start?" "Does it radiate or travel anywhere?" "What is the pain like?" If the patient has trouble describing the pain, try a multiple-choice question such as "Is it aching, burning, gnawing, or what?"

Cramping colicky pain often is related to peristalsis.

You need to ask "How severe is the pain?" "How about on a scale of 1 to 10?" Find out if it is bearable and if it interferes with the patient's usual activities. Does it make the patient lie down?

The description of the *severity of the pain* may tell you something about the patient's responses to pain and its effects on the patient's life, but it is not consistently helpful in assessing the pain's cause. Sensitivity to abdominal pain varies widely and tends to diminish over the later years, masking acute abdominal problems in older people, especially those in or beyond their 70s.

Careful *timing of the pain,* on the other hand, is particularly helpful. Did it start suddenly or gradually? When did the pain begin? How long does it last? What is its pattern over a 24-hour period? Over weeks and months? Are you dealing with an acute illness or a chronic or recurring one?

Determine *what factors aggravate or relieve the pain,* with special reference to meals, antacids, alcohol, medications (including aspirin and aspirinlike drugs and any over-the-counter drugs), emotional factors, and body position. Also, is the pain related to defecation, urination, or menstruation? You also need to elicit any *symptoms associated with the pain,* such as fever or chills, and their sequence.

Citrus fruits may aggravate the pain of *reflux esophagitis;* lactase deficiency is possible if abdominal discomfort is linked to milk ingestion.

Dysphagia and/or Odynophagia. Less commonly, patients may report difficulty swallowing, or *dysphagia,* the sense that food or liquid is sticking, hesitating, or "won't go down right." Dysphagia may result from esophageal disorders or from difficulty transferring food from the mouth to the esophagus. The sensation of a lump in the throat or in the retrosternal area, unassociated with swallowing, is not true dysphagia.

For types of dysphagia, see Table 10-2, Dysphagia, p. 396.

Ask the patient to point to where the dysphagia occurs and describe with what types of food it occurs. Does it occur with relatively solid foods such as meat, with softer foods such as ground meat and mashed potatoes, or with hot or cold liquids? Has the pattern changed?

Pointing to the throat suggests a transfer or esophageal disorder; pointing to the chest suggests an esophageal disorder.

Establish the timing. When did it start? Is it intermittent or persistent? Is it progressing? If so, over what period? What are the associated symptoms and medical conditions?

Dysphagia with solid food in mechanical narrowing of the esophagus; dysphagia related to both solids and liquids suggests a disorder of esophageal motility.

Odynophagia, or pain on swallowing, may occur in two forms. A sharp, burning pain suggests mucosal inflammation, whereas a squeezing, cramping pain suggests a muscular cause. Odynophagia may accompany dysphagia, but either symptom may occur independently.

Mucosal inflammation in reflux esophagitis or infection from *Candida*, herpes virus, or cytomegalovirus.

Change in Bowel Function. With respect to the lower gastrointestinal tract, you will frequently need to assess *bowel function*. Start with open-ended questions: "How are your bowel movements?" "How frequent are they?" "Do you have any difficulties?" "Have you noticed any change in your bowel habits?" Frequency of bowel movements normally ranges from about three times a day to twice a week. A change in pattern within these limits, however, may be significant for an individual patient.

Constipation or Diarrhea. Patients vary widely in their views of constipation and diarrhea. Be sure to clarify what the patient means by these terms. For example, is *constipation* . . . a decrease in frequency of bowel movements? . . . The passage of hard and perhaps painful stools? . . . The need to strain unusually hard? . . . A sense of incomplete defecation or pressure in the rectum? Ask if the patient actually looks at the stool. If yes, what does the stool look like in terms of color and bulk? What remedies has the patient tried? Do medications, stress, unrealistic ideas about normal bowel habits, or time and setting allotted for defecation play a role? Occasionally there is complete constipation with no passage of either feces or gas, or *obstipation*.

See Table 10-3, Constipation (p. 397) and Table 10-4, Diarrhea (pp. 398–399).

Thin pencil-like stool in an obstructing "apple-core" lesion of the sigmoid colon

Obstipation in *intestinal obstruction*

Inquire about the color of the stools and ask about any *black tarry stools*, suggesting *melena*, or *red blood in the stools*, known as *hematochezia*. If either condition is present, find out how long and how often. If the blood is red, how much is there? Is it pure blood mixed in with stool or on the surface of the stool? Is there blood on the toilet paper?

See Table 10-5, Black and Bloody Stools, p. 400.

Blood on the stool surface and on toilet paper in *hemorrhoids*

Diarrhea is an excessive frequency in the passage of stools that are usually unformed or watery. Ask about size, frequency, and volume. Are the stools bulky or small? How many episodes of diarrhea occur each day?

Consistently large diarrheal stools often in small bowel or proximal colon disorders; small frequent stools with urgency of defecation in left colon or rectal disorders

Ask for descriptive terms. Are the stools greasy or oily? Frothy? Foul smelling? Floating on the surface because of excessive gas, making them difficult to flush? Accompanied by mucus, pus, or blood?

Large yellowish or gray greasy foul-smelling stools, sometimes frothy or floating, in *steatorrhea*, or fatty stools—seen in malabsorption

Assess the course of diarrhea over time. Is it acute, chronic, or recurrent? Or is your patient experiencing the first acute episode of a chronic or recurrent illness?

Look into other factors as well. Does the diarrhea awaken the patient at night? What seem to be the aggravating or relieving factors? Does the patient get relief from a bowel movement, or is there an intense urge with

Nocturnal diarrhea suggests a pathophysiologic cause.

straining but little or no result, known as *tenesmus.* What is the setting? Does t entail travel, stress, or a new medication? Do family members or companions have similar symptoms? Are there associated symptoms?

Relief after passing feces or gas suggests left colon or rectal disorders; *tenesmus* in rectal conditions near the anal sphincter

Jaundice. In some patients, you will be struck by *jaundice* or *icterus*, the yellowish discoloration of the skin and sclerae from increased levels of bilirubin, a bile pigment derived chiefly from the breakdown of hemoglobin. Normally the hepatocytes conjugate, or combine, unconjugated bilirubin with other substances, making the bile water soluble, and then excrete it into the bile. The bile passes through the cystic duct into the common bile duct, which also drains the extrahepatic ducts from the liver. More distally the common bile duct and the pancreatic ducts empty into the duodenum at the ampulla of Vater. Mechanisms of jaundice include the following:

- Increased production of bilirubin
- Decreased uptake of bilirubin by the hepatocytes
- Decreased ability of the liver to conjugate bilirubin

Predominantly unconjugated bilirubin from the first three mechanisms, as in *hemolytic anemia* (increased production) and *Gilbert's syndrome*

- Decreased excretion of bilirubin into the bile, resulting in absorption of *conjugated* bilirubin back into the blood.

Impaired excretion of conjugated bilirubin in *viral hepatitis, cirrhosis, primary biliary cirrhosis*, drug-induced cholestasis, as from oral contraceptives, methyl testosterone, chlorpromazine

Intrahepatic jaundice can be *hepatocellular*, from damage to the hepatocytes, or *cholestatic*, from impaired excretion as a result of damaged hepatocytes or intrahepatic bile ducts. *Extrahepatic* jaundice arises from obstruction of the extrahepatic bile ducts, most commonly the cystic and common bile ducts.

Obstruction of the common bile duct by gallstones or *pancreatic carcinoma*

As you assess the patient with jaundice, pay special attention to the associated symptoms and the setting in which the illness occurred. What was the *color of the urine* as the patient became ill? When the level of conjugated bilirubin increases in the blood, it may be excreted into the urine, turning the urine a dark yellowish brown or tea color. Unconjugated bilirubin is not water-soluble, so it is not excreted into urine.

Dark urine from bilirubin indicates impaired excretion of bilirubin into the gastrointestinal tract.

Ask also about the *color of the stools.* When excretion of bile into the intestine is completely obstructed, the stools become gray or light colored, or *acholic*, without bile.

Acholic stools briefly in *viral hepatitis*, common in obstructive jaundice

Does the skin itch without other obvious explanation? Is there associated pain? What is its pattern? Has it been recurrent in the past?

Itching in cholestatic or obstructive jaundice; pain from a distended liver capsule, *biliary cholic, pancreatic cancer*

Ask about risk factors for liver diseases, such as:

- *Hepatitis:* Travel or meals in areas of poor sanitation, ingestion of contaminated water or foodstuffs (hepatitis A); parenteral or mucous membrane exposure to infectious body fluids such as blood, serum, semen, and saliva, especially through sexual contact with an infected partner or use of shared needles for injection drug use (hepatitis B); intravenous illicit drug use or blood transfusion (hepatitis C)
- *Alcoholic hepatitis* or *alcoholic cirrhosis* (interview the patient carefully about alcohol use)
- *Toxic liver damage* from medications, industrial solvents, or environmental toxins
- *Gallbladder disease* or *surgery* that may result in extrahepatic biliary obstruction
- *Hereditary disorders* in the Family History

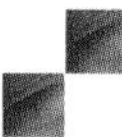

THE URINARY TRACT

General questions for a urinary history include: "Do you have any difficulty passing your urine?" "How often do you go?" "Do you have to get up at night? How often?" "How much urine do you pass at a time?" "Is there any pain or burning?" "Do you ever have trouble getting to the toilet in time?" "Do you ever leak any urine? Or wet yourself involuntarily?" Does the patient sense when the bladder is full and when voiding occurs?

See Table 10-6, Frequency, Nocturia, and Polyuria (p. 401).

Involuntary voiding or lack of awareness suggests cognitive or neurosensory deficits.

Ask women if sudden coughing, sneezing, or laughing makes them lose urine. Roughly half of young women report this experience even before bearing children. Occasional leakage is not necessarily significant. Ask older men, "Do you have trouble starting your stream?" "Do you have to stand close to the toilet to void?" "Is there a change in the force or size of your stream, or straining to void?" "Do you hesitate or stop in the middle of voiding?" "Is there dribbling when you're through?"

Stress incontinence from decreased intraurethral pressure (see pp. 402–403).

Common in men with partial bladder outlet obstruction from *benign prostatic hyperplasia;* also seen with *urethral stricture*

Suprapubic Pain. Disorders in the urinary tract may cause pain in either the abdomen or the back. Bladder disorders may cause *suprapubic pain.* In *bladder infection,* pain in the lower abdomen is typically dull and pressure-like. In sudden overdistention of the bladder, pain is often agonizing; in contrast, chronic bladder distention is usually painless.

Pain of sudden overdistention in acute urinary retention

Dysuria, Urgency, or Frequency. Infection or irritation of either the bladder or urethra often provokes several symptoms. Frequently there is *pain on urination,* usually felt as a burning sensation. Some clinicians refer to this as *dysuria,* whereas others reserve the term dysuria for difficulty voiding. Women may report internal urethral discomfort, sometimes described as a pressure, or an external burning from the flow of urine across irritated

Painful urination with cystitis or urethritis

Also consider bladder stones, foreign bodies, tumors; also *acute prostatitis.* In women, internal

or inflamed labia. Men typically feel a burning sensation proximal to the glans penis. In contrast, *prostatic pain* is felt in the perineum and occasionally in the rectum.

burning in urethritis, external burning in *vulvovaginitis*

Other associated symptoms are common. Urinary *urgency* is an unusually intense and immediate desire to void, sometimes leading to involuntary voiding or *urge incontinence*. Urinary *frequency*, or abnormally frequent voiding, may occur. Ask about any related fever or chills, blood in the urine, or any pain in the abdomen, flank, or back (see illustration on next page). Men with partial obstruction to urinary outflow often report *hesitancy* in starting the urine stream, *straining to void, reduced caliber and force of the urinary stream*, or *dribbling* as voiding is completed.

Urgency in bladder infection or irritation. In men, painful urination without frequency or urgency suggests urethritis.

Polyuria or Nocturia. Three additional terms describe important alterations in the pattern of urination. *Polyuria* refers to a significant increase in 24-hour urine volume, roughly defined as exceeding 3 liters. It should be distinguished from urinary frequency, which can involve voiding in high amounts, seen in polyuria, or in small amounts, as in infection. *Nocturia* refers to urinary frequency at night, sometimes defined as awakening the patient more than once; urine volumes may be large or small. Clarify any change in nocturnal voiding patterns and the number of trips to the bathroom.

Abnormally high renal production of urine in polyuria. Frequency without polyuria during the day or night in bladder disorder or impairment to flow at or below the bladder neck

Urinary Incontinence. Up to 30% of older patients are concerned about *urinary incontinence*, an involuntary loss of urine that may become socially embarrassing or cause problems with hygiene. If the patient reports incontinence, ask when it happens and how often. Find out if the patient has leaking of small amounts of urine with increased intra-abdominal pressure from coughing, sneezing, laughing, or lifting. Or, is it difficult for the patient to hold the urine once there is an urge to void, and loss of large amounts of urine? Is there a sensation of bladder fullness, frequent leakage or voiding of small amounts but difficulty emptying the bladder?

See Table 10-7, Urinary Incontinence (pp. 402–403).

As described earlier, bladder control involves complex neuroregulatory and motor mechanisms (see p. 361). A number of central or peripheral nerve lesions may affect normal voiding. Can the patient sense when the bladder is full? And when voiding occurs? Although there are four broad categories of incontinence, a patient may have a combination of causes.

Stress incontinence with increased intra-abdominal pressure from decreased contractility of urethral sphincter or poor support of bladder neck; *urge incontinence* if unable to hold the urine, from detrusor overactivity; *overflow incontinence* when the bladder cannot be emptied until bladder pressure exceeds urethral pressure, from anatomical obstruction by prostatic hypertrophy or stricture, also neurogenic abnormalities

In addition, the patient's functional status may significantly affect voiding behaviors even when the urinary tract is intact. Is the patient mobile? Alert? Able to respond to voiding cues and reach the bathroom? Is alertness or voiding affected by medications?

Functional incontinence from impaired cognition, musculoskeletal problems, immobility

Hematuria. Blood in the urine, or *hematuria*, is an important cause for concern. When visible to the naked eye, it is called *gross hematuria*. The urine may appear frankly bloody. Blood may be detected only during microscopic urinalysis, known as *microscopic hematuria*. Smaller amounts of blood may tinge the urine with a pinkish or brownish cast. In women, be sure to distinguish menstrual blood from hematuria. If the urine is reddish,

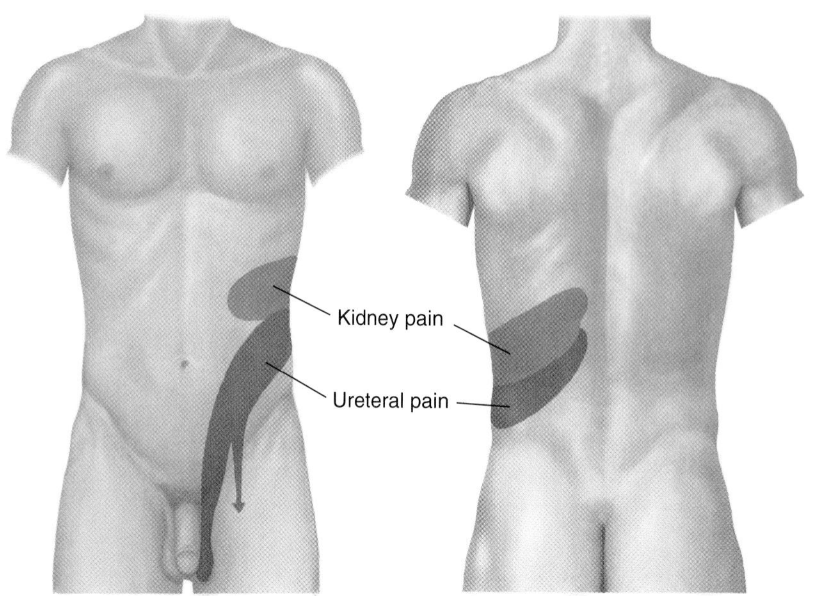

ask about ingestion of beets or medications that might discolor the urine. Test the urine with a dipstick and microscopic examination before you settle on the term hematuria.

Kidney or Flank Pain; Ureteral Colic. Disorders of the urinary tract may also cause *kidney pain*, often reported as *flank pain* at or below the posterior costal margin near the costovertebral angle. It may radiate anteriorly toward the umbilicus. Kidney pain is a visceral pain usually produced by distention of the renal capsule and typically dull, aching, and steady. *Ureteral pain* is dramatically different. It is usually severe and colicky, originating at the costovertebral angle and radiating around the trunk into the lower quadrant of the abdomen, or possibly into the upper thigh and testicle or labium. Ureteral pain results from sudden distention of the ureter and associated distention of the renal pelvis. Ask about any associated fever or chills, or hematuria.

Kidney pain occurs in *acute pyelonephritis*.

Renal or ureteral colic is caused by sudden obstruction of a ureter, as by urinary stones or blood clots.

HEALTH PROMOTION AND COUNSELING

Important Topics for Health Promotion and Counseling

- Screening for alcohol and substance abuse
- Risk factors for hepatitis A, B, and C
- Screening for colon cancer

Health promotion and counseling relevant to the abdomen include screening for alcoholism, for risk of infectious hepatitis, and for risk of colon cancer.

Clues from social patterns and behavioral problems in the history and findings of liver enlargement or tenderness on physical examination often alert the clinician to possible alcoholism or risk for infectious hepatitis. Past medical history and family history are important when assessing risk for colon cancer.

The effects of addiction to *alcohol* on public health may be even greater than those of addiction to illicit drugs. More than 10 million Americans currently abuse alcohol. Lifetime prevalence of alcohol abuse or dependence is approximately 13.5%.[1] Alcohol abuse is highly correlated with fatal car accidents, suicide and other comorbid mental health disorders, hypertension, family disruption, violence, and malignancies of the upper gastrointestinal tract and liver, to name but a few of its sequelae.

Assessing patients for use of alcohol and other substances is a prime clinical responsibility. The clinician should focus on detection, counseling, and, for significant impairment, specific recommendations for treatment. When asking about alcohol use, recall current definitions of risky or hazardous drinking and harmful drinking.[2]

- *Risky or hazardous drinking:* For *women*—more than 7 drinks per week or more than 3 drinks per occasion; for *men*—more than 14 drinks per week or more than 4 drinks per occasion

- *Harmful drinking*—drinking that causes physical, social, or psychological harm from alcohol use but does not meet the criteria for dependence

Use the four CAGE questions, validated across many studies, to screen for alcohol dependence or abuse[2,3] (see Chapter 2, Interviewing and the Health History, pp. 50–51). Effective interventions about misuse can be brief. Initial counseling of approximately 15 minutes, with intermittent follow-up by trained office staff for feedback, advice, and goal setting, reduces consumption by 13%–34% over 6 to 12 months.[2,4–6] Motivational interviewing has also been successful in promoting abstinence.[7] One model for brief interventions is FRAMES: **F**eedback based on thorough assessment; **R**esponsibility; **A**dvice on behavior change; a **M**enu of options for making change; **E**mpathy about the difficulty of changing; and support for **S**elf-efficacy in achieving change.[8] Tailor recommendations for treatment to the severity of the problem, ranging from support groups to inpatient detoxification to more extended rehabilitation.

Protective measures against infectious hepatitis include counseling about how the viruses are spread and the need for immunization. Transmission of hepatitis A is fecal–oral: fecal shedding in food handlers leads to contamination of water and foods. Illness occurs approximately 30 days after exposure. Hepatitis A vaccine is recommended for travelers to endemic areas, food handlers, military personnel, caretakers of children, Native Americans and Alaskan natives, and selected health care, sanitation, and laboratory workers. Vaccination is also recommended for homosexual contacts and injection drug users. For immediate protection and prophylaxis for household contacts and travelers, consider administering immune serum globulin.

Hepatitis B poses more serious threats to patients' health, including risk for fulminant hepatitis as well as chronic infection and subsequent cirrhosis and hepatocellular carcinoma. Transmission occurs during contact with infected body fluids, such as blood, semen, saliva, and vaginal secretions. Adults between the ages of 20 and 39 are most affected, especially injection drug users and sex workers. Up to one tenth of infected adults become chronically infected asymptomatic carriers. Behavioral counseling and serologic screening are advised for patients at risk. Because up to 30% of patients have no identifiable risk factors, hepatitis B vaccine is recommended for all young adults not previously immunized, injection drug users and their sexual partners, people at risk for sexually transmitted diseases, travelers to endemic areas, recipients of blood products as in hemodialysis, and health care workers with frequent exposure to blood products. Many of these groups should also be screened for HIV infection. The U.S. Preventive Services Task Force currently recommends screening for only pregnant women at their first prenatal visit because 30%–40% of infected individuals have no identifiable risk factors.[9]

Hepatitis C is transmitted by repeated percutaneous exposures to blood and is present in approximately 2% of U.S. adults. Infected patients are often asymptomatic; some experience fatigue, malaise, anorexia, nausea, and reduced quality of life. More than 70% develop chronic liver disease. Because of its low prevalence and low rate of progression to cirrhosis, routine screening of the general or even high-risk populations is currently not recommended.[10] Risk factors include injection drug use, transfusion before 1990, an HCV-infected mother, and unsafe sex.

It is also important to screen patients for *colorectal cancer*, the fourth most common U.S. malignancy and the second leading cause of death from cancer.[11] Lifetime risk for diagnosis at age 50 is approximately 5%. Roughly 80% of colorectal cancers originate from adenomatous polyps, usually those larger than 1 cm. Prevalence increases from approximately 20% at age 50 to 50% at age 75.[12] For men and women at average risk, the American Cancer Society recommends one of the following tests beginning at age 50:[13]

- Fecal occult blood test (FOBT) annually
- Flexible sigmoidoscopy every 5 years
- Annual FOBT plus flexible sigmoidoscopy every 5 years
- Double-contrast barium enema every 5 years
- Colonoscopy every 10 years

The U.S. Preventive Services Task Force finds strong evidence in support of screening beginning at age 50.

Most colorectal cancers are sporadic, but approximately 20% occur in patients with specific risk factors: prior adenomatous polyps or colorectal cancer; ulcerative colitis; colorectal cancer in a first-degree relative; and family history of adenomatous polyps before age 60. Familial adenomatous polyposis or hereditary nonpolyposis colorectal cancer accounts for approximately 6% of colorectal malignancies. Screening in these groups should begin at age 40 or earlier. Note that the FOBT has a highly variable sensitivity (26%–92%), but good specificity (90%–99%).[14] It produces many false-positive results related to diet, selected medications, and gastrointestinal conditions such as ulcer disease, diverticulosis, and hemorrhoids. The benefits of sigmoidoscopy are linked to the length of the sigmoidoscope and its depth of insertion. Detection rates for colorectal cancer and insertion depths are roughly as follows: 25%–30% at 20 cm; 50%–55% at 35 cm; 40%–65% at 40–50 cm. Full colonoscopy or air contrast barium enema detects 80%–95% of colorectal cancers, but these procedures are more uncomfortable, and colonoscopy is more expensive. When counseling patients about prevention, there is preliminary but inconsistent evidence that diets high in fiber may reduce risk for colorectal malignancy.

TECHNIQUES OF EXAMINATION

For a skilled abdominal examination, you need good light, a relaxed patient, and full exposure of the abdomen from above the xiphoid process to the symphysis pubis. The groin should be visible. The genitalia should remain draped. The abdominal muscles should be relaxed to enhance all aspects of the examination, but especially palpation.

Tips for Enhancing Examination of the Abdomen

- Check that the patient has an empty bladder.
- Make the patient comfortable in the supine position, with a pillow for under the head and perhaps another for under the knees. Slide your hand under the low back to see if the patient is relaxed and lying flat on the table.
- Ask the patient to keep the arms at the sides or folded across the chest. If the arms are above the head, the abdominal wall stretches and tightens, making palpation difficult.
- Before you begin palpation, ask the patient to point to any areas of pain and examine these areas last.
- Warm your hands and stethoscope. To warm your hands, rub them together or place them under hot water. You can also palpate through the patient's gown to absorb warmth from the patient's body before exposing the abdomen.
- Approach the patient calmly and avoid quick unexpected movements. *Watch the patient's face for any signs of pain or discomfort.* Make sure you avoid long fingernails.
- Distract the patient if necessary with conversation or questions. If the patient is frightened or ticklish, begin palpation with the patient's hand under yours. After a few moments, slip your hand underneath to palpate directly.

An arched back thrusts the abdomen forward and tightens the abdominal muscles.

Visualize each organ in the region you are examining. Stand at the patient's right side and proceed in an orderly fashion with inspection, auscultation, percussion, and palpation. Assess the liver, spleen, kidneys, and aorta.

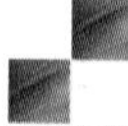

THE ABDOMEN

INSPECTION

Starting from your usual standing position at the right side of the bed, inspect the abdomen. As you look at the contour of the abdomen, watch for peristalsis. It is helpful to sit or bend down so that you can view the abdomen tangentially.

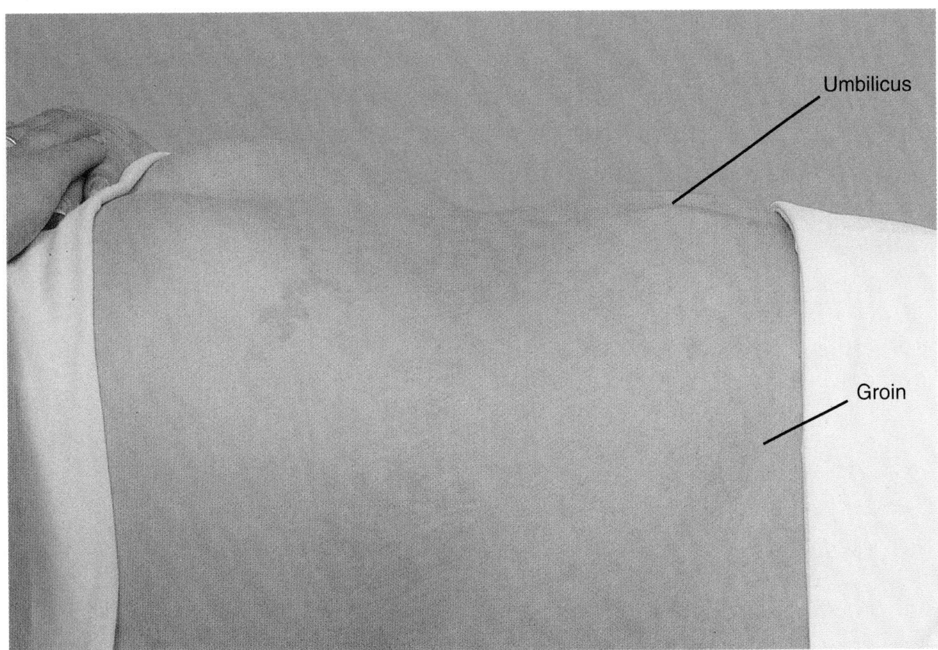

Inspect the surface, contours, and movements of the abdomen, including the following:

- *The skin,* note:

  Scars. Describe or diagram their location.

  Striae. Old silver striae or stretch marks are normal.

  Pink–purple striae of *Cushing's syndrome*

  Dilated veins. A few small veins may be visible normally.

  Dilated veins of *hepatic cirrhosis* or of *inferior vena cava obstruction*

  Rashes and lesions

- *The umbilicus.* Observe its contour and location and any inflammation or bulges suggesting a hernia.

  See Table 10-8, Localized Bulges in the Abdominal Wall (p. 404).

- *The contour of the abdomen*

  Is it flat, rounded, protuberant, or scaphoid (markedly concave or hollowed)?

  See Table 10-9, Protuberant Abdomens (p. 405).

  Do the flanks bulge, or are there any local bulges? Also survey the inguinal and femoral areas.

  Bulging flanks of *ascites;* suprapubic bulge of a distended bladder or pregnant uterus; hernias

  Is the abdomen symmetric?

  Asymmetry from an enlarged organ or mass

  Are there visible organs or masses? Look for an enlarged liver or spleen that has descended below the rib cage.

  Lower abdominal mass of an ovarian or a uterine tumor

- *Peristalsis.* Observe for several minutes if you suspect intestinal obstruction. Peristalsis may be visible normally in very thin people.

  Increased peristaltic waves of *intestinal obstruction*

- *Pulsations.* The normal aortic pulsation is frequently visible in the epigastrium.

Increased pulsation of an *aortic aneurysm* or of *increased pulse pressure*

AUSCULTATION

Auscultation provides important information about bowel motility. *Listen to the abdomen before performing percussion or palpation because these maneuvers may alter the frequency of bowel sounds.* Practice auscultation until you are thoroughly familiar with variations in normal bowel sounds and can detect changes suggestive of inflammation or obstruction. Auscultation may also reveal *bruits*, or vascular sounds resembling heart murmurs, over the aorta or other arteries in the abdomen. Bruits suggest vascular occlusive disease.

Place the diaphragm of your stethoscope gently on the abdomen. Listen for bowel sounds and note their frequency and character. Normal sounds consist of clicks and gurgles, occurring at an estimated frequency of 5 to 34 per minute. Occasionally you may hear *borborygmi*—long prolonged gurgles of hyperperistalsis—the familiar "stomach growling." Because bowel sounds are widely transmitted through the abdomen, listening in one spot, such as the right lower quadrant, is usually sufficient.

Bowel sounds may be altered in diarrhea, intestinal obstruction, *paralytic ileus,* and *peritonitis.* See Table 10-10, Sounds in the Abdomen (p. 406).

If the patient has high blood pressure, listen in the epigastrium and in each upper quadrant for *bruits.* Later in the examination, when the patient sits up, listen also in the costovertebral angles. Epigastric bruits confined to systole may be heard normally.

A bruit in one of these areas that has both systolic and diastolic components strongly suggests *renal artery stenosis* as the cause of hypertension.

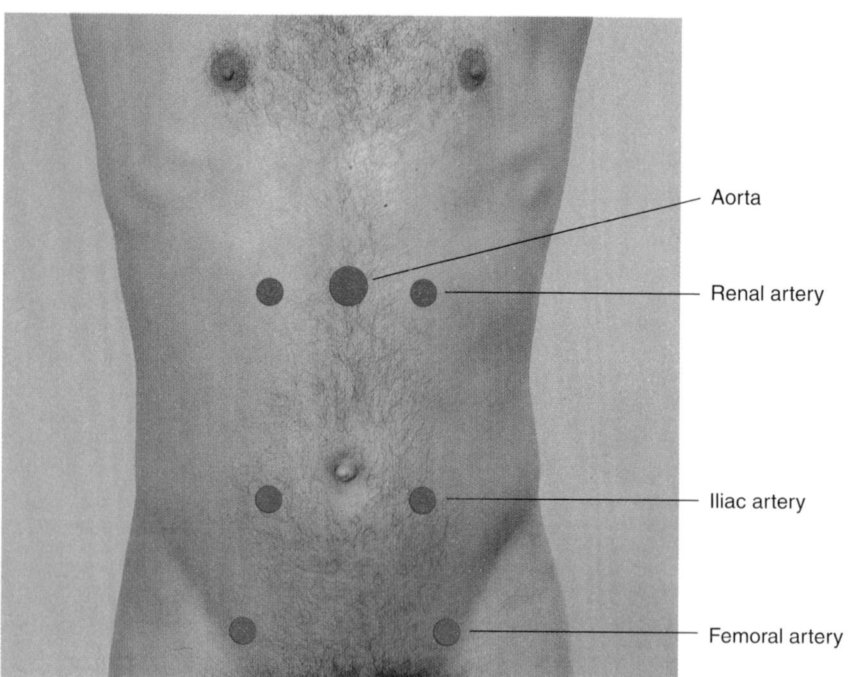

Listen for bruits over the aorta, the iliac arteries, and the femoral arteries. Bruits confined to systole are relatively common, however, and do not necessarily signify occlusive disease.

Listening points for bruits in these vessels are illustrated above.

Bruits with both systolic and diastolic components suggest the turbulent blood flow of *partial arterial occlusion* or *arterial insufficiency.* See Table 10-10, Sounds in the Abdomen (p. 406).

Listen over the liver and spleen for *friction rubs.*

See Table 10-10, Sounds in the Abdomen (p. 406).

Friction rubs in liver tumor, gonococcal infection around the liver, splenic infarction

PERCUSSION

Percussion helps you to assess the amount and distribution of gas in the abdomen and to identify possible masses that are solid or fluid filled. Its use in estimating the size of the liver and spleen will be described in later sections.

Percuss the abdomen lightly in all four quadrants to assess the distribution of *tympany* and *dullness.* Tympany usually predominates because of gas in the gastrointestinal tract, but scattered areas of dullness from fluid and feces there are also typical.

A protuberant abdomen that is tympanitic throughout suggests *intestinal obstruction.* See Table 10-9, Protuberant Abdomens (p. 405).

- Note any large dull areas that might indicate an underlying mass or enlarged organ. This observation will guide your palpation.

Pregnant uterus, ovarian tumor, distended bladder, large liver or spleen

- On each side of a protuberant abdomen, note where abdominal tympany changes to the dullness of solid posterior structures.

Dullness in both flanks indicates further assessment for ascites (see pp. 387–389).

Briefly percuss the lower anterior chest, between lungs above and costal margins below. On the right, you will usually find the dullness of liver; on the left, the tympany that overlies the gastric air bubble and the splenic flexure of the colon.

In *situs inversus* (rare), organs are reversed: air bubble on the right, liver dullness on the left.

PALPATION

Light Palpation. Feeling the abdomen gently is especially helpful for identifying abdominal tenderness, muscular resistance, and some superficial organs and masses. It also serves to reassure and relax the patient.

Keeping your hand and forearm on a horizontal plane, with fingers together and flat on the abdominal surface, palpate the abdomen with a light, gentle, dipping motion. When moving your hand from place to place, raise it just off the skin. Moving smoothly, feel in all quadrants.

Identify any superficial organs or masses and any area of tenderness or increased resistance to your hand. If resistance is present, try to distinguish voluntary guarding from involuntary muscular spasm. To do this:

- Try all the relaxing methods you know (see p. 374).

Involuntary rigidity (muscular spasm) typically persists despite these maneuvers. It indicates *peritoneal inflammation.*

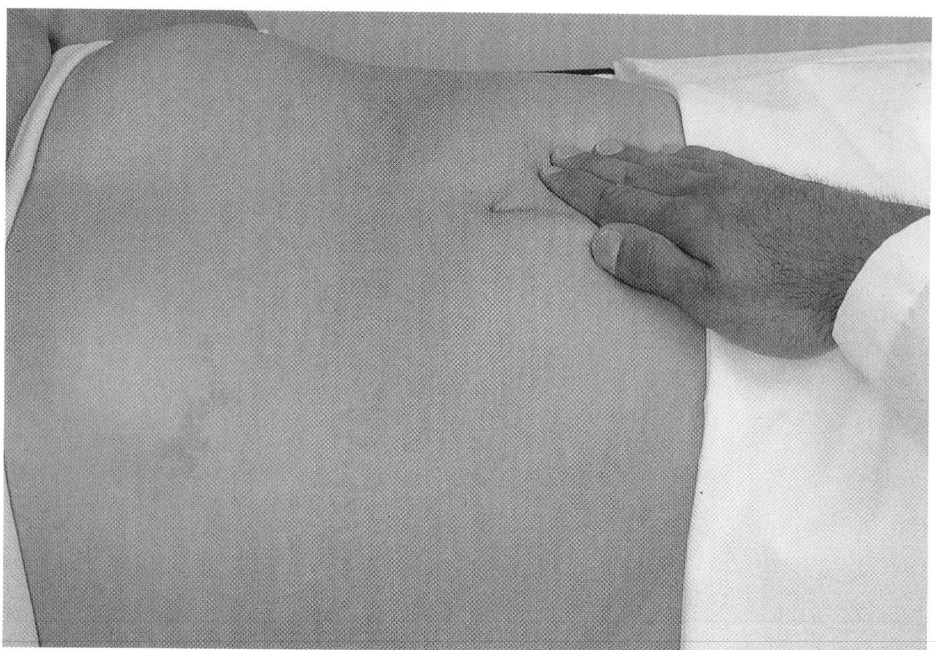

- Feel for the relaxation of abdominal muscles that normally accompanies exhalation.
- Ask the patient to mouth-breathe with jaw dropped open.

Voluntary guarding usually decreases with these maneuvers.

Deep Palpation. This is usually required to delineate abdominal masses. Again using the palmar surfaces of your fingers, feel in all four quadrants. Identify any masses and note their location, size, shape, consistency, tenderness, pulsations, and any mobility with respiration or with the examining hand. Correlate your palpable findings with their percussion notes.

Abdominal masses may be categorized in several ways: physiologic (pregnant uterus), inflammatory (diverticulitis of the colon), vascular (an aneurysm of the abdominal aorta), neoplastic (carcinoma of the colon), or obstructive (a distended bladder or dilated loop of bowel).

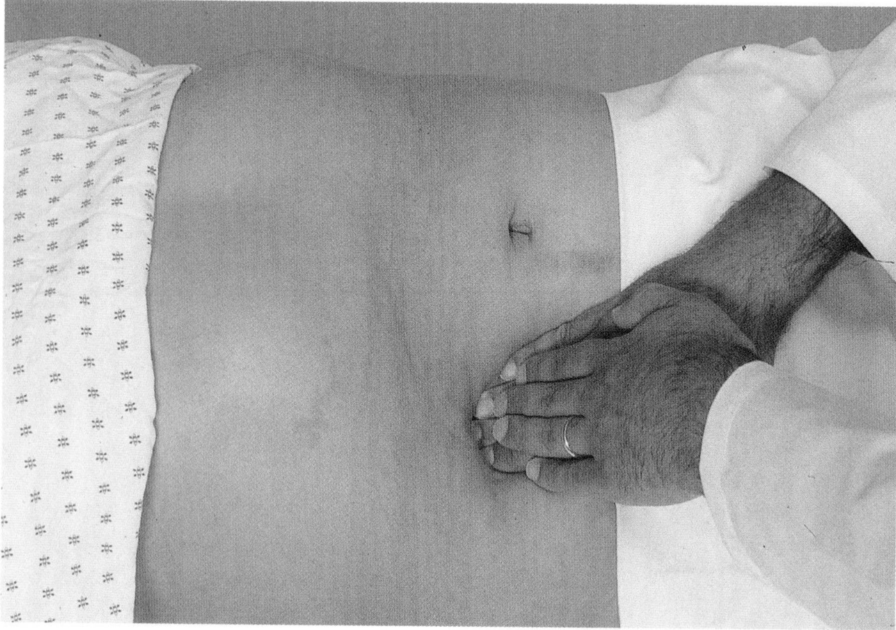

TWO-HANDED DEEP PALPATION

Assessment for Peritoneal Inflammation. Abdominal pain and tenderness, especially when associated with muscular spasm, suggest inflammation of the parietal peritoneum. Localize the pain as accurately as possible. First, even before palpation, *ask the patient to cough* and determine where the cough produced pain. Then, *palpate gently with one finger* to map the tender area. Pain produced by light percussion has similar localizing value. These gentle maneuvers may be all you need to establish an area of peritoneal inflammation.

Abdominal pain when coughing or with light percussion suggests peritoneal inflammation. See Table 10-11, Tender Abdomens (pp. 407–408).

If not, look for *rebound tenderness.* Press down with your fingers firmly and slowly, then withdraw them quickly. Watch and listen to the patient for signs of pain. Ask the patient "Which hurts more, when I press or let go?" Have the patient locate the pain exactly. Pain induced or increased by quick withdrawal constitutes *rebound tenderness* caused by rapid movement of an inflamed peritoneum.

Rebound tenderness suggests peritoneal inflammation. If tenderness is felt elsewhere than where you were trying to elicit rebound, that area may be the real source of the problem.

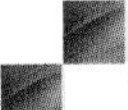

THE LIVER

Because the rib cage shelters most of the liver, assessment is difficult. Liver size and shape can be estimated by percussion and perhaps palpation, however, and the palpating hand helps you to evaluate its surface, consistency, and tenderness.

PERCUSSION

Measure the vertical span of liver dullness in the right midclavicular line. Starting at a level below the umbilicus (in an area of tympany, not dullness), lightly percuss upward toward the liver. Ascertain the *lower border of liver dullness* in the midclavicular line.

Next, identify the *upper border of liver dullness* in the midclavicular line. Lightly percuss from lung resonance down toward liver dullness. Gently displace a woman's breast as necessary to be sure that you start in a resonant area. The course of percussion is shown below.

The span of liver dullness is *increased* when the liver is enlarged.

The span of liver dullness is *decreased* when the liver is small, or when free air is present below the diaphragm, as from a *perforated hollow viscus.* Serial observations may show a decreasing span of dullness with resolution of *hepatitis* or *congestive heart failure* or, less commonly, with progression of *fulminant hepatitis.*

Liver dullness may be displaced downward by the low diaphragm of *chronic obstructive pulmonary disease.* Span, however, remains normal.

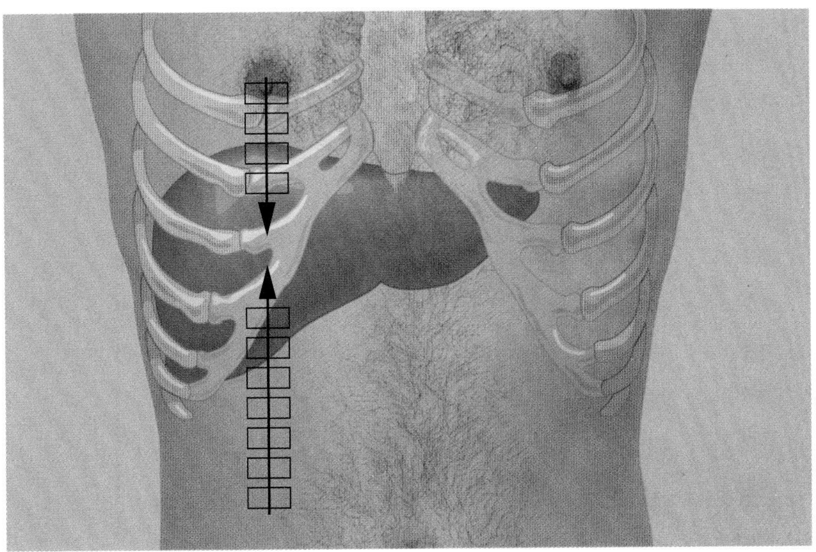

PERCUSSING LIVER SPAN

Now measure in centimeters the distance between your two points—the vertical span of liver dullness. Normal liver spans, shown below, are generally greater in men than in women, in tall people than in short. If the liver seems to be enlarged, outline the lower edge by percussing in other areas.

Dullness of a right pleural effusion or consolidated lung, if adjacent to liver dullness, may falsely *increase* the estimate of liver size.

Gas in the colon may produce tympany in the right upper quadrant, obscure liver dullness, and falsely *decrease* the estimate of liver size.

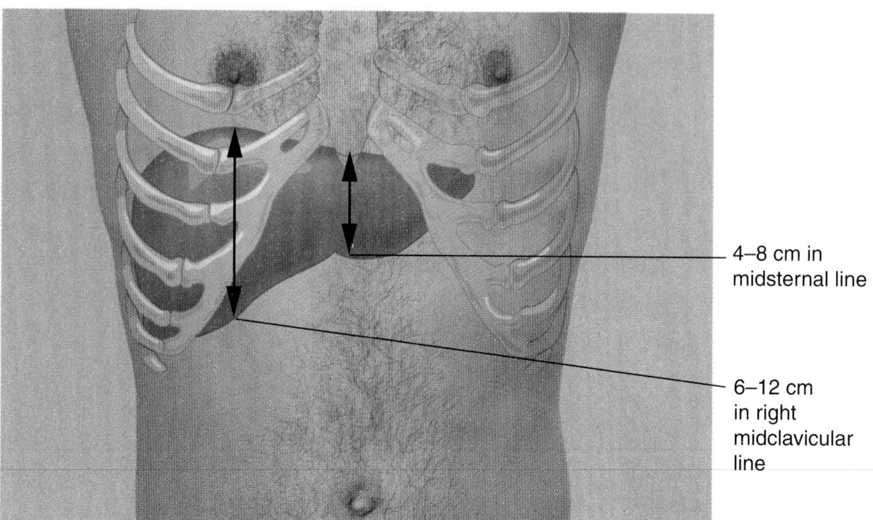

NORMAL LIVER SPANS

Although percussion is probably the most accurate clinical method for estimating the vertical size of the liver, it typically leads to underestimation.

PALPATION

Place your left hand behind the patient, parallel to and supporting the right 11th and 12th ribs and adjacent soft tissues below. Remind the patient to relax on your hand if necessary. By pressing your left hand forward, the patient's liver may be felt more easily by your other hand.

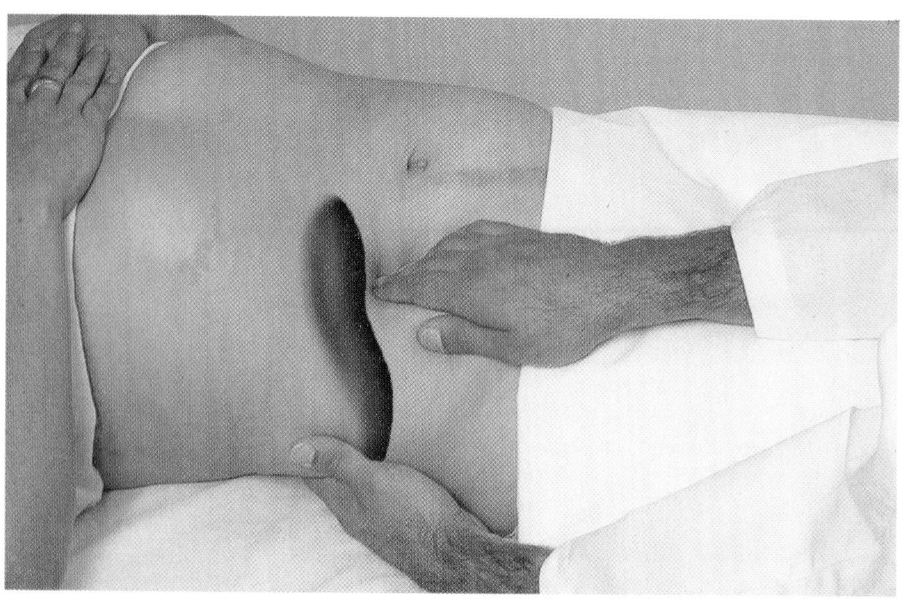

Place your right hand on the patient's right abdomen lateral to the rectus muscle, with your fingertips well below the lower border of liver dullness. Some examiners like to point their fingers up toward the patient's head, whereas others prefer a somewhat more oblique position, as shown below. In either case, press gently in and up.

Ask the patient to take a deep breath. Try to feel the liver edge as it comes down to meet your fingertips. If you feel it, lighten the pressure of your palpating hand slightly so that the liver can slip under your finger pads and you can feel its anterior surface. Note any tenderness. If palpable at all, the normal liver edge is soft, sharp, and regular, with a smooth surface. The normal liver may be slightly tender.

Firmness or hardness of the liver, bluntness or rounding of its edge, and irregularity of its contour suggest an abnormality of the liver.

On inspiration, the liver is palpable about 3 cm below the right costal margin in the midclavicular line. Some people breathe more with their chests than with their diaphragms. It may be helpful to train such a patient to "breathe with the abdomen," thus bringing the liver, as well as the spleen and kidneys, into a palpable position during inspiration.

An obstructed, distended gallbladder may form an oval mass below the edge of the liver and merging with it. It is dull to percussion.

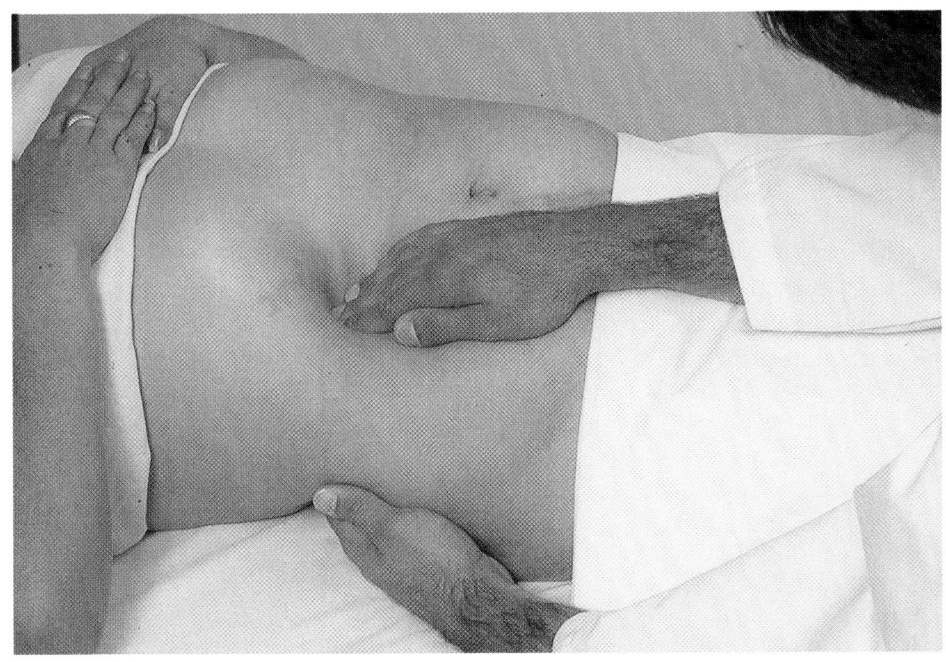

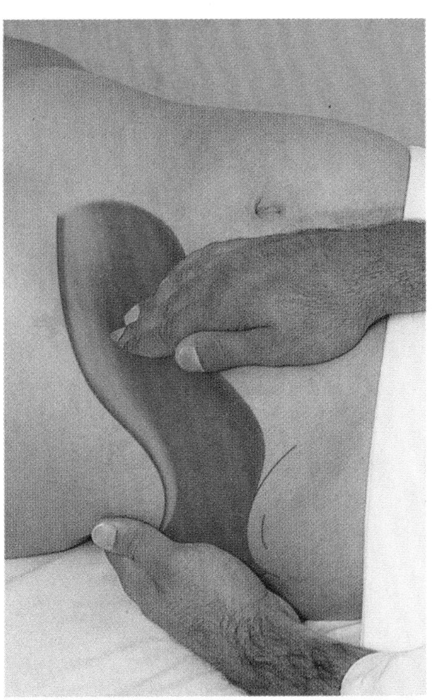

In order to feel the liver, you may have to alter your pressure according to the thickness and resistance of the abdominal wall. If you cannot feel it, move your palpating hand closer to the costal margin and try again.

The edge of an enlarged liver may be missed by starting palpation too high in the abdomen.

Try to trace the liver edge both laterally and medially. Palpation through the rectus muscles, however, is especially difficult. Describe or sketch the liver edge, and measure its distance from the right costal margin in the midclavicular line.

See Table 10-12, Liver Enlargement: Apparent and Real (p. 409).

The "hooking technique" may be helpful, especially when the patient is obese. Stand to the right of the patient's chest. Place both hands, side by side, on the right abdomen below the border of liver dullness. Press in with your fingers and up toward the costal margin. Ask the patient to take a deep breath. The liver edge shown below is palpable with the fingerpads of both hands.

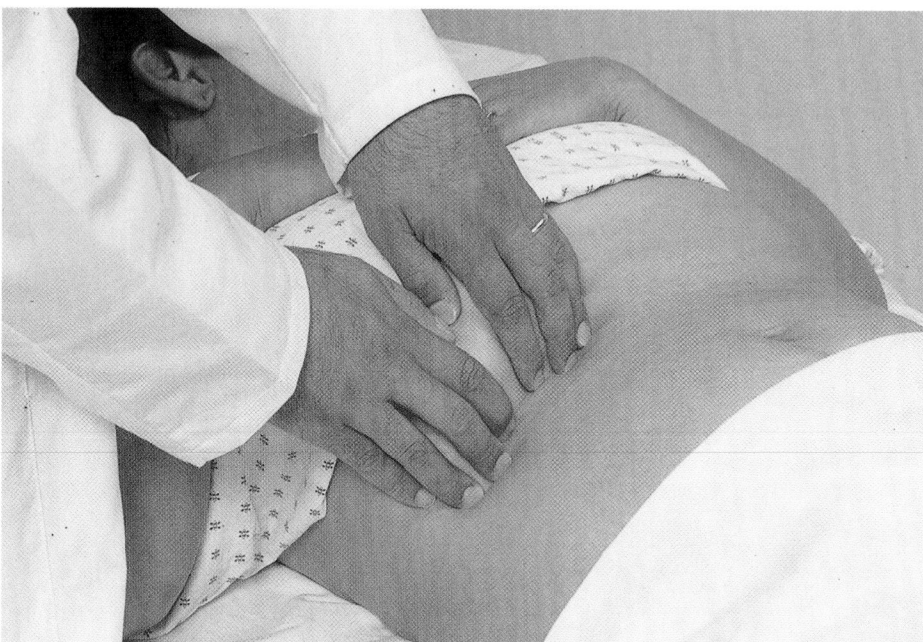

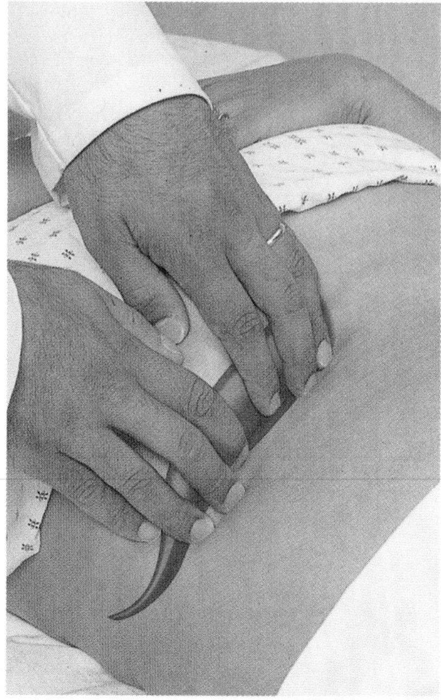

Assessing Tenderness of a Nonpalpable Liver. Place your left hand flat on the lower right rib cage and then gently strike your hand with the ulnar surface of your right fist. Ask the patient to compare the sensation with that produced by a similar strike on the left side.

Tenderness over the liver suggests inflammation, as in *hepatitis*, or congestion, as in *heart failure.*

THE SPLEEN

When a spleen enlarges, it expands anteriorly, downward, and medially, often replacing the tympany of stomach and colon with the dullness of a solid organ. It then becomes palpable below the costal margin. Percussion cannot confirm splenic enlargement but can raise your suspicions of it. Palpation can confirm the enlargement, but often misses large spleens that do not descend below the costal margin.

PERCUSSION

Two techniques may help you to detect *splenomegaly*, an enlarged spleen:

- *Percuss the left lower anterior chest wall* between lung resonance above and the costal margin, an area termed *Traube's space*. As you percuss along the routes suggested by the arrows in the following figures, note the lateral extent of tympany.

Dullness, as shown on the following page, raises the question of splenomegaly.

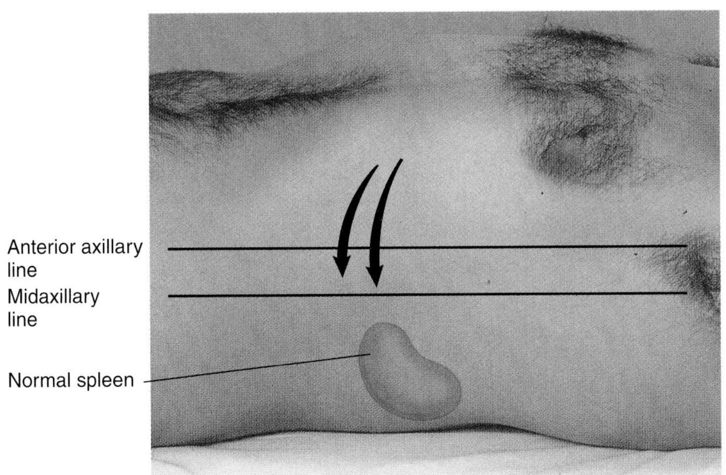

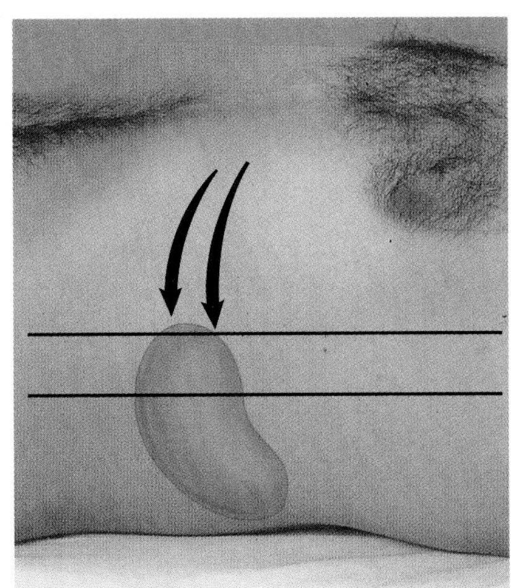

This is variable, but if tympany is prominent, especially laterally, splenomegaly is not likely. The dullness of a normal spleen is usually hidden within the dullness of other posterior tissues.

Fluid or solids in the stomach or colon may also cause dullness in Traube's space.

- *Check for a splenic percussion sign.* Percuss the lowest interspace in the left anterior axillary line, as shown below. This area is usually tympanitic. Then ask the patient to take a deep breath, and percuss again. When spleen size is normal, the percussion note usually remains tympanitic.

A change in percussion note from tympany to dullness on inspiration suggests splenic enlargement. This is a *positive splenic percussion sign.*

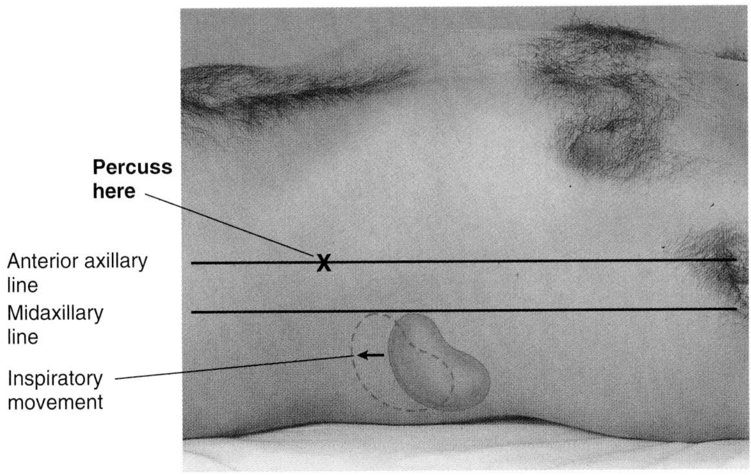

NEGATIVE SPLENIC PERCUSSION SIGN

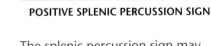

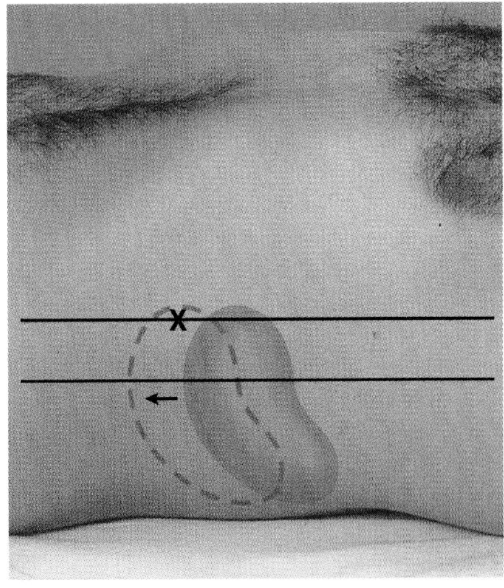

POSITIVE SPLENIC PERCUSSION SIGN

If either or both of these tests is positive, pay extra attention to palpation of the spleen.

The splenic percussion sign may also be positive when spleen size is normal.

PALPATION

With your left hand, reach over and around the patient to support and press forward the lower left rib cage and adjacent soft tissue. With your right hand below the left costal margin, press in toward the spleen. Begin palpation low

An enlarged spleen may be missed if the examiner starts too high in the abdomen to feel the lower edge.

enough so that you are below a possibly enlarged spleen. (If your hand is close to the costal margin, moreover, it is not sufficiently mobile to reach up under the rib cage.) Ask the patient to take a deep breath. Try to feel the tip or edge of the spleen as it comes down to meet your fingertips. Note any tenderness, assess the splenic contour, and measure the distance between the spleen's lowest point and the left costal margin. In a small percentage of normal adults, the tip of the spleen is palpable. Causes include a low, flat diaphragm, as in chronic obstructive pulmonary disease, and a deep inspiratory descent of the diaphragm.

A palpable spleen tip, though not necessarily abnormal, may indicate splenic enlargement. The spleen tip below is just palpable deep to the left costal margin.

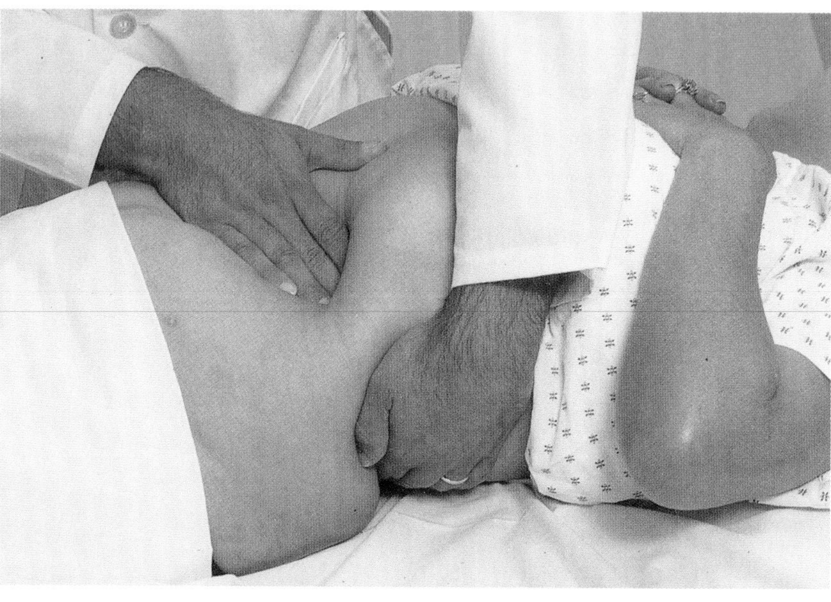

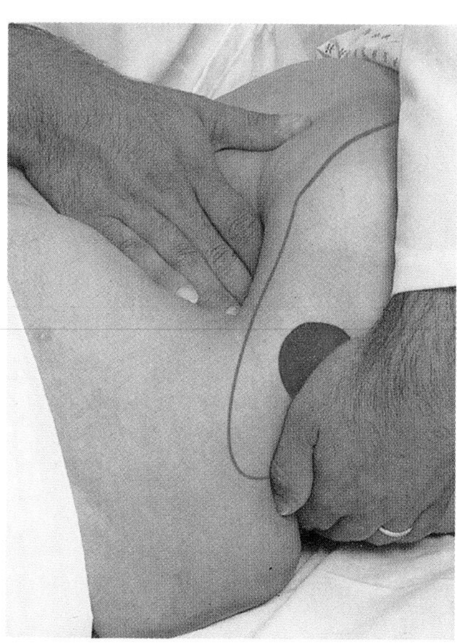

Repeat with the patient lying on the right side with legs somewhat flexed at hips and knees. In this position, gravity may bring the spleen forward and to the right into a palpable location.

The enlarged spleen is palpable about 2 cm below the left costal margin on deep inspiration.

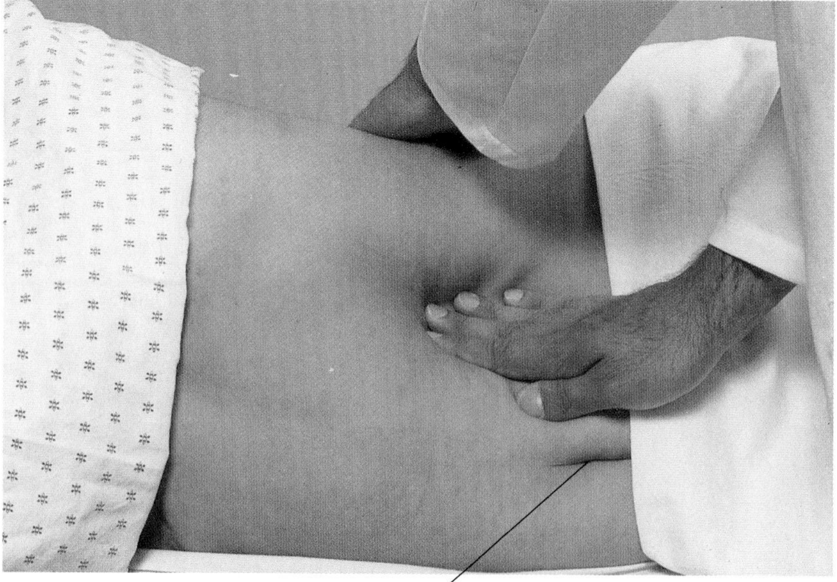

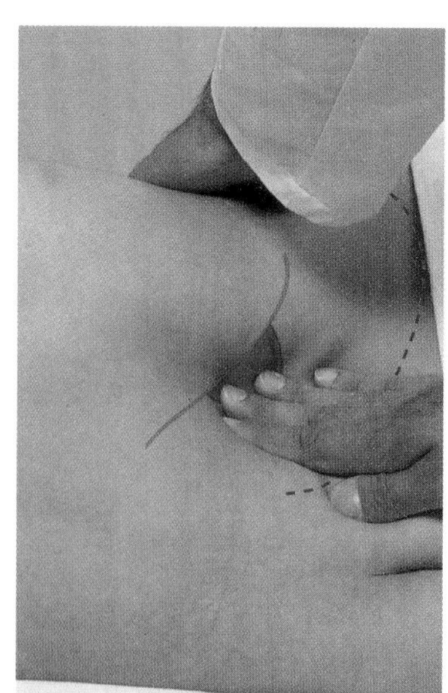

PALPATING THE SPLEEN—PATIENT LYING ON RIGHT SIDE

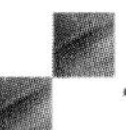

THE KIDNEYS

PALPATION

Although kidneys are not usually palpable, you should learn and practice the techniques for examination. Detecting an enlarged kidney may prove to be very important.

A left flank mass (see the solid line on photo on previous page) may represent marked *splenomegaly* or an enlarged left kidney. Suspect *splenomegaly* if notch is palpated on medial border, edge extends beyond the midline, percussion is dull, and your fingers can probe deep to the medial and lateral borders but not between the mass and the costal margin. Confirm findings with further evaluation.

Palpation of the Left Kidney. Move to the patient's left side. Place your right hand behind the patient just below and parallel to the 12th rib, with your fingertips just reaching the costovertebral angle. Lift, trying to displace the kidney anteriorly. Place your left hand gently in the left upper quadrant, lateral and parallel to the rectus muscle. Ask the patient to take a deep breath. At the peak of inspiration, press your left hand firmly and deeply into the left upper quadrant, just below the costal margin, and try to "capture" the kidney between your two hands. Ask the patient to breathe out and then to stop breathing briefly. Slowly release the pressure of your left hand, feeling at the same time for the kidney to slide back into its expiratory position. If the kidney is palpable, describe its size, contour, and any tenderness.

Attributes favoring an *enlarged kidney* over an enlarged spleen include preservation of normal tympany in the left upper quadrant and the ability to probe with your fingers between the mass and the costal margin, but not deep to its medial and lower borders.

Alternatively, try to feel for the left kidney by a method similar to feeling for the spleen. With your left hand, reach over and around the patient to lift the left loin, and with your right hand feel deep in the left upper quadrant. Ask the patient to take a deep breath, and feel for a mass. A normal left kidney is rarely palpable.

Palpation of the Right Kidney. To capture the right kidney, return to the patient's right side. Use your left hand to lift from in back, and your right hand to feel deep in the left upper quadrant. Proceed as before.

A normal right kidney may be palpable, especially in thin, well-relaxed women. It may or may not be slightly tender. The patient is usually aware of a capture

Causes of kidney enlargement include hydronephrosis, cysts, and tumors. Bilateral enlargement suggests *polycystic kidney disease.*

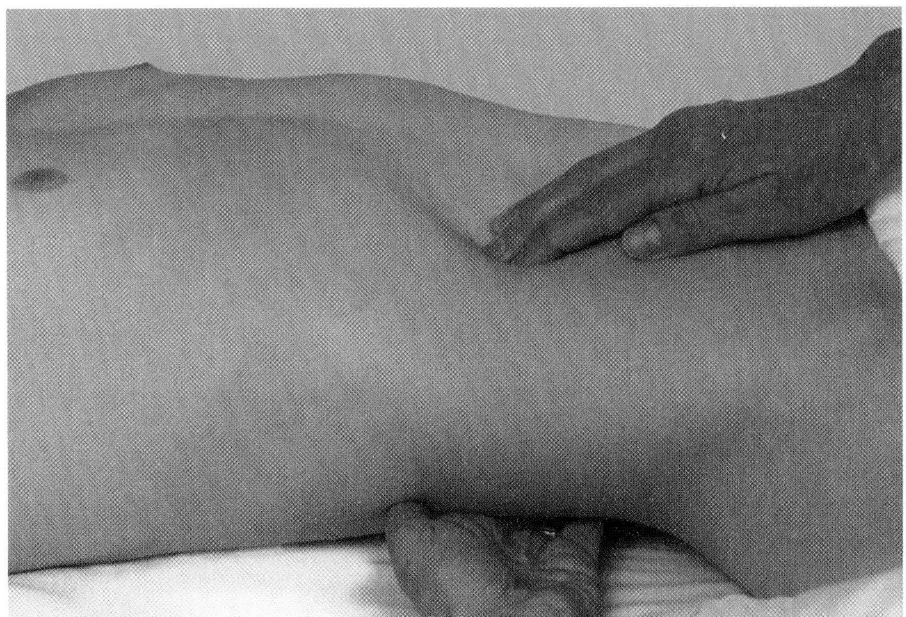

and release. Occasionally, a right kidney is located more anteriorly than usual and then must be distinguished from the liver. The edge of the liver, if palpable, tends to be sharper and to extend farther medially and laterally. It cannot be captured. The lower pole of the kidney is rounded.

Assessing Kidney Tenderness. You may note tenderness when examining the abdomen, but also search for it at each costovertebral angle. Pressure from your fingertips may be enough to elicit tenderness, but if not, use fist percussion. Place the ball of one hand in the costovertebral angle and strike it with the ulnar surface of your fist. Use enough force to cause a perceptible but painless jar or thud in a normal person.

Pain with pressure or fist percussion suggests *pyelonephritis* but may also have a musculoskeletal cause.

To save the patient needless exertion, integrate this assessment with your examination of the back (see p. 10).

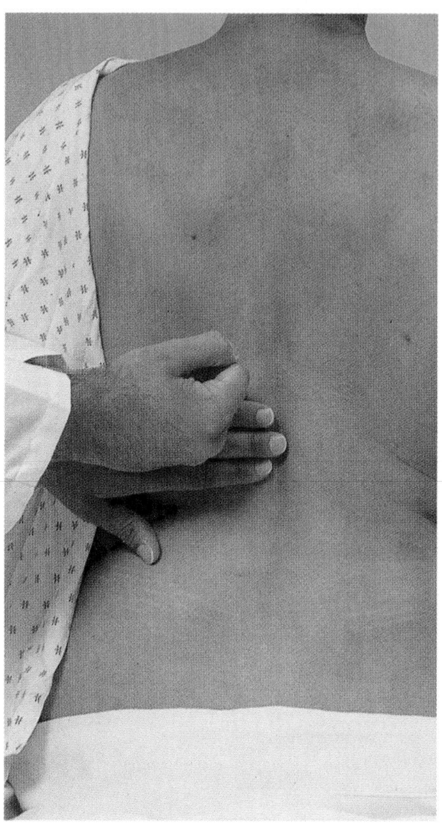

ASSESSING COSTOVERTEBRAL ANGLE TENDERNESS

THE BLADDER

The bladder normally cannot be examined unless it is distended above the symphysis pubis. On palpation, the dome of the distended bladder feels smooth and round. Check for tenderness. Use percussion to check for dullness and to determine how high the bladder rises above the symphysis pubis.

Bladder distention from outlet obstruction due to *urethral stricture, prostatic hyperplasia;* also from medications and neurologic disorders such as *stroke, multiple sclerosis.*

Suprapubic tenderness in *bladder infection*

THE AORTA

Press firmly deep in the upper abdomen, slightly to the left of the midline, and identify the aortic pulsations. In people older than age 50, try to assess the width of the aorta by pressing deeply in the upper abdomen with one hand on each side of the aorta, as illustrated. In this age group, a normal aorta is not more than 3.0 cm wide (average 2.5 cm). This measurement does not include the thickness of the abdominal wall. The ease of feeling

In an older person, a periumbilical or upper abdominal mass with expansile pulsations suggests an *aortic aneurysm.*

aortic pulsations varies greatly with the thickness of the abdominal wall and with the anteroposterior diameter of the abdomen.

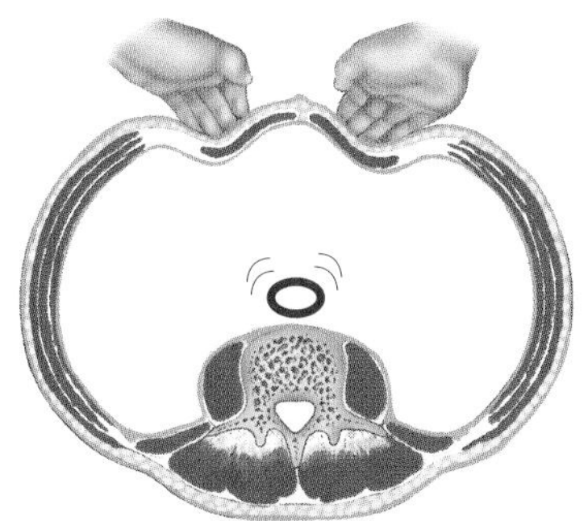

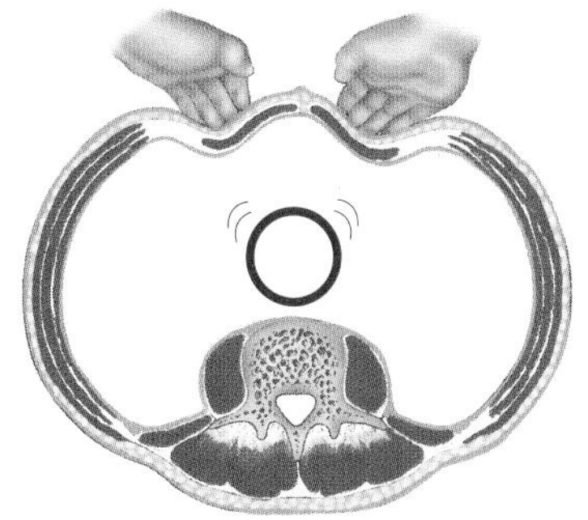

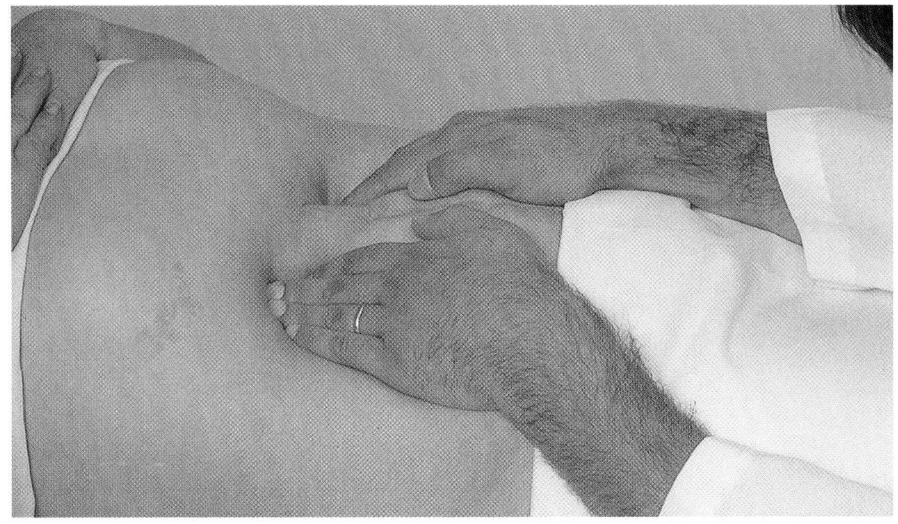

An *aortic aneurysm* is a pathologic dilatation of the aorta, usually due to arteriosclerosis. A merely tortuous abdominal aorta, however, may be difficult to distinguish from an aneurysm on clinical grounds.

Although an aneurysm is usually painless, pain may herald its most dreaded and frequent complication—rupture of the aorta.

Apparent enlargement of the aorta indicates assessment by ultrasound.

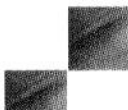

SPECIAL TECHNIQUES

Assessment Techniques for:

- Ascites
- Appendicitis
- Acute cholecystitis
- Ventral hernia
- Mass in abdominal wall

ASSESSING POSSIBLE ASCITES

A protuberant abdomen with bulging flanks suggests the possibility of ascitic fluid. Because ascitic fluid characteristically sinks with gravity, whereas gas-filled loops of bowel float to the top, percussion gives a dull note in dependent areas of the abdomen. Look for such a pattern by percussing outward in several directions from the central area of tympany. Map the border between tympany and dullness.

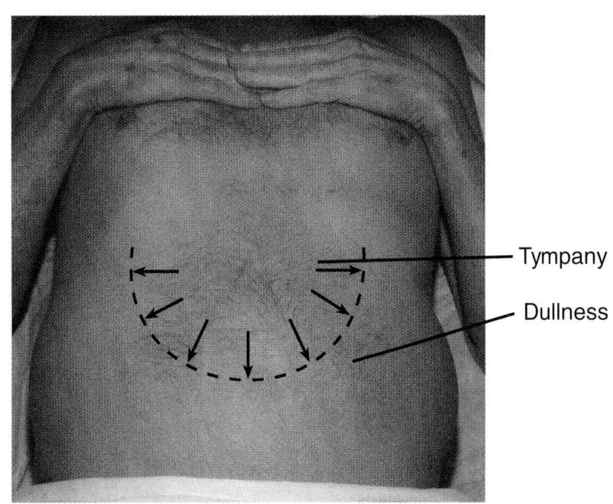

Two further techniques help to confirm ascites, although both signs may be misleading.

- *Test for shifting dullness.* After mapping the borders of tympany and dullness, ask the patient to turn onto one side. Percuss and mark the borders again. In a person without ascites, the borders between tympany and dullness usually stay relatively constant.

In ascites, dullness shifts to the more dependent side, whereas tympany shifts to the top.

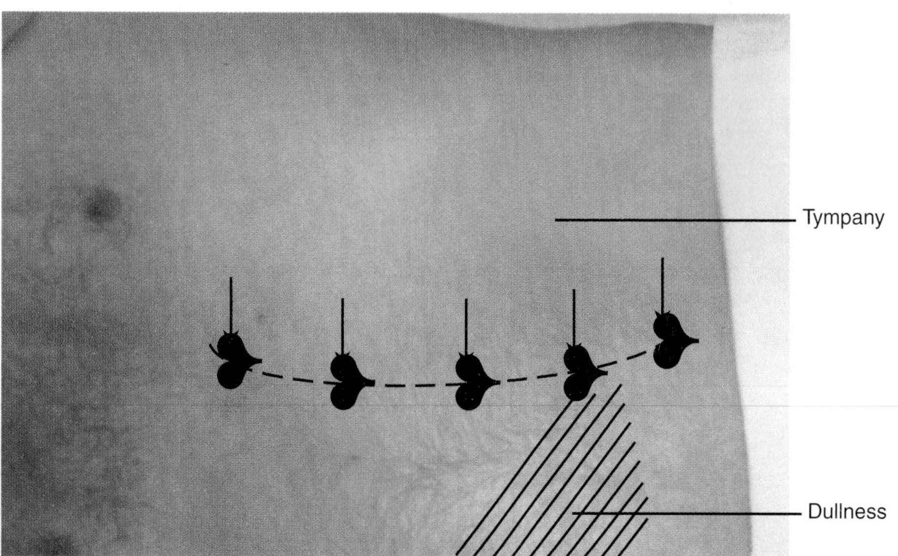

- *Test for a fluid wave.* Ask the patient or an assistant to press the edges of both hands firmly down the midline of the abdomen. This pressure helps to stop the transmission of a wave through fat. While you tap one flank sharply with your fingertips, feel on the opposite flank for an impulse trans-

An easily palpable impulse suggests ascites.

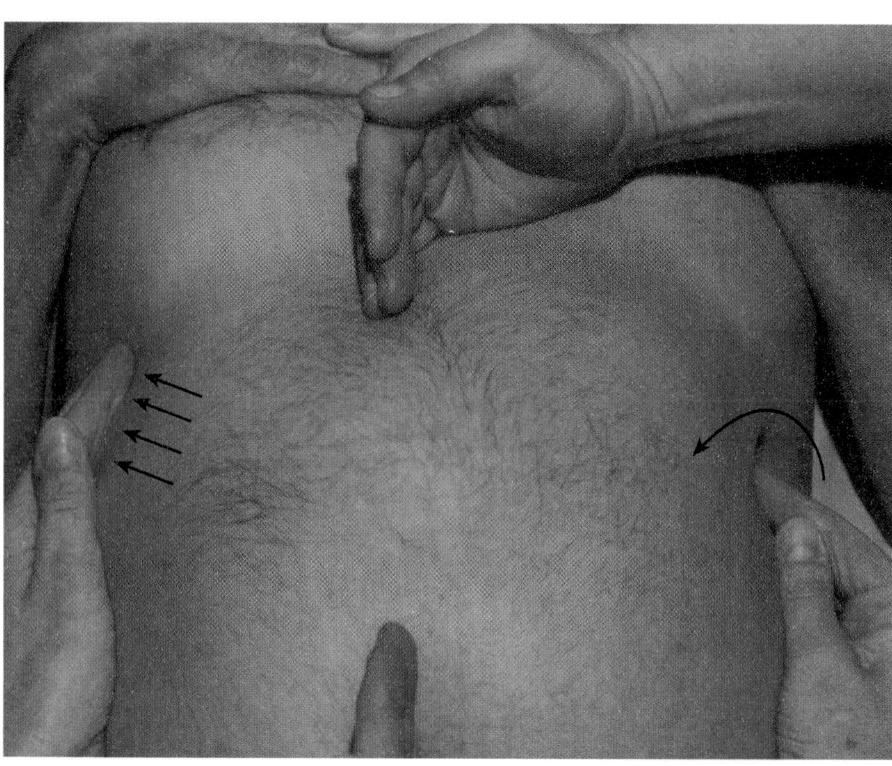

mitted through the fluid. Unfortunately, this sign is often negative until ascites is obvious, and it is sometimes positive in people without ascites.

Identifying an Organ or a Mass in an Ascitic Abdomen. Try to *ballotte* the organ or mass, exemplified here by an enlarged liver. Straighten and stiffen the fingers of one hand together, place them on the abdominal surface, and make a brief jabbing movement directly toward the anticipated structure. This quick movement often displaces the fluid so that your fingertips can briefly touch the surface of the structure through the abdominal wall.

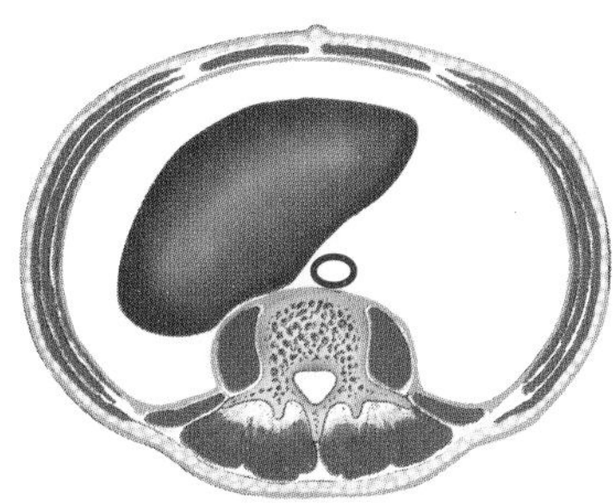

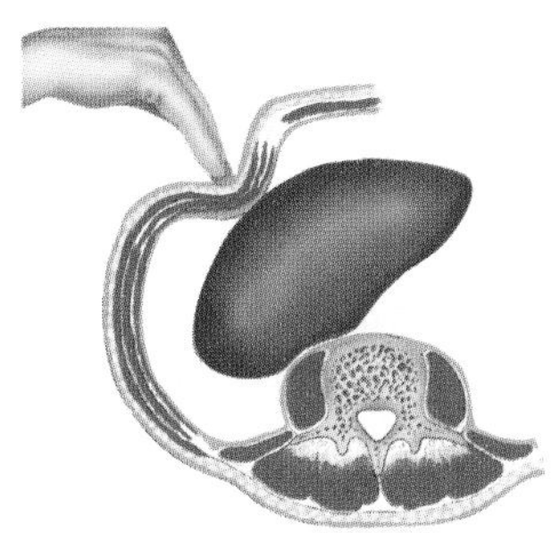

ASSESSING POSSIBLE APPENDICITIS

- Ask the patient to point to where the pain began and where it is now. Ask the patient to cough. Determine whether and where pain results.

The pain of appendicitis classically begins near the umbilicus, then shifts to the right lower quadrant, where coughing increases it. Older patients report this pattern less frequently than younger ones.

- Search carefully for an area of local tenderness.

Localized tenderness anywhere in the right lower quadrant, even in the right flank, may indicate appendicitis.

- Feel for muscular rigidity.

Early voluntary guarding may be replaced by involuntary muscular rigidity.

- *Perform a rectal examination and, in women, a pelvic examination.* These maneuvers may not help you to discriminate between a normal and an inflamed appendix, but they may help to identify an inflamed appendix atypically located within the pelvic cavity. They may also suggest other causes of the abdominal pain.

Right-sided rectal tenderness may be caused by, for example, inflamed adnexa or an inflamed seminal vesicle, as well as by an inflamed appendix.

Additional techniques are sometimes helpful:

- Check the tender area for rebound tenderness. (If other signs are typically positive, you can save the patient unnecessary pain by omitting this test.)

Rebound tenderness suggests peritoneal inflammation, as from appendicitis.

- Check for *Rovsing's sign* and for referred rebound tenderness. Press deeply and evenly in the *left* lower quadrant. Then quickly withdraw your fingers.

Pain in the *right* lower quadrant during *left*-sided pressure suggests appendicitis (a positive Rovsing's sign). So does right lower quadrant pain on quick withdrawal (*referred rebound tenderness*).

- Look for a *psoas sign*. Place your hand just above the patient's right knee and ask the patient to raise that thigh against your hand. Alternatively, ask the patient to turn onto the left side. Then extend the patient's right leg at the hip. Flexion of the leg at the hip makes the psoas muscle contract; extension stretches it.

Increased abdominal pain on either maneuver constitutes a *positive psoas* sign, suggesting irritation of the psoas muscle by an inflamed appendix.

- Look for an *obturator sign*. Flex the patient's right thigh at the hip, with the knee bent, and rotate the leg internally at the hip. This maneuver stretches the internal obturator muscle. (Internal rotation of the hip is described on p. 542.)

Right hypogastric pain constitutes a positive obturator sign, suggesting irritation of the obturator muscle by an inflamed appendix.

- Test for *cutaneous hyperesthesia*. At a series of points down the abdominal wall, gently pick up a fold of skin between your thumb and index finger, without pinching it. This maneuver should not normally be painful.

Localized pain with this maneuver, in all or part of the right lower quadrant, may accompany appendicitis.

ASSESSING POSSIBLE ACUTE CHOLECYSTITIS

When right upper quadrant pain and tenderness suggest acute cholecystitis, look for *Murphy's sign*. Hook your left thumb or the fingers of your right hand under the costal margin at the point where the lateral border of the rectus muscle intersects with the costal margin. Alternatively, if the liver is enlarged, hook your thumb or fingers under the liver edge at a comparable point below. Ask the patient to take a deep breath. Watch the patient's breathing and note the degree of tenderness.

A sharp increase in tenderness with a sudden stop in inspiratory effort constitutes a *positive Murphy's sign* of *acute cholecystitis.* Hepatic tenderness may also increase with this maneuver, but is usually less well localized.

ASSESSING VENTRAL HERNIAS

Ventral hernias are hernias in the abdominal wall exclusive of groin hernias. If you suspect but do not see an umbilical or incisional hernia, ask the patient to raise both head and shoulders off the table.

The bulge of a hernia will usually appear with this action (see p. 419).

Inguinal and femoral hernias are discussed in the next chapter. They can give rise to important abdominal problems and must not be overlooked.

The cause of intestinal obstruction or peritonitis may be missed by overlooking a strangulated femoral hernia.

MASS IN THE ABDOMINAL WALL

To Distinguish an Abdominal Mass From a Mass in the Abdominal Wall. An occasional mass is in the abdominal wall rather than inside the abdominal cavity. Ask the patient either to raise the head and shoulders or to strain down, thus tightening the abdominal muscles. Feel for the mass again.

A mass in the abdominal wall remains palpable; an intra-abdominal mass is obscured by muscular contraction.

RECORDING YOUR FINDINGS

Note that initially you may use sentences to describe your findings; later you will use phrases. The style below contains phrases appropriate for most write-ups.

Recording the Physical Examination—The Abdomen

"Abdomen is protuberant with active bowel sounds. It is soft and nontender; no masses or hepatosplenomegaly. Liver span is 7 cm in the right midclavicular line; edge is smooth and palpable 1 cm below the right costal margin. Spleen and kidneys not felt. No costovertebral angle (CVA) tenderness."

OR

"Abdomen is flat. No bowel sounds heard. It is firm and boardlike, with increased tenderness, guarding, and rebound in the right midquadrant. Liver percusses to 7 cm in the midclavicular line; edge not felt. Spleen and kidneys not felt. No CVA tenderness.

Suggests peritonitis from possible appendicitis (see pp. 389–400 and pp. 387–388)

Bibliography

CITATIONS

1. Regier DA, Farmer ME, Rae DS, et al. Comorbidity of mental disorders with alcohol and other drug abuse. Results from the Epidemiologic Catchment Area (ECA) Study. JAMA 264(19): 2511–2518, 1990.
2. U.S. Preventive Services Task Force. Screening and Behavioral Counseling Interventions in Primary Care to Reduce Alcohol Misuse: Recommendation Statement. Rockville, MD, Agency for Healthcare Research and Quality, April 2004. Available at: http://www.ahrq.gov/clinic/3rduspstf/alcohol/alcomisrs.htm. Accessed December 4, 2004.
3. Ewing JA. Detecting alcoholism: the CAGE questionnaire. JAMA 252(14):1905–1907, 1984.
4. Whitlock EP, Green CA, Polen MR. Behavioral Counseling Interventions in Primary Care to Reduce Risky/Harmful Alcohol Use, Systematic Evidence Review. No. 30. (Prepared by the Oregon Evidence-based Practice Center under Contract No. 290-97-0018). Rockville, MD, Agency for Healthcare Research and Quality, April 2004. Available at www.ahrq/gov/clinic/serfiles.htm.
5. Whitlock EP, Orleans CT, Pender N., Allan J. Evaluating primary care behavioral counseling interventions. An evidence-based approach. Am J Prev Med 22(4):267–284, 2002.
6. Fiellin DA, Reid MC, O'Connor PG. Screening for alcohol problems in primary care: a systematic review. Arch Intern Med 160(13):1977–1989, 2000.
7. Miller WR, Rollnick S, Con K. Motivational Interviewing: Preparing People for Change, 2nd ed. New York, Guilford Press, 2002.
8. Miller WR, Sanchez VC. Motivating Young Alcoholics for Treatment and Lifestyle Changes. In Howard G (ed): Issues in Alcohol Use and Misuse by Young Adults. Notre Dame, IN, University of Notre Dame Press, 1993.
9. U.S. Preventive Services Task Force. Screening for Hepatitis B Infection: Recommendation Statement. Rockville, MD, Agency for Healthcare Research and Quality, February 2004. Available at: http://www.ahrq.gov/clinic/3rduspstf/hepbscr/hepbrs.htm. Accessed December 4, 2004.
10. U.S. Preventive Services Task Force. Screening for Hepatitis C Infection: Recommendation Statement. Rockville, MD, Agency for Healthcare Research and Quality, March 2004. Available at: http://www.ahrq.gov/clinic/uspstf/uspshepc.htm. Accessed December 4, 2004.
11. U.S. Preventive Services Task Force Screening for Colorectal Cancer: Recommendations and Rationale. Rockville, MD, Agency for Healthcare Research and Quality, July 2002. Available at: http://www.ahrq.gov/clinic/3rduspstf/colorectal/colorr.htm. Accessed December 4, 2004.
12. Winawer SJ, Shike M. Prevention and control of colorectal cancer. In Greenwald P, Kramer BS, Weed DL, eds. Cancer Prevention and Control. New York, Marcel-Dekker, 537–560, 1995.
13. American Cancer Society. ACS cancer detection guidelines. Available at: www.cancer.org. Accessed November 18, 2004.
14. U.S. Preventive Services Task Force. Screening for colorectal cancer. In Guide to Clinical Preventive Services, 2nd ed. Baltimore, Williams & Wilkins, 89–103, 1996.

ADDITIONAL REFERENCES

Examination of the Abdomen

Fink HA, Lederle FA, Rptj CS. The accuracy of physical examination to detect abdominal aortic aneurysm. Arch Intern Med 160(6):833–836, 2000.

Lederle FA, Simel DL. Does the patient have abdominal aortic aneurysm? JAMA 281(1):77–82, 1999.

McGee SR. Percussion and physical diagnosis: separating myth from science. Dis Mon 41(10):641–688, 1995.

Silen W, Cope Z. Cope's Early Diagnosis of the Acute Abdomen, 21st ed. Oxford, UK, and New York, Oxford University Press, 2005.

Sleisenger MH, Feldman M, Griedman LS, et al (eds). Sleisenger and Fortran's Gastrointestinal and Liver Disease: Pathophysiology, Diagnosis, Management, 8th ed. Philadelphia, WB Saunders, 2006.

Turnbull JM. Is listening for abdominal bruits useful in the evaluation of hypertension? JAMA 274(16):1299–1301, 1995.

Yamamoto W, Kono H, Maekawa H, et al. The relationship between abdominal pain regions and specific diseases: an epidemiologic approach to clinical practice. J Epidemiol 7(1):27–32, 1997.

Examination of the Liver

Meidl EJ, Ende J. Evaluation of liver size by physical examination. J Gen Intern Med 8(11):635–637, 1993.

Naylor CD. Physical examination of the liver. JAMA 271(23): 1859–1865, 1994.

Williams JW, Simel DL. Does this patient have ascites? How to divine fluid in the abdomen. JAMA 267(19):2645–2648, 1992.

Zoli M, Magliotti D, Drimaldi M, et al. Physical examination of the liver: is it still worth it? Am J Gastroenterol 90(9):1428–1432, 1995.

Examination of the Spleen

Barkun ANB, Camus M, Green L, et al. The bedside assessment of splenic enlargement. Am J Med 91(5):512–518, 1991.

Barkun AN, Camus M, Meagher T, et al. Splenic enlargement and Traube's space: how useful is percussion? Am J Med 87(5): 562–566, 1989.

Grover SA, Barkun AN, Sackett DL. Does this patient have splenomegaly? JAMA 270(18):2218–1121, 1993.

Tamayo SG, Rickman LS, Matthews WC, et al. Examiner dependence on physical diagnostic tests of splenomegaly: a prospective study with multiple observers. J Gen Intern Med 8(2):69–75, 1993.

Gastrointestinal Conditions

Craig AS, Schaffner W. Prevention of hepatitis A with the hepatitis A vaccine. N Engl J Med 350(5):476–480, 2004.

Lembo A, Camilleri M. Chronic constipation. N Engl J Med 349(14):1360–1368, 2003.

Mertz HR. Irritable bowel syndrome. N Engl J Med 349(22): 2136–2146, 2003.

Thielman NM, Guerrant RL. Acute infectious diarrhea. N Engl J Med 350(1):38–47, 2004.

TABLE 10-1 Abdominal Pain

Problem	Process	Location	Quality
Peptic Ulcer and Dyspepsia *(These disorders cannot be reliably differentiated by symptoms and signs.)*	Peptic ulcer refers to a demonstrable ulcer, usually in the duodenum or stomach. Dyspepsia causes similar symptoms but no ulceration. Infection by *Helicobacter pylori* is often present.	Epigastric, may radiate to the back	Variable: gnawing burning, boring, aching, pressing, or hungerlike
Cancer of the Stomach	A malignant neoplasm	Epigastric	Variable
Acute Pancreatitis	An acute inflammation of the pancreas	Epigastric, may radiate to the back or other parts of the abdomen; may be poorly localized	Usually steady
Chronic Pancreatitis	Fibrosis of the pancreas secondary to recurrent inflammation	Epigastric, radiating through to the back	Steady, deep
Cancer of the Pancreas	A malignant neoplasm	Epigastric and in either upper quadrant; often radiates to the back	Steady, deep
Biliary Colic	Sudden obstruction of the cystic duct or common bile duct by a gallstone	Epigastric or right upper quadrant; may radiate to the right scapula and shoulder	Steady, aching; *not* colicky
Acute Cholecystitis	Inflammation of the gallbladder, usually from obstruction of the cystic duct by a gallstone	Right upper quadrant or upper abdominal; may radiate to the right scapular area	Steady, aching
Acute Diverticulitis	Acute inflammation of a colonic diverticulum, a saclike mucosal outpouching through the colonic muscle	Left lower quadrant	May be cramping at first, but becomes steady
Acute Appendicitis	Acute inflammation of the appendix with distention or obstruction	▪ Poorly localized *periumbilical pain,* followed usually by ▪ *Right lower quadrant pain*	▪ Mild but increasing, possibly cramping ▪ Steady and more severe
Acute Mechanical Intestinal Obstruction	Obstruction of the bowel lumen, most commonly caused by (1) adhesions or hernias (small bowel), or (2) cancer or diverticulitis (colon)	▪ *Small bowel:* periumbilical or upper abdominal ▪ *Colon:* lower abdominal or generalized	▪ Cramping ▪ Cramping
Mesenteric Ischemia	Blood supply to the bowel and mesentery blocked from thrombosis or embolus (acute arterial occlusion), or reduced from hypoperfusion	May be periumbilical at first, then diffuse	Cramping at first, then steady

Timing	Factors That May Aggravate	Factors That May Relieve	Associated Symptoms and Setting
Intermittent. Duodenal ulcer is more likely than gastric ulcer or dyspepsia to cause pain that (1) wakes the patient at night, and (2) occurs intermittently over a few weeks, then disappears for months, and then recurs.	Variable	Food and antacids may bring relief, but not necessarily in any of these disorders and least commonly in gastric ulcer.	Nausea, vomiting, belching, bloating; heartburn (more common in duodenal ulcer); weight loss (more common in gastric ulcer). Dyspepsia is more common in the young (20–29 yrs), gastric ulcer in those over 50 yrs, and duodenal ulcer in those from 30–60 yrs.
The history of pain is typically shorter than in peptic ulcer. The pain is persistent and slowly progressive.	Often food	*Not* relieved by food or antacids	Anorexia, nausea, early satiety, weight loss, and sometimes bleeding. Most common in ages 50–70
Acute onset, persistent pain	Lying supine	Leaning forward with trunk flexed	Nausea, vomiting, abdominal distention, fever. Often a history of previous attacks and alcohol abuse or gallstones
Chronic or recurrent course	Alcohol, heavy or fatty meals	Possibly leaning forward with trunk flexed; often intractable	Symptoms of decreased pancreatic function may appear: diarrhea with fatty stools (steatorrhea) and diabetes mellitus.
Persistent pain; relentlessly progressive illness		Possibly leaning forward with trunk flexed; often intractable	Anorexia, nausea, vomiting, weight loss, and jaundice. Emotional symptoms, including depression
Rapid onset over a few minutes, lasts one to several hours and subsides gradually. Often recurrent			Anorexia, nausea, vomiting, restlessness
Gradual onset; course longer than in biliary colic	Jarring, deep breathing		Anorexia, nausea, vomiting, fever
Often a gradual onset			Fever, constipation. There may be initial brief diarrhea.
▪ Lasts roughly 4–6 hr ▪ Depends on intervention	▪ Movement or cough	▪ If it subsides temporarily, suspect perforation of the appendix.	Anorexia, nausea, possibly vomiting, which typically follow the onset of pain; low fever
▪ Paroxysmal; may decrease as bowel mobility is impaired			▪ Vomiting of bile and mucus (high obstruction) or fecal material (low obstruction). Obstipation develops.
▪ Paroxysmal, though typically milder			▪ Obstipation early. Vomiting late if at all. Prior symptoms of underlying cause.
Usually abrupt in onset, then persistent			Vomiting, diarrhea (sometimes bloody), constipation, shock

TABLE 10-2 Dysphagia

Process and Problem	Timing	Factors That Aggravate	Factors That Relieve	Associated Symptoms and Conditions
Transfer Dysphagia, *due to motor disorders affecting the pharyngeal muscles*	Acute or gradual onset and a variable course, depending on the underlying disorder	Attempts to start the swallowing process		Aspiration into the lungs or regurgitation into the nose with attempts to swallow. Neurologic evidence of stroke, bulbar palsy, or other neuromuscular conditions
Esophageal Dysphagia				
Mechanical Narrowing				
▪ Mucosal rings and webs	Intermittent	Solid foods	Regurgitation of the bolus of food	Usually none
▪ Esophageal stricture	Intermittent, may become slowly progressive	Solid foods	Regurgitation of the bolus of food	A long history of heartburn and regurgitation
▪ Esophageal cancer	May be intermittent at first; progressive over months	Solid foods, with progression to liquids	Regurgitation of the bolus of food	Pain in the chest and back and weight loss, especially late in the course of illness
Motor Disorders				
▪ Diffuse esophageal spasm	Intermittent	Solids or liquids	Maneuvers described below; sometimes nitroglycerin	Chest pain that mimics angina pectoris or myocardial infarction and lasts minutes to hours; possibly heartburn
▪ Scleroderma	Intermittent, may progress slowly	Solids or liquids	Repeated swallowing, movements such as straightening the back, raising the arms, or a Valsalva maneuver (straining down against a closed glottis)	Heartburn. Other manifestations of scleroderma
▪ Achalasia	Intermittent, may progress	Solids or liquids		Regurgitation, often at night when lying down, with nocturnal cough; possibly chest pain precipitated by eating

TABLE 10-3 Constipation

Problem	Process	Associated Symptoms and Setting
Life Activities and Habits		
Inadequate Time or Setting for the Defecation Reflex	Ignoring the sensation of a full rectum inhibits the defecation reflex.	Hectic schedules, unfamiliar surroundings, bed rest
False Expectations of Bowel Habits	Expectations of "regularity" or more frequent stools than a person's norm	Beliefs, treatments, and advertisements that promote the use of laxatives
Diet Deficient in Fiber	Decreased fecal bulk	Other factors such as debilitation and constipating drugs may contribute.
Irritable Bowel Syndrome	A common disorder of bowel motility	Small, hard stools, often with mucus. Periods of diarrhea. Cramping abdominal pain. Stress may aggravate.
Mechanical Obstruction		
Cancer of the Rectum or Sigmoid Colon	Progressive narrowing of the bowel lumen	Change in bowel habits; often diarrhea, abdominal pain, and bleeding. In rectal cancer, tenesmus and pencil-shaped stools
Fecal Impaction	A large, firm, immovable fecal mass, most often in the rectum	Rectal fullness, abdominal pain, and diarrhea around the impaction. Common in debilitated, bedridden, and often elderly patients
Other Obstructing Lesions (such as diverticulitis, volvulus, intussusception, or hernia)	Narrowing or complete obstruction of the bowel	Colicky abdominal pain, abdominal distention, and in intussusception, often "currant jelly" stools (red blood and mucus)
Painful Anal Lesions	Pain may cause spasm of the external sphincter and voluntary inhibition of the defecation reflex.	Anal fissures, painful hemorrhoids, perirectal abscesses
Drugs	A variety of mechanisms	Opiates, anticholinergics, antacids containing calcium or aluminum, and many others
Depression	A disorder of mood. See Table 16-1, Disorders of Mood.	Fatigue, feelings of depression, and other somatic symptoms
Neurologic Disorders	Interference with the autonomic innervation of the bowel	Spinal cord injuries, multiple sclerosis, Hirschsprung's disease, and other conditions
Metabolic Conditions	Interference with bowel motility	Pregnancy, hypothyroidism, hypercalcemia

TABLE 10-4 Diarrhea

Problem	Process	Characteristics of Stool
Acute Diarrhea		
Secretory Infections	Infection by viruses, preformed bacterial toxins (such as *Staphylococcus aureus, Clostridium perfringens,* toxigenic *Escherichia coli, Vibrio cholerae*), cryptosporidium, *Giardia lamblia*	Watery, without blood, pus, or mucus
Inflammatory Infections	Colonization or invasion of intestinal mucosa (nontyphoid *Salmonella, Shigella, Yersinia, Campylobacter,* enteropathic *E. coli, Entamoeba histolytica*)	Loose to watery, often with blood, pus, or mucus
Drug-Induced Diarrhea	Action of many drugs, such as magnesium-containing antacids, antibiotics, antineoplastic agents, and laxatives	Loose to watery
Chronic Diarrhea		
Diarrheal Syndromes		
▪ Irritable bowel syndrome	A disorder of bowel motility with alternating diarrhea and constipation	Loose; may show mucus but no blood. Small, hard stools with constipation
▪ Cancer of the sigmoid colon	Partial obstruction by a malignant neoplasm	May be blood-streaked
Inflammatory Bowel Disease		
▪ Ulcerative colitis	Inflammation of the mucosa and submucosa of the rectum and colon with ulceration; cause unknown	Soft to watery, often containing blood
▪ Crohn's disease of the small bowel (regional enteritis) or colon (granulomatous colitis)	Chronic inflammation of the bowel wall, typically involving the terminal ileum and/or proximal colon	Small, soft to loose or watery, usually free of gross blood (enteritis) or with less bleeding than ulcerative colitis (colitis)
Voluminous Diarrheas		
▪ Malabsorption syndromes	Defective absorption of fat, including fat-soluble vitamins, with steatorrhea (excessive excretion of fat) as in pancreatic insufficiency, bile salt deficiency, bacterial overgrowth	Typically bulky, soft, light yellow to gray, mushy, greasy or oily, and sometimes frothy; particularly foul-smelling; usually floats in the toilet
▪ Osmotic diarrheas		
Lactose intolerance	Deficiency in intestinal lactase	Watery diarrhea of large volume
Abuse of osmotic purgatives	Laxative habit, often surreptitious	Watery diarrhea of large volume
▪ Secretory diarrheas from bacterial infection, secreting villous adenoma, fat or bile salt malabsorption, hormone-mediated conditions (gastrin in Zollinger–Ellison syndrome, vasoactive intestinal peptide [VIP])	Variable	Watery diarrhea of large volume

Timing	Associated Symptoms	Setting, Persons at Risk
Duration of a few days, possibly longer. Lactase deficiency may lead to a longer course.	Nausea, vomiting, periumbilical cramping pain. Temperature normal or slightly elevated	Often travel, a common food source, or an epidemic
An acute illness of varying duration	Lower abdominal cramping pain and often rectal urgency, tenesmus; fever	Travel, contaminated food or water. Men and women who have had frequent anal intercourse.
Acute, recurrent, or chronic	Possibly nausea; usually little if any pain	Prescribed or over-the-counter medications
Often worse in the morning. Diarrhea rarely wakes the patient at night.	Crampy lower abdominal pain, abdominal distention, flatulence, nausea, constipation	Young and middle-aged adults, especially women
Variable	Change in usual bowel habits, crampy lower abdominal pain, constipation	Middle-aged and older adults, especially older than 55 yrs
Onset ranges from insidious to acute. Typically recurrent, may be persistent. Diarrhea may wake the patient at night.	Crampy lower or generalized abdominal pain, anorexia, weakness, fever	Often young people
Insidious onset, chronic or recurrent. Diarrhea may wake the patient at night.	Crampy periumbilical or right lower quadrant (enteritis) or diffuse (colitis) pain, with anorexia, low fever, and/or weight loss. Perianal or perirectal abscesses and fistulas	Often young people, especially in the late teens, but also in the middle years. More common in people of Jewish descent
Onset of illness typically insidious	Anorexia, weight loss, fatigue, abdominal distention, often crampy lower abdominal pain. Symptoms of nutritional deficiencies such as bleeding (vitamin K), bone pain and fractures (vitamin D), glossitis (vitamin B), and edema (protein)	Variable, depending on cause
Follows the ingestion of milk and milk products; is relieved by fasting	Crampy abdominal pain, abdominal distention, flatulence	African Americans, Asians, Native Americans
Variable	Often none	Persons with anorexia nervosa or bulimia nervosa
Variable	Weight loss, dehydration, nausea, vomiting, and cramping abdominal pain	Variable depending on cause

TABLE 10-5 Black and Bloody Stools

Problem	Selected Causes	Associated Symptoms and Setting
Melena Melena refers to the passage of black, tarry (sticky and shiny) stools. Tests for occult blood are positive. Melena signifies the loss of at least 60 ml of blood into the gastrointestinal tract (less in infants and children), usually from the esophagus, stomach, or duodenum. Less commonly, when intestinal transit is slow, the blood may originate in the jejunum, ileum, or ascending colon. In infants, melena may result from swallowing blood during the birth process.	Peptic ulcer	Often, but not necessarily, a history of epigastric pain
	Gastritis or stress ulcers	Recent ingestion of alcohol, aspirin, or other anti-inflammatory drugs; recent bodily trauma, severe burns, surgery, or increased intracranial pressure
	Esophageal or gastric varices	Cirrhosis of the liver or other cause of portal hypertension
	Reflux esophagitis	History of heartburn
	Mallory-Weiss tear, a mucosal tear in the esophagus due to retching and vomiting	Retching, vomiting, often recent ingestion of alcohol
Black, Nonsticky Stools Black stools may result from other causes and then usually give negative results when tested for occult blood. (Ingestion of iron or other substances, however, may cause a positive test result in the absence of blood.) These stools have no pathologic significance.	Ingestion of iron, bismuth salts as in Pepto-Bismol, licorice, or even commercial chocolate cookies	
Red Blood in the Stools Red blood usually originates in the colon, rectum, or anus, and much less frequently in the jejunum or ileum. Upper gastrointestinal hemorrhage, however, may also cause red stools. The amount of blood lost is then usually large (more than a liter). Transit time through the intestinal tract is accordingly rapid, giving insufficient time for the blood to turn black.	Cancer of the colon	Often a change in bowel habits
	Benign polyps of the colon	Often no other symptoms
	Diverticula of the colon	Often no other symptoms
	Inflammatory conditions of the colon and rectum	
	▪ Ulcerative colitis, Crohn's disease	See Table 10-4, Diarrhea.
	▪ Infectious dysenteries	See Table 10-4, Diarrhea.
	▪ Proctitis (various causes) in men or women who have had frequent anal intercourse	Rectal urgency, tenesmus
	Ischemic colitis	Lower abdominal pain and sometimes fever or shock in persons older than age 50 yrs
	Hemorrhoids	Blood on the toilet paper, on the surface of the stool, or dripping into the toilet
	Anal fissure	Blood on the toilet paper or on the surface of the stool; anal pain
Reddish but Nonbloody Stools	Ingestion of beets	Pink urine, which usually precedes the reddish stool

TABLE 10-6 Frequency, Nocturia, and Polyuria

Problem	Mechanisms	Selected Causes	Associated Symptoms
Frequency	Decreased capacity of the bladder		
	▪ Increased bladder sensitivity to stretch because of inflammation	*Infection*, stones, tumor, or foreign body in the bladder	Burning on urination, urinary urgency, sometimes gross hematuria
	▪ Decreased elasticity of the bladder wall	Infiltration by scar tissue or tumor	Symptoms of associated inflammation (see above) are common.
	▪ Decreased cortical inhibition of bladder contractions	Motor disorders of the central nervous system, such as a stroke	Urinary urgency; neurologic symptoms such as weakness and paralysis
	Impaired emptying of the bladder, with residual urine in the bladder		
	▪ Partial mechanical obstruction of the bladder neck or proximal urethra	Most commonly, benign prostatic hyperplasia; also urethral stricture and other obstructive lesions of the bladder or prostate	Prior obstructive symptoms: hesitancy in starting the urinary stream, straining to void, reduced size and force of the stream, and dribbling during or at the end of urination
	▪ Loss of peripheral nerve supply to the bladder	Neurologic disease affecting the sacral nerves or nerve roots, e.g., diabetic neuropathy	Weakness or sensory defects
Nocturia			
With High Volumes	Most types of polyuria (see p. 369)		
	Decreased concentrating ability of the kidney with loss of the normal decrease in nocturnal urinary output	Chronic renal insufficiency due to a number of diseases	Possibly other symptoms of renal insufficiency
	Excessive fluid intake before bedtime	Habit, especially involving alcohol and coffee	
	Fluid-retaining, edematous states. Dependent edema accumulates during the day and is excreted when the patient lies down at night.	Congestive heart failure, nephrotic syndrome, hepatic cirrhosis with ascites, chronic venous insufficiency	Edema and other symptoms of the underlying disorder. Urinary output during the day may be reduced as fluid reaccumulates in the body. See Table 14-4, Some Peripheral Causes of Edema.
With Low Volumes	Frequency		
	Voiding while up at night without a real urge, a "pseudo-frequency"	Insomnia	Variable
Polyuria	Deficiency of antidiuretic hormone (diabetes insipidus)	A disorder of the posterior pituitary and hypothalamus	Thirst and polydipsia, often severe and persistent; nocturia
	Renal unresponsiveness to antidiuretic hormone (nephrogenic diabetes insipidus)	A number of kidney diseases, including hypercalcemic and hypokalemic nephropathy; drug toxicity, e.g., from lithium	Thirst and polydipsia, often severe and persistent; nocturia
	Solute diuresis		
	▪ Electrolytes, such as sodium salts	Large saline infusions, potent diuretics, certain kidney diseases	Variable
	▪ Nonelectrolytes, such as glucose	Uncontrolled diabetes mellitus	Thirst, polydipsia, and nocturia
	Excessive water intake	Primary polydipsia	Polydipsia tends to be episodic. Thirst may not be present. Nocturia is usually absent.

TABLE 10-7 Urinary Incontinence*

Problem	Mechanisms
Stress Incontinence The urethral sphincter is weakened so that transient increases in intra-abdominal pressure raise the bladder pressure to levels that exceed urethral resistance.	In women, most often a weakness of the pelvic floor with inadequate muscular support of the bladder and proximal urethra and a change in the angle between the bladder and the urethra. Suggested causes include childbirth and surgery. Local conditions affecting the internal urethral sphincter, such as postmenopausal atrophy of the mucosa and urethral infection, may also contribute. In men, stress incontinence may follow prostatic surgery.
Urge Incontinence Detrusor contractions are stronger than normal and overcome the normal urethral resistance. The bladder is typically *small.*	▪ Decreased cortical inhibition of detrusor contractions, as by strokes, brain tumors, dementia, and lesions of the spinal cord above the sacral level ▪ Hyperexcitability of sensory pathways, as in bladder infections, tumors, and fecal impaction ▪ Deconditioning of voiding reflexes, as in frequent voluntary voiding at low bladder volumes
Overflow Incontinence Detrusor contractions are insufficient to overcome urethral resistance. The bladder is typically *large,* even after an effort to void.	▪ Obstruction of the bladder outlet, as by benign prostatic hyperplasia or tumor ▪ Weakness of the detrusor muscle associated with peripheral nerve disease at the sacral level ▪ Impaired bladder sensation that interrupts the reflex arc, as from diabetic neuropathy
Functional Incontinence This is a functional inability to get to the toilet in time because of impaired health or environmental conditions.	Problems in mobility resulting from weakness, arthritis, poor vision, or other conditions. Environmental factors such as an unfamiliar setting, distant bathroom facilities, bed rails, or physical restraints
Incontinence Secondary to Medications Drugs may contribute to any type of incontinence listed.	Sedatives, tranquilizers, anticholinergics, sympathetic blockers, and potent diuretics

*Patients may have more than one kind of incontinence.

Symptoms	Physical Signs
Momentary leakage of small amounts of urine concurrent with stresses such as coughing, laughing, and sneezing while the person is in an upright position. A desire to urinate is not associated with pure stress incontinence.	The bladder is not detected on abdominal examination. Stress incontinence may be demonstrable, especially if the patient is examined before voiding and in a standing position. Atrophic vaginitis may be evident.
Incontinence preceded by an urge to void. The volume tends to be moderate. Urgency Frequency and nocturia with small to moderate volumes If acute inflammation is present, pain on urination Possibly "pseudo-stress incontinence"—voiding 10–20 sec after stresses such as a change of position, going up or down stairs, and possibly coughing, laughing, or sneezing	The bladder is not detectable on abdominal examination. When cortical inhibition is decreased, mental deficits or motor signs of central nervous system disease are often, though not necessarily, present. When sensory pathways are hyperexcitable, signs of local pelvic problems or a fecal impaction may be present.
A continuous dripping or dribbling incontinence Decreased force of the urinary stream Prior symptoms of partial urinary obstruction or other symptoms of peripheral nerve disease may be present.	An enlarged bladder is often found on abdominal examination and may be tender. Other possible signs include prostatic enlargement, motor signs of peripheral nerve disease, a decrease in sensation including perineal sensation, and diminished to absent reflexes.
Incontinence on the way to the toilet or only in the early morning	The bladder is not detectable on physical examination. Look for physical or environmental clues to the likely cause.
Variable. A careful history and chart review are important.	Variable

TABLE 10-8 Localized Bulges in the Abdominal Wall

Localized bulges in the abdominal wall include *ventral hernias* (defects in the wall through which tissue protrudes) and subcutaneous tumors such as *lipomas.* The more common ventral hernias are umbilical, incisional, and epigastric. Hernias and a rectus diastasis usually become more evident when the patient raises head and shoulders from a supine position.

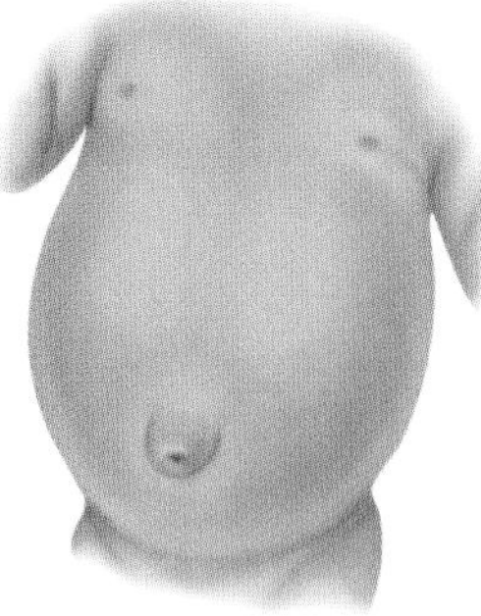

INFANT

Umbilical Hernia

A protrusion through a defective umbilical ring is most common in infants but also occurs in adults. In infants, but not in adults, it usually closes spontaneously within 1 to 2 years.

Diastasis Recti

Separation of the two rectus abdominis muscles, through which abdominal contents form a midline ridge when the patient raises head and shoulders. Often is seen in repeated pregnancies, obesity, and chronic lung disease. It has no clinical consequences.

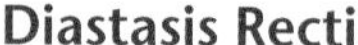

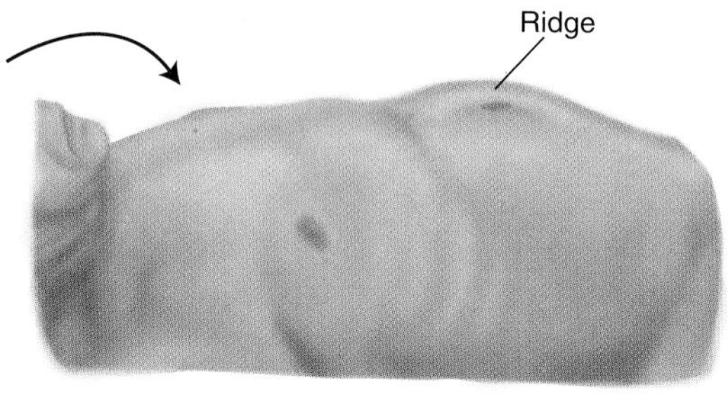

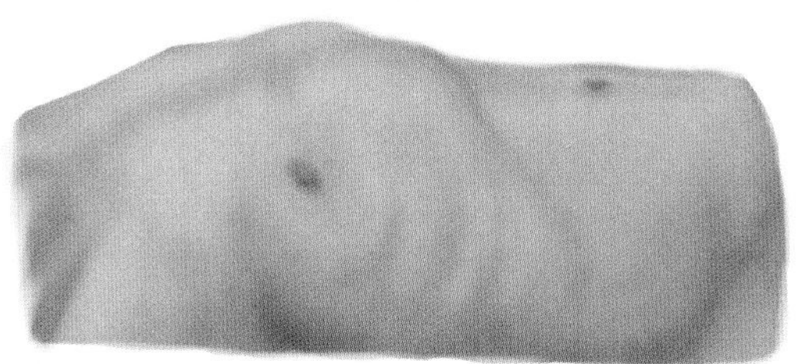

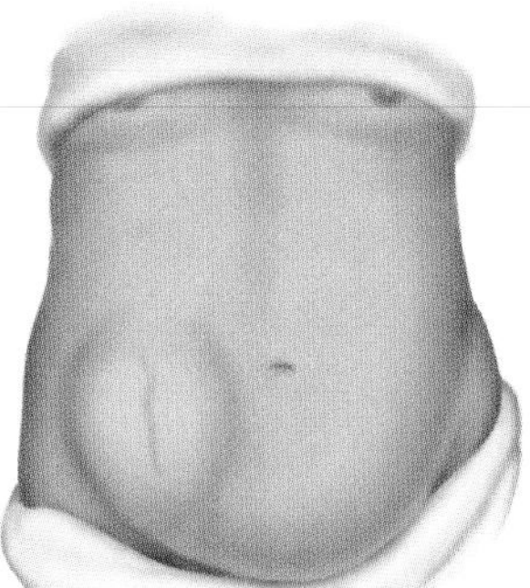

Incisional Hernia

This is a protrusion through an operative scar. Palpate to detect the length and width of the defect in the abdominal wall. A small defect, through which a large hernia has passed, has a greater risk for complications than a large defect.

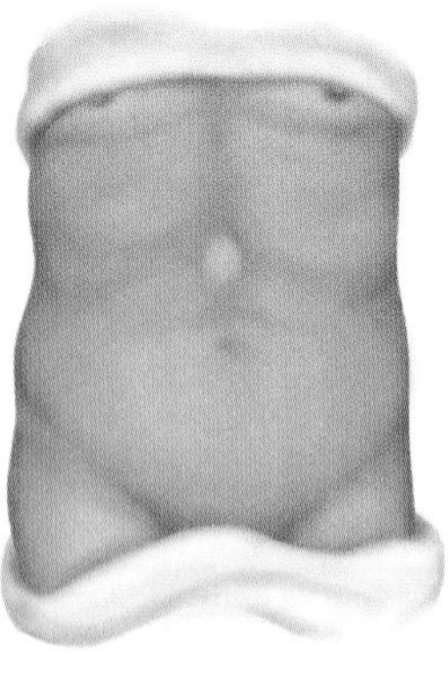

Epigastric Hernia

A small midline protrusion through a defect in the linea alba occurs between the xiphoid process and the umbilicus. With the patient's head and shoulders raised (or with the patient standing), run your fingerpad down the linea alba to feel it.

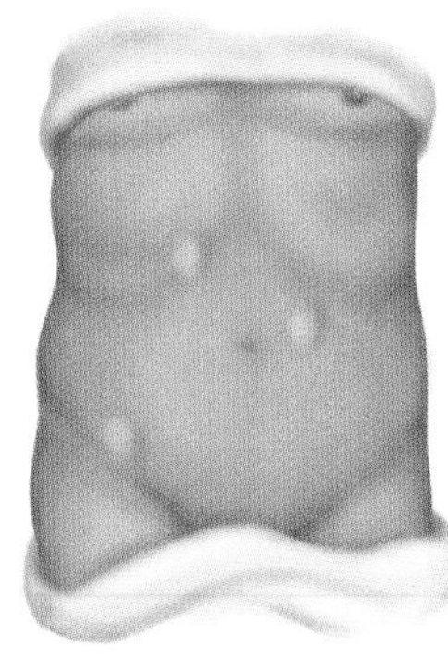

Lipoma

Common, benign, fatty tumors usually occur in the subcutaneous tissues almost anywhere in the body, including the abdominal wall. Small or large, they are usually soft and often lobulated. Press your finger down on the edge of a lipoma. The tumor typically slips out from under it.

TABLE 10-9 Protuberant Abdomens

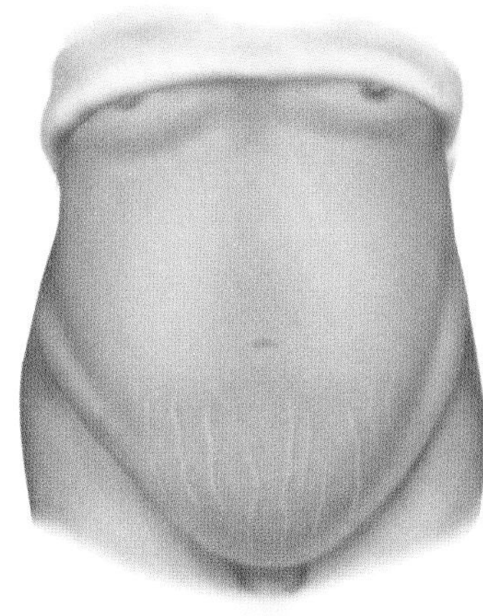

Fat

Fat is the most common cause of a protuberant abdomen. Fat thickens the abdominal wall, the mesentery, and omentum. The umbilicus may appear sunken. A *pannus*, or apron of fatty tissue, may extend below the inguinal ligaments. Lift it to look for inflammation in the skin folds or even for a hidden hernia.

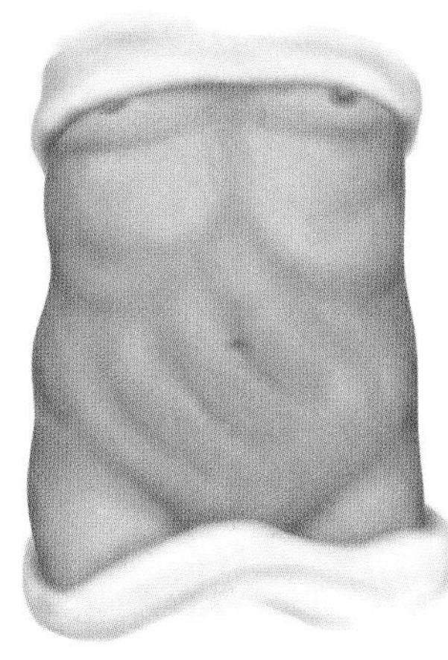

Gas

Gaseous distention may be localized or generalized. It causes a tympanitic percussion note. Increased intestinal gas production from certain foods may cause mild distention. More serious are intestinal obstruction and adynamic (paralytic) ileus. Note the location of the distention. Distention becomes more marked in colonic than in small bowel obstruction.

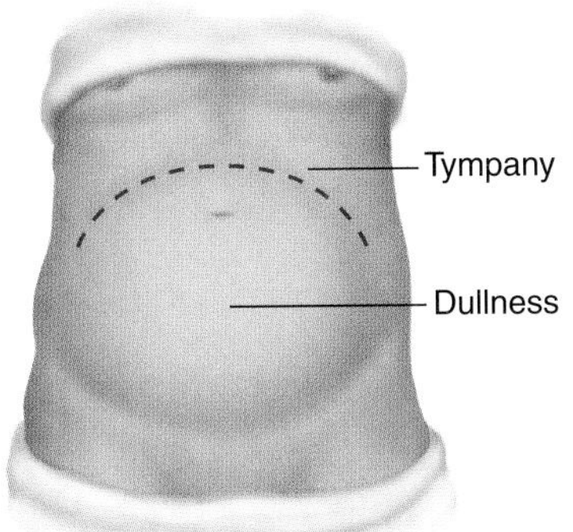

Tumor

A large, solid tumor, usually rising out of the pelvis, is dull to percussion. Air-filled bowel is displaced to the periphery. Causes include ovarian tumors and uterine myomata. Occasionally a markedly distended bladder may be mistaken for such a tumor.

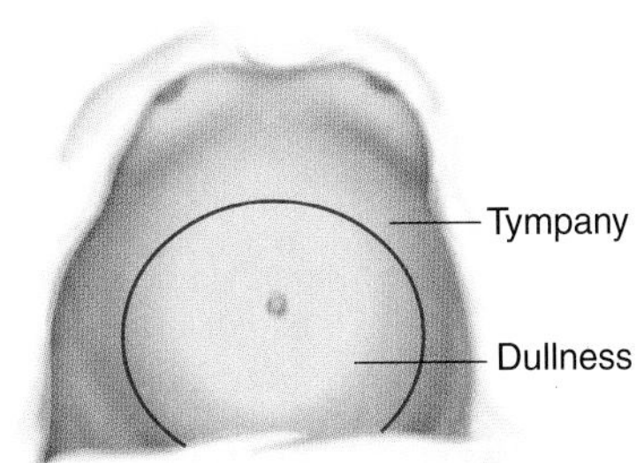

Pregnancy

Pregnancy is a common cause of a pelvic "mass." Listen for the fetal heart (see pp. 830–831).

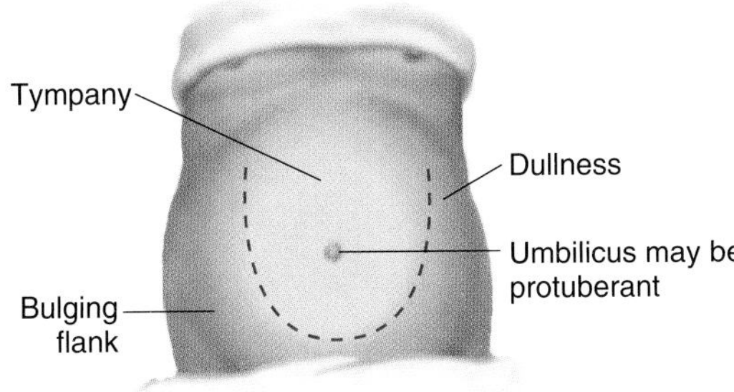

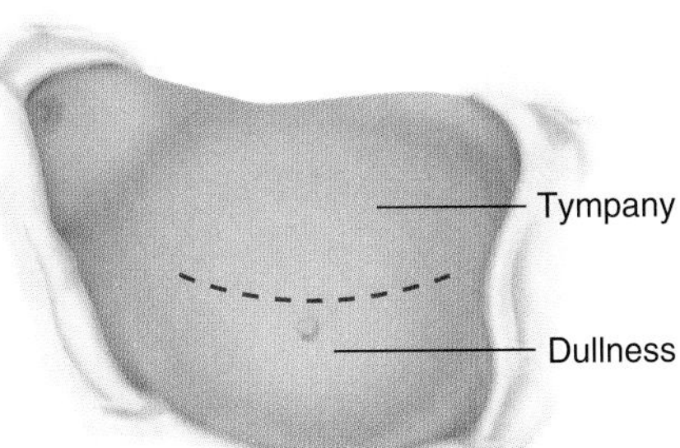

Ascitic Fluid

Ascitic fluid seeks the lowest point in the abdomen, producing bulging flanks that are dull to percussion. The umbilicus may protrude. Turn the patient onto one side to detect the shift in position of the fluid level (shifting dullness). (See pp. 387–389 for the assessment of ascites.)

TABLE 10-10 Sounds in the Abdomen

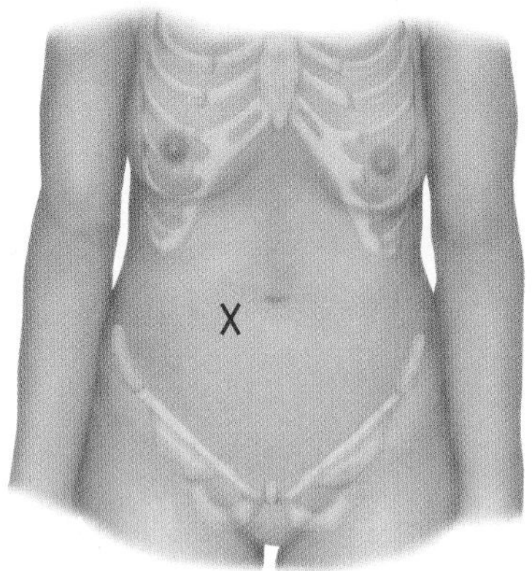

Bowel Sounds

Bowel sounds may be:

- *Increased*, as from diarrhea or *early intestinal obstruction*
- *Decreased*, then absent, as in *adynamic ileus and peritonitis.* Before deciding that bowel sounds are absent, sit down and listen where shown for 2 min or even longer.

High-pitched tinkling sounds suggest intestinal fluid and air under tension in a dilated bowel. *Rushes of high-pitched sounds* coinciding with an abdominal cramp indicate intestinal obstruction.

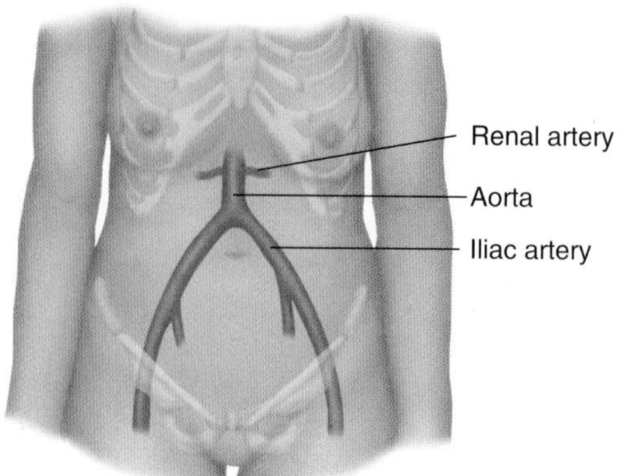

Bruits

A *hepatic bruit* suggests carcinoma of the liver or alcoholic hepatitis. *Arterial bruits* with both systolic and diastolic components suggest partial occlusion of the aorta or large arteries. Partial occlusion of a renal artery may explain hypertension.

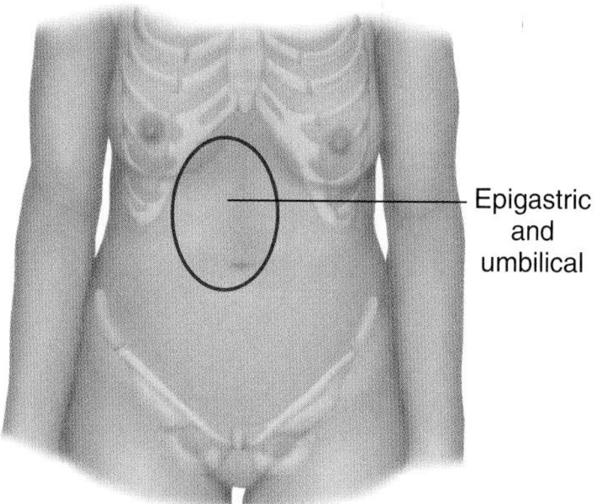

Venous Hum

A venous hum is rare. It is a soft humming noise with both systolic and diastolic components. It indicates increased collateral circulation between portal and systemic venous systems, as in hepatic cirrhosis.

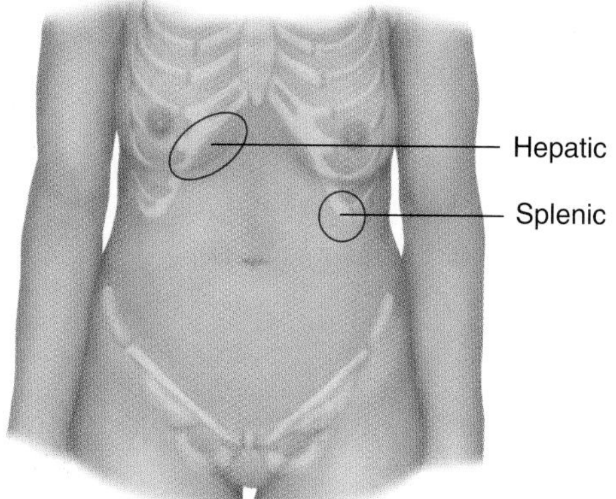

Friction Rubs

Friction rubs are rare. They are grating sounds with respiratory variation. They indicate inflammation of the peritoneal surface of an organ, as from a liver tumor, chlamydial or gonococcal perihepatitis, recent liver biopsy, or splenic infarct. When a systolic bruit accompanies a hepatic friction rub, suspect carcinoma of the liver.

TABLE 10-11 Tender Abdomens

Abdominal Wall Tenderness

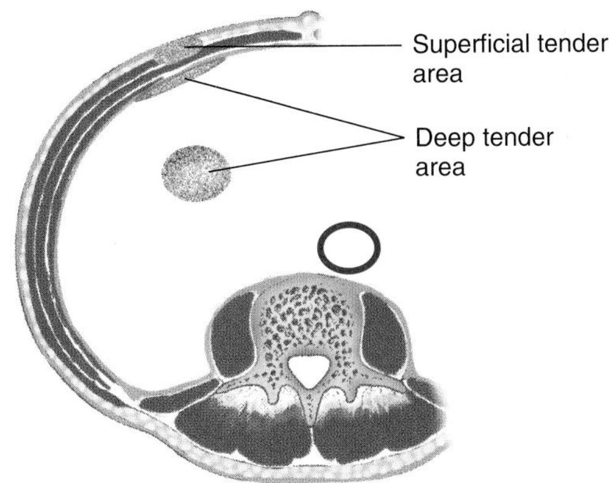

Tenderness may originate in the abdominal wall. When the patient raises head and shoulders, this tenderness persists, whereas tenderness from a deeper lesion (protected by the tightened muscles) decreases.

Visceral Tenderness

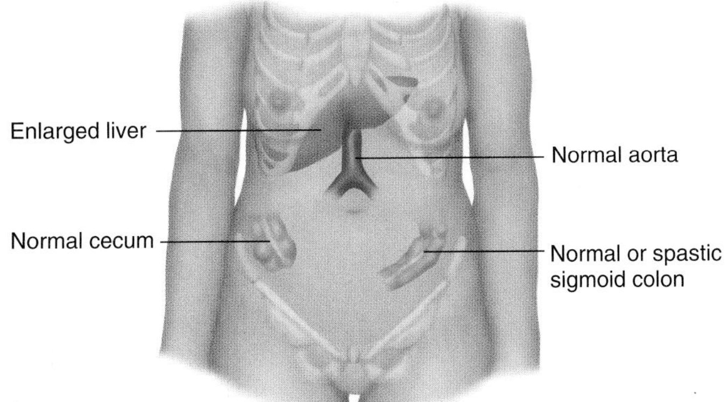

The structures shown may be tender to deep palpation. Usually the discomfort is dull with no muscular rigidity or rebound tenderness. A reassuring explanation to the patient may prove quite helpful.

Tenderness From Disease in the Chest and Pelvis

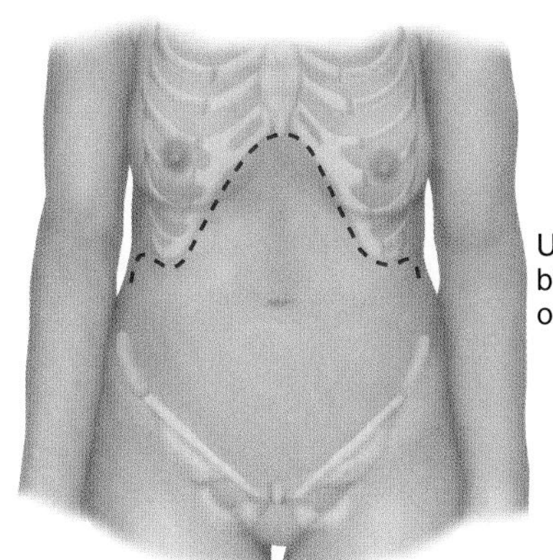

Acute Pleurisy

Abdominal pain and tenderness may result from acute pleural inflammation. When unilateral, it may mimic acute cholecystitis or appendicitis. Rebound tenderness and rigidity are less common; chest signs are usually present.

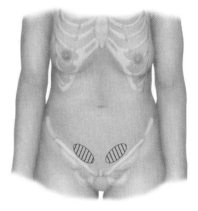

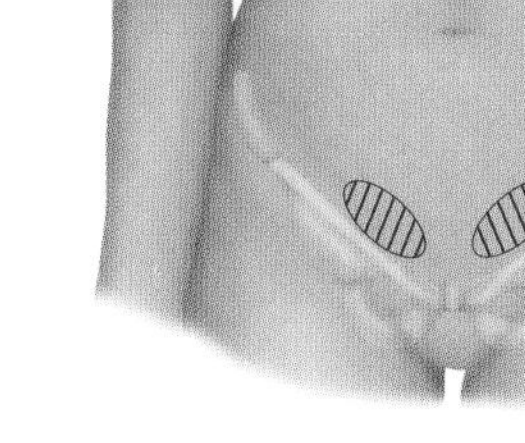

Acute Salpingitis

Frequently bilateral, the tenderness of acute salpingitis (inflammation of the fallopian tubes) is usually maximal just above the inguinal ligaments. Rebound tenderness and rigidity may be present. On pelvic examination, motion of the uterus causes pain.

(table continues next page)

Tenderness of Peritoneal Inflammation

Tenderness associated with peritoneal inflammation is more severe than visceral tenderness. Muscular rigidity and rebound tenderness are frequently but not necessarily present. Generalized peritonitis causes exquisite tenderness throughout the abdomen, together with boardlike muscular rigidity. Local causes of peritoneal inflammation include:

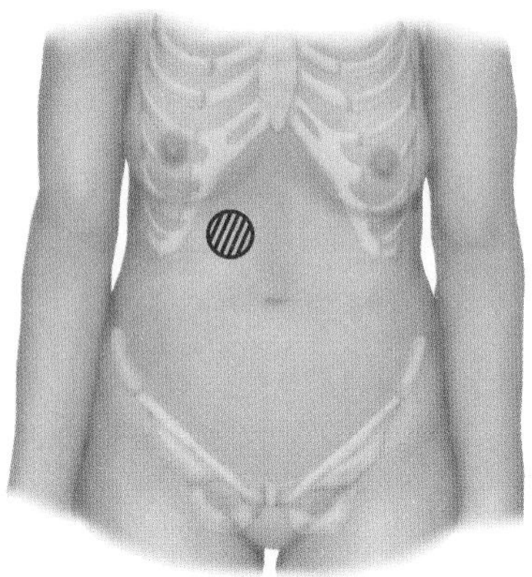

Acute Cholecystitis

Signs are maximal in the right upper quadrant. Check for Murphy's sign (see p. 400).

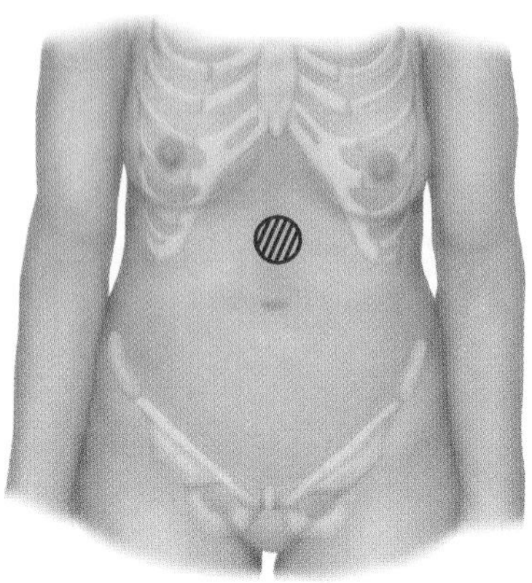

Acute Pancreatitis

In acute pancreatitis, epigastric tenderness and rebound tenderness are usually present, but the abdominal wall may be soft.

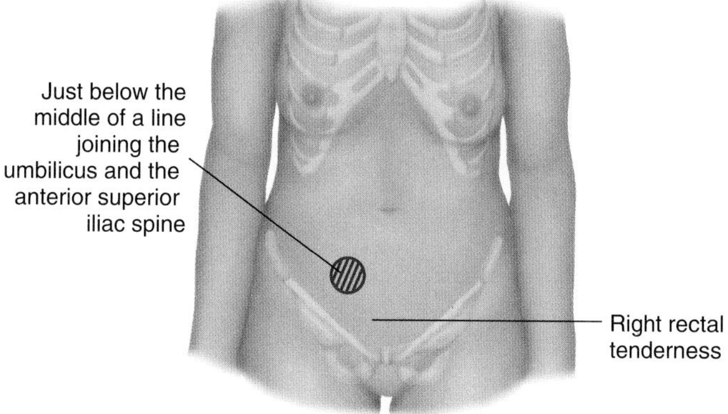

Acute Appendicitis

Right lower quadrant signs are typical of acute appendicitis, but may be absent early in the course. The typical area of tenderness is illustrated. Explore other portions of the right lower quadrant as well as the right flank.

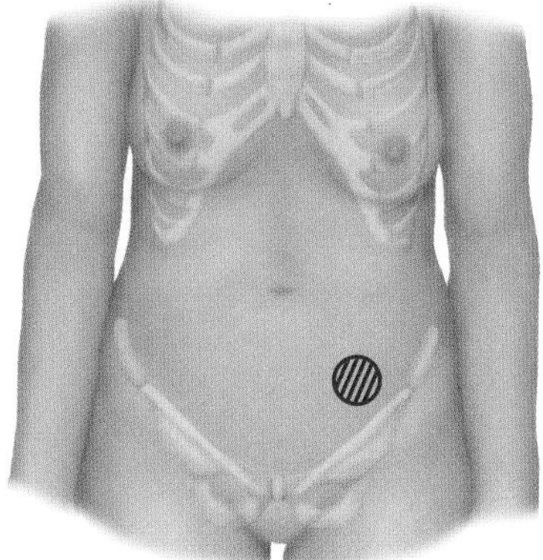

Acute Diverticulitis

Acute diverticulitis most often involves the sigmoid colon and then resembles a left-sided appendicitis.

TABLE 10-12 Liver Enlargement: Apparent and Real

A palpable liver does not necessarily indicate hepatomegaly (an enlarged liver), but more often results from a change in consistency—from the normal softness to an abnormal firmness or hardness, as in cirrhosis. Clinical estimates of liver size should be based on both percussion and palpation, although even these techniques are far from perfect.

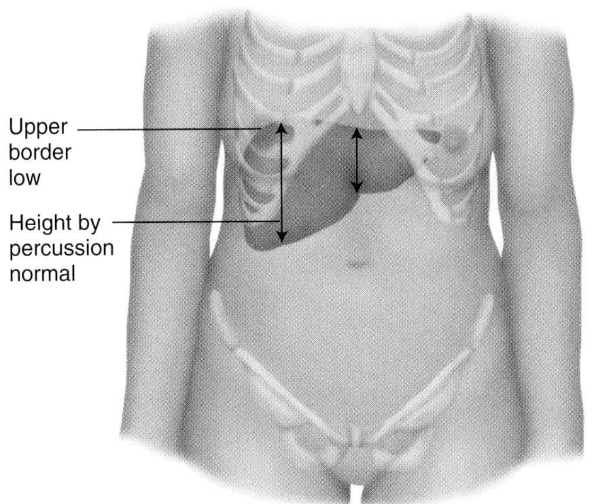

Downward Displacement of the Liver by a Low Diaphragm

This finding is common when the diaphragm is low (e.g., in emphysema). The liver edge may be readily palpable well below the costal margin. Percussion, however, reveals a low upper edge also, and the vertical span of the liver is normal.

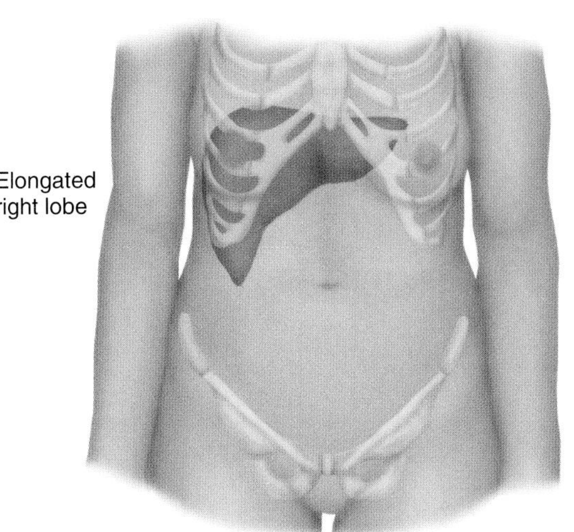

Normal Variations in Liver Shape

In some people, especially those with a lanky build, the liver tends to be elongated so that its right lobe is easily palpable as it projects downward toward the iliac crest. Such an elongation, sometimes called *Riedel's lobe*, represents a variation in shape, not an increase in liver volume or size. Examiners can only estimate the upper and lower borders of an organ with three dimensions and differing shapes. Some error is unavoidable.

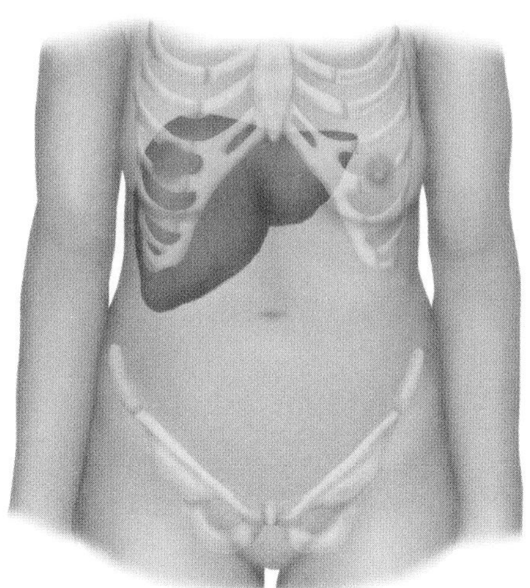

Smooth Large Liver

Cirrhosis may produce an enlarged liver with a firm *nontender* edge. The liver is not always enlarged in this condition, however, and many other diseases may produce similar findings. An enlarged liver with a smooth *tender* edge suggests inflammation, as in hepatitis, or venous congestion, as in right-sided heart failure.

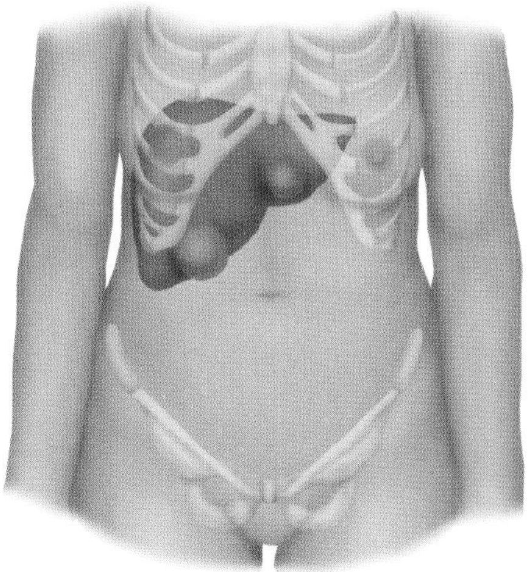

Irregular Large Liver

An enlarged liver that is firm or hard and has an irregular edge or surface suggests malignancy. There may be one or more nodules. The liver may or may not be tender.

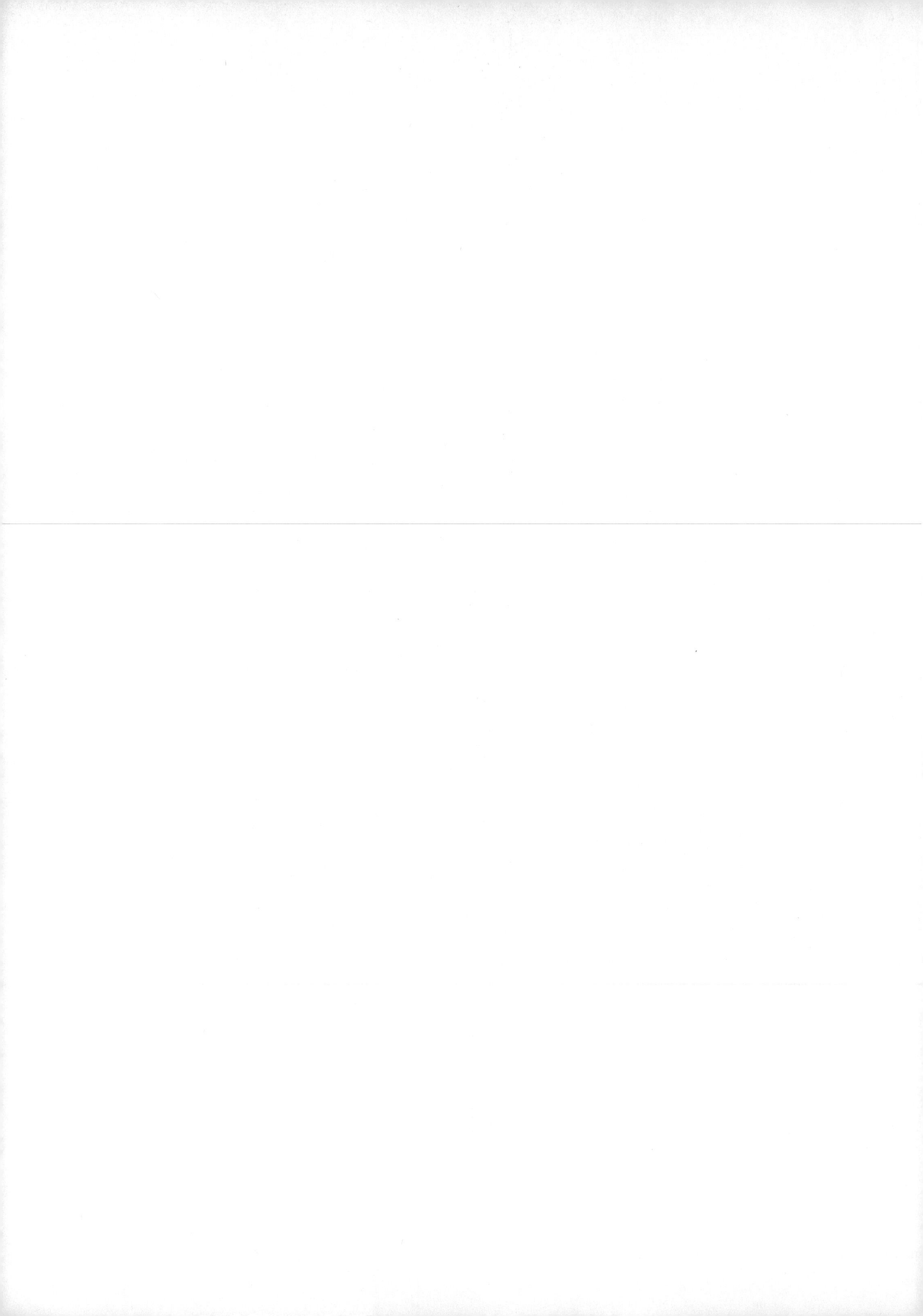

CHAPTER

11

Male Genitalia and Hernias

ANATOMY AND PHYSIOLOGY

Review the anatomy of the male genitalia.

The *shaft of the penis* is formed by three columns of vascular erectile tissue: the *corpus spongiosum*, containing the urethra, and two *corpora cavernosa*. The corpus spongiosum forms the bulb of the penis, ending in the cone-

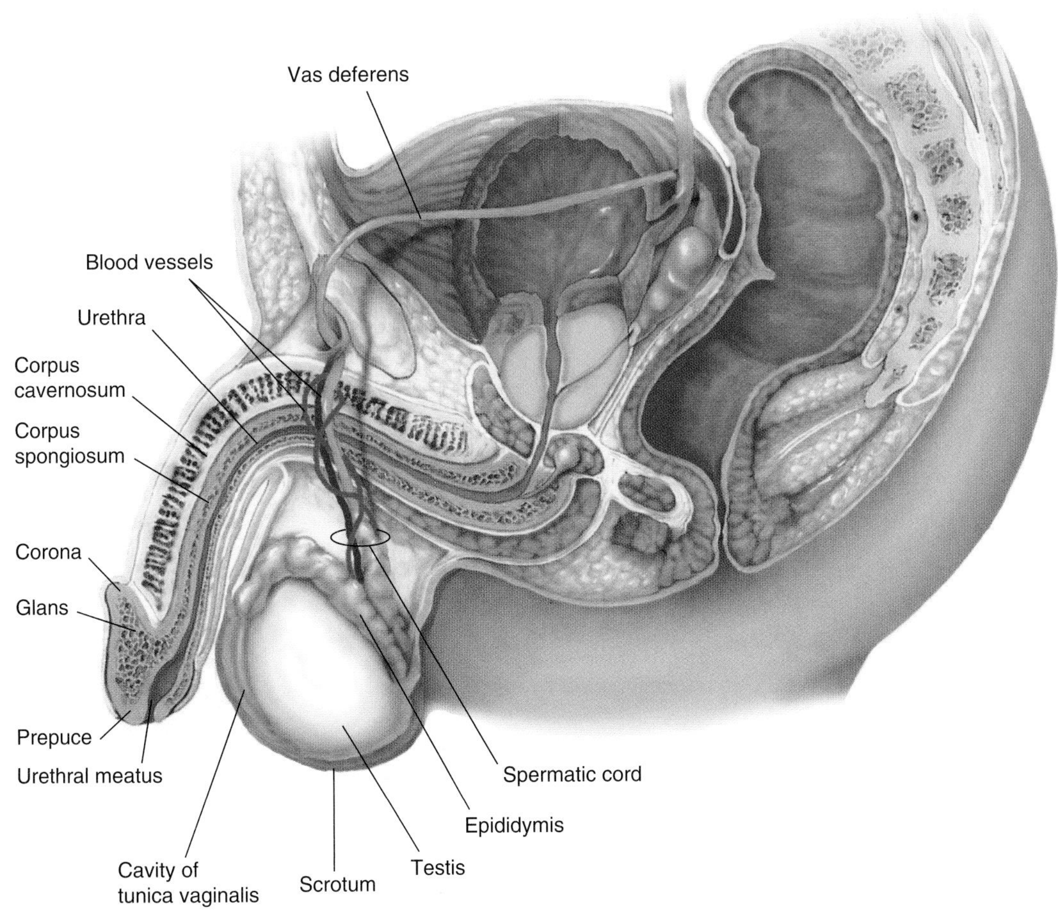

shaped *glans* with its expanded base, or *corona.* In uncircumsized men, the glans is covered by a loose, hoodlike fold of skin called the *prepuce* or *foreskin* where *smegma,* or secretions of the glans, may collect. The urethra is located ventrally in the shaft of the penis; urethral abnormalities may sometimes be felt there. The urethra opens into the vertical, slitlike *urethral meatus,* located somewhat ventrally at the tip of the glans.

The *testes* are ovoid, somewhat rubbery structures approximately 4.5 cm long, although their size ranges from 3.5 cm to 5.5 cm. The left testis usually lies somewhat lower than the right. The testes produce spermatozoa and testosterone. Testosterone stimulates the pubertal growth of the male genitalia, prostate, and seminal vesicles. It also stimulates the development of masculine secondary sex characteristics, including facial hair, body hair, musculoskeletal growth, and enlargement of the larynx, with its associated low-pitched voice.

Surrounding or appended to the testes are several structures. The *scrotum* is a loose wrinkled pouch divided into two compartments, each containing a testis or testicle. Covering the testis, except posteriorly, is the serous membrane of the *tunica vaginalis.* On the posterolateral surface of each testis is the softer comma-shaped *epididymis,* consisting of tightly coiled spermatic ducts that provide a reservoir for storage, maturation, and transport of sperm from the testis to the *vas deferens.*

The *vas deferens,* a cordlike structure, begins at the tail of the epididymis, ascends within the scrotal sac, and passes through the external inguinal ring on its way to the abdomen and pelvis. Behind the bladder, it is joined by the duct from the seminal vesicle and enters the urethra within the prostate gland. Sperm thus passes from the testis and the epididymis through the vas deferens into the urethra. Secretions from the vasa deferentia, the seminal vesicles, and the prostate all contribute to the semen. Within the scrotum, each vas is closely associated with blood vessels, nerves, and muscle fibers. These structures make up the *spermatic cord.*

Male sexual function depends on normal levels of testosterone, adequate arterial blood flow to the inferior epigastric artery and its cremasteric and pubic branches, and intact neural innervation from α-adrenergic and cholinergic pathways. Erection from venous engorgement of the corpora cavernosa results from two types of stimuli. Visual, auditory, or erotic cues trigger sympathetic outflow from higher brain centers to the T11 through L2 levels of the spinal cord. Tactile stimulation initiates sensory impulses from the genitalia to S_2 to S_4 reflex arcs and parasympathetic pathways through the pudendal nerve. Both sets of stimuli appear to increase levels of nitric oxide and cyclic GMP, resulting in local vasodilation.

Lymphatics. Lymphatics from the penile and scrotal surfaces drain into the inguinal nodes. *When you find an inflammatory or possibly malignant lesion* on these surfaces, *assess the inguinal nodes especially carefully* for enlargement or tenderness. The lymphatics of the testes, however, drain into the abdomen, where enlarged nodes are clinically undetectable. See page 477 for further discussion of the inguinal nodes.

Anatomy of the Groin. Because hernias are relatively common, it is important to understand the anatomy of the groin. The basic landmarks are the anterior superior iliac spine, the pubic tubercle, and the inguinal ligament that runs between them. Find these on yourself or a colleague.

The *inguinal canal,* which lies above and approximately parallel to the inguinal ligament, forms a tunnel for the vas deferens as it passes through the abdominal muscles. The exterior opening of the tunnel—the *external inguinal ring*—is a triangular, slitlike structure palpable just above and lateral to the pubic tubercle. The internal opening of the canal—or *internal inguinal ring*—is approximately 1 cm above the midpoint of the inguinal ligament. Neither canal nor internal ring is palpable through the abdominal wall. When loops of bowel force their way through weak areas of the inguinal canal, they produce *inguinal hernias,* as illustrated on pp. 426–427.

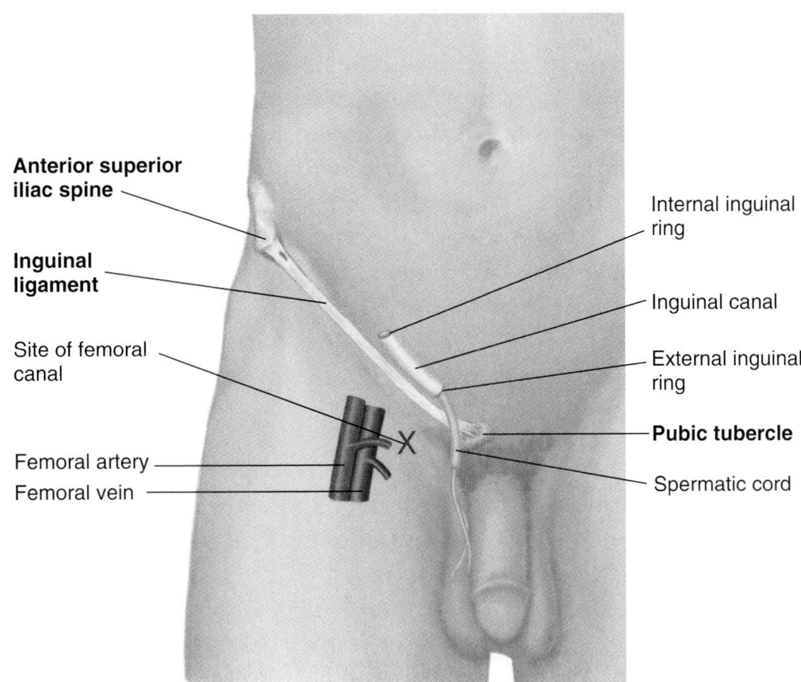

Another potential route for a herniating mass is the *femoral canal.* This lies below the inguinal ligament. Although you cannot see it, you can estimate its location by placing your right index finger, from below, on the right femoral artery. Your middle finger will then overlie the femoral vein; your ring finger, the femoral canal. Femoral hernias protrude here.

THE HEALTH HISTORY

Common or Concerning Symptoms

- Changes in sexual function and response
- Penile discharge or lesions
- Scrotal pain, swelling, or lesions

For men, questions about the genitalia follow naturally after those dealing with the urinary system. You will need to review sexual function and screen for symptoms of infection. Begin with general questions such as "How is sexual function for you?" "Are you satisfied with your sexual life?" "What about your ability to perform sexually?" If the patient reports a sexual problem, ask him to tell you about it. Ask if there has been any change in desire or level of sexual activity recently. What does he think has caused it, what has he tried to do about it, and what are his hopes? Identify the patient's sexual preference as to partners (male, female, or both). Find out if the patient's partner has any concerns.

Direct questions help you to assess each phase of the sexual response. To assess *libido,* or desire, ask "Have you maintained interest in sex?" For the *arousal phase,* ask "Can you achieve and maintain an erection?" Explore the timing, severity, setting, and any other factors that may be contributing to problems. Have any changes in the relationship with his partner or in his life circumstances coincided with onset of a problem? Are there circumstances when erection is normal? On awakening in the early morning or during the night? With other partners? With masturbation?

Lack of libido may arise from psychogenic causes such as depression, endocrine dysfunction, or side effects of medications.

Erectile dysfunction may be from psychogenic causes, especially if early morning erection is preserved; also from decreased testosterone, decreased blood flow in the hypogastric arterial system, or impaired neural innervation.

Other questions relate to the phase of *orgasm* and *ejaculation* of semen. If ejaculation is premature, or early and out of control, ask "About how long does intercourse last?" "Do you climax too soon?" "Do you feel like you have any control over climaxing?" "Do you think your partner would like intercourse to last longer?" For reduced or absent ejaculation, "Do you find that you cannot have orgasm even though you can have an erection?" Try to determine whether the problem involves the pleasurable sensation of orgasm, the ejaculation of seminal fluid, or both. Review the frequency and setting of the problem, medications, surgery, and neurologic symptoms.

Premature ejaculation is common, especially in young men. Less common is reduced or absent ejaculation affecting middle-aged or older men. Possible causes are medications, surgery, neurologic deficits, or lack of androgen. Lack of orgasm with ejaculation is usually psychogenic.

To assess the possibility of genital infection from sexually transmitted diseases (STDs), ask about any *discharge from the penis,* dripping, or staining of underwear. If penile discharge is present, assess the amount, its color and consistency, and any fever, chills, rash, or associated symptoms.

Penile discharge may accompany gonococcal (usually yellow) and nongonococcal urethritis (may be clear or white).

Inquire about *sores or growths on the penis,* and any *pain or swelling in the scrotum.* Ask about previous genital symptoms or a past history of infections from herpes, gonorrhea, or syphilis. A patient who has multiple partners, is homosexual, uses illicit drugs, or has a prior history of STDs is at increased risk for subsequent STDs.

See Table 11-1, Abnormalities of the Penis (p. 422), Table 11-2, Abnormalities of the Scrotal Sac (p. 423), and Table 11-3, Abnormalities of the Testis (p. 424). In addition to STDs, many skin conditions affect the genitalia; likewise, some STDs have minimal symptoms or signs.

Because STDs may involve other parts of the body, additional questions are often indicated. An introductory explanation may be useful. "Sexually transmitted diseases can involve any body opening where you have sex. It's important for you to tell me which openings you use." And further, as needed, "Do you have oral sex? Anal sex?" If the patient's answers are affirmative, ask about symptoms such as sore throat, diarrhea, rectal bleeding, and anal itching or pain.

Infections from oral–penile transmission include gonorrhea, *Chlamydia*, syphilis, and herpes. Symptomatic or asymptomatic proctitis may follow anal intercourse.

For the many patients without symptoms or known risk factors, it is wise to ask, "Do you have any concerns about HIV infection?" as an important screening question and to continue with the more general questions suggested on pp. 48–49.

HEALTH PROMOTION AND COUNSELING

Important Topics for Health Promotion and Counseling

- Prevention of STDs and HIV
- Testicular self-examination

Each clinician must address the high burden of *STDs* on the U.S. population that warrants direct engagement with patients in disease prevention, especially adolescents and young adults. The U.S. Preventive Services Task Force registers an estimated 12 million new infections each year from *Chlamydia* (approximately 4 million cases), gonorrhea (approximately 800,000 cases), and *Trichomas* vaginitis and nonspecific urethritis ("several million cases" annually).[1] More than 1 million Americans are currently infected with HIV, with approximately 40,000 new infections annually. Additional infections that can be transmitted sexually include syphilis, human papillomavirus (HPV), hepatitis B, and genital herpes. Clinicians should educate patients about STD infections and HIV, practice early detection during history-taking and physical examination, and identify and treat infected patients and their partners.

Health promotion and counseling should address patient education about STDs and HIV, early detection of infection during history taking and physical examination, and identification and treatment of infected partners. Discussion of risk factors for STDs and HIV is especially important for adolescents and younger patients, the age groups most adversely affected. Clinicians must be comfortable with eliciting the sexual history and with asking frank but tactful questions about sexual practices. A minimal history includes identifying the patient's sexual orientation, the number of sexual partners in the past month, and any history of STDs (see Chap. 2, p. 48). Questions should be clear and nonjudgmental. You should also identify use of alcohol and drugs, particularly injection drugs. Counsel patients at risk about limiting the number of partners, using condoms, and establishing regular medical care for treatment of STDs and HIV. It is important for men to seek prompt attention for any genital lesions or penile discharge.

The U.S. Preventive Services Task Force recommends counseling and testing for HIV infection in the following groups: all persons at increased risk for infection with HIV, STDs, or both; men with male partners; past or present injection drug users; any past or present partners of people with HIV infection, bisexual practices, or injection drug use; and patients with a history of transfusion between 1978 and 1985.

In addition, encourage men, especially those between the ages of 15 and 35, to perform monthly *testicular self-examinations* and to seek physician evaluation for the following findings: any painless lump, swelling, or enlargement in either testicle; pain or discomfort in a testicle or the scrotum; a feeling of heaviness or a sudden fluid collection in the scrotum; or a dull ache in the lower abdomen or the groin. (See p. 420 for instructions to patients.)[2]

TECHNIQUES OF EXAMINATION

Many students feel uneasy about examining a man's genitalia. "How will the patient react?" "Will he have an erection?" "Will he let me examine him?" It may be reassuring to explain each step of the examination so that the patient knows what to expect. Requesting an assistant to accompany you is common practice. Occasionally, male patients have erections during the examination. If this happens, you should explain to the patient that this is a normal response, finish your examination, and proceed with an unruffled demeanor. If the man refuses to be examined, you should respect his wishes.

A good genital examination can be done with the patient either standing or supine. To check for hernias or varicoceles, however, the patient should stand, and you should sit comfortably on a chair or stool. A gown conveniently covers the patient's chest and abdomen. Wear *gloves* throughout the examination. Expose the genitalia and inguinal areas. For younger patients, review the sexual maturity ratings on page 781.

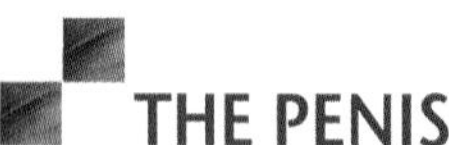

THE PENIS

INSPECTION

Inspect the penis, including:

See Table 11-1, Abnormalities of the Penis (p. 422).

- The *skin*
- The *prepuce* (foreskin). If it is present, retract it or ask the patient to retract it. This step is essential for the detection of many chancres and carcinomas. Smegma, a cheesy, whitish material, may accumulate normally under the foreskin.

Phimosis is a tight prepuce that cannot be retracted over the glans. *Paraphimosis* is a tight prepuce that, once retracted, cannot be returned. Edema ensues.

- The *glans*. Look for any ulcers, scars, nodules, or signs of inflammation.

Balanitis (inflammation of the glans); *balanoposthitis* (inflammation of the glans and prepuce)

Check the skin around the base of the penis for excoriations or inflammation. Look for nits or lice at the bases of the pubic hairs.

Pubic or genital excoriations suggest the possibility of lice (crabs) or sometimes scabies.

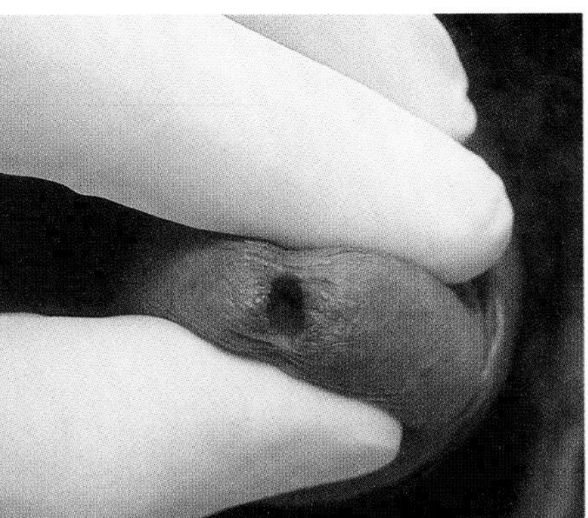

Note the location of the urethral meatus.

Hypospadias is a congenital, ventral displacement of the meatus on the penis (p. 422).

Compress the glans gently between your index finger above and your thumb below. This maneuver should open the urethral meatus and allow you to inspect it for discharge. Normally there is none.

Profuse yellow discharge in gonococcal urethritis; scanty white or clear discharge in nongonococcal urethritis. Definitive diagnosis requires Gram stain and culture.

If the patient has reported a discharge that you are unable to see, ask him to strip, or milk, the shaft of the penis from its base to the glans. Alternatively, do it yourself. This maneuver may bring some discharge out of the urethral meatus for appropriate examination. Have a glass slide and culture materials ready.

PALPATION

Palpate any abnormality of the penis, noting any tenderness or induration. Palpate the shaft of the penis between your thumb and first two fingers, noting any induration. Palpation of the shaft may be omitted in a young, asymptomatic male patient.

If you retract the foreskin, replace it before proceeding on to examine the scrotum.

Induration along the ventral surface of the penis suggests a urethral stricture or possibly a carcinoma. Tenderness of such an indurated area suggests periurethral inflammation secondary to a urethral stricture.

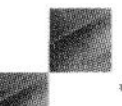

THE SCROTUM AND ITS CONTENTS

INSPECTION

Inspect the scrotum, including:

See Table 11-2, Abnormalities of the Scrotal Sac (p. 423).

- The *skin*. Lift up the scrotum so that you can see its posterior surface.

Rashes, epidermoid cysts, rarely skin cancer

- The *scrotal contours*. Note any swelling, lumps, or veins.

A poorly developed scrotum on one or both sides suggests *cryptorchidism* (an undescended testicle). Common scrotal swellings include indirect inguinal hernias, hydroceles, and scrotal edema. Tender, painful scrotal swelling in acute epididymitis, acute orchitis, torsion of the spermatic cord, or a strangulated inguinal hernia.

See Table 11-3, Abnormalities of the Testis (p. 425) and Table 11-4, Abnormalities of the Epididymis and Spermatic Cord (p. 425).

PALPATION

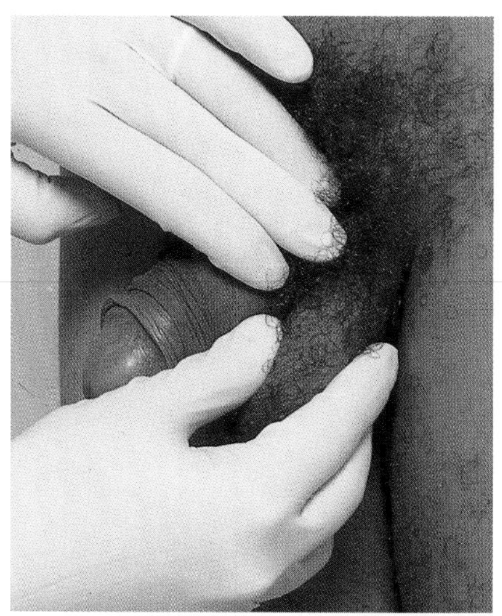

Palpate each testis and epididymis between your thumb and first two fingers. Locate the epididymis on the superior posterior surface of each testicle. It feels nodular and cordlike and should not be confused with an abnormal lump.

Note size, shape, consistency, and tenderness; feel for any nodules. Pressure on the testis normally produces a deep visceral pain.

Any painless nodule in the testis must raise the possibility of *testicular cancer,* a potentially curable cancer with a peak incidence between the ages of 15 and 35 years.

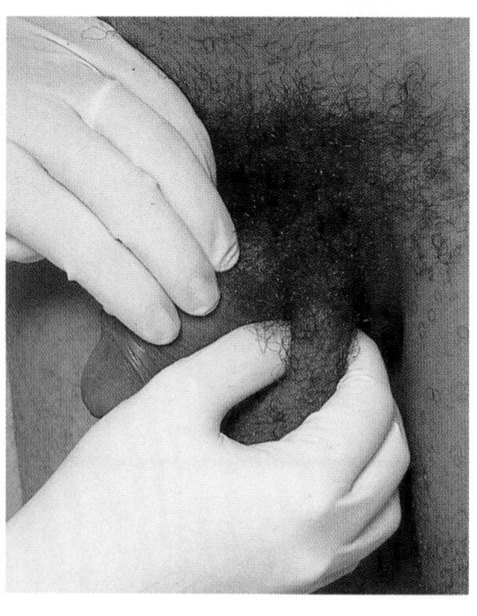

Palpate each spermatic cord, including the vas deferens, between your thumb and fingers from the epididymis to the superficial inguinal ring.

Note any nodules or swellings.

Multiple tortuous veins in this area, usually on the left, may be palpable and even visible. They indicate a *varicocele* (p. 425).

The vas deferens, if chronically infected, may feel thickened or beaded. A cystic structure in the spermatic cord suggests a hydrocele of the cord.

Swelling in the scrotum other than the testicles can be evaluated by transillumination. After darkening the room, shine the beam of a strong flashlight from behind the scrotum through the mass. Look for transmission of the light as a red glow.

Swellings containing serous fluid, as in hydroceles, light up with a red glow, or transilluminate. Those containing blood or tissue, such as a normal testis, a tumor, or most hernias, do not.

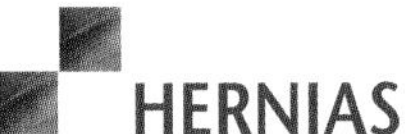

HERNIAS

INSPECTION

Inspect the inguinal and femoral areas carefully for bulges. While you continue your observation, ask the patient to strain and bear down, as if having a bowel movement (the Valsalva maneuver) to enhance detection of hernias.

A bulge that appears on straining suggests a hernia.

PALPATION

Palpate for an inguinal hernia. With the patient still standing, and using in turn your right hand for the patient's right side and your left hand for the patient's left side, invaginate loose scrotal skin with your index finger. Start at a point low enough to be sure that your finger will have enough mobility to reach as far as the internal inguinal ring if this proves possible. Follow the spermatic cord upward to above the inguinal ligament and find the triangular, slitlike opening of the external inguinal ring. This is just above and lateral to the pubic tubercle. If the ring is somewhat enlarged, it may admit your index finger. If possible, gently follow the inguinal canal laterally in its oblique course. With your finger located either at the external ring or within the canal, ask the patient to strain down or cough. Note any palpable herniating mass as it touches your finger.

See Table 11-5, Course and Presentation of Hernias in the Groin (p. 426).

See Table 11-6, Differentiation of Hernias in the Groin (p. 427).

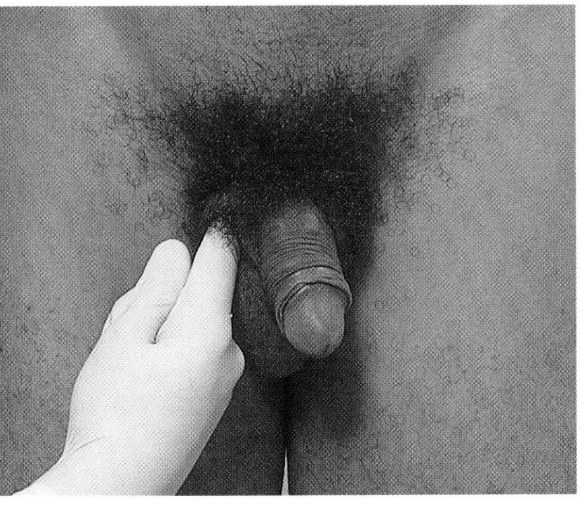

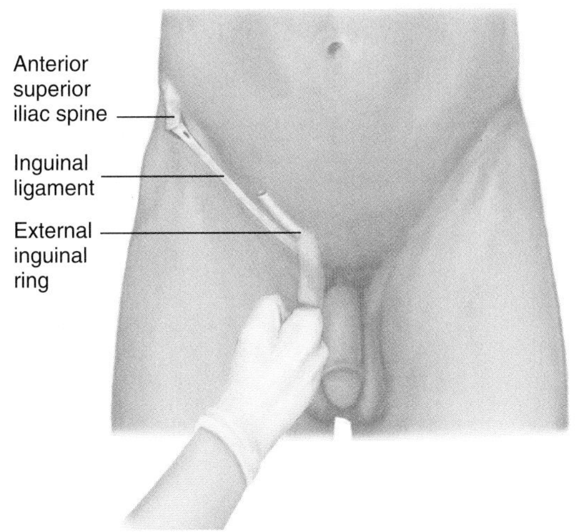

Palpate for a femoral hernia by placing your fingers on the anterior thigh in the region of the femoral canal. Ask the patient to strain down again or cough. Note any swelling or tenderness.

Evaluating a Possible Scrotal Hernia. If you find a large scrotal mass and suspect that it may be a hernia, ask the patient to lie down. The mass may return to the abdomen by itself. If so, it is a hernia. If not:

- Can you get your fingers above the mass in the scrotum?

If you can, suspect a hydrocele.

- Listen to the mass with a stethoscope for bowel sounds.

Bowel sounds may be heard over a hernia, but not over a hydrocele.

If the findings suggest a hernia, gently try to reduce it (return it to the abdominal cavity) by sustained pressure with your fingers. Do not attempt this maneuver if the mass is tender or the patient reports nausea and vomiting.

A hernia is *incarcerated* when its contents cannot be returned to the abdominal cavity. A hernia is *strangulated* when the blood supply to the entrapped contents is compromised. Suspect strangulation in the presence of tenderness, nausea, and vomiting and consider surgical intervention.

History may be helpful here. The patient can usually tell you what happens to his swelling on lying down and may be able to demonstrate how he reduces it himself. Remember to ask him.

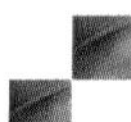

SPECIAL TECHNIQUES

THE TESTICULAR SELF-EXAMINATION

The incidence of testicular cancer is low, about 4 per 100,000 men, but it is the most common cancer of young men between ages 15 and 35. Although the testicular self-examination (TSE) has not been formally endorsed as a screen for testicular carcinoma, you may wish to teach your patient the TSE to enhance health awareness and self-care. When detected early, testicular carcinoma has an excellent prognosis. Risk factors include cryptorchidism, which confers a high risk for testicular carcinoma in the undescended testicle; a history of carcinoma in the contralateral testicle; mumps orchitis; an inguinal hernia; and a hydrocele in childhood.

PATIENT INSTRUCTIONS FOR THE TESTICULAR SELF-EXAMINATION*

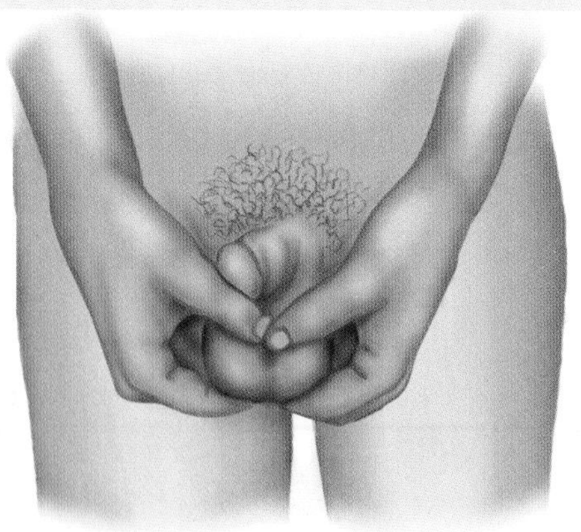

This examination is best performed after a warm bath or shower. The heat relaxes the scrotum and makes it easier to find anything unusual.

- Standing in front of a mirror, check for any swelling on the skin of the scrotum.
- Examine each testicle with both hands. Cup the index and middle fingers under the testicle and place the thumbs on top.
- Roll the testicle gently between the thumbs and fingers. One testicle may be larger than the other . . . that's normal, but be concerned about any lump or area of pain.
- Find the epididymis. This is a soft, tubelike structure at the back of the testicle that collects and carries sperm, not an abnormal lump.
- If you find any lump, don't wait. See your doctor. The lump may just be an infection, but if it is cancer, it will spread unless stopped by treatment.

* Medline Plus. U.S. National Library of Medicine and National Cancer Institute. Medical Encyclopedia—Testicular self-examination. Available at: www.nlm.nih.gov/medlineplus/ency/article/003909.htm. Accessed October 31, 2004.

RECORDING YOUR FINDINGS

Note that initially you may use sentences to describe your findings; later you will use phrases. The style below contains phrases appropriate for most write-ups.

Recording the Physical Examination—Male Genitalia and Hernias

"Circumsized male. No penile discharge or lesions. No scrotal swelling or discoloration. Testes descended bilaterally, smooth, without masses. Epididymis nontender. No inguinal or femoral hernias."

OR

"Uncircumsized male; prepuce easily retractible. No penile discharge or lesions. No scrotal swelling or discoloration. Testes descended bilaterally; right testicle smooth; 1 × 1 cm firm nodule on left lateral testicle. It is fixed and nontender. Epididymis nontender. No inguinal or femoral hernias."

Suspicious for testicular carcinoma, the most common form of cancer in men between the ages of 15 and 35

Bibliography

CITATIONS

1. Agency for Healthcare Research and Quality. Electronic Archive. Guide to Clinical Preventive Services, 2nd ed. 1996. Available at: www.ahrq.gov/clinic/cpsix.htm#counseling. Accessed October 31, 2004. (For the *Guide to Clinical Preventive Services,* 3rd ed., periodic updates, see www.ahrq/gov/clinic/cps3dix.htm. Accessed October 31, 2004.)
2. National Cancer Institute. Cancer Facts. Available at: http://cis.nih.gov/fact/6_34.htm. Accessed October 31, 2004.

ADDITIONAL REFERENCES

Barry MJ. Prostate-specific antigen testing for early diagnosis of prostate cancer. N Engl J Med 344(18):1373–1377, 2001.

Campbell MF, Walsh PC, Patrick C, Retik AB (eds). Campbell's Urology, 8th ed. Philadelphia, WB Saunders, 2002.

DeBusk RF. Sexual activity in patients with angina. JAMA 290(23):3129–3132, 2003.

Delancey JOL, Ashton-Miller JA. Pathophysiology of adult urinary incontinence. Gastroenterology 126(Suppl 1):S23–S32, 2004.

Eubanks S. Hernias (Chapter 42). In Townsend CM, Sabiston DC (eds). Sabiston Textbook of Surgery: The Biological Basis of Modern Surgical Practice, 17th ed. Philadelphia, Elsevier Saunders, 2004.

Fitzgibbons RJ, Filipi CJ, Quinn TH. Inguinal hernias (Chapter 36). In Brunicardi FC, Andersen DK, Billiar TR, et al (eds). Schwartz's Principles of Surgery, 8th ed. New York, McGraw-Hill, 2005.

Gillenwater JY. Adult and Pediatric Urology, 4th ed. Philadelphia, Lippincott Williams & Wilkins, 2002.

Handsfield HH. Color Atlas and Synopsis of Sexually Transmitted Diseases, 2nd ed. New York, McGraw-Hill, 2001.

Laumann EO, Paik A, Rosen RC. Sexual function in the United States: prevalence and predictors. JAMA 281(6):537–544, 1999.

Tanagho EA, McAninch JW (eds). Smith's General Urology, 16th ed. New York, Lange Medical Books, McGraw-Hill, 2004.

Teunissen TAM, de Jonge A, van Weel C, et al. Treating urinary incontinence in the elderly—conservative measures that work: a systematic review. J Fam Pract 53(1):25–30, 2004.

TABLE 11-1 Abnormalities of the Penis

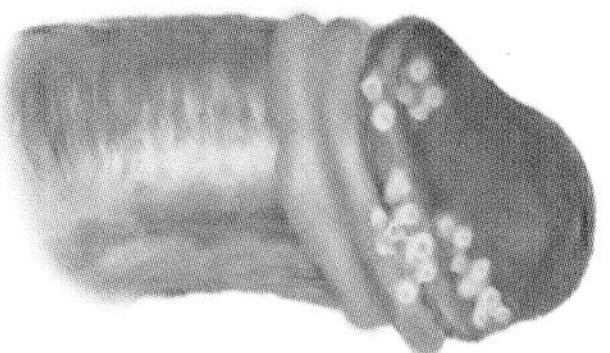

Venereal Wart
(Condyloma acuminatum)
Venereal warts are rapidly growing excrescences that are moist and often malodorous. They result from infection by human papillomavirus.

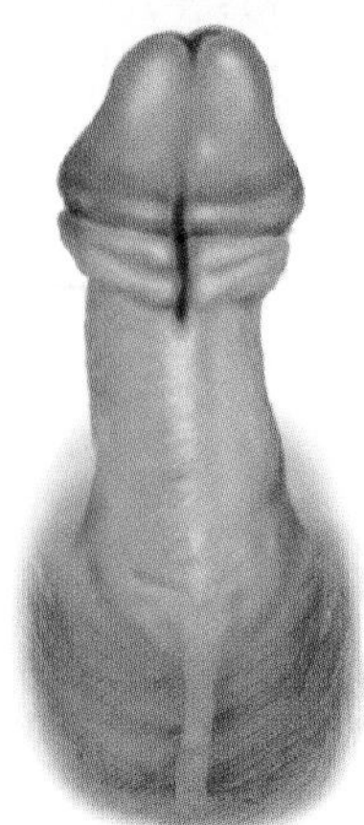

Hypospadias
Hypospadias is a congenital displacement of the urethral meatus to the inferior surface of the penis. A groove extends from the actual urethral meatus to its normal location on the tip of the glans.

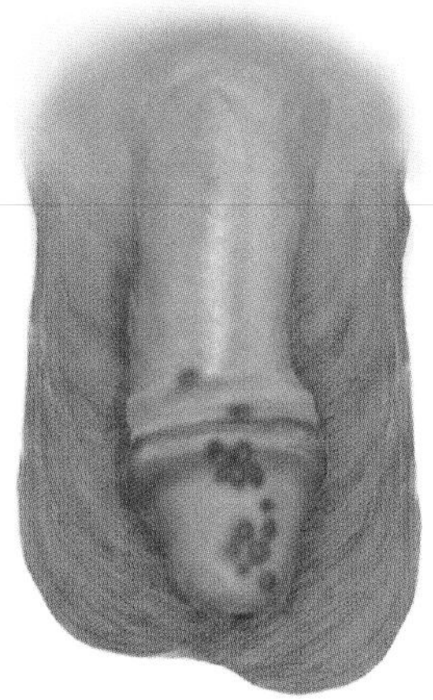

Genital Herpes
A cluster of small vesicles, followed by shallow, painful, nonindurated ulcers on red bases, suggests a herpes simplex infection. The lesions may occur anywhere on the penis. Usually there are fewer lesions when the infection recurs.

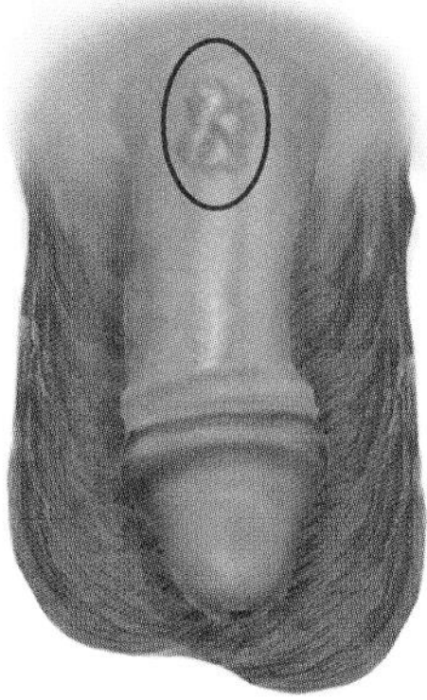

Peyronie's Disease
In Peyronie's disease, palpable nontender hard plaques are found just beneath the skin, usually along the dorsum of the penis. The patient complains of crooked, painful erections.

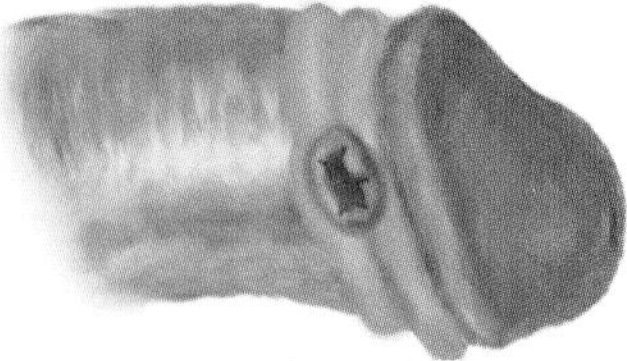

Syphilitic Chancre
A syphilitic chancre usually appears as an oval or round, dark red, painless erosion or ulcer with an indurated base. Nontender enlarged inguinal lymph nodes are typically associated. Chancres may be multiple and, when secondarily infected, may be painful. They may then be mistaken for the lesions of herpes. Chancres are infectious.

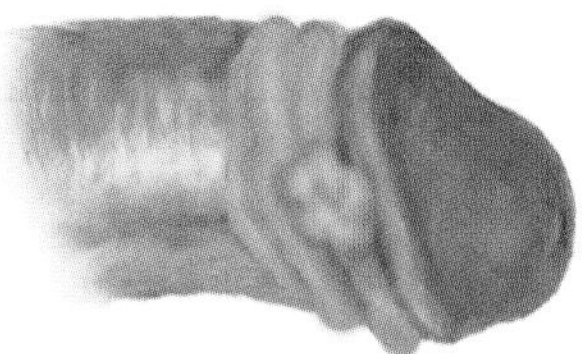

Carcinoma of the Penis
Carcinoma may appear as an indurated nodule or ulcer that is usually nontender. Limited almost completely to men who are not circumcised in childhood, it may be masked by the prepuce. Any persistent penile sore must be considered suspicious.

TABLE 11-2 Abnormalities of the Scrotal Sac

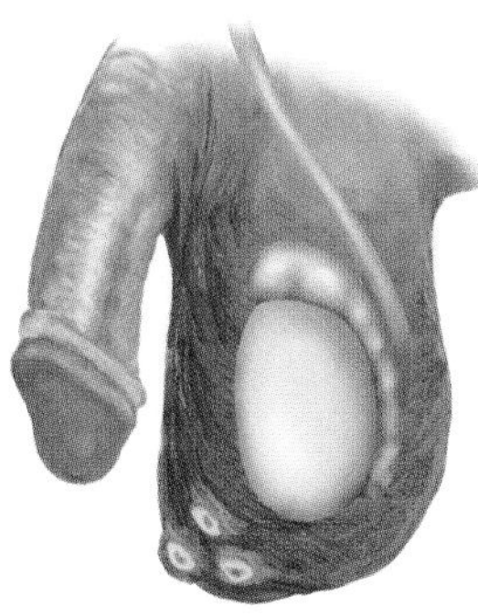

Epidermoid Cysts
These are firm, yellowish, nontender, cutaneous cysts up to about 1 cm in diameter. They are common and frequently multiple.

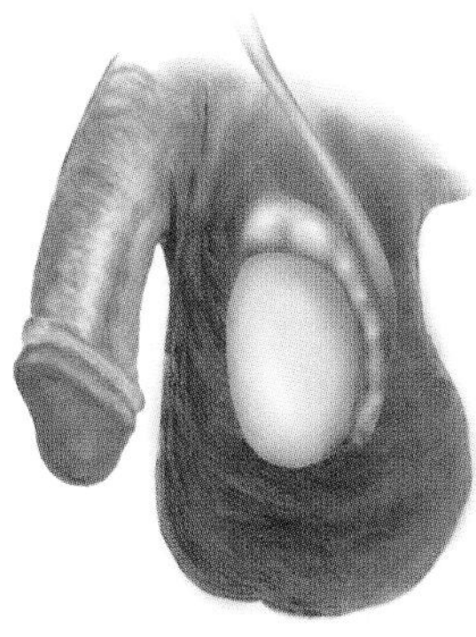

Scrotal Edema
Pitting edema may make the scrotal skin taut. This may accompany the generalized edema of congestive heart failure or nephrotic syndrome.

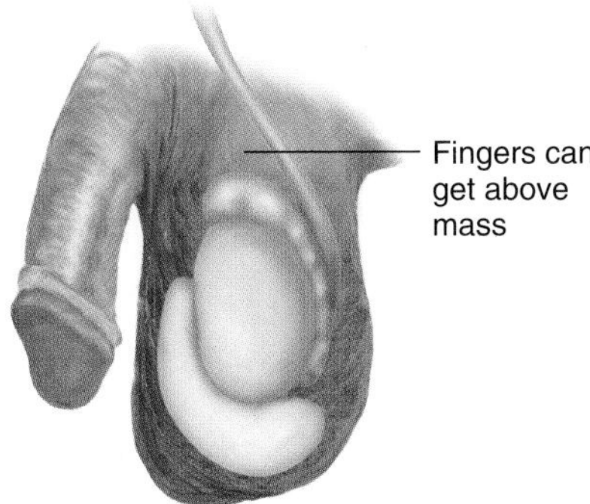

Hydrocele
A hydrocele is a nontender, fluid-filled mass within the tunica vaginalis. It transilluminates, and the examining fingers can get above the mass within the scrotum.

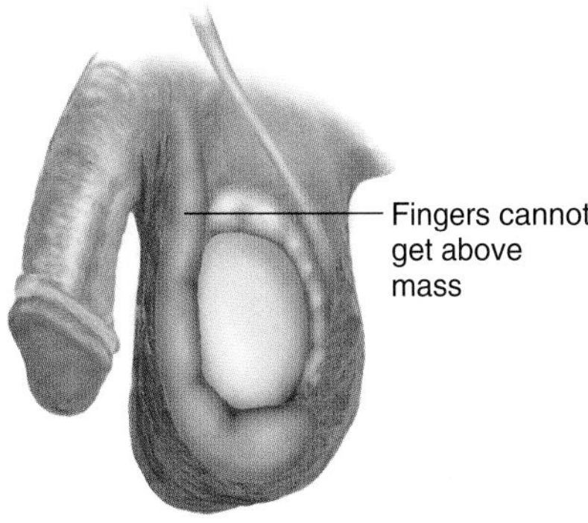

Scrotal Hernia
A hernia within the scrotum is usually an *indirect inguinal hernia*. It comes through the external inguinal ring, so the examining fingers cannot get above it within the scrotum.

TABLE 11-3 Abnormalities of the Testis

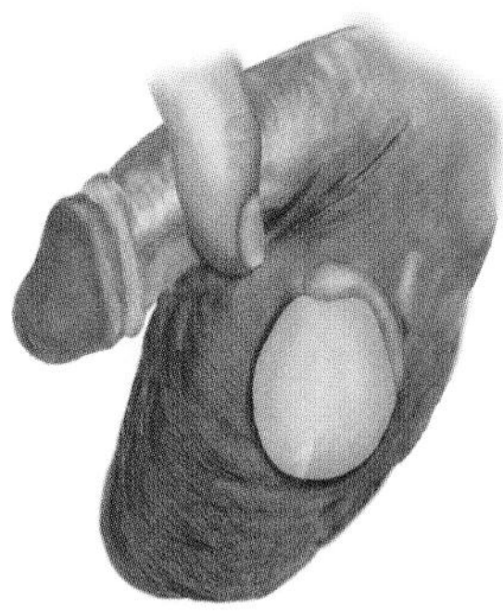

Cryptorchidism

In cryptorchidism, the testis is atrophied and may lie in the inguinal canal or the abdomen, resulting in an undeveloped scrotum, as above. There is no palpable left testis or epididymis. Cryptorchidism markedly raises the risk for testicular cancer.

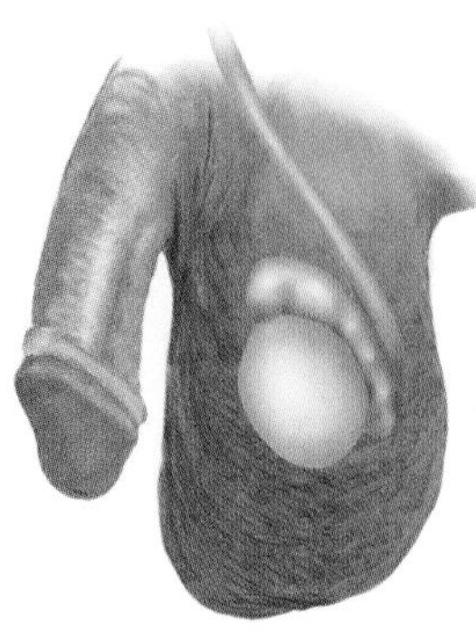

Small Testis

In adults, the length is usually ≤ 3.5 cm. Small firm testes in *Klinefelter's syndrome,* usually ≤ 2 cm. Small soft testes suggesting atrophy seen in cirrhosis, myotonic dystrophy, use of estrogens, and hypopituitarism; may also follow orchitis.

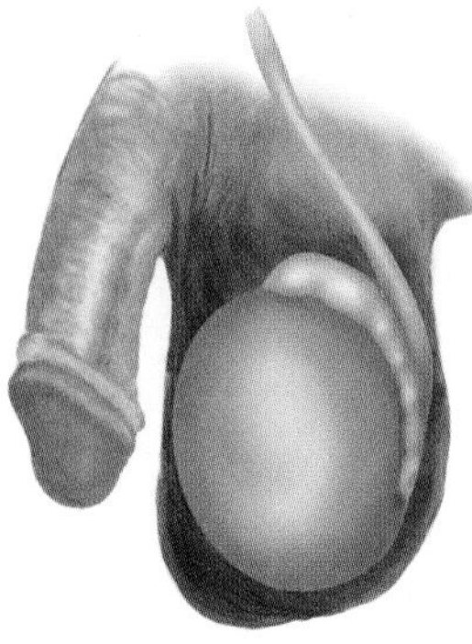

Acute Orchitis

The testis is acutely inflamed, painful, tender, and swollen. It may be difficult to distinguish from the epididymis. The scrotum may be reddened. Seen in mumps and other viral infections; usually unilateral.

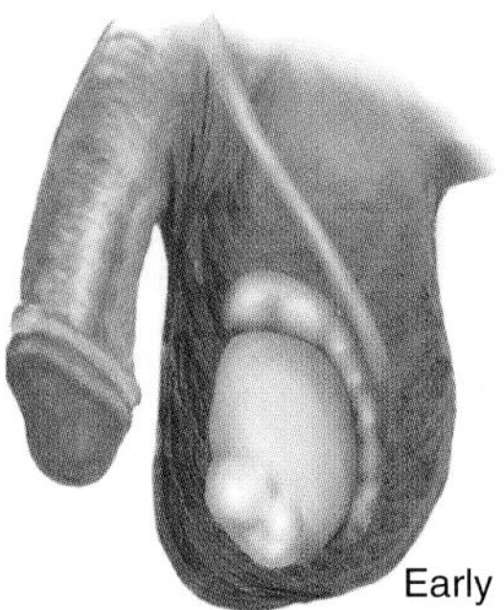

Tumor of the Testis

Usually appears as a painless nodule. Any nodule within the testis warrants investigation for malignancy.

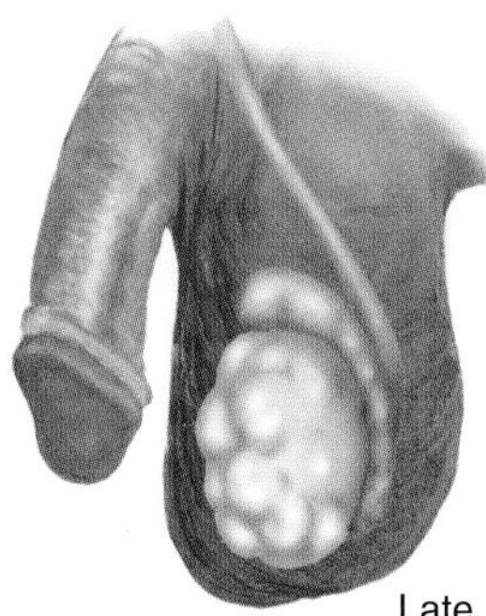

As a testicular neoplasm grows and spreads, it may seem to replace the entire organ. The testicle characteristically feels heavier than normal.

TABLE 11-4 Abnormalities of the Epididymis and Spermatic Cord

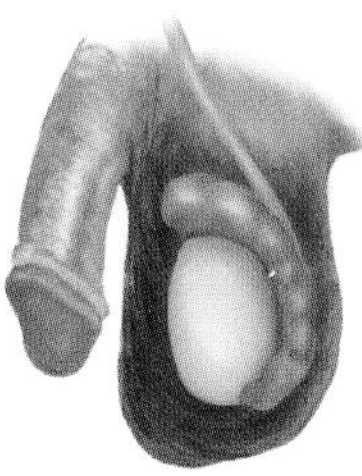

Acute Epididymitis

An acutely inflamed epididymis is tender and swollen and may be difficult to distinguish from the testis. The scrotum may be reddened and the vas deferens inflamed. It occurs chiefly in adults. Coexisting urinary tract infection or prostatitis supports the diagnosis.

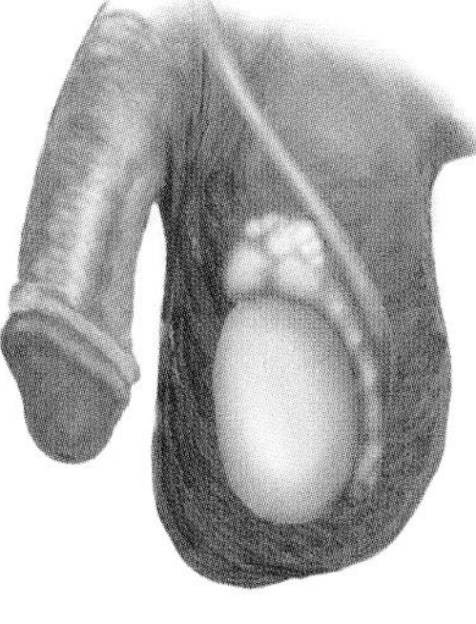

Spermatocele and Cyst of the Epididymis

A painless, movable cystic mass just above the testis suggests a spermatocele or an epididymal cyst. Both transilluminate. The former contains sperm, and the latter does not, but they are clinically indistinguishable.

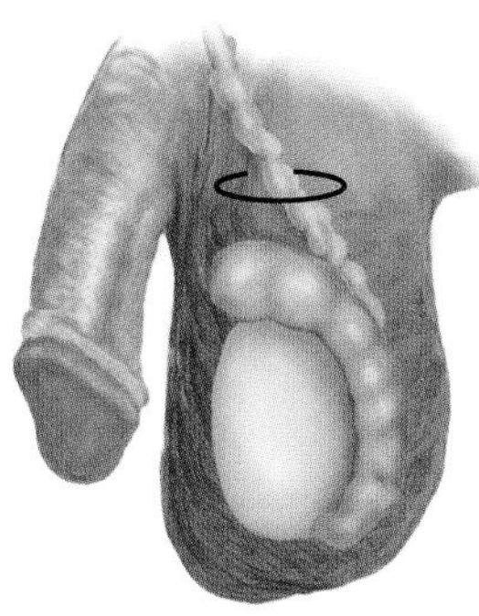

Tuberculous Epididymitis

The chronic inflammation of tuberculosis produces a firm enlargement of the epididymis, which is sometimes tender, with thickening or beading of the vas deferens.

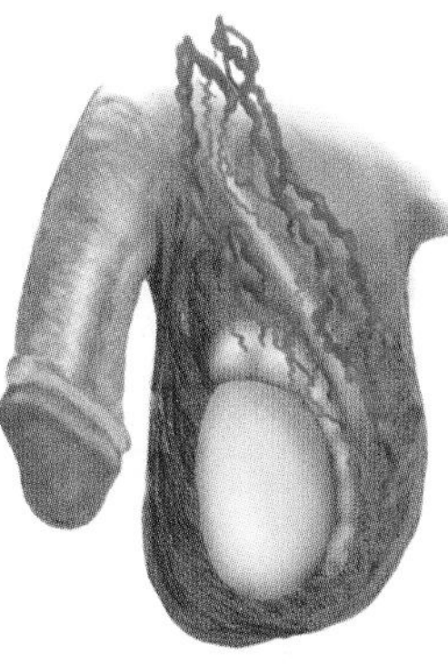

Varicocele

Varicocele refers to varicose veins of the spermatic cord, usually found on the left. It feels like a soft " bag of worms" separate from the testis, and slowly collapses when the scrotum is elevated in the supine patient. Infertility may be associated.

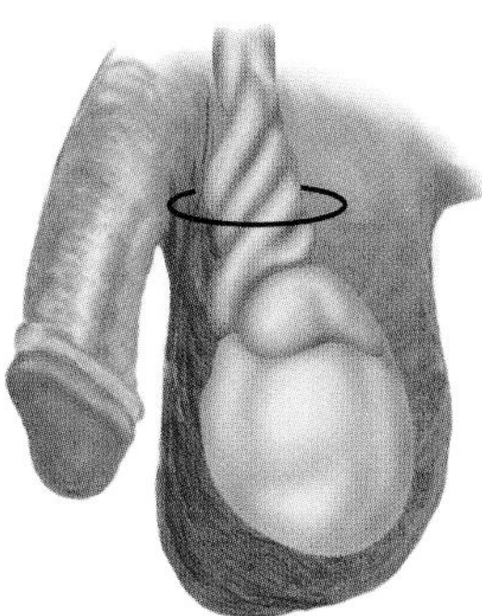

Torsion of the Spermatic Cord

Torsion, or twisting, of the testicle on its spermatic cord produces an acutely painful, tender, and swollen organ that is retracted upward in the scrotum. The scrotum becomes red and edematous. There is no associated urinary infection. Torsion, most common in adolescents, is a surgical emergency because of obstructed circulation.

TABLE 11-5 Course and Presentation of Hernias in the Groin

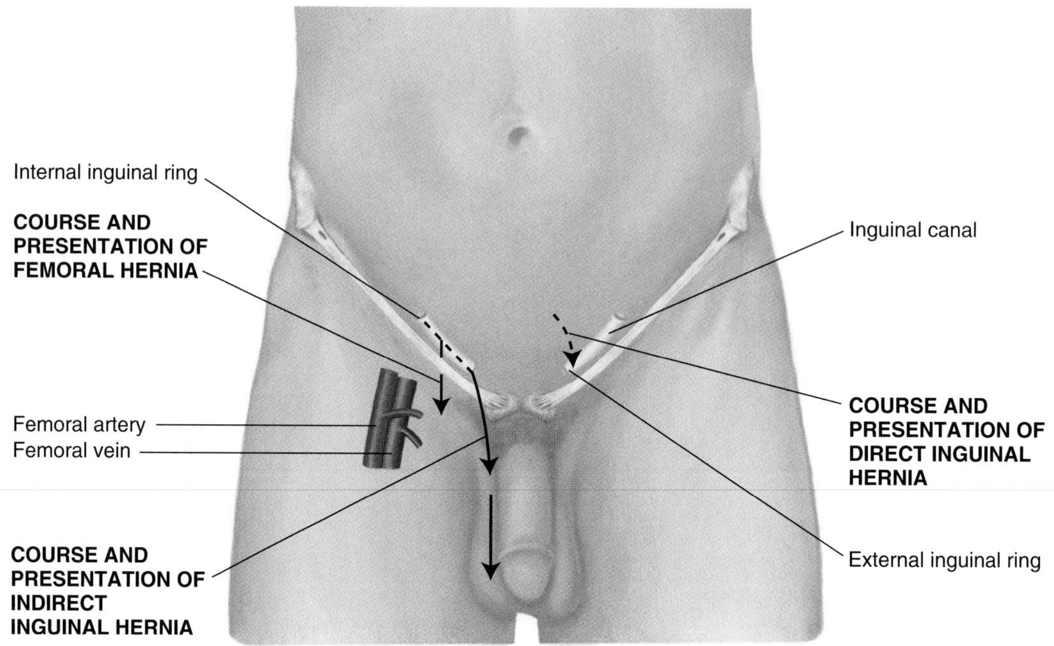

TABLE 11-6 Differentiation of Hernias in the Groin

Differentiation among these hernias is not always clinically possible. Understanding their features, however, improves your observation.

	Inguinal		
	Indirect	*Direct*	**Femoral**
Frequency	Most common, all ages, both sexes	Less common	Least common
Age and Sex	Often in children, may be in adults	Usually in men older than 40, rare in women	More common in women than in men
Point of Origin	Above inguinal ligament, near its midpoint (the internal inguinal ring)	Above inguinal ligament, close to the pubic tubercle (near the external inguinal ring)	Below the inguinal ligament; appears more lateral than an inguinal hernia and may be hard to differentiate from lymph nodes
Course	Often into the scrotum	Rarely into the scrotum	Never into the scrotum
With the examining finger in the inguinal canal during straining or cough	The hernia comes down the inguinal canal and touches the fingertip.	The hernia bulges anteriorly and pushes the side of the finger forward.	The inguinal canal is empty.

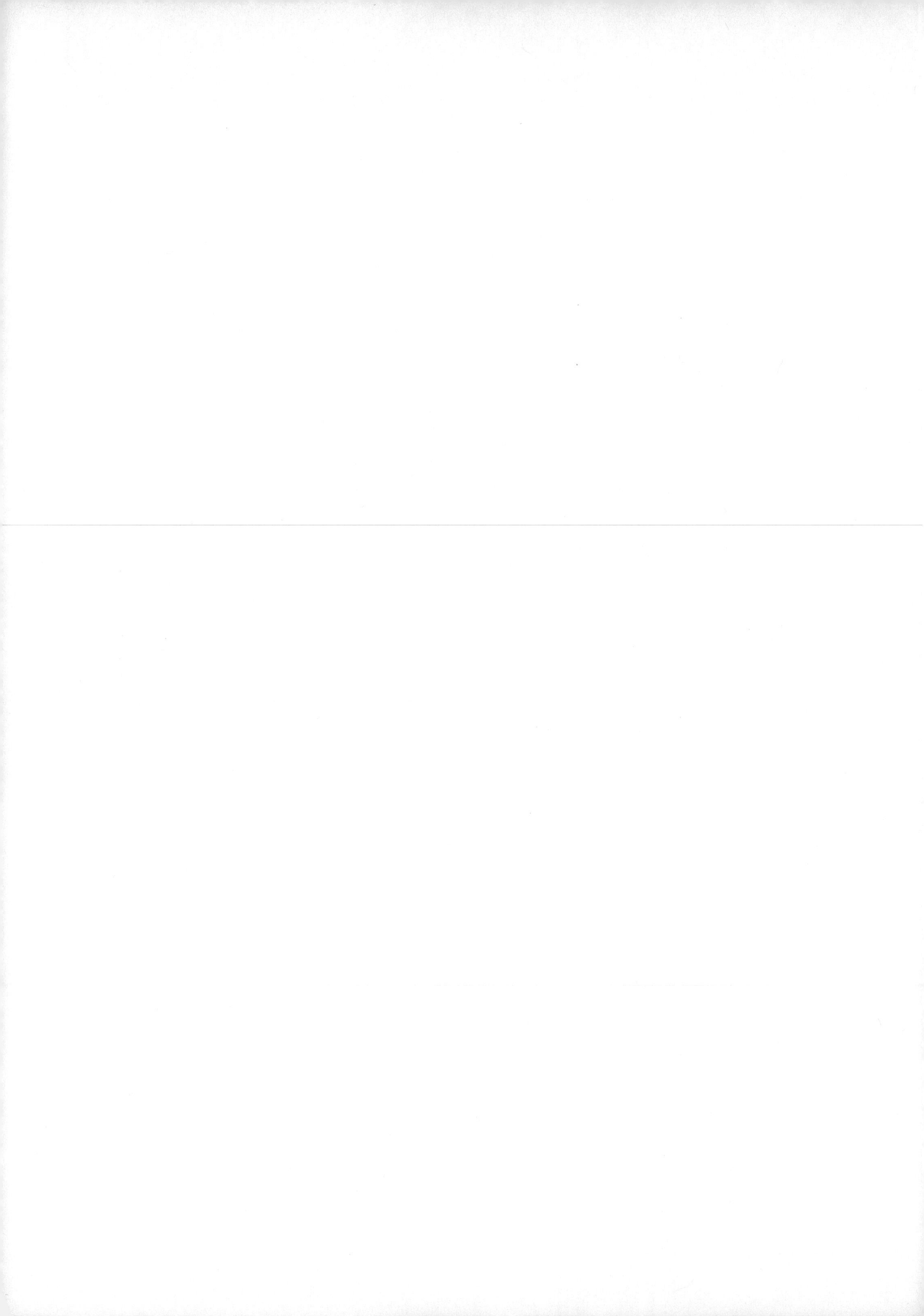

CHAPTER

12

Female Genitalia

ANATOMY AND PHYSIOLOGY

Review the anatomy of the external female genitalia, or *vulva*, including the *mons pubis*, a hair-covered fat pad overlying the symphysis pubis; the *labia majora*, rounded folds of adipose tissue; the *labia minora*, thinner pinkish red folds that extend anteriorly to form the *prepuce;* and the *clitoris*. The *vestibule* is the boat-shaped fossa between the labia minora. In its posterior portion lies the vaginal opening, the *introitus*, which in virgins may be hidden by the *hymen*. The term *perineum*, as commonly used clinically, refers to the tissue between the introitus and the anus.

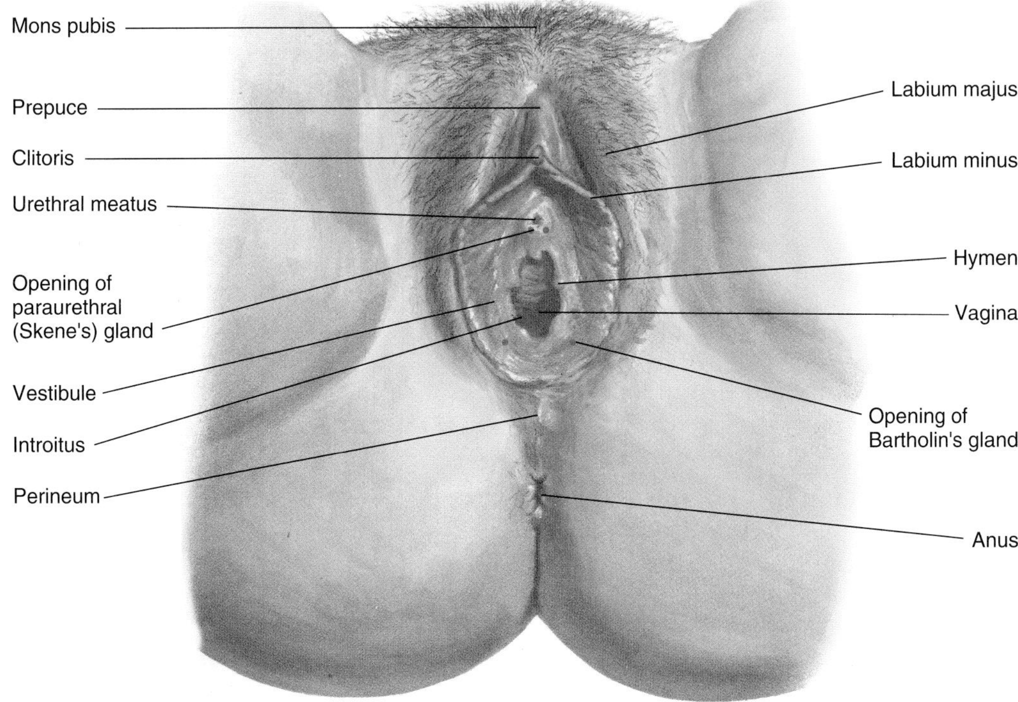

The *urethral meatus* opens into the vestibule between the clitoris and the vagina. Just posterior to it on either side lie the openings of the *paraurethral* (Skene's) *glands*.

The openings of *Bartholin's glands* are located posteriorly on either side of the vaginal opening, but are not usually visible. Bartholin's glands themselves are situated more deeply.

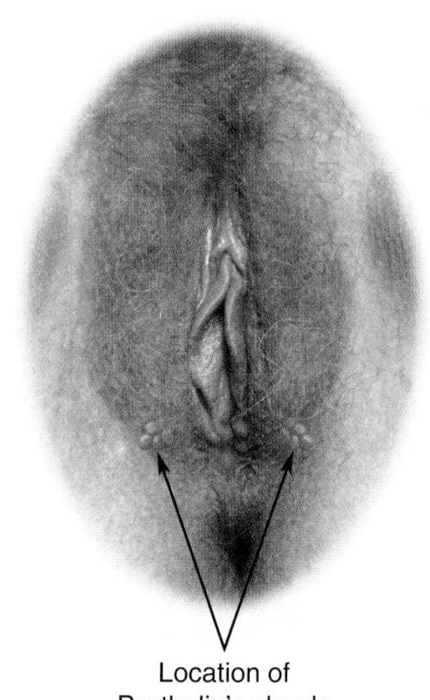

Location of Bartholin's glands

The *vagina* is a musculomembranous tube extending upward and posteriorly between the urethra and the rectum. Its upper third takes a horizontal plane and terminates in the cup-shaped *fornix*. The vaginal mucosa lies in transverse folds, or rugae.

At almost right angles to the vagina lies the *uterus*, a flattened fibromuscular structure shaped like an inverted pear. The uterus has two parts: the body (corpus) and the cervix, which are joined together by the isthmus. The convex upper surface of the body is called the *fundus* of the uterus. The lower part of the uterus, the *cervix*, protrudes into the vagina, dividing the fornix into anterior, posterior, and lateral fornices.

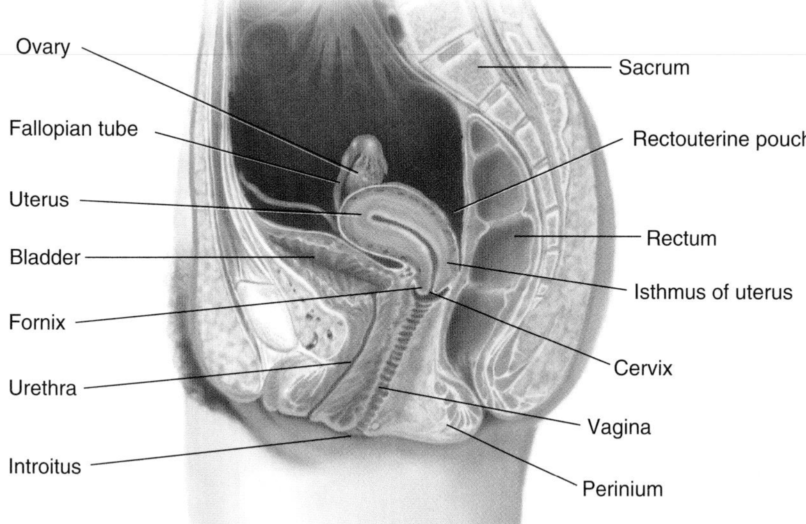

The vaginal surface of the cervix, the *ectocervix*, is seen easily with the help of a speculum. At its center is a round, oval, or slitlike depression, the *external os* of the cervix, which marks the opening into the endocervical canal. The ectocervix is covered by epithelium of two possible types: a plushy, red columnar epithelium surrounding the os, which resembles the lining of the endocervical canal; and a shiny pink squamous epithelium continuous with the vaginal lining. The *squamocolumnar junction* forms the boundary between these two types of epithelium. During puberty, the broad band of columnar epithelium encircling the os, called *ectropion*, is gradually replaced by columnar epithelium. The squamocolumnar junction migrates toward the os, creating the *transformation zone*. This is the area at risk for later dysplasia, which is sampled by the Papanicolaou, or Pap, smear.

A *fallopian tube* with a fanlike tip extends from each side of the uterus toward the ovary. The two ovaries are almond-shaped structures that vary con-

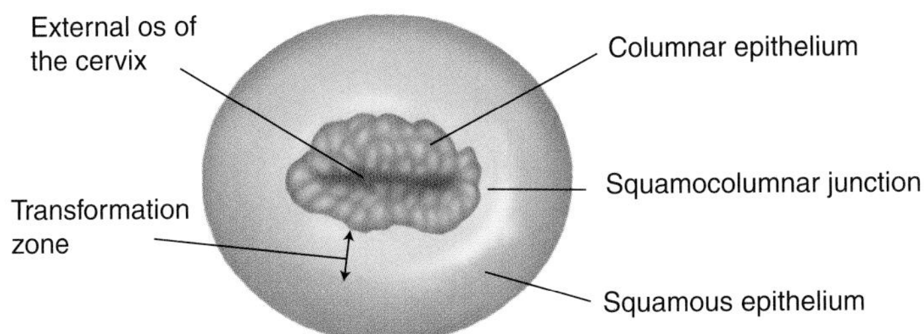

siderably in size but average about 3.5 × 2 × 1.5 cm from adulthood through menopause. The ovaries are palpable on pelvic examination in roughly half of women during the reproductive years. Normally, fallopian tubes cannot be felt. The term *adnexa*, a plural Latin word meaning appendages, refers to the ovaries, tubes, and supporting tissues.

The ovaries have two primary functions: the production of ova and the secretion of hormones, including estrogen, progesterone, and testosterone. Increased hormonal secretions during puberty stimulate the growth of the uterus and its endometrial lining. They stimulate enlargement of the vagina and thicken its epithelium. They also stimulate the development of secondary sex characteristics, including the breasts and pubic hair.

The parietal peritoneum extends downward behind the uterus into a cul de sac called the *rectouterine pouch* (pouch of Douglas). You can just reach this area on rectovaginal examination.

The pelvic organs are supported by a sling of tissues composed of muscle, ligaments, and fascia, through which the urethra, vagina, and rectum all pass.

Assessment of sexual maturity in girls, as classified by Tanner, depends not on internal examination, but on the growth of pubic hair and the development of breasts. Tanner's stages, or sexual maturity ratings, as they relate to pubic hair and breasts are shown in Chapter 18, Assessing Children: Infancy Through Adolescence.

In most women, pubic hair spreads downward in a triangular pattern, pointing toward the vagina. In 10% of women, it may form an inverted triangle, pointing toward the umbilicus. This growth is usually not completed until the middle 20s or later.

Just before menarche, there is a physiologic increase in vaginal secretions—a normal change that sometimes worries a girl or her mother. As menses become established, increased secretions (*leukorrhea*) coincide with ovulation. They also accompany sexual arousal. These normal kinds of discharges must be differentiated from those of infectious processes.

Lymphatics. Lymph from the vulva and the lower vagina drains into the inguinal nodes. Lymph from the internal genitalia, including the upper vagina, flows into the pelvic and abdominal lymph nodes, which are not palpable.

THE HEALTH HISTORY

Common Concerns

- Menarche, menstruation, menopause, postmenopausal bleeding
- Pregnancy
- Vulvovaginal symptoms
- Sexual activity

Questions in this section focus on menstruation, pregnancy and related topics, vulvovaginal symptoms, and sexual function.

Menarche, Menstruation, Menopause. For the menstrual history, ask the patient how old she was when her monthly, or menstrual, periods began, or age at *menarche*. When did her last period start, and, if possible, the one before that? How often does she have periods, as measured by the interval between the first days of successive periods? How regular or irregular are they? How long do they last? How heavy is the flow? What color is it? Flow can be assessed roughly by the number of pads or tampons used daily. Because women vary in their practices for sanitary measures, however, ask the patient whether she usually soaks a pad or tampon, spots it lightly, etc. Further, does she use more than one at a time? Does she have any bleeding between periods? Any bleeding after intercourse?

The dates of previous periods signal possible pregnancy or menstrual irregularities.

Unlike the normal dark red menstrual discharge, excessive flow tends to be bright red and may include "clots" (not true fibrin clots).

Does the patient have any discomfort or pain before or during her periods? If so, what is it like, how long does it last, and does it interfere with her usual activities? Are there other associated symptoms? Ask a middle-aged or older woman if she has stopped menstruating. When? Did any symptoms accompany her change? Has she had any bleeding since?

Questions about *menarche, menstruation,* and *menopause* often give you an opportunity to explore the patient's need for information and her attitude toward her body. When talking with an adolescent girl, for example, opening questions might include: "How did you first learn about monthly periods? How did you feel when they started? Many girls worry when their periods aren't regular or come late. Has anything like that bothered you?" You can explain that girls in the United States usually begin to menstruate between the ages of 9 and 16 years, and often take 1 year or more before they settle into a reasonable, regular pattern. Age at menarche is variable, depending on genetic endowment, socioeconomic status, and nutrition. The interval between periods ranges roughly from 24 to 32 days; the flow lasts from 3 to 7 days.

Menopause, the absence of menses for 12 consecutive months, usually occurs between the ages of 48 and 55 years.[1] Associated symptoms include hot flashes, flushing, sweating, and disturbances of sleep. Often you will ask, "How do (did) you feel about not having your periods anymore? Has it af-

Postmenopausal bleeding raises the question of endometrial cancer, although it also has other causes.